HANDBOOK OF CRITICAL CARE NURSING

HANDBOOK OF CRITICAL CARE NURSING

Edited by

Kathy Lynn Emanuelsen, RN, CCRN, MEd

Clinical Coordinator of Medicine
Hartford Hospital
Hartford, Connecticut

and

Jacqueline McQuay Rosenlicht, RN, BSN, MS

Clinical Instructor, Division of Nursing
St. Joseph College
West Hartford, Connecticut

A WILEY MEDICAL PUBLICATION
JOHN WILEY & SONS
New York • Chichester • Brisbane • Toronto • Singapore
FLESCHNER PUBLISHING CO.
Bethany, Connecticut

Library of Congress Cataloging in Publication Data:

Main entry under title:

Handbook of critical care nursing.

(A Wiley medical publication)

1. Intensive care nursing—Handbooks, manuals, etc.
I. Emanuelsen, Kathy Lynn. II. Rosenlicht, Jacqueline McQuay.
III. Series. [DNLM: 1. Critical Care—handbooks
2. Critical Care—nurses' instruction. WY 39 H2345]
RT120.I5H36 1986 616'.028 85–31456
ISBN 0-471-80418-5

Printed in the United States of America

10 9 8 7 6 5 4 3 2 1

Copy editor: Elizabeth D. Crawford
Illustrator: Robert Tutsky
Indexer: Wendy Green
Compositor: Advanced Typographic Services

This book is dedicated with love
to our families and friends whose understanding and
support made it all possible.

Although many persons have contributed to the success of this project we would like to specifically thank R. Craig Percy for his knowledge, patience, and friendship throughout the entire process.

CONTRIBUTORS

Deborah Chyun, RN, BSN, MSN
Bristol, Connecticut

Joyce B. Comer, Pharm D.
Associate Professor
School of Nursing
The University of Connecticut
Storrs, Connecticut

Linda C. Degutis, RN, MSN
Trauma Coordinator
Yale University School of Medicine
New Haven, Connecticut

Mary Jane Densmore, RN, BA
Clinical Research Coordinator
Hartford Hospital Pulmonary Laboratory
Hartford, Connecticut

Margaret A. O'Neill DeVito, RN, BSN, MS
Head Nurse
Surgical Unit
Hartford Hospital
Hartford, Connecticut

Mary Alice Higgins Donius, RN, BSN MEd
Associate in Nursing
School of Nursing
Columbia University
New York, New York

Susan DeGroot Emanuelsen, RN, BSN
Gadsden, Alabama

Linda J. Frigon, RN, BA
Head Nurse
Medical Intensive Care Unit
Hartford Hospital
Hartford, Connecticut

Barbara A. Goldrick, RN, MS
Nurse Epidemiologist
Instructor of Nursing
The University of Connecticut
Storrs, Connecticut

Anita Rubbo Gorman, RN, MS
Diabetes Nurse Clinician
Hartford Hospital
Hartford, Connecticut

Antoinette E. Grenier, RN, JD
Trial Attorney
New Haven, Connecticut

Michael P. Hickey, RN, MS.
Clinical Coordinator of Surgery
Hartford Hospital
Hartford, Connecticut

Thomas W. Hijeck, RN, MS
Clinical Coordinator
Hartford Hospital
Hartford, Connecticut

Sally Walton Hills, RN, MS
District Manager Nurse Clinicians
Abbott Laboratories
West Hartford, Connecticut

Melissa Mesick Meth, RN, MSN, CS
Clinical Specialist in Psychiatric/Mental Health Nursing
Hartford Hospital
Hartford, Connecticut

Marsha Evans Orr, RN, MS, CNSN
Patient Education Coordinator
St. Joseph's Hospital Health Center
Syracuse, New York

Lani Wasserman Smith, RN, BA, BSN, MEd
Nurse Research Fellow
Louisiana State University Medical Center
New Orleans, Louisiana

Sylvia Talkington, RN, CCRN
Critical Care Practitioner
Faculty Consultant
Resource Applications, Inc.
Baltimore, Maryland

Constance S. Weiskopf, RN, MSN
Director of Psychiatric Nursing
University of Connecticut Health Center
Farmington, Connecticut

Celeste B. Williams, RN, BSN, CCRN
Critical Care and Emergency Room Clinical Supervisor
Waterbury Hospital Health Center
Waterbury, Connecticut

CONTENTS

PREFACE

The number of critically ill patients admitted to acute care facilities continues to escalate. The complexity of these patients' problems necessitates that the critical care nurse be able to rapidly assess the constantly changing physical and/or psychosocial needs of the patient. In meeting the demands of the patient in the critical care environment, the nurse is confronted both by the impending potential crisis of the patient's condition and the increasing technological sophistication of the patient's environment. These nurses, therefore, need to possess and utilize a broad knowledge base in the provision of patient care.

Many of the currently available general and specialized critical care texts focus on the problems and management of acutely ill patients. The general texts are expanding in content but also in size. Although these texts can provide in-depth information, they are frequently cumbersome for use in a critical care setting. Specialized texts also provide in-depth knowledge but are limited in their range.

This handbook is designed to serve as a complete, concise resource for use in the critical care setting. Its compact, ready-to-use information enhances its value for critical care nurses, students, and educators as well as for all others who provide care for critically ill adults.

The handbook discusses the philosophy of critical care and incorporates the components of the nursing process as it relates to the deliverance and documentation of patient care. The patient-problem-oriented format easily lends itself to the development of nursing care plans.

The handbook is divided into two sections. The first section presents information about the major body systems (cardiovascular, respiratory, hematologic, nervous, endocrine, renal, and gastrointestinal). A review of each system includes anatomy and physiology, assessment of the patient, pathophysiology of the associated major disorders, and the medical and nursing interventions. The second section examines the special considerations in critical care nursing as follows: burns, multiple trauma, nutritional aspects of critical care, arterial blood gases, oxygen therapy, hemodynamic monitoring, advanced life support, infection control, shock, legal issues, and psychosocial aspects of critical care. Finally, two appendices provide information on interpretation of ECG rhythms and arrhythmias and pharmacology in critical care.

This book will, we believe, fulfill an important need for critical care nurses.

KLE AND JMR
Hartford, Connecticut

ABBREVIATIONS AND SYMBOLS

ACTH	adrenocorticotrophic hormone
ADH	antidiuretic hormone
ADP	adenosine diphosphate
AMP	adenosine monophosphate
ANS	autoncmic nervous system
ATP	adenosine triphosphate
BCG	Bacillus Calmette-Guéin (vaccine)
bid	2 times a day
BP	blood pressure
bpm	beats per minute
BUN	blood urea nitrogen
CAT	computerized axial tomography
CBC	complete blood count
CHF	congestive heart failure
CNS	central nervous system
CO	cardiac output
COPD	chronic obstructive pulmonary disease
CPR	cardiopulmonary resuscitation
CSF	cerebrospinal fluid
DNA	deoxyribonucleic acid
DW	dextrose in water
ECF	extracellular fluid
ECG	electrocardiogram
EEG	electroencephalogram
ER	emergency room
GFR	glomerular filtration rate
GI	gastrointestinal
GU	genitourinary
Hb	hemoglobin
Hct	hematocrit
ICF	intracellular fluid
ICU	intensive care unit
IgA, etc.	immunoglobulin A, etc.
IM	intramuscular(ly)
IQ	intelligence quotient
IU	international unit(s)
IV	intravenous(ly)
MI	myocardial infarction

NPO	nothing by mouth
OR	operating room
$PaCO_2$	arterial carbon dioxide pressure
$PACO_2$	alveolar carbon dioxide pressure
PAO_2	alveolar oxygen pressure
PCO_2	carbon dioxide pressure
PO	oral(ly)
PO_2	oxygen pressure
prn	as needed
q	every
q 4 hr, etc.	every 4 hours, etc.
qid	4 times a day
RBC	red blood cell
RDA	Recommended Daily Allowance(s)
RNA	ribonucleic acid
SC	subcutaneous(ly)
SGOT	serum glutamic oxaloacetic transaminase
SGPT	serum glutamic pyruvic transaminase
SLE	systemic lupus erythematosus
sp gr	specific gravity
TB	tuberculosis
tid	3 times a day
TPN	total parenteral nutrition
VD	venereal disease
WBC	white blood cell

CHAPTER 1

CRITICAL CARE PRACTICE STANDARDS

Kathy Lynn Emanuelsen and Jacqueline McQuay Rosenlicht

For any practice to be described as professional, several features must be inherent in its framework and be accepted by its membership. A philosophy incorporating the basic beliefs and ethical principles of the practice is an essential feature, along with accepted standards of practice, educational requirements, and a method for documenting and evaluating the outcomes of the practice.

Nurses who practice in critical care units can be confident of their professional status. Enormous effort has been devoted to the establishment of a philosophy of critical care, the development of standards of critical care, and the maintenance of quality through the use of appropriate evaluative criteria and documentation.

PHILOSOPHY

The underlying professional, moral, and ethical principles that guide an individual's actions can be considered to be that person's philosophy. Just as individual nurses incorporate their ethical principles into their own practice, a formal philosophy of nursing practice exists at most institutions. Time and effort should be taken to demonstrate what is meant by the institutional philosophy and how to implement it, because it forms the basis for the expected practice outcomes.

The philosophy of the critical care division must reflect and support the nursing service philosophy just as the nurse service department philosophy must reflect and support the administrative philosophy. The critical care environment encourages a unique interpretation of the general philosophy.

SCOPE OF NURSING PRACTICE

The American Association of Critical Care Nurses has developed a statement regarding the scope of practice for critical care nursing that includes a definition of the critically ill patient, the critical care nurse, and the environment in which critical care nursing is delivered.

The critically ill patient is identified as having real or potential life-threatening health problems that require continuous observation and appropriate interventions to prevent complications and restore health. This concept includes concern for the patient's family and/or significant other.

The critical care nurse is a registered professional nurse committed to the concept that all critically ill patients receive optimal care. This individual's practice is based upon personal professional accountability; knowledge of the interrelatedness of the body systems; recognition of the individual's wholeness, uniqueness, and significant social relationships; and appreciation of the collaborative role of all members of the health-care team.

To develop and maintain this practice, the critical care nurse participates in ongoing educational activities. Theoretical knowledge of psychosocial, physiologic, and therapeutic aspects of critical care practice is essential. Clinical competence and the ability to interact effectively with patients' families and other members of the health-care team must be developed. In addition, she develops an awareness of the responsibility for practicing in a safe environment.

The critical care environment is any geographically designated area that is designed to facilitate the care of the critically ill patient by critical care nurses. It is an area where safety, organizational, and ethical standards are maintained for patient welfare. This can occur in any setting that meets the established standards by providing a supportive environment for the patients and families, adequate functioning equipment and supplies, available emergency equipment, facilities for the staff's needs, and access to support departments.

STANDARDS OF PRACTICE

The purpose for the development of critical care standards of practice is to improve the quality of care delivered to the critically ill. This can only be achieved when the determined standards have become incorporated into the practice of the individual nurse. Accountability for one's own personal practice is a key concept, along with the obligation to reevaluate oneself and others in an ongoing effort to improve quality care.

The American Association of Critical Care Nurses published its Standards for Nursing Care of the Critically Ill in 1981. These standards are listed in Figure 1–1. They are subject to evaluation and subsequent modification, reflecting the dynamic nature of critical care nursing.

Structure standards

1. The critical care unit shall be designed to ensure a safe and supportive environment for critically ill patients and for the personnel who care for them.
2. The critical care unit shall be constructed, equipped, and operated in a manner which protects patients, visitors, and personnel from electrical hazards.
3. The critical care unit shall be constructed, equipped, and operated in a manner which protects patients, visitors, and personnel from fire hazard.
4. The critical care unit shall have essential equipment and supplies immediately available at all times.
5. The critical care unit shall have a comprehensive infection control program.
6. The critical care unit shall be managed in a manner which ensures the delivery of safe and effective care to the critically ill.
7. The critical care unit shall have appropriately qualified staff to provide care on a twenty-four-hour basis.
8. The critical care nurse shall be competent and current in critical care nursing.
9. The critical care nurse's performance appraisal shall be based upon the roles and responsibilities identified in the job description.
10. The critical care unit shall have a well-defined, organized, written program to evaluate care of the critically ill.
11. Critical care nursing practice shall include both the conduct and utilization of clinical research.
12. The critical care nurse shall ensure the delivery of safe nursing care to patients, being cognizant of the various "causes of action" for which the nurse may be liable.

Process standards

The critical care nurse shall utilize the nursing process in the delivery of patient care.

1. Data shall be collected continuously on all critically ill patients wherever they may be located.
2. The identification of patient problems/needs and their priority shall be based upon collected data.
3. An appropriate plan of nursing care shall be formulated.
4. The plan of nursing care shall be implemented according to the priority of identified problems/needs.
5. The results of nursing care shall be continuously evaluated.

Figure 1–1. American Association of Critical Care Nurses' Standards for Nursing Care of the Critically Ill. *Reprinted with permission from* the American Association of Critical Care Nurses.

The Joint Commission on Accreditation of Hospitals (JCAH) also published its Standards for Special Care Units in 1983. These standards are presented in Figure 1–2. In each of the above publications, the specific standard is defined and interpreted so that its application to practice can be identified and its outcome measured.

1. Each special care unit shall be well organized and integrated with other units and departments/services of the hospital. The scope of services provided in each special care unit shall be specified.
2. Each special care unit shall be properly directed and staffed according to the nature of the special patient care needs anticipated and the scope of services offered.
3. All personnel shall be prepared for their responsibilities in the special care unit through appropriate orientation, in-service training, and continuing education programs.
4. The provision of patient care in special care units shall be guided by written policies and procedures.
5. Special care units shall be designed and equipped to facilitate the safe and effective care of patients.
6. As part of the hospital's quality assurance program, the quality and appropriateness of the patient care provided by special care units are monitored and evaluated, and identified problems are resolved.
7. Specific-purpose special care units may be established by the patient needs of the community and only as supported by the resources available to the hospital.

Figure 1–2. Standards for special care units established by the Joint Commission on Accreditation of Hospitals. *Reprinted with permission from* the Joint Commission on Accreditation of Hospitals.

DOCUMENTATION

The role of the professional nurse is expanding in areas of critical care. Nurses in ICUs are assuming greater responsibilities for managing patient care in acute settings. Along with these responsibilities comes the demand for increased accountability and the need for improved documentation. Also, as the prevalence of malpractice cases increases, the nursing care documented is defined, legally and professionally, as the nursing care given.

Traditionally, documentation in critical care areas is maintained with flow sheets and narrative notes, representing an evaluative approach to the patient's condition and care rendered. Based on isolated and fragmented actions or technical skills, this method does not reflect the nurse's ability to utilize the nursing process and problem-solving skills. Documentation of this type tends to represent noncommunication among the disciplines involved and often results in fragmented or uncoordinated patient care.

Documentation in the narrative format delivers evidence that the nurse has assessed the patient but does not reflect what the nurse planned to do with this information. It tends to be lengthy because nurses feel obligated to document every action of the patient. Consequently, nursing progress notes are read infrequently by other health-care professionals because to uncover scattered pertinent information about the patient in a long, narrative note is time-consuming. This type of situation also leads to reliance on verbal communication of individual patient needs via nursing reports, which results in unreliability of the importance of the information and a further decreased emphasis on documentation of the patient's response to care.

The best method for reflecting individualization of patient care is through use of nursing care plans. The nurse is thus enabled to provide patient care based on principles of the nursing process. Decision-making and problem-solving skills are reflected through the nurse's abilities to assess, diagnose, plan, implement, and evaluate the nursing care she delivers.

Unfortunately, in many critical care units, the development of nursing care plans is not routine because they are not viewed as a priority by the nurses. Care plans are seen as time-consuming for the critical care nurse, but there are many advantages to their use. Nursing care plans developed with a corresponding problem list provide an opportunity for documentation of in-depth assessment. Problem lists provide an index to the patient's actual and potential problems; progress notes and plans illustrate the nurse's ability to analyze and determine care requirements.

The problem-oriented record (POR)

The POR is the tool developed by Dr. Lawrence Weed as a structured method of documentation. It is based on concepts of a health-care system that focuses on the total patient in all phases of health care (preventive, curative, and restorative) and encompasses utilization of all health professionals. The POR method of documentation is also congruent with the nursing process because it provides a logical data-organizing system and facilitates thorough communication of patient needs. It delineates nursing interventions that are directed at eliminating or decreasing the severity of the problem and provides a method for evaluation of care.

Using the POR as a structured method of documentation in the critical care unit has the following advantages:

1. It is patient-oriented and focuses on actual and potential problems.
2. Interventions directed at eliminating or decreasing the severity of the problem are delineated.
3. Its format increases efficiency in information gathering and clustering of data.
4. It facilitates communication among health-care professionals involved in patient care.
5. It promotes confidence and trust among those providing care.

6. Continuous evaluation and revision of the plan of care improve the quality of care.
7. Patient-care rounds are enhanced, with the problem list being the outline and agenda for evaluation and planning.
8. It promotes the use of the nursing process.

The POR consists of four basic steps: (1) data collection; (2) development of the problem list; (3) plans in the SOAP format; (4) progress notes in the SOAP format. *S* represents subjective data, for information stated by the patient/significant other; *O* represents objective data, for information and data obtained through observation, auscultation, percussion, and palpation; *A* represents assessment, a statement of one's best judgment of the patient's problem; *P* represents plan of care, which is subdivided into three components: (1) diagnostic: studies necessary to confirm suspected problem; (2) therapeutic: measures indicated to assist the patient in dealing with the problem; (3) education: measures taken to enhance the level of understanding of the patient/significant other.

Data collection is the first component of the POR and corresponds to the initial assessment of the patient. It is the basis from which actual and potential problems are identified and the plan of care is developed. There are many formats that can be used for a data base, and most hospitals have one that has been developed as their own. The data is collected in a systematic way, often within a specific time frame, such as the shift during which the patient was admitted, or within the first 24 hours of admission.

From the data base, a **problem list** is formulated by analyzing items and grouping them according to management requirements. The list is modified as problems develop or resolve, or as more information is obtained. The problem list is the basis for organizing the patient care plan and documentation within the progress notes.

The **initial plan of care** for each actual or potential problem is the third component of the POR. It consists of expected outcomes and specific interventions directed toward helping the patient achieve those results. Plans should be patient-centered, realistic, and measurable and can be developed in terms of short-term and/or long-term goals.

Finally, using the data base and plans as a reference, patient response and status are **documented in the progress notes** at certain intervals, as determined by policies or objectives for the particular problem. The frequency of documentation is regulated by the nature of the problem, goals, and status of the patient as well as by the specific guidelines established by individual institutions.

POR is a method well-suited to the documentation needs of the ICU because it provides a means of thorough recording of nursing care while allowing ongoing evaluation of that care. Figure 1–3 outlines the POR method and how it is utilized within the critical care setting.

The POR can also be used in conjunction with flow sheets to document frequently monitored parameters and repetitive nursing interventions. In the ICU, flow sheets are designed to allow frequent recording of such data

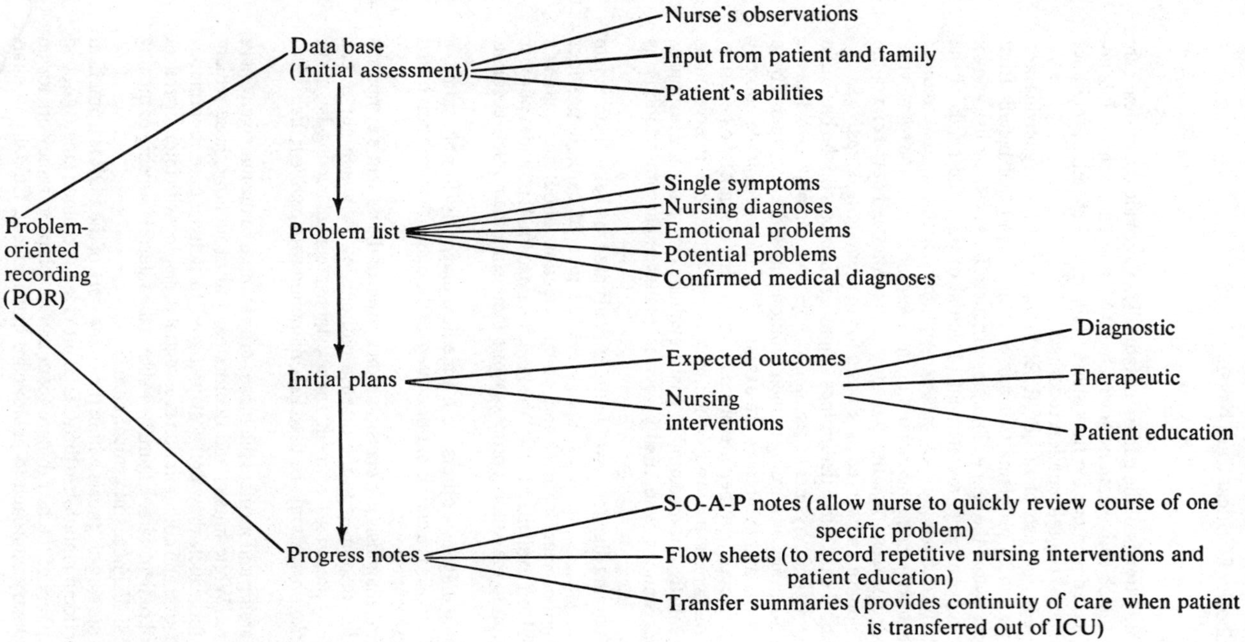

Figure 1–3. Outline of the problem-oriented recording method. S, subjective data; O, objective data; A, assessment; P, plan of care. *Reprinted with permission from* Merkel, S. Problem-oriented recording in the intensive care unit. *Dimensions of Critical Care Nursing* (July-August 1982). p. 239.

and to identify trends in the patient's status. They provide the critical care nurse with the objective data from which SOAP notes are written. It is not necessary to redocument the flow sheet in the note, but rather, reference may be made to the information recorded.

Inherent in the use of the POR is the potential for organizing and developing a list of problems that nurses identify and that benefit from interventions within the scope of nursing practice. This problem list, known as nursing diagnoses, is a statement of actual or potential needs of the patient, derived from nursing assessment and judgment, that require management from independent nursing interventions within the framework of the nursing process. A nursing diagnosis is formulated at the end of the assessment phase and serves as a basis for the remaining steps.

The critical care nurse determines a nursing diagnosis on the basis of a nursing history and physical assessment. Subjective and objective data are clustered into groups according to their relationship with each other. These clusters of signs and symptoms are examined for the appropriate etiology for each set of cues and then are placed into nursing diagnostic categories. Once the diagnoses are established, the nurse prescribes interventions based on realistic and measurable goals, evaluates the patient's responses to the interventions, and finally revises management prescriptions as necessary.

Use of nursing diagnoses within the critical care area helps to designate priorities in patient problems and direct the plan of care. It provides standardization, clarification, and communication about the patient's health problems to all members of the health-care team. It provides purpose and direction to the nursing process while increasing the nurse's accountability.

A nursing diagnosis differs from a medical diagnosis. Simply stated, a medical diagnosis is a classification system of the patient's symptoms based on a disease pathology.

A nursing diagnosis is a classification system of the patient's symptoms based on his responses to the disease pathologies for which nurses can independently prescribe treatment. In the establishment of nursing diagnosis, the word *diagnosis* should be used in conjunction with *problem identification.*

Both nursing and medical diagnoses are essential to the management of patient care. While nurses and doctors each must identify those patient problems for which they are best prepared to deliver care, continuous communication and collaboration is essential in dealing with interdependent functions of patient care. Figure 1–4 shows the interrelationship of nursing and medical diagnoses in critical care.

Use of nursing diagnosis within the framework of the POR is a practical method for documentation in the ICU. It provides a common language bond for all members of the health-care team and develops a framework for an interdisciplinary approach to health-care management. Concurrent chart

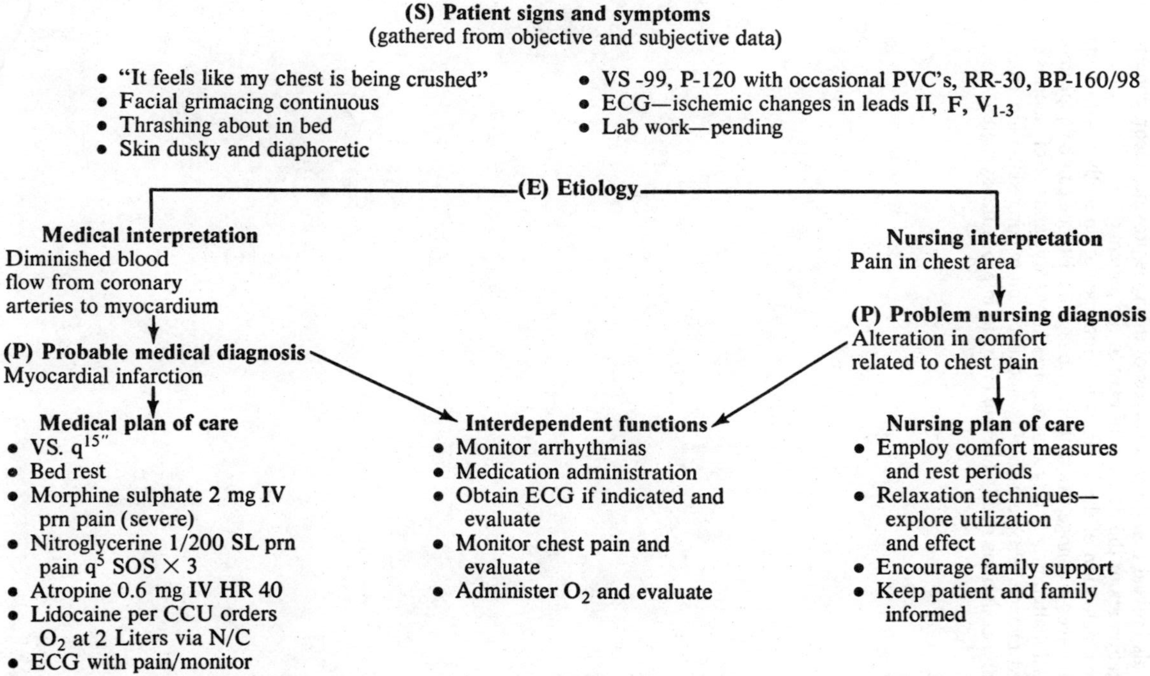

Figure 1–4. Interrelationship of nursing diagnosis and medical diagnosis in critical care. CCU, coronary care unit; HR, heart rate; N/C, nasal cannula; RR, respiration rate; P, pulse; PVC, premature ventricular contractions; SL, sublingual; SOS, if necessary; VS, vital signs. *Reprinted with permission from* Hickey, M. Nursing diagnosis in the critical care unit. *Dimensions of Critical Care Nursing* (March-April 1984). p. 96.

audits also reveal that documentation of this type provides clear, concise information about the delivery of care to the patient.

Implementation of the POR as the documentation method within the ICU involves a change. As with any change, resistance can be expected. Successful alteration of a system requires knowledge and use of theories of planned change. Problem-solving and decision-making skills are called upon in a conscious and deliberate effort to improve the system.

CHAPTER 2

THE CARDIOVASCULAR SYSTEM

Lani W. Smith

ANATOMY AND PHYSIOLOGY REVIEW

The function of the cardiovascular system is to circulate blood to all regions of the body, thus delivering O_2 and nutrients and removing wastes. The distribution of blood flow must be regulated to meet the varying demands of different tissues; e.g., there is increased blood flow to the gut after eating, and to skeletal muscle with exercise. Because the circulation of blood is absolutely essential for life, the cardiovascular system must have built-in safeguards that protect its ability to carry out its function under almost any conditions.

The cardiovascular system consists of three main components. The most important is the **pump,** the heart itself. The heart is actually two pumps: the low-pressure right-side pump and the high-pressure left-side pump. The function of the pump is to generate pressure for the circulation of blood. The second component is the high-pressure peripheral or **systemic circulation,** consisting of the aorta, systemic arteries, arterioles, capillaries, venules, veins, and the venae cavae. The function of the peripheral circulation is to circulate blood containing O_2 and nutrients throughout the tissues of the body. The third component of the cardiovascular system is the low-pressure **pulmonary circulation,** consisting of the pulmonary artery, arterioles, capillaries, venules, and pulmonary veins. The main function of the pulmonary circulation is the oxygenation of blood and removal of CO_2.

THE PUMP

The heart is a complex structure, consisting of three layers. The innermost layer, the endocardium, is continuous with the vascular endothelium of the great vessels (the aorta, venae cavae, pulmonary artery, and pulmonary veins). It covers the heart valves and the chordae tendineae. The middle layer is the myocardium. This layer contains myocytes, the contractile cells of the heart. The outermost layer is the epicardium, which is actually part of the pericardium. The pericardium is a double-layered sac in which the heart lies: the inner layer is the epicardium, and the outer layer is fibrous tissue that protects the heart. Normally, there is a small amount of fluid between the two layers of the pericardium.

The heart itself is a four-chambered organ that lies in the anterior thoracic cavity, slightly to the left of the midline. The heart is so oriented in the thorax that the right atrium and ventricle lie anterior to the left atrium and ventricle.

Structures

The two two-chambered pumps of the heart operate in series. Deoxygenated blood returning to the heart from the peripheral circulation enters the right side of the heart via the superior and inferior venae cavae (Fig. 2–1). The mean right atrial pressure (RAP), sometimes referred to as central venous pressure (CVP), is normally ~0 to 3 mmHg. From the right atrium, the blood flows past the tricuspid valve into the right ventricle, a chamber with a normal pressure of ~25 mmHg during contraction (systole) and ~2 mmHg during relaxation (diastole). The right ventricle pumps

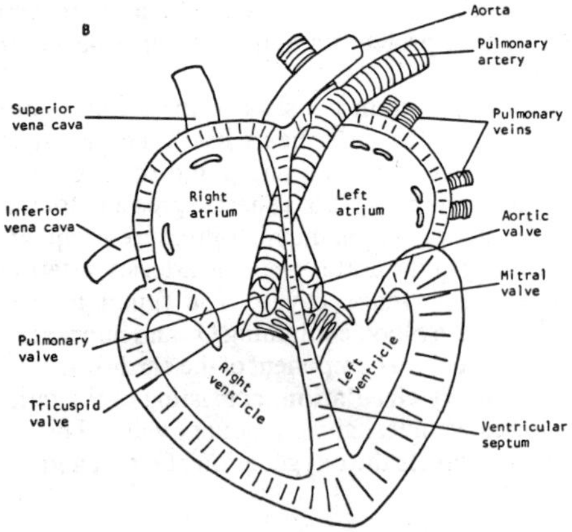

Figure 2–1. Structure of the heart. *Reprinted from* Mahoney, E. A., and J. P. Flynn, editors. Handbook of Medical-Surgical Nursing. John Wiley & Sons, Inc., New York. 1983. p. 384.

blood into the pulmonary artery, via the pulmonary valve. The normal pressure in the pulmonary artery is ~25 mmHg during systole and ~10 mmHg during diastole. The blood then flows through the lungs, picking up O_2 and giving up CO_2. The oxygenated blood from the lungs returns to the left heart via the pulmonary veins, emptying into the left atrium, where the mean pressure (LAP) is normally ~12 mmHg. From the left atrium, the blood flows into the left ventricle via the mitral valve. In the left ventricle, the pressure is normally ~120 mmHg during systole and ~10 mmHg during diastole. Finally, the left ventricle pumps blood into the aorta, via the aortic valve. In the aorta, the pressure is normally 120 mmHg during systole and 80 mmHg during diastole (*see* Fig. 2–1).

At a heart rate of 70 bpm, the **cardiac cycle** lasts ~850 milliseconds. At the start of the cycle, the mitral and tricuspid valves are open and blood returning to the heart enters the atria and ventricles. Following electrical excitation of the atria, as manifested by the P wave of the ECG, the atria contract, pumping the final bolus of blood into the ventricles before ventricular systole. Following electrical excitation of the ventricles, represented by the QRS complex on the ECG, the ventricles begin to contract, forcing shut the mitral and tricuspid valves. This valve closure causes turbulence of blood flow, which is heard as the S_1 heart sound. As the ventricles continue to contract, intraventricular pressure rises above the pressure in the aorta and pulmonary artery, forcing open the aortic and pulmonary valves. Blood is then ejected into these great arteries. The ventricles then begin to relax, allowing intraventricular pressures to fall below the pressure in the great arteries and allowing passive closure of the aortic and pulmonary valves. This closure can be seen on pressure tracings from the aorta and pulmonary artery as the dicrotic notch, and the related blood turbulence can be heard as the S_2 heart sound.

Electrical function

Electrical excitation of the heart is essential for its normal mechanical function and is ensured by the presence of a specialized **electrical conduction** system. The normal pacemaker of the heart is the sinoatrial (SA) node, a small group of cells that lie in the posterior-superior portion of the right atrium. A spontaneously arising impulse from the SA node spreads through the right atrium via local conduction and to the left atrium via Bachmann's bundle. Depolarization of the atria is seen on the surface ECG as the P wave.

The impulse also spreads to the atrioventricular (AV) node via the internodal pathways. The AV node, also referred to as the AV junction, is located in the lower right atrium, close to the interatrial septum. Conduction velocity is extremely slow through the AV node; thus, the impulse is delayed there, allowing time for the atria to be fully depolarized before the onset of ventricular depolarization.

From the AV node, the impulse travels inferiorly via the common bundle, also referred to as the bundle of His, and then on to the right and left bundle branches. The right bundle branch travels down the right side of the interventricular septum, giving rise to Purkinje fibers, which allow the impulse to be spread throughout the right ventricle. The left bundle branch travels only a short distance before it branches into its two primary divisions, the posteroinferior fascicle and the anterosuperior fascicle. Both fascicles further divide, eventually giving rise to Purkinje fibers, allowing the impulse to spread throughout the left ventricle. Conduction velocity is extremely rapid through the ventricular conduction system; thus, both the right and left ventricles are depolarized almost instantaneously and simultaneously. Ventricular depolarization is seen on the surface ECG as the QRS complex. The electrical system of the heart can be seen in Figure 2–2.

Like all other cells in the body, the cardiac cell exhibits a **resting membrane potential.** The magnitude of this resting potential is ~−90

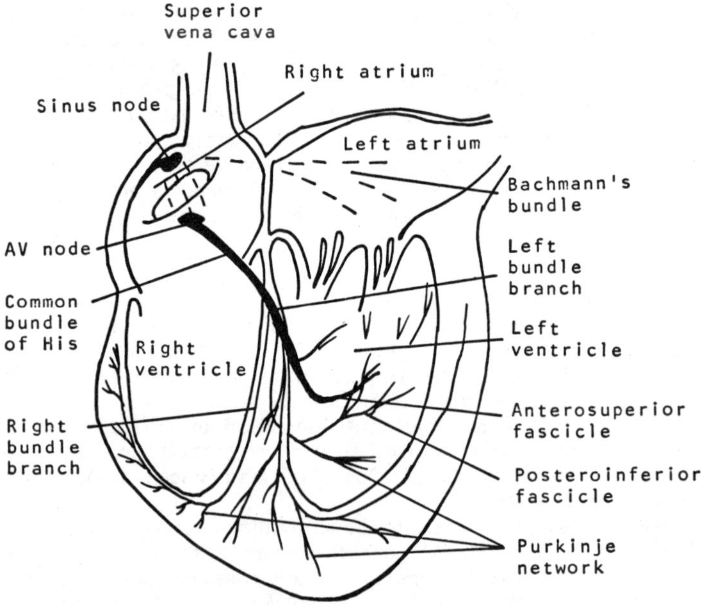

Figure 2–2. Electrical system of the heart. *Reprinted from* Mahoney, E. A., and J. P. Flynn, editors. Handbook of Medical Surgical Nursing. John Wiley & Sons, Inc., New York. 1983. p. 387.

millivolts (mV), the interior of the cell being negative with respect to the exterior. This resting membrane potential exists primarily because the resting cell membrane is impermeable to proteins, essentially impermeable to sodium ions (Na^+), and relatively permeable to potassium ions (K^+). A small contribution to the resting membrane potential is made by the sodium-potassium ATPase located on the cell membrane. This ATPase pumps Na^+ out of the cardiac cell in exchange for K^+ being pumped back into the cell. When the cell is at rest, the concentration of Na^+ is higher outside the cell and the concentration of K^+ is higher inside the cell.

When a cardiac cell is electrically excited, there is a characteristic alteration in the permeability of the cell membrane to various ions, resulting in what is referred to as an **action potential.** Initially, there is an influx of Na^+, entering via "fast channels" in most cells of the heart. This Na^+ influx causes the membrane potential to become less negative. This early Na^+ influx occurs during what is termed phase 0 of the cardiac action potential, when the membrane potential changes from its resting level of −90 mV to ~+20 mV. During the next phase, phase 1, there is an influx of chloride ions (Cl^-), which tends to make the membrane potential a little more negative, bringing the membrane potential back to ~0 mV. During the next phase, phase 2, or the plateau phase, there is an influx of calcium ions (Ca^{++}) through the so-called "slow channels." During this phase, the membrane potential is fairly stable at ~0 mV. Because the heart is dependent upon extracellular Ca^{++} for contraction and because the intracellular Ca^{++} concentration is an important determinant of myocardial contractility, the amount of Ca^{++} that can enter the cell during the plateau is extremely important in determining the mechanical function of the heart. During the next phase of the cardiac action potential, phase 3, there is efflux of K^+. This returns the membrane potential to its resting level of ~−90 mV. Finally, during phase 4, the resting state, the membrane potential is maintained at ~−90 mV.

The configuration of the action potential varies in different areas of the heart. In the atria, there is a typical fast action potential, with rapid influx of Na^+ through fast channels during phase 0. The plateau phase is relatively short, resulting in little Ca^{++} influx during this period. In contrast, the ventricles also have a fast action potential, but with a long plateau phase, thus allowing for greater Ca^{++} entry during the action potential. In pacemaker cells—for instance, the SA node—there is a slow action potential, with the influx of Na^+ during phase 0 being much slower. Another characteristic of slow action potentials is that there is diastolic depolarization, also referred to as a prepotential or phase 4 drift, probably occurring because of increased Na^+ permeability or decreased K^+ permeability in the resting state. This diastolic depolarization causes the resting potential to drift upward to that threshold value that elicits an action potential. The inherent rate of the pacemaker can be varied by altering the rate at which the membrane potential changes during phase 4, by altering the threshold value at which the action potential will be elicited, or by altering the membrane potential at the start of phase 4. Any cell in the heart that normally has a fast action potential can be converted to a slow-action-potential cell under various pathologic situations, such as ischemia, and thus act as an ectopic pacemaker.

At certain times in the electrical cycle, the heart is refractory to further stimulation. During the absolute refractory period, which lasts from the beginning of phase 0 and extends about halfway through phase 3, not even a strong stimulus can elicit another action potential. This is due to inactivation of the Na^+ fast channels. The relative refractory period follows and lasts until almost the end of phase 3. During this period, a stronger-than-normal stimulus could elicit an action potential. Finally, during the supranormal period, which lasts until the end of phase 3, a weaker-than-normal stimulus can elicit an action potential. It is during the supranormal period that ventricular ectopic activity can lead to ventricular fibrillation or ventricular tachycardia.

Mechanical function

The amount of blood that is ejected from either ventricle of the heart during one minute is termed the **CO.** In normal humans, the resting CO in liters equals 7 to 8% of the body weight in kg. Thus, a normal 70-kg man has a resting CO of ~5 liters/min.

Normally, the COs of the left and right ventricles are equal. A change in the CO from one ventricle will cause a change in the CO of the other ventricle within a few contractions. For instance, if the CO from the right ventricle suddenly decreases, there will be decreased venous return to the left heart. This will result in decreased ejection of blood from the left ventricle during the next contraction.

CO is sometimes expressed as the **cardiac index.** The cardiac index equals the CO divided by the body surface area. A 70-kg man has a body surface area of ~1.6 square meters; thus, his normal resting cardiac index is ~3 liters/min.

The output of the heart can also be expressed on a per beat basis. The **stroke volume** is the amount of blood that is ejected from either ventricle during a single contraction; it normally equals ~70 ml. CO equals the stroke volume times the heart rate. The **stroke index** equals the stroke volume divided by the body surface area; it is normally ~40 ml in a 70-kg man.

The heart's mechanical function is closely regulated, both by influences extrinsic to the heart and by intrinsic properties of the heart. A main controller of the function of the heart is the **Frank-Starling**—or **length-tension—relationship,** which describes the correlation between CO and end-diastolic ventricular volume—i.e., the amount of blood in the ventricle just prior to contraction, the **preload,** is a determinant of the amount of blood that will be ejected from the heart on the succeeding contraction. Under normal conditions, the end-diastolic ventricular volume is proportional to end-diastolic ventricular pressure; in turn, left ventricular end-diastolic pressure can be estimated by the pulmonary artery wedge pressure (PAWP) (in the absence of pulmonary hypertension or mitral valve disease). Thus, PAWP is a good estimator of preload. In health, the normal PAWP is 5 to 10 mmHg.

The basis of the length-tension relationship is that, like skeletal muscle, cardiac cells consist of interdigitating contractile fibers made up of actin and myosin, organized into repeating units known as sarcomeres. When the cardiac cell is electrically excited, there is an influx of Ca^{++}, which binds to a regulatory protein (troponin) on the actin filament, shifting the tropomyosin molecule, which also sits on the actin filament, and thereby uncovering the myosin binding site. This allows the actin and myosin to form cross-bridges and, at the expense of metabolic energy, to effect shortening of the sarcomere.

There is maximal ability to effect sarcomere shortening at a resting sarcomere length of ~2.2 microns (μ). At shorter lengths, there is overlap of some of the filaments and further shortening is less effective. At longer sarcomere lengths, there is too little overlap of the contractile filaments and thus there is decreased ability to form cross-bridges and effect shortening. In the intact heart, sarcomere length is proportional to end-diastolic ventricular volume. At optimal end-diastolic ventricular volumes, corresponding to optimal resting sarcomere lengths, the heart is able to develop the greatest tension during contraction and thus is able to pump the most blood. At both larger and smaller ventricular volumes, the ventricle is less able to develop pressure and pump blood.

A second controller of heart function is the pressure against which the heart must pump in order to eject blood; this pressure is termed the **afterload.** At higher afterloads, the heart must work harder to eject the same volume of blood. The afterload of the left ventricle is estimated by the mean aortic pressure (MABP), normally ~90 to 95 mmHg. For the right ventricle, the afterload is estimated by the mean pulmonary artery pressure (PAM), which normally is ~15 mmHg.

Another controller of the function of the heart is its inotropic, or contractile, state. A change in **contractility** is defined as a change in CO without a change in preload or afterload. Contractility is determined primarily by Ca^{++} availability, since it is Ca^{++} binding to troponin that allows the actin and myosin filaments to bind to each other and cause actual muscle shortening. Thus, anything that increases Ca^{++} availability during contraction will increase contractility. For instance, catecholamines such as epinephrine and norepinephrine increase the contractility of the heart by increasing Ca^{++} influx during phase 2 of the cardiac action potential. Digitalis increases Ca^{++} availability in part by increasing the activity of a calcium-sodium exchange pump on the cell membrane; this exchange pump, active during diastole, brings Ca^{++} into the cell in exchange for moving Na^{+} out of the cell.

The ANS controls not only the inotropic state of the heart but other myocardial functions as well. Sympathetic stimulation, arising from the vasomotor center in the medulla, causes an increase in heart rate and conductivity. Parasympathetic stimulation, arising from the cardioinhibitory center in the medulla, causes a decrease in heart rate and conductivity. Normally, the heart is under predominantly parasympathetic control.

As a working tissue, the heart requires O_2 and nutrients. In fact, the heart is an obligatory aerobe, i.e., it cannot function in the absence of a continuous supply of O_2. The amount of O_2 that the heart requires, the **myocardial O_2 consumption** or myocardial O_2 demand (MVO_2) is determined by ventricular-wall tension, heart rate, the velocity of contraction (which is primarily determined by the contractile state), and the pressure against which the heart ejects blood (the afterload).

THE PERIPHERAL CIRCULATION

Structures

The peripheral circulation functions to deliver nutrients and oxygenated blood to working tissues and to remove CO_2 and metabolic wastes. Its function is closely regulated to ensure that all tissues receive an adequate supply of blood under varying physiologic conditions.

The aorta and large arteries have elastic properties that allow them to store some of the energy generated during ventricular contraction and release the energy during diastole. This function, known as the Windkessel function, allows the blood flow to be fairly continuous, rather than intermittent, during the cardiac cycle. Pressure in the aorta and large arteries is the highest pressure in the systemic circulation. The velocity of blood flow is also the highest in the aorta and large arteries.

The arterioles are highly muscular, allowing them to function as resistance vessels. Their tone, or resistance, is determined by the interplay of two factors: ANS activity (primarily sympathetic vasoconstriction) and local factors (whereby a lack of O_2 or an excess of certain metabolic wastes can cause vasodilation). Certain tissues, such as the heart and brain, can autoregulate, i.e., they can maintain adequate blood flow in the event of major changes in the perfusion pressure generated in the systemic circulation.

The capillaries are the site of gas and nutrient exchange with the tissues and thus are the actual working part of the circulatory system. Although each individual capillary is small, ~7 to 10 μ in diameter, the total capillary cross-sectional area is large.

Exchange of fluid across the capillary wall is determined by the balance between forces that tend to hold fluid in the capillary and those forces that tend to move fluid out of the capillary. The most important force tending to move fluid out of the capillary is the capillary oncotic pressure; this is the portion of the capillary osmotic pressure that results from the presence of plasma proteins. Capillary oncotic pressure can be low in conditions such as hypoalbuminemia, resulting in peripheral edema. The most important force that tends to move fluid out of the capillary is the capillary hydrostatic pressure; this pressure is determined primarily by venous pressure. For instance, in left-ventricular heart failure, elevation of pulmonary venous pressure can raise pulmonary capillary hydrostatic pressure and thus result in pulmonary edema. Fluid that leaves the capillary is usually returned to the circulation via the lymphatic system; in the lungs, the fluid fills the alveoli and cannot be removed by the lymphatic system.

The venous system is primarily a capacitance system, with the ability to store large amounts of blood. Normally, ~60% of the blood in the systemic circulation is in the venous system. Venous tone, or capacitance, is also primarily under sympathetic nervous system control.

Expressed in liters, the average **circulating blood volume** in humans is 7 to 8% of the body weight in kg. Thus, in a 70-kg man, blood volume is ~5 liters. At any time, about two-thirds of this volume is in the systemic venous circulation, one-sixth is in the systemic arterial circulation, and the remainder is divided between the systemic capillaries and the pulmonary circulation.

The **coronary circulation** is a special branch of the peripheral circulation, of primary importance for maintaining the nutrient and O_2 supply to the heart itself. The coronary vessels arise off the ascending aorta, just behind the cusps of the aortic valve. The right coronary artery descends to the groove (coronary sulcus) located between the atria and ventricles; posteriorly it gives rise to the posterior descending coronary artery. In ~90% of people, the right coronary artery supplies blood to the SA node and atria and to the right ventricle, to the AV node, and the bundle of His; in ~50% of people, it also supplies blood to the SA node and atria. The posterior descending branch supplies the inferior, or diaphragmatic, wall of the left ventricle and the posterior papillary muscle in most people. The left coronary artery divides into the left anterior descending and circumflex coronary arteries. The left anterior descending coronary artery travels inferiorly in the interventricular sulcus, supplying blood to the anterior septum and walls of the right and left ventricles, the anterior papillary muscle, the right bundle branch, and the anterior portion of the left bundle branch. The circumflex coronary artery travels posteriorly in the sulcus separating the left atrium and ventricle. In ~50% of people, it supplies the SA node and atria; in ~10% of people, it supplies the AV node and the bundle of His. The circumflex coronary artery also supplies the lateral wall and part of the inferior wall of the left ventricle. Diagonal branches off the left coronary artery supply the anterior and lateral walls of the left ventricle. Figure 2–3 depicts the arteries of the coronary circulation.

Control of the peripheral circulation

As the heart ejects blood, it encounters resistance to flow. CO equals the pressure drop across the circulation divided by the resistance to flow. For the systemic circulation, the pressure drop is from the aorta (with a mean pressure of ~90 mmHg) to the right atrium (with a pressure of ~0 mmHg).

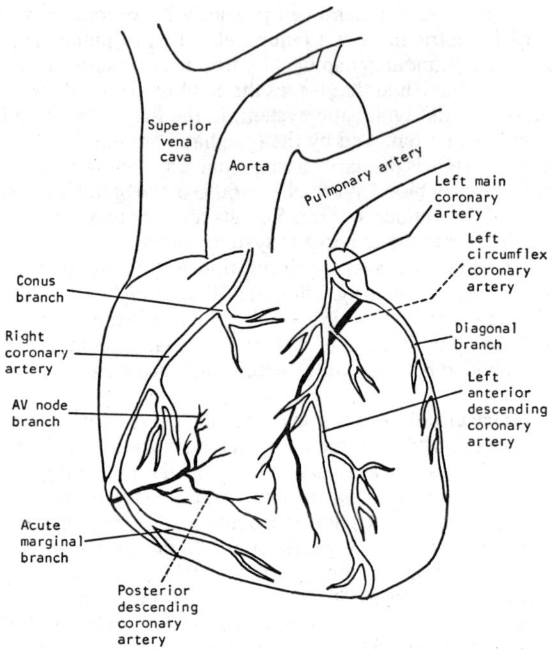

Figure 2–3. Coronary circulation—arteries. *Reprinted from* Mahoney, E. A., and J. P. Flynn, editors. Handbook of Medical Surgical Nursing. John Wiley & Sons, Inc., New York. 1983. p. 385.

Thus, with a normal CO of ~5 liters/min, the calculated systemic resistance is 90/5, or 18 mmHg/liter/min. Peripheral resistance is usually expressed in dyne-sec/cm^5; this value is obtained by multiplying mmHg/liter/min by 80. Thus, the normal systemic resistance is 1440 dyne-sec/cm^5. For the pulmonary circulation, the pressure drop is from the pulmonary artery (with a mean pressure of ~15 mmHg) to the left atrium (with a pressure of ~5 mmHg). At the same CO of 5 liters/min, the calculated pulmonary resistance is 2 mmHg/liter/min, or 160 dyne-sec/cm^5.

Vascular resistance is determined primarily by the radius of blood vessels, primarily arterioles, in the circulation. As the vessel radius decreases, vascular resistance increases. In most tissues, blood vessel radius is primarily under control of the sympathetic nervous system.

In some tissues, blood vessels have the ability to autoregulate, i.e., they can maintain constant blood flow in the face of changes in perfusion pressure. Tissues that are the most capable of autoregulation are the vital organs: the heart, kidneys, and brain. An additional property of blood vessels in many organs is the ability to vasodilate in response to increased O_2 demand by the tissue. Of particular importance is the ability of the coronary arteries to dilate in response to increased MVO_2.

Control of arterial BP

Arterial BP is closely regulated because it provides the pressure head for perfusion of the various organ beds of the body. Arterial BP is sensed by baroreceptors in the aortic arch and carotid sinus. These stretch receptors increase their firing rate as arterial pressure rises. In a healthy person they are most sensitive to pressure changes in the range of 60 to 160 mmHg. The sensitivity of the baroreceptors can be altered, e.g., in hypertension, where the most sensitive range may be 100 to 200 mmHg.

Impulses from the carotid sinus and aortic arch travel via the glossopharyngeal and vagus nerves, respectively. Impulses are processed in the cardiovascular centers of the medulla, and efferent impulses are emitted from the vasomotor (sympathetic) and cardioinhibitory (parasympathetic) centers. Increasing sympathetic outflow from the medulla will cause an increase in BP by increasing vasomotor tone in arterioles, increasing venous tone—and thus decreasing venous capacitance and increasing venous return to the heart—and by directly affecting the heart to increase contractility, conductivity, and heart rate. There is little parasympathetic enervation to the vasculature; increasing parasympathetic outflow exerts effects primarily by inhibiting sympathetic outflow. In addition, the parasympathetic nervous system can affect the heart directly, causing decreased heart rate, contractility, and conductivity.

THE PULMONARY CIRCULATION

The pulmonary circulation is anatomically analogous to the peripheral circulation. Physiologically, however, it is different because the pulmonary vessels have little elastic or muscular content. The pulmonary circulation will be considered only briefly in this chapter.

ASSESSMENT OF THE PATIENT

Health history

Relevant areas about which information should be obtained for individuals with actual or potential cardiovascular disease are outlined in Table 2–1.

Physical examination

Inspection. General inspection of the patient may reveal nonspecific signs of cardiovascular disease such as anxiety, pain, and general distress.

TABLE 2–1
Health History

Assessment	Possible abnormality
Pain Location Precipitating factors Alleviating factors Severity Quality Associated signs and symptoms	Angina pectoris Substernal pressure or dull ache, usually mild to moderate in intensity, rarely with associated signs or symptoms, often precipitated by exercise or stress, usually relieved by nitroglycerin MI Substernal pressure or dull ache, may radiate to left arm, back, mild to severe in intensity, may be accompanied by shortness of breath, diaphoresis, nausea, vomiting, not usually precipitated by exercise or stress, not usually relieved by nitroglycerin Pericarditis Sharp, stabbing pain in left anterior chest, often aggravated by deep inspiration Anxiety May mimic angina pectoris or acute MI
Dyspnea Duration Occurrence at rest or with exertion Correlated with body position (orthopnea) Occurrence at night (paroxysmal nocturnal dyspnea)	CHF Anxiety secondary to angina pectoris, acute MI
Palpitations	Arrhythmias Premature ventricular contractions Premature atrial contractions Paroxysmal atrial tachycardia Anxiety
Headache	Hypertension
Epistaxis	Hypertension
Edema Weight gain Rings or shoes fit too tightly	CHF
Syncope	Arrhythmias Anxiety
Family history of cardiovascular disease	May predispose to cardiovascular disease
Current medications Compliance with therapeutic regimen	Poor compliance may increase risk of cardiovascular complications

Assessment	Possible abnormality
Exercise habits Recreational activity Type Frequency Duration Occupational activity	Sedentary life-style predisposes to coronary artery disease and hypertension
Occupation	Stressful occupation increases risk of coronary artery disease and hypertension
Usual diet Salt intake Saturated fat intake Cholesterol intake Alcohol consumption	High intake of salt, saturated fat, and cholesterol may predispose to coronary artery disease and hypertension Moderate alcohol intake may decrease risk of coronary artery disease; high intake may lead to heart failure
Cigarette smoking Amount Years smoked Type of tobacco product used	May predispose to coronary artery disease and hypertension
Other diseases Diabetes mellitus Thyroid disease	May predispose to coronary artery disease and hypertension

Body build and physique should be noted, as obesity and the lack of physical exercise may be indicators of coronary artery disease (CAD) risk factors. In addition, there are several specific signs that may be detected on inspection of the patient.

Ophthalmoscopic examination of the retina may aid in the medical diagnosis of hypertension.

The skin, particularly in the extremities, lips, and mucosa, should be examined for color (cyanosis), turgor (indicative of fluid balance), and temperature (indicative of peripheral vasomotor tone).

Capillary refill time may be estimated by blanching the finger- or toenails with brief pressure and watching for the return of normal coloration. Delayed return indicates sluggish circulation to that extremity.

The CVP may be estimated by inspecting the jugular veins. The patient should be positioned in a relaxed position with the head turned away from the examiner; the head of the bed should then be raised until the upper level of venous pulsation can be seen in the neck. The vertical height from that point to the suprasternal notch is a good estimator of CVP, or RAP. The normal CVP is $<$3cm of water pressure.

With the patient lying in semi-Fowler's position, the chest should be examined for the position of the apical impulse, normally located at the fifth intercostal space at the midclavicular line. In addition, the presence of any abnormal lifts or heaves on the anterior chest should be noted. These abnormal movements may be more easily detected at the end of expiration.

The presence or absence of peripheral edema should be noted and graded on a five-point scale, with 0 representing no edema and 4+ representing severe, pitting edema. Areas to be examined include the legs (ankles and pretibial area), hands, and sacrum.

Palpation. The pulse rate and rhythm should be initially evaluated over a full minute. To determine the pulse deficit, the radial pulse rate should be compared to a simultaneously determined apical pulse rate, determined by auscultation. A pulse deficit may be indicative of hypovolemia or certain arrhythmias.

All major arterial pulses (radial, brachial, carotid, femoral, popliteal, posterior tibial, dorsalis pedis) should be evaluated bilaterally for quality and symmetry. Pulses are graded on a five-point scale on which 0 represents an absent pulse, 2+ represents a normal pulse, and 4+ represents a bounding pulse. If the pulse is weak in a given artery, its location should be marked on the skin so that it may be more easily located for serial comparisons. Weak or apparently absent pulses may also be assessed with the use of a Doppler detection device.

Systolic BP may be determined by palpation. This technique is particularly useful when the pulse volume is too small to allow detection of turbulent flow by auscultation. In order to determine the systolic BP by palpation, the brachial artery is palpated while pressure is released from the sphygmomanometer cuff. The systolic BP is recorded as being that point at which pulsations are first felt.

The presence of hepatojugular reflux may be determined by positioning the patient as for inspection of the jugular venous pulse. If firm, sustained pressure over the right upper quadrant, directly below the costal margin, increases jugular venous pressure by >1 cm of water pressure, then reflux is said to be present and may indicate the presence of CHF.

Percussion. Percussion may be used to outline the lateral border of the heart. However, this determination is more readily made from the chest x-ray and therefore is not commonly used.

Auscultation. Basic measurement of arterial BP by auscultation will not be discussed here. Certain cardiovascular abnormalities may, however, be detected by careful BP auscultation. First, BP should be measured in both arms and both legs; a difference of >10 mmHg is consistent with aortic disease.

Pulsus paradoxus is a drop in systolic BP on inspiration. In order to detect this drop by auscultation, the BP cuff is inflated above the systolic BP and then slowly deflated until intermittent Korotkoff sounds are heard, while the patient breathes quietly. The cuff is then further deflated very slowly until Korotkoff sounds are heard with every heartbeat. If the point at which the sounds are first heard and the point at which they are consistently heard are >10 mmHg apart, then pulsus paradoxus is said to be present. Pulsus paradoxus may also be detected with intra-arterial pressure monitoring; again, it is the difference in systolic BP between inspiration and expiration. Pulsus paradoxus is a clinical finding in constrictive pericardial disease and in COPD.

Auscultation of the heart is useful primarily in the diagnosis of valvular heart disease. It can, however, also be useful in diagnosing and following the clinical progression of certain arrhythmias, pericarditis, and CHF. Proper auscultation of the heart in the ICU may be difficult, because it requires a quiet environment and adequate time. A stethoscope with both a bell (for lower-pitched sounds) and a diaphragm (for higher-pitched sounds) should be used.

S_1 is a normal sound, created by turbulent blood flow at the time of closure of the mitral and tricuspid valves. It occurs at the onset of systole. It is heard simultaneously with the apical impulse and slightly before the carotid impulse. It is best heard at the apex of the heart (fifth intercostal space at the midclavicular line) with the diaphragm of the stethoscope. S_1 should be evaluated in terms of its intensity. A loud S_1 may be associated with mitral stenosis, a short PR interval on the ECG, tachycardia, or hyperthyroidism. A soft S_1 may be associated with a thick chest wall or first-degree heart block. Variations in the intensity of S_1 are heard with atrial fibrillation and complete heart block.

S_2 is the sound created by turbulent blood flow at the time of closure of the aortic and pulmonary valves. It occurs at the end of systole and is best heard at the pulmonic area (second intercostal space at the left sternal border) using the diaphragm of the stethoscope. S_2 should be evaluated in terms of splitting into its aortic and pulmonic components.

Physiologic splitting of S_2 is a delay in the pulmonary component that is usually detectable only on inspiration. The delay occurs because on inspiration there is greater venous return to the right heart, resulting in a greater stroke volume. It takes a fraction of a second longer to pump out this additional amount of blood, and thus there is a slight delay in closure of the pulmonary valve, detectable as a split S_2 on inspiration. Physiologic splitting is a normal variation, often heard in healthy people.

On the other hand, **paradoxic splitting** of S_2, an abnormal finding, is detectable only on expiration. This condition is most commonly seen in left bundle branch block, in which there is delayed closure of the aortic valve. On expiration, this delayed closure, occurring later than closure of the pulmonary valve, may be detected as paradoxic splitting of S_2. On inspiration, however, as discussed above, there is also delayed closure of the pulmonary valve. Thus, on inspiration, there is nearly simultaneous closure of the aortic and pulmonary valves; a single S_2 is then heard.

Fixed splitting of S_2 is splitting that does not vary with respiration. It is most commonly seen with right ventricular failure.

Wide splitting of S_2 is splitting that is heard on expiration and is accentuated on inspiration. It may be due to delayed pulmonary valve closure, as in pulmonary stenosis, right ventricular pacing, and right bundle branch block, or early closure of the aortic valve, as in aortic stenosis.

S_3 is a heart sound that is heard normally only in people under the age of 30. In older people, it indicates decreased ventricular compliance and is often referred to as a ventricular gallop. It is commonly heard in individuals with CHF. S_3 occurs just after S_2 and is a low-pitched sound, best heard with the bell of the stethoscope over the apex of the heart, with the patient lying on the left side.

S_4, also referred to as an atrial gallop, occurs just before S_1. It is also a low-pitched sound, heard with the bell of the stethoscope over the apex of the heart with the patient lying on the left side. Although S_4 may be heard in normal people, more commonly it is caused by increased resistance to ventricular filling. It is found in patients with hypertension, CAD, and aortic stenosis.

When both S_3 and S_4 are heard in a patient, it is referred to as a summation gallop. This finding is consistent with CHF.

Murmurs are abnormal heart sounds that most commonly occur because of turbulence associated with blood flow past a partial obstruction or irregular valve or increased blood flow past normal structures. Murmurs are evaluated in terms of timing, intensity, location, radiation, configuration, pitch, and quality.

Timing refers to whether the murmur occurs during systole (between S_1 and S_2) or during diastole (between S_2 and S_1).

Intensity is usually graded on a six-point scale, as follows: (1) a faint murmur heard only with special efforts; (2) a faint but readily heard murmur; (3) a prominent but not loud murmur; (4) a loud murmur with thrill; (5) a very loud murmur with thrill; (6) an exceptionally loud murmur with thrill, best heard with the stethoscope just removed from the chest.

Location and *radiation* of the murmur refer to the anatomic area where the murmur can be heard best and the limits of the area where it can be even minimally detected. Location is often described in the following terms: aortic—2nd intercostal space, right sternal border; pulmonary—2nd intercostal space, left sternal border; tricuspid—5th intercostal space, left sternal border; mitral (apical)—5th intercostal space, midclavicular line.

Configuration refers to whether the murmur increases or decreases in intensity during the cardiac cycle. A crescendo murmur becomes louder over the cycle while a decrescendo murmur becomes softer. Other configurations include crescendo-decrescendo and decrescendo-crescendo murmurs. A plateau murmur does not change in intensity during the cardiac cycle.

Pitch refers to the tonal frequency of the sound and is usually described as being high, medium, or low.

Quality refers to the nature of the sound. Words such as blowing, rumbling, harsh, and musical are used to describe the quality of the murmur.

A few common murmurs are described in Table 2–2.

A pericardial friction rub is a three-component sound that is heard over the entire cardiac cycle. The first component occurs with atrial systole, the second with ventricular systole, and the third with ventricular diastole.

TABLE 2–2
Common Heart Murmurs

	AS	AI	PS	MI	MS	TI
Timing	Systolic	Diastolic	Systolic	Systolic	Diastolic	Systolic
Intensity	Variable	Variable	Variable	Variable	Variable	Variable
Location	Aortic area	Aortic area	Pulmonary area	Mitral area	Mitral area	Tricuspid area
Radiation	To neck, apex	To apex, right sternal border	To left shoulder, neck	To left axilla	Little radiation	To apex, right sternal border
Configuration	C/D	D	C/D	Plateau	D/C	Plateau
Pitch	Medium	High	Medium	High	Low	High
Quality	Harsh	Blowing	Harsh	Blowing	Rumbling	Blowing

AI, aortic insufficiency; AS, aortic stenosis; C/D, crescendo-decresendo; D, decresendo; D/C, decresendo-cresendo; MI, mitral insufficiency; MS; mitral stenosis; PS, pulmonary stenosis; TI, tricuspid insufficiency.

TABLE 2–3

Cardiovascular Diagnostic Measures

Name	Procedure	Associated care	Possible findings
ECG	Measurement of electrical activity of heart, as detected by skin surface electrodes.	None required	Arrhythmias MI Chamber enlargement Pericarditis
Vectrocardiogram	Similar to ECG, but graphic output is in terms of loops representing instantaneous changes in vectors of electrical activity of heart.	None required	Same as ECG
Holter monitoring	Continuous one- or two-lead ECG monitoring over extended time period (12–24 hr), recorded onto magnetic tape. Patient maintains diary of activity during recording period, to allow correlation with arrhythmias.	Patient teaching about diary maintenance	Arrhythmias May pick up arrhythmias that are not detected by routine ICU monitoring
Chest x-ray	Usually anterior-posterior and lateral roentgenograms.	None required	Cardiomegaly CHF Identification of pacemaker lead placement
Cardiac catheterization	Insertion of catheter(s) into heart chambers. Right heart catheterization: catheter inserted via femoral or brachial vein. Left heart catheterization: catheter inserted transseptally or via carotid, brachial, or femoral artery. May include: Coronary arteriography via injection of dye into coronary arteries, via aortic catheter. May also administer drugs or have patient exercise to induce angina. Ventriculography by injecting dye into ventricles. Blood gas measurements. Pressure measurements.	Preprocedure: NPO Void on call Informed consent Patient teaching about procedure and sensation that will probably be experienced during procedure Postprocedure: Monitor vital signs Check color, sensation, and movement of affected extremity Check for bleeding from catheter insertion sites Bed rest for 24 hr Sandbag to arterial puncture	Coronary artery disease Variant angina Abnormal ventricular wall motion Ventricular aneurysm Septal defects Valvular lesions

Electrophysiologic study (His bundle ECG)	Insertion of one or more catheters into heart; may be left in place for several days. May involve administration of various antiarrhythmic agents. May involve repeated induction of ventricular tachycardia, with possible need for cardioversion or resuscitation.	Preprocedure: As for cardiac catherization Postprocedure: As for cardiac catheterization If catheters are left in place: bed rest, arrhythmia monitoring	Location of irritable electrical focus or source of recurrent lethal arrhythmias Selection of optimal antiarrhythmic therapy
Phonocardiogram	Sensitive microphone applied to chest wall; graphic recording of sound intensity during cardiac cycle.	None required	Evaluation of cardiac murmurs
Echocardiogram	Microphone-transducer applied to chest wall; skin contact increased by application of mineral oil or other lubricant. May be M-mode or two-dimensional; difference is in type of instrument applied to chest and type of recording produced.	None required	Infective endocarditis Valvular lesions Pericardial effusion
Exercise ECG (stress test)	Evaluation of resting ECG, followed by incremental exercise on bicycle or treadmill ergometer with constant ECG and intermittent BP monitoring. Test is stopped when angina or undue fatigue or dyspnea occur, heart rate reaches given percentage of predicted maximum, BP exceeds normal range, or ECG abnormalities are seen. May involve adminstration of thallium just prior to end of exercise, followed by chest scanning immediately and 6–8 hr later.	Preprocedure: NPO for 2–4 hr Avoid nicotine and caffeine for 2–4 hr before test Instruct patient to wear comfortable clothes for exercise (shoes, brassiere) Postprocedure: Monitor vital signs until back to base line and patient is asymptomatic When monitoring is complete, instruct patient that he may take warm (not hot) shower	Diagnosis of angina Exercise prescription or follow-up of therapy
Gated blood pool study (MUGA scan)	Labeling of RBCs with technetium-99m (requires two venipunctures), then scintillation camera placed over chest wall at varying angles; patient positioned supine for 15–30 min; ECG monitoring leads attached	Teach patient about sensations that will probably be experienced during procedure	Measurement of ejection fraction

All components may not always be heard. A friction rub is usually best heard in the third intercostal space at the left sternal border; it usually does not radiate. The intensity is variable but may be increased on expiration, with the patient sitting forward. The pitch is high, and the quality is scratchy.

Diagnostic tests

A variety of invasive and noninvasive tests may be performed on patients with known or suspected cardiovascular disease. Basic information about many of these tests is presented in Table 2–3. Additional information on electrocardiography is presented in Appendix A and on hemodynamic monitoring in Chapter 14.

MAJOR DISORDERS

ANGINA PECTORIS

Angina pectoris is chest pain that occurs when MVO_2 exceeds O_2 supply.

Pathophysiology

The primary cause of angina pectoris is a decrease in blood supply to the heart, below the level required to meet its metabolic demands. Disease processes that can decrease blood supply to the heart include CAD and coronary vasospasm. Chest pain of cardiac origin may also be caused by increased MVO_2, as in severe exercise or in certain forms of valvular heart disease. It may also be caused by decreased MABP, which causes decreased coronary perfusion pressure and thus decreased myocardial blood supply. These two latter causes of cardiac pain will not be discussed further in this chapter.

CAD, also referred to as coronary atherosclerosis, is the most common cause of death in the USA today. The earliest lesion of coronary atherosclerosis is the fatty streak. This is a smooth, yellow lesion in the intima, or innermost layer, of the vessel wall. It does not extend into the vessel lumen and thus does not decrease flow through the vessel. The lesion results from the accumulation of lipids, primarily cholesterol and cholesterol esters, in the cells of the intima. Fatty streaks have been observed in people of all ages and are universally found in people >1 yr. Whether or not they are the precursors of later lesions in the progression of CAD is unknown. It is known, however, that the fatty streak occurs at the same location in the vascular tree as do subsequent lesions.

The fibrous plaque is the typical lesion of CAD. Unlike the fatty streak, the fibrous plaque extends into the vessel lumen and may reduce or completely obstruct blood flow through the vessel. The fibrous plaque consists of smooth muscle cells, collagen, and lipid, accumulating in the intimal layer of the vessel.

The complicated lesion is the most advanced lesion of **CAD**. **It is a** fibrous plaque that has been worsened by thrombus formation, hemorrhage, or calcification. Complicated lesions typically are seen in the setting of MI.

Development of atherosclerotic lesions has been correlated with the presence of certain coronary risk factors. These risk factors have been identified by large epidemiologic studies, such as the Framingham study. The incidence of atherosclerotic CAD is higher than average in males, postmenopausal females, older individuals, individuals with a family history of atherosclerosis, individuals with hypertension or diabetes mellitus, overweight individuals, sedentary individuals, individuals who lead a stressful life, in individuals who smoke or who consume a diet high in cholesterol, saturated fatty acids and salt, and in individuals with hypertriglyceridemia, hyperlipoproteinemia, or hypercholesterolemia.

There are several hypotheses that have been advanced to explain why CAD occurs. One such hypothesis, the Virchow response-to-injury hypothesis, holds that damage to the vascular endothelium leads to platelet aggregation, smooth muscle proliferation, and lipid deposition. If the damage is not allowed to heal, permanent changes characteristic of atherosclerosis may occur. This hypothesis can explain the observed link between CAD and certain coronary risk factors such as hypertension, smoking, hypercholesterolemia, hypertriglyceridemia, and hyperlipoproteinemia.

A second hypothesis that may explain the pathogenesis of CAD is the monoclonal hypothesis. Briefly, this hypothesis holds that following exposure to certain mutagens, smooth muscle cells in the vessel wall begin to proliferate abnormally, eventually resulting in an atherosclerotic lesion. This hypothesis can explain the observed link between coronary atherosclerosis and cigarette smoking and hypercholesterolemia.

A third hypothesis is the lipid insudation hypothesis, which posits that atherosclerotic lesions result when lipids taken up from the blood act as irritants in the vessel wall. This hypothesis is consistent with the observation that hypercholesterolemia, hypertriglyceridemia, and hyperlipoproteinemia are correlated with an increased incidence of CAD.

A second cause of angina pectoris is **coronary vasospasm;** the resulting syndrome is referred to as Prinzmetal's or variant angina. Coronary vasospasm can occur either in the presence or absence of CAD. In coronary vasospasm, there is increased coronary vascular resistance, most likely resulting from excessive sympathetic stimulation or from excessive responsiveness to sympathetic stimulation.

Regardless of the cause of the angina pectoris, the result is inadequate blood flow to meet the metabolic demands of the myocardium. There are two possible ways that the vascular system can compensate for O_2 insufficiency in peripheral tissues: increase O_2 extraction or increase coronary flow. Even at rest, however, the heart normally extracts a maximal amount of O_2 from the blood that nourishes it. Thus, the only way that O_2 supply to the heart can be increased is to decrease coronary vascular resistance. Coronary vascular resistance is under local control, i.e., vasodilation occurs in response to local demands and despite extrinsic controllers of vascular tone. In the individual with CAD, coronary vasodilation may occur at low levels of MVO_2; in the face of increased demand, further vasodilation cannot occur, and angina pectoris results.

A second possible response to relatively insufficient blood flow to the myocardium is decreased MVO_2. This demand is dependent upon heart rate, MABP, inotropic state, and ventricular wall tension. Decreasing any of these factors can help balance the relationship between supply and demand.

There is usually no permanent damage to the heart in individuals with angina pectoris. During episodes of ischemia, however, arrhythmias and contractile dysfunction may occur. Repeated episodes of myocardial ischemia may lead to microscopic changes in the heart; the significance of these changes is not fully understood.

Clinical picture

Signs and symptoms of angina pectoris are present only during the episodes of chest pain. The pain may be mild to severe in intensity, substernal in location, rarely radiating to other areas, usually precipitated by physical or emotional stress, and usually alleviated by rest or nitroglycerin. Pain quality is often described in terms such as "squeezing," "pressing," or "tightening." In the ICU, there may be some patients in whom it is difficult to distinguish angina pain from that of MI. Alternatively, in the ICU, there may be patients in whom the frequency of pain is increasing (crescendo or unstable angina). Unlike patients with MI, during episodes of chest pain, patients with angina pectoris are less likely to complain of symptoms such as nausea, diaphoresis, and shortness of breath.

ECG evidence of angina pectoris is usually obtainable only during the episodes of chest pain. Such evidence includes arrhythmias and ST-segment and T-wave changes. Downward-sloping ST segments are most common in angina pectoris of atherosclerotic origin, whereas in coronary vasospasm, ST-segment elevation may be seen.

The diagnosis of angina pectoris is based on the clinical history and the presence of coronary risk factors. In some cases, it is necessary to perform exercise ECGs (stress tests), possibly with thallium scanning, or cardiac catheterization with coronary angiography to confirm the diagnosis.

Determination of the angina threshold can be accomplished either during ECG or during cardiac catheterization by atrial pacing. The threshold is usually described by the double product (the product of the heart rate and systolic BP) at the point at which anginal pain occurs. The threshold is relatively constant in patients with CAD; therefore determination of the angina threshold can be useful in following the progression of the disease and in prescribing exercise regimens.

In coronary vasospasm, the diagnosis is often confirmed by elicitation of characteristic pain, for instance by the administration of ergonovine. This is usually performed in the cardiac catheterization laboratory.

Medical interventions

Medical therapy for the patient with angina pectoris consists of measures to prevent the progression of the disease, to decrease MVO_2, and to increase myocardial perfusion.

Measures to prevent progression of the disease include identification of coronary risk factors and their elimination wherever possible. This includes drug and/or diet therapy for hypertension, hyperlipoproteinemia, hypertriglyceridemia, hypercholesterolemia, obesity, and diabetes mellitus. An exercise regimen may be prescribed, on the basis of the results of an exercise ECG.

To reduce MVO_2, the mainstay of therapy in atherosclerotic angina pectoris is nitroglycerin. In the patient with coronary atherosclerosis, nitroglycerin exerts its antianginal effect primarily by causing peripheral vasodilation and thereby reducing the MVO_2. Other, long-acting nitrates, such as isosorbide dinitrate, may also be used in angina pectoris. Alternatively, beta-adrenergic blockers, such as propranolol, may be prescribed; these agents also decrease MVO_2.

To increase coronary perfusion, medical interventions include drug therapy, percutaneous transluminal coronary angioplasty (PTCA), and coronary artery bypass graft surgery (CABG). Drug therapy to increase coronary perfusion is usually not effective in atherosclerotic angina pectoris, although in healthy individuals nitroglycerin is a coronary vasodilator. In coronary vasospasm, the mainstay of pharmacologic therapy is nifedipine, a calcium channel blocker that prevents coronary vasoconstriction.

PTCA is a nonsurgical procedure in which a balloon catheter is inserted into the heart in a technique similar to that used in cardiac catheterization. Under fluoroscopy, the balloon is positioned at the site of the stenosis. It is then briefly inflated, resulting in an increased vessel lumen. PTCA is most commonly performed in individuals with atherosclerotic CAD who are unresponsive to pharmacologic therapy and in whom there is a single proximal lesion. It is rarely performed in individuals with left anterior descending lesions. Advantages of PTCA include the fact that it may be performed under local anesthesia; thus, the incidence of immediate postprocedure morbidity is low. Disadvantages of PTCA include intraprocedure complications such as vessel damage and frequent recurrence of the lesion within 6 mo.

CABG is a surgical procedure, performed under general anesthesia, in which coronary stenoses are bypassed by inserting a segment of blood vessel between the aorta and the myocardium distal to the lesion. The grafted segment is usually isolated from the saphenous veins of the legs. Following thoracotomy, cardiopulmonary bypass is initiated, the heart is arrested, and the graft is performed. The incidence of immediate postoperative complications is correlated with the duration of cardiopulmonary bypass, with longer times associated with a higher incidence of complications. The most frequent complications post-CABG include arrhythmias, hypotension, perioperative MI, or cerebral vascular accident (CVA), cardiac tamponade, respiratory insufficiency ("pump lung"), altered mentation ("postpericardiectomy syndrome"), and low CO syndrome. In addition, complications similar to those seen following any major surgical procedure may occur.

The question of which patients with angina pectoris will benefit from CABG is controversial. Patients with unstable or crescendo angina, with left main (anterior descending) lesions, and those with triple-vessel disease and left ventricular dysfunction are generally considered good candidates for surgical therapy. Individuals with coronary vasospasm are not usually treated with CABG unless there is also underlying atherosclerosis. Advantages of CABG include its effectiveness in reducing the severity and frequency of chest pain and in improving the quality of life for individuals with CAD. The main disadvantage is significant postoperative morbidity similar to that subsequent to any type of major surgery.

In individuals with unstable angina, CABG may be preceded by stabilization with intra-aortic balloon counterpulsation (*see* Chapter 14).

Nursing interventions

Nursing interventions for the patient with angina pectoris are described below.

Life-style. (1) Be a role model for a healthy life-style. (2) Interview patient and family to identify coronary risk factors. (3) Request appropriate consultations from dieticians, exercise therapists, smoking cessation clinics. (4) Teach patient and family about the pathogenesis of CAD. (5) Teach patient and family about the importance of coronary-risk-factor modification. (6) Offer patient and family practical suggestions for risk-factor modification.

Lack of knowledge of medications. (1) Teach patients on nitroglycerin when and how to take medication; about side effects that may occur; what to do in the event that chest pain continues despite nitroglycerin use; teach patient and family about proper handling and storage of unused medication. (2) Teach patients on other antianginal medications the reason for using particular medication; how and when to take medication; about side effects that may occur.

Anxiety related to planned PTCA. (1) Provide information about sensory experiences common during PTCA; about related diagnostic studies that may be done; about postprocedure care. (2) Inform patient about the possibility of coronary bypass surgery immediately post PTCA if complications arise. (3) Allow patient to verbalize fears and encourage realistic expectations for procedure.

Possible complications following PTCA. (1) Assess patient frequently for presence of chest pain. (2) Frequently monitor hemodynamic status (vital signs, PAM). (3) Monitor ECG for arrhythmias. (4) Postrecovery, attempt coronary risk factor modification (*see above*).

Anxiety related to planned CABG. (1) Provide information about sensory experiences common during perioperative period, (ICU environment; presence of lines, tubes, and drains). (2) Prepare family for probable physical appearance of patient immediately postsurgery. (3) Instruct patient in respiratory hygiene techniques. (4) Allow patient to verbalize fears and encourage realistic expectations for recovery.

Possible complications following CABG. (1) Monitor continuously for arrhythmias. (2) Obtain frequent 12-lead ECGs. (3) Monitor hemodynamic status (MABP, PAM, PAWP, LAP, RAP, CO, physical assessment). (4) Monitor pulmonary status (physical assessment, arterial and venous blood gases, chest x-rays). (5) Monitor renal function (urine output, urine specific gravity, serum creatinine, BUN). (6) Monitor GI function (physical assessment, testing of stool and nasogastric aspirate for occult blood). (7) Monitor hematologic function (measurement of clotting parameters, CBC, physical assessment). (8) Institute vigorous pulmonary hygiene. (9) Provide frequent wound care. (10) Reduce environmental stressors in ICU (lights, noise, awareness of other acutely ill patients). (11) Prepare patient emotionally for transfer to regular nursing unit and eventual discharge home.

MYOCARDIAL INFARCTION

MI is irreversible destruction of heart muscle tissue secondary to a prolonged or permanent interruption in blood flow to the tissue.

Pathophysiology

MI is most commonly the result of atherosclerotic CAD (*see above*). Other, less frequent causes of MI include embolization and severe shock.

Because the heart is dependent upon a continual supply of O_2 to maintain functioning, an interruption in the supply of oxygenated blood to the myocardium results in decreased energy production, which, in turn, leads to decreased contractile function and eventually to cell death.

Surrounding the infarcted, or irreversibly damaged, tissue is tissue that is ischemic, i.e., tissue that is damaged but is receiving enough O_2 to prevent cellular death. The ischemic zone may be electrically unstable, however, giving rise to arrhythmias. Furthermore, the ischemic zone usually exhibits contractile dysfunction. The salvage of this "twilight zone"—i.e., its recovery to full functioning—is the focus of many clinical interventions during the postinfarction period.

Because of the decreased contractility of the infarcted and ischemic zones, there is decreased mechanical functioning of the heart postinfarction. The decrease in function is correlated with the size of the infarcted area, with larger infarctions possibly resulting in CHF or cardiogenic shock.

The left ventricle is the chamber of the heart that is most commonly affected by MI because of its large mass and associated large blood supply. Infarctions of the left ventricle are the most significant hemodynamically because of its important mechanical functions. The specific signs and symptoms of **left ventricular infarction** depend on the affected coronary artery. Occlusion of the left anterior descending coronary artery results in infarction of the anterior wall of the left ventricle. Occlusion of the right coronary artery results in inferior or posterior wall infarctions. Occlusion of the left circumflex coronary artery results in lateral wall infarction. The frequency and significance of **right ventricular infarctions** is increasingly being recognized by clinicians. Right ventricular infarctions are most commonly the result of occlusion of the right coronary artery and thus are commonly seen in conjunction with inferior and posterior left ventricular wall infarctions.

Coronary arteries lie on the epicardial surface, sending off smaller vessels into the myocardium. The endocardium is the most sensitive to reductions in coronary flow, both because it is most distant from the larger vessels and because its O_2 demand is slightly higher than that of the epicardium. When there is an interruption in coronary blood flow, the result may be a transmural or a subendocardial MI. In a subendocardial infarction, only the innermost layer of the myocardium is damaged, and mechanical dysfunction may not occur. With more severe reduction in coronary flow, a transmural infarction occurs, resulting in damage to both the endocardium and epicardium. A classical MI is transmural, giving rise to classical ECG changes and mechanical dysfunction.

In addition to the cardiovascular effects of MI, there is usually a nonspecific stress response, manifested primarily as increased levels of circulating catecholamines. This results in increased MVO_2 and increased left ventricular afterload, thus increasing the work load of the heart at a time when its capacity is diminished. Elevated catecholamine levels can also be arrhythmogenic. Other nonspecific responses to MI include elevation in circulating levels of glucocorticoids and aldosterone and decreased levels of insulin.

Clinical picture

The clinical picture seen in acute MI is dependent upon the size and location of the infarction as well as the time elapsed postinfarction. The primary symptom is severe substernal chest pain, often radiating to the neck, back, or left arm, not usually precipitated by exercise or stress and not relieved with nitroglycerin. It is, however, possible for an individual to have an acute MI without experiencing chest pain. Other classical signs and symptoms of acute MI include nausea, vomiting, shortness of breath, diaphoresis, a sense of impending doom, and anxiety.

On ECG, early manifestations of acute MI are ST-segment elevation, T-wave inversion, and the appearance of abnormal Q waves. These indicative changes are seen in those leads that overlie the infarcted area. In inferior or diaphragmatic wall infarctions of the left ventricle, these indicative changes are seen in leads II, III, and aVF. In anterior wall infarctions, indicative changes are seen in leads V_1 through V_3. In lateral wall infarction, these indicative changes are seen in leads I, aVL, and V_4 through V_6. No leads of the standard twelve-lead ECG overlie the posterior wall of the left ventricle; therefore, there are no leads that will show indicative changes of posterior wall infarction.

Reciprocal changes are seen in leads that lie behind the infarcted area. Such reciprocal changes include depressed ST segments, elevated T waves, and tall R waves. Reciprocal changes seen in infarctions of the inferior wall of the left ventricle are seen in those leads that overlie the lateral wall, i.e., leads I, aVL, V_4, V_5, and V_6. In lateral wall infarctions, reciprocal changes are seen in leads II, III, and aVF. Posterior wall infarctions are manifested as reciprocal changes in leads V_1 through V_3. There are no leads that show reciprocal changes in anterior wall infarctions.

ECG changes postinfarction are time-dependent. Q waves are permanent indicators of transmural infarctions, whereas ST-segment changes are very transient. T-wave inversions are usually transient but may take days to weeks to revert to normal.

Blood tests postinfarction classically show elevation of certain enzymes. Serum creatine phosphokinase (CPK) levels rise early following infarction, peaking at ~24 hr postinfarction. CPK-MB is an isozyme of CPK that, unlike other forms of CPK, arises primarily from cardiac muscle. The extent of the CPK-MB elevation is correlated with the size of the infarction. SGOT, also known as aspartate transaminase (AST), rises somewhat later than does CPK, peaking at ~36 hr postinfarction. It is not, however, specific for MI, because the liver and certain other tissues are rich sources of SGOT, and isozyme fractionation to determine the source of the serum enzymes is not possible. Lactate dehydrogenase (LDH) is the last enzyme to rise following MI, peaking between 48 and 72 hr. As it is for CPK, it is possible to measure levels of LDH isozymes. Normally, there is less of the LDH-1 isozyme than of the LDH-2 isozyme; postinfarction, this ratio flips, with LDH-1 levels increasing more than the LDH-2 levels. Other abnormal findings on blood analysis following MI are nonspecific and include an elevation in the WBC and an increased erythrocyte sedimentation rate (ESR).

The diagnosis of MI is usually made on the basis of the clinical history of chest pain, ECG changes, and serum enzyme levels. Other diagnostic procedures may, however, be performed to confirm the diagnosis. Radioisotopic studies of myocardial perfusion may be carried out to define the necrotic area. Hemodynamic assessment, using pulmonary artery catheterization, may provide information about left ventricular function.

Complications of acute MI include arrhythmias, CHF, cardiogenic shock, pericarditis (Dressler's syndrome), aneurysm formation, mitral insufficiency (secondary to papillary muscle infarction), arterial embolization, pulmonary embolization, cerebral infarction, ventricular rupture, renal failure, and death.

The most common arrhythmias following MI include sinus tachycardia and premature ventricular contractions (PVCs). Lethal arrhythmias, including ventricular tachycardia, ventricular fibrillation, idioventricular rhythm, and asystole, are not infrequent. In anterior wall infarctions of the left ventricle, bundle branch blocks are common, while in posterior and inferior wall infarction, sinus arrhythmias and AV blocks are more common.

Medical interventions

Medical treatment for MI is usually carried out in the coronary care unit (CCU). The aim of medical treatment in the acute phase is to stabilize the patient hemodynamically, allow the patient physical and emotional rest, and to prevent or treat complications.

Hemodynamic stabilization is dependent upon knowledge of current hemodynamic status and thus often involves the insertion of hemodynamic monitoring lines, particularly pulmonary artery catheters. Cardiac failure following infarction may be treated with diuretics (furosemide, ethacrynic acid, hydrochlorothiazide), positive inotropic agents (digitalis or dobutamine), provision of a low-sodium diet, vasopressors (dopamine or, less commonly, norepinephrine), and vasodilators (nitroprusside or nitroglycerin). Cardiogenic shock may require intra-aortic balloon counterpulsation (*see* Chapter 14); however, since this is palliative therapy rather than curative, it is most commonly used only for those MI patients in whom the cause of the cardiogenic shock can be effectively treated, e.g., for papillary muscle infarction.

The provision of rest following MI is very important in reducing MVO_2 and thereby optimizing conditions for salvage of the ischemic zone. Medical interventions to ensure rest include administration of analgesics (usually morphine), sedatives (commonly diazepam), and hypnotics (such as chloral hydrate or secobarbital).

Prevention of complications following acute MI includes administration of O_2, antiarrhythmic therapy, maintenance of an IV line, administration of stool softeners, and anticoagulation. O_2 is routinely administered to patients with suspected MI because of the possibility that it improves O_2 delivery to the ischemic zone and thus prevents extension of the infarction. Prophylactic antiarrhythmic therapy involves the IV administration of lidocaine or, less commonly, procainamide. Arrhythmia prophylaxis may be initiated on all patients who are admitted to the CCU with a suspected MI or only on those patients exhibiting frequent or malignant PVCs. Anticoagulation is usually accomplished with small doses of heparin, administered SC.

Should malignant arrhythmias occur, prompt treatment is essential. Lethal ventricular arrhythmias are usually managed with defibrillation, while AV conduction defects may require pacemaker therapy (*see below*).

Pericarditis postinfarction is usually managed conservatively, with analgesics and rest. Steroids or nonsteroidal anti-inflammatory agents may be given but may increase the risk of aneurysm formation. Pericarditis is usually a late complication of MI.

Aneurysm formation may be managed conservatively by treating the resultant arrhythmias and CHF. In more severe cases, aneurysmectomy may be required, although this is usually delayed until ≥4 to 6 wk postinfarction.

Mitral insufficiency, secondary to papillary muscle infarction, may also require surgery. As with aneurysmectomy, surgery is delayed for 4 to 6 wk postinfarction if possible. In the interim, the resultant CHF may be managed conservatively.

Ventricular rupture is difficult to treat because of its rapid onset. In a few patients, however, surgical repair may be possible.

Streptokinase may be given via direct intracoronary infusion, in an attempt to dissolve coronary thromboses that caused or were caused by the MI. Patients in whom streptokinase therapy may be useful are those who can be treated within a few hours of the onset of chest pain; streptokinase therapy is contraindicated in individuals who are pregnant, have recently suffered surgical or other trauma, have recently suffered CVA, or who have bleeding disorders. Because of the antigenicity of streptokinase, diphenhydramine and steroids may be given pretreatment; in addition, the use of streptokinase is contraindicated in individuals who have received it in the past, because of the risk of allergic reactions on repeated contact with the substance.

Nursing interventions

Nursing interventions for the patient who has suffered a MI are described below.

Inability to tolerate physical activity. (1) Immediately postinfarction, maintain patient on bed rest, in semi-Fowler's position, with commode privileges. (2) Immediately postinfarction, allow self-feeding. (3) Gradually increase physical activity during the first 10 to 14 days postinfarction. (4) Monitor physiologic response to increased activity: BP, pulse, respiratory rate, occurrence of chest pain. (5) By hospital discharge, patient should be able to climb one flight of stairs without undue side effects.

Inability to tolerate emotional stress. (1) Judiciously restrict visiting hours while in ICU; allow liberal visiting if it seems to reduce anxiety. (2) Minimize mentally upsetting influences while in the ICU (lights, noise, awareness of other acutely ill patients). (3) Provide emotional support to patient and family.

Complications postinfarction. (1) Monitor patient for early indicators of complications (pain, fatigue, untoward response to activity, arrhythmias). (2) Teach patient to notify nurse immediately should pain occur. (3) Should pain occur, administer analgesic immediately. (4) Monitor hemodynamic status for indicators of impending CHF. (5) Monitor body wieght daily. (6) Record intake and output. (7) Prevent the hazards of immobility: provide range-of-motion exercises, leg exercises, promote coughing and deep breathing. (8) Implement "coronary precautions" (although efficacy is unproven): restrict cold fluids, caffeine, avoid rectal temperature measurement.

Need to adjust to new health status. (1) Assess patient's understanding of what a MI is. (2) Assess patient's ability to learn/manage self-care postdischarge. (3) Teach patient about coronary-risk-factor modification (*see above*).

Possible complications of streptokinase therapy. (1) Preprocedure management is like that for other patients with MI. Provide information about sensory experiences that are common during procedure. (2) During procedure, monitor patient for arrhythmias, allergic reaction, excessive bleeding, chest pain. (3) Postprocedure, monitor patient for chest pain, increased serum cardiac enzymes, ECG changes.

ATRIOVENTRICULAR CONDUCTION SYSTEM DEFECTS

Pathophysiology

Electrical excitation of the heart normally begins at the SA node in the upper right atrium and proceeds down a specialized conduction system to the rest of the heart (*see* Anatomy and Physiology Review). If there is abnormal conduction through this system, various arrhythmias can occur. The most common conduction defects involve conduction between the atria and ventricles via the AV node and related structures.

AV conduction defects can be the result of anatomic lesions or pathophysiologic abnormalities. **Anatomic lesions** may be congenital or may result from accidental or surgical trauma. **Pathophysiologic abnormalities** that may result in AV conduction defects include myocardial ischemia or necrosis, electrolyte abnormalities, such as hypokalemia, and connective tissue diseases that affect the heart. In addition, many cardiac drugs, including digitalis, can interfere with AV conduction.

AV conduction defects are classified according to the degree of impairment. In **first degree AV block,** all supraventricular impulses are conducted to the ventricles, but the conduction time through the AV node is prolonged. This condition is manifested on the ECG as a prolonged PR interval. In **second-degree AV block**, only a fraction of the supraventricular impulses are conducted to the ventricles. This is manifested on the ECG by normally occurring P waves that are not followed by QRS complexes. In **complete,** or **third degree AV block,** there is no conduction of supraventricular impulses to the ventricles; ventricular excitation is the result of impulses arising in the ventricles themselves. Permanent pacemakers are most often implanted for the treatment of complete heart block.

Clinical picture

The individual with **first-degree** AV block is usually asymptomatic, although on ECG, typical prolongation of the PR interval is seen.

The individual with **second-degree** heart block is also usually asymptomatic, although supraventricular beats that are not conducted to the ventricles may be detected by the individual as "skipped" beats. This is because the ventricle has a longer time to fill during the interval between succeeding conducted beats; according to the Frank-Starling relationship, the CO on the next conducted beat is larger than usual.

In **third-degree** AV block, the individual may be asymptomatic. More commonly, the individual complains of dizziness, light-headedness, syncope, fatigability, forgetfulness, confusion, and poor exercise tolerance. The peripheral pulse rate is slow and the pulse pressure is widened, the result of both an elevated systolic pressure and a decreased diastolic pressure. On auscultation, an S_3 may be heard and the intensity of S_1 may vary.

Medical interventions

In **first-degree AV block,** medical therapy is aimed at determining the cause of the block and preventing progression to a higher-degree block by eliminating, if possible, any causative factors. Pacemaker insertion is usually not indicated in first-degree AV block.

In **second-degree AV block,** medical therapy is also aimed at determining the cause of the block and preventing its progression to a higher degree of block. In some cases, however, pacemaker insertion may be indicated. Depending on the probable cause of the AV block, either a temporary or a permanent pacemaker may be inserted.

In **third-degree AV block,** pacemaker insertion is almost always indicated. Depending upon the clinical situation, therapy with isoproterenol may be indicated, to maintain adequate heart rate until the pacemaker can be inserted. Isoproterenol increases MVO_2 and thus should be used cautiously in individuals with CAD.

Temporary pacemaking electrodes may be inserted transvenously or may be attached to the heart at the time of open-chest surgery. The electrical unit is externally situated. Permanent pacemaking electrodes may be inserted transvenously, usually via the subclavian vein, or may be directly implanted in the epicardium of the ventricle. Venous pacemaker electrodes usually terminate in the right atrium of the heart; in certain pacing modalities, electrodes may also be implanted in the right atrium.

Pacing modes include demand (also known as chamber-sensed) and fixed-rate. In the demand-pacing mode, the pacemaker senses the intrinsic electrical activity of the heart. Depending upon the type of pacemaker, it may sense the R wave or the P wave. If no activity occurs within a predetermined period of time, the pacemaker will discharge. If, on the other hand, intrinsic electrical activity does occur, then no pacemaker discharge will occur. Demand pacemaking is the most common pacemaking mode.

Synchronous pacemaking is a type of demand pacemaking in which the pacemaker senses the intrinsic electrical activity of the heart but is stimulated, rather than inhibited; e.g., the pacemaker may sense electrical activity in the atria and, in response, pace the ventricles.

In fixed-rate pacemaking, also referred to as asynchronous and as chamber-paced pacemaking, the pacemaker discharges electrically whether or not there is any intrinsic electrical activity. A typical fixed-rate pacemaker does not contain any sensing circuitry. Fixed-rate pacemakers are not commonly used, although they may occasionally be implanted in individuals with complete heart block.

Bifocal pacemakers have electrodes in both the atrium and ventricle; electrical discharge in the two chambers is sequential. This type of pacing is usually indicated for individuals in whom there is both abnormal impulse formation in the atria and abnormal AV conduction.

In many types of pacemakers, it is possible to alter pacemaking characteristics by manipulation of an external programmer or by percutaneous insertion of a needle into a control device in the pacemaker. In addition, a magnet applied to the exterior of the chest wall can convert a demand pacemaker into a fixed-rate mode.

Nursing interventions

Nursing interventions for patients with AV conduction system defects are described below.

Hemodynamic compromise caused by conduction defects. (1) Monitor ECG. (2) Assess patient for evidence of clinical deterioration (chest pain, dizziness, altered level of consciousness, decreased BP).

Anxiety. Teach patient about sensory experiences common during procedure. (2) Teach patient about postprocedure care. (3) Allow patient to verbalize fears and encourage realistic expectations about recovery.

Complications of temporary pacemaker therapy. (1) Monitor ECG. (2) Assess pacing and sensing function of pacemaker. (3) Restrict movement of involved extremity. (4) Provide wound care at insertion site. (5) Check stimulation threshold of pacemaker (increase pacemaker firing rate until continuously pacing heart, then decrease electrical output in milliamperes until pacing is no longer occuring). (6) Set pacemaker to deliver 2 to 3 time threshold current. (7) If stimulation threshold changes significantly, notify physician of possible electrode placement problems. (8) Ensure electrical safety: ensure grounding of all electrical equipment in contact with patient; electrically isolate pacing unit.

Complications of permanent pacemaker insertion. (1) Monitor ECG for evidence of proper pacemaker function. (2) Monitor patient for evidence of hemodynamic stability (BP, level of consciousness, chest pain, dizziness). (3) Provide wound care.

Patient education. (1) Teach patient how to monitor pacemaker function (pulse rate measurement). (2) Teach patient about precautions necessary in everyday life. (3) Teach patient how to care for incision until healed.

CONGESTIVE HEART FAILURE

CHF is a descriptive term for a condition in which the CO is insufficient to meet the metabolic demands of the body. In more severe form, CHF can result in pulmonary edema, which is discussed in below. In most severe form, CHF results in cardiogenic shock (*see* Chapter 17).

Pathophysiology

Classically, there are three stages in the pathogenesis of CHF. In the first stage, there is a pathologic inability of the heart to meet the demands imposed upon it. In the second stage, the heart compensates for these demands. In the third and final stage, the heart becomes unable to meet the demands and decompensation occurs.

In the **first stage** of the pathogenesis of CHF, there is pathologic cardiac overloading, resulting in increased myocardial work. This, in turn, results in increased MVO_2.

Cardiac overloading may be caused by intrinsic cardiac disease, such as in cardiomyopathy or after MI. Alternatively, the overloading may be the result of increased myocardial work. This increased work may be the result of an increase in afterload, the pressure in the pulmonary artery or aorta against which the right or left ventricle must pump. The ventricles also have to pump more forcibly to eject blood across a stenotic valve; thus, aortic or pulmonary valve stenosis can result in cardiac overload. Alternatively, the increased work might result from increased preload, the volume in the ventricle prior to systole. When preload increases, ventricular wall stress increases and thus increases MVO_2. Increased preload can result from increased venous return or from regurgitant aortic or pulmonary valves.

In the **second stage** of the pathogenesis of CHF, the heart and vascular system compensate for the increased myocardial work imposed upon the heart. The involved compensatory mechanisms include (1) cardiac dilation, which, according to the Frank-Starling relationship, increases stroke volume and CO; (2) increased sympathetic nervous system activity, resulting in increased heart rate, increased myocardial contractility, increased venous return to the heart, redistribution of blood flow away from nonessential tissues, and increased salt and water retention by the kidneys; and (3) cardiac hypertrophy, which results in a greater mass of contractile tissue to accomplish the work of the heart. The net result is the ability of the heart to meet the metabolic demands of the body, at the cost to the heart of increasing its MVO_2.

In the **third**, or final, **stage**, the heart decompensates, becoming unable to meet the demands imposed upon it. Reasons for the decompensation include (1) a disruption of the Frank-Starling relationship, whereby increased preload no longer results in increased stroke volume, but rather in a decreased stroke volume; (2) relative ischemia of the heart, i.e., an inability of the heart to obtain adequate O_2 and nutrients to meet the increased demands imposed upon it; (3) an inability to respond appropriately to sympathetic stimulation, either from depletion of sympathetic neurotransmitters or from down-regulation of sympathetic receptors; and (4) subcellular defects in myocardial contractile mechanisms, resulting from dilation, hypertrophy, or relative ischemia. The result of this decompensation is an inability of the heart to respond to the demands imposed upon it and manifestations of the clinical syndrome of CHF.

Clinical picture

CHF produces a range of signs and symptoms. The particular manifestations that are seen depend upon both the stage and the cause of the CHF.

In the **first stage**, there are no indicators of CHF, although careful clinical examination may reveal the presence of factors, such as hypertension, that may lead to failure.

In the **second**, or **compensatory**, **stage** of CHF, signs and symptoms indicative of increased sympathetic nervous system activity may be evident. Sympathetic nervous system effects on the heart are primarily manifested as an increased heart rate. Sympathetically mediated sodium and fluid retention may be manifested as gradually increasing weight gain.

In the **third**, or **decompensated**, stage, the typical clinical picture of CHF is seen. Manifestations occur both downstream from the failing chamber of the heart, secondary to decreased ejection of blood from that chamber (forward failure), and upstream from the failing chamber, secondary to increased volume in the chamber at the end of systole (backward failure).

In left-sided failure, the predominant problem is an inability of the left ventricle to pump adequately. This results in inadequate perfusion of the systemic vasculature because of forward failure and pulmonary venous distension because of backward failure. The signs and symptoms of the inadequate systemic perfusion include fatigue, weakness, irritability, restlessness, mental confusion, and cool and pale extremities. Pulmonary venous distension is manifested as shortness of breath, dyspnea on exertion, orthopnea, paroxysmal nocturnal dyspnea, and by the presence of adventitious lung sounds (rales and rhonchi). Blood gas analysis may reveal decreased $PaCO_2$ and an increased pH. On chest x-ray, pulmonary vascular congestion may be evident as haziness of the lung fields and vascular distension. Cardiac enlargement may also be evident. PAM and PAWP are usually elevated. On auscultation, an S_3 and an S_4 may be heard.

In right-sided failure, the predominant problem is an inability of the right ventricle to pump adequately. The primary signs and symptoms are the result of systemic venous distension secondary to backward failure. This is manifested as peripheral edema, hepatomegaly, ascites, anorexia, and distended neck veins. CVP (RAP) is elevated. No specific signs of right-sided failure are seen on chest x-ray. On auscultation, an S_3 and an S_4 may be heard.

Although there are no specific ECG manifestations of heart failure, there are specific indicators of ventricular hypertrophy. In left ventricular hypertrophy, there is increased R-wave voltage in the lateral leads (I, aVL, V_4, V_5, and V_6) and increased S-wave voltage in the anterior leads (V_1, V_2, and V_3), left axis deviation, slight prolongation of the QRS duration, and ST-segment and T-wave changes. Left atrial enlargement may also be seen on the ECG of patients with left ventricular failure; this is manifested as wide and notched P waves. In right ventricular hypertrophy, there are relatively large R waves in the anterior leads and relatively large S waves in the lateral leads. Other manifestations are right axis deviation and ST-segment and T-wave changes. Right atrial enlargement may also be seen on the ECG of patients with right ventricular failure; this is manifested as narrow and peaked P waves.

Right- and left-sided failure may coexist. The clinical syndrome is then referred to as biventricular failure.

Medical interventions

Although the symptoms of right- and left-sided heart failure differ, the treatment is essentially the same. Aims of medical therapy in CHF are to treat any factors that contribute to or cause the failure, to increase myocardial contractility, and to correct fluid and electrolyte balance in the body.

Treatable factors that may contribute to or cause the failure include increased afterload and increased preload. Vasodilators such as nitroglycerin, isosorbide dinitrate, minoxidil, nifedipine, nitroprusside, and hydralazine may be used for their ability to decrease both afterload and preload. The mainstay of positive inotropic therapy is digitalis, which acts to increase myocardial contractility by increasing calcium availability. A newer positive inotropic agent is dobutamine, a $beta_1$ agonist that increases myocardial contractility by stimulating sympathetic receptors in the heart. Other positive inotropic agents, such as norepinephrine, dopamine, isoproterenol, and epinephrine, may be given parenterally in acute CHF.

Diuretics are administered to correct the fluid retention secondary to sympathetic-nervous-system-induced sodium and fluid retention. Commonly administered diuretics in the acute stages of CHF include furosemide and ethacrynic acid. In more chronic stages, other diuretics such as hydrochlorothiazide and chlorthalidone may be used. Concomitantly, sodium and water intake may be limited.

Nursing interventions

Nursing interventions for the patient with CHF are described below.

Lack of knowledge about medications. (1) Teach patient why particular drugs are being used. (2) Teach patient about side effects of drugs. (3) For patients on digitalis compounds, teach how to monitor own pulse and about side effects (slow heart rate, nausea, yellow-green vision).

Potential digitalis toxicity. (1) Monitor patient for evidence of arrhythmias, especially AV blocks, ventricular ectopy. (2) Monitor patient for evidence of nausea, vomiting, yellow-green vision. (3) Monitor serum digitalis levels. (4) Monitor serum potassium levels.

Potential fluid and electrolyte imbalance. (1) Obtain daily body weights. (2) Monitor patient for physical evidence of volume overload or deficit (skin turgor, peripheral edema, dry mucous membranes). (3) Record intake and output. (4) Monitor serum electrolytes.

Lack of knowledge of dietary restrictions. (1) Consult with dietician. (2) Allow patient and/or family to select allowed foods while in hospital.

Reduced exercise tolerance. (1) Teach patient how to monitor own physical response to activity (pulse rate). (2) After stabilization of physical condition in hospital, discuss how home environment might be modified to allow patient to carry out the activities of daily living without untoward stress.

PULMONARY EDEMA

Pulmonary edema results from the accumulation of excess fluid in the pulmonary interstitium, thereby interfering with normal lung function, particularly with gas exchange. Pulmonary edema is an acute condition, most commonly the result of CHF.

Pathophysiology

The movement of fluid across the capillary endothelium is dependent upon the permeability of the capillary and the balance of forces that hold fluid in the capillary (capillary osmotic and tissue hydrostatic pressures) and forces that tend to hold fluid in the tissue (tissue osmotic and capillary hydrostatic pressures). Pulmonary edema occurs when the balance of these forces results in increased fluid accumulation in the tissues. The most common causes are increased capillary permeability, decreased capillary osmotic pressure, and increased capillary hydrostatic pressure.

Increased capillary permeability can result in pulmonary edema by allowing more rapid movement of fluid across the capillary wall. Conditions that may affect capillary permeability and thus result in pulmonary edema include infections, certain toxins, and O_2 toxicity.

Capillary osmotic pressure is the pressure exerted by particles in solution within the vascular space. These particles include crystalloids (electrolytes and other small, water-soluble molecules) and colloids (primarily proteins). Decreased capillary osmotic pressure can result in pulmonary edema. This can be the result of decreased colloid osmotic pressure, as in hyproproteinemia, or decreased total osmotic pressure, as in water intoxication following excessive administration of IV fluids.

Capillary hydrostatic pressure is primarily dependent upon pressure in the veins, or, in the case of the lungs, the PAM. As PAM increases, capillary hydrostatic pressure increases and thus increases the forces favoring fluid movement from the intravascular space into the pulmonary interstitium. Causes of increased PAM include left ventricular heart failure, pulmonary venous occlusion, and water intoxication (fluid overload).

Other causes of pulmonary edema include heroin overdose, head injury, and high altitude. The pathophysiologic mechanism responsible for the development of pulmonary edema in these conditions is not well understood.

As pulmonary edema develops, fluid accumulates in the pulmonary interstitium. This increases tissue hydrostatic pressure and thus limits further fluid accumulation.

Clinical picture

The signs and symptoms of acute pulmonary edema resemble those of severe, abrupt-onset left-sided CHF (*see above*). They include shortness of breath, productive cough, hemoptysis (pink, frothy sputum), severe orthopnea, tachypnea, anxiety, cyanosis, tachycardia, and hypotension. On auscultation of the lungs, rales and rhonchi are heard. If the cause of the pulmonary edema is left-sided CHF, an S_3 and an S_4 may be heard on auscultation of the heart. Blood gas analysis may reveal hypoxemia and mixed metabolic and respiratory acidosis. On chest x-ray, pulmonary vascular congestion may be seen, as well as indicators of CHF if present.

Untreated, pulmonary edema may lead to arrhythmias, shock, and death.

Medical interventions

The aims of medical therapy in acute pulmonary edema are to treat the underlying cause and to support the patient until recovery can occur. If the **underlying cause** of the problem is CHF, then positive inotropic agents, vasodilators, and diuretics are administered (*see above*). Infectious causes of pulmonary edema may be treated with antibiotics. Water intoxication may be treated with diuretics and fluid restriction. Hypoproteinemia may be treated with the IV administration of salt-poor albumin or other colloid solutions. Pulmonary venous occlusion, as in pulmonary embolism, may be treated with anticoagulation (*see* Chapter 3). Heroin overdose is often treated with naloxone, although whether or not this reverses the acute pulmonary edema is unclear. Head injuries are managed with agents that reduce soft-tissue swelling, e.g., mannitol and dexamethasone (*see* Chapter 5). High-altitude pulmonary edema is best managed with return to a lower altitude.

Supportive care of the patient with pulmonary edema includes O_2 administration, guided by blood gas analysis. Bronchodilators, such as aminophylline, may be used both for their positive effects on the work of breathing and because of their mild diuretic side effects. Morphine sulfate is often used in acute pulmonary edema because of its antianxiety effects. Morphine also causes venous dilation, thereby reducing venous return to the heart.

In pulmonary edema, measures may be taken to reduce circulating blood volume. Such measures include the use of rotating tourniquets and phlebotomy. Blood removed during phlebotomy is usually saved and the packed RBCs reinfused once the patient has stabilized.

Nursing interventions

Nursing interventions for the patient with pulmonary edema are described below. In addition, when the patient's physical condition has stabilized, nursing interventions as described for the patient with CHF may be indicated (*see above*).

Anxiety. (1) Maintain a quiet environment when possible. (2) Provide as much information about disease and therapy as is appropriate for patient's emotional and physical state. (3) Provide for uninterrupted periods of physical rest.

Risk of complications due to rotating tourniquets. (1) Maintain tourniquet pressure above venous pressure but below arterial pressure. (2) Rotate tourniquet locations q 15 min. (3) Assess distal tissue frequently for evidence of damage (pulse, skin color, sensation). (4) Use extra caution in individuals with underlying peripheral vascular disease.

PERICARDITIS

Pericarditis is an inflammation of the pericardium, the double-layered sac that surrounds the heart. The most common clinical manifestations of pericardial inflammation that are seen in the ICU are acute pericarditis and pericardial effusion with or without tamponade.

Pathophysiology

Inflammation of the pericardium may result from many factors. Systemic infections or infections arising in the lungs or mediastinum, particularly viral infections, may spread to the pericardium, resulting in pericarditis. Pericarditis may also result from trauma to the heart, as a sequela of MI (Dressler's syndrome) or cardiac surgery (postpericardiotomy syndrome), in certain malignancies (especially lymphoma), or as a complication of radiation therapy. Pericarditis may also occur as a complication of several connective tissue diseases including SLE, rheumatoid arthritis, and progressive systemic sclerosis (scleroderma). Certain metabolic diseases, such as uremia and hypothyroidism, may be complicated by pericarditis. Finally, pericarditis may occur as an untoward effect of therapy with agents such as procainamide or hydralazine.

Regardless of the cause, pericarditis can result in fluid accumulation in the space surrounding the heart. This can, if severe enough, affect the mechanical performance of the heart, because it can restrict ventricular filling during diastole. Decreased ventricular filling results in decreased ejection and thus a lower stroke volume and lower CO. Significant hemodynamic compromise can occur if filling is seriously compromised, as in cardiac tamponade.

Clinical picture

The classical signs and symptoms of acute pericarditis are chest pain, pericardial friction rub, and ECG changes. Chest pain in acute pericarditis is characteristically sharp and stabbing, substernal in location, with radiation to the neck, back, shoulders, and possibly upper arms. The pain is usually worsened with respiration, coughing, swallowing, or movement, although in certain positions the pain may lessen. Characteristic ECG changes seen in acute pericarditis are ST-segment elevation or depression and T-wave inversion, reflecting a current of injury in the underlying myocardium. Arrhythmias may also be present.

Other signs and symptoms that may be seen in acute pericarditis include dyspnea and general indicators of systemic disease: fatigue, weakness, malaise, anorexia, and weight loss. If the underlying cause is an infectious process, signs and symptoms such as fever and chills may also be seen.

In pericardial effusion culminating in cardiac tamponade, the collection of fluid around the heart results in diminished cardiac filling and hemodynamic compromise. The characteristic signs and symptoms of tamponade are decreased arterial BP, increased venous BP, increased heart rate, increased pulsus paradoxus, and diminished heart sounds. An enlarged cardiac silhouette may be seen on chest x-ray, although this is not always present. On ECG, in addition to those changes seen in acute pericarditis, electrical alternans may be seen. This is manifested as changes in the amplitude or polarity of the QRS complex with each heartbeat. On echocardiogram, there may be evidence of fluid accumulation around the heart.

Medical interventions

Medical therapy in pericarditis is directed toward treatment of the underlying cause whenever possible, supportive care while healing occurs, and surgical intervention should significant hemodynamic compromise occur.

Surgical intervention ranges from pericardiocentesis to pericardiectomy. Pericardiocentesis is the removal of fluid from the pericardium, usually by needle aspiration, under local anesthesia. A catheter may be left in place for a few days if fluid accumulation is likely to rapidly recur. In cases of chronic recurring cardiac tamponade, a pericardial window may be created or pericardiectomy performed to prevent the hemodynamic consequences of fluid accumulation around the heart.

Pharmacologic pain management may be indicated in pericarditis. Because of the inflammatory nature of the pericarditis, aspirin or other nonsteroidal anti-inflammatory agents are often used as analgesics. Steroids may be given but are associated with a higher-than-average risk of recurrence or complications.

Hemodynamic support in cardiac tamponade involves the administration of relatively large volumes of IV fluids.

Nursing interventions

Nursing interventions for the patient with pericarditis are described below.

Potential complications of immobility. (1) Instruct patient in coughing and deep breathing. (2) Provide range-of-motion exercises and leg exercises.

Pain. (1) Administer analgesics. (2) Instruct patient in stress-reduction techniques (visualization, controlled breathing). (3) Provide calm, quiet environment.

Potential worsening of hemodynamic status. (1) Monitor patient's hemodynamic status (venous pressure, jugular venous distension). (2) Postpericardiocentesis, monitor BP, pulse, venous pressure, jugular venous distension for evidence of iatrogenic hemopericardium or rapid recurrence of the tamponade.

MALIGNANT HYPERTENSION

Malignant hypertension, also referred to as accelerated hypertension or hypertensive crisis, is a form of high BP in which there is a rapid increase in arterial BP over a short period of time.

Pathophysiology

The causes and mechanisms responsible for the development of malignant hypertension are not well understood, but it can develop in any individual with idiopathic or secondary hypertension. At times, it may be precipitated by stress or noncompliance with hypertensive therapy.

Although the causes of malignant hypertension are not clear, the effects on many organ systems are clear. The effects are related more to the rate of elevation of BP than to the absolute level of BP. Target organs that may be damaged by rapid elevation of BP include the kidneys, heart, brain, and peripheral vasculature. Acute effects of the kidney include renal failure. In the brain, hypertensive encephalopathy may occur, primarily because of damage to the brainstem and basal ganglia. Cardiovascular effects include cardiac failure and dissecting aortic aneurysm.

Clinical picture

The cardinal sign of malignant hypertension is an elevation of diastolic BP, usually to >130 mmHg. Concurrently, patients often exhibit visual impairment, headache, hematuria, and signs and symptoms of CHF.

Renal failure from malignant hypertension is usually manifested by azotemia, proteinuria, oliguria or anuria, uremia, and hematuria. Hypertensive encephalopathy is manifested by a decreased level of consciousness, seizures, increased intracranial pressure, nausea, headache, and coma. Hematologic abnormalities that may be seen in malignant hypertension include anemia, thrombocytopenia, and an elevated reticulocyte count.

Without treatment, there is ~80% mortality within one year and 100% mortality within two years. Death is usually from cardiovascular or renal complications.

Medical interventions

Effective therapy for all individuals with systemic hypertension is important to prevent the progression of the disease to the malignant form. Prompt therapy of patients with malignant hypertension can prevent renal failure.

Pharmacologic therapy for malignant hypertension usually consists of IV administration of rapidly acting antihypertensives such as nitroprusside, diazoxide, or trimethaphan. In less severe cases, agents such as hydralazine, reserpine, methyldopa, or minoxidil may be used.

Dialysis may be used in malignant hypertension, both to decrease blood volume in fluid-overloaded patients and to alleviate manifestations of renal failure.

Nursing interventions

Nursing interventions for the patient with malignant hypertension are described below.

Potential deterioration of clinical condition. (1) Monitor arterial pressure frequently with arterial line. (2) Titrate BP medications to BP.

Potential complications of sudden lowering of BP. (1) Monitor patient for the development of angina pectoris, circulatory shock, cerebral ischemia. (2) Observe for complications of drug therapy (hyperglycemia with diazoxide, elevated serum thiocyanate levels with sodium nitroprusside).

VALVULAR HEART DISEASE

In the adult, valvular heart disease is most often an acquired dysfunction, resulting from either rheumatic fever or infective endocarditis. Any of the four heart valves may be affected, but the most common problems seen in the ICU involve the aortic and mitral valves.

Pathophysiology

Rheumatic fever is a systemic disease that sometimes develops following infections produced by beta-hemolytic streptococci. Rheumatic fever is most commonly seen in children between the ages of 5 and 15. Among the complications of rheumatic fever is carditis, resulting in rheumatic heart disease.

Rheumatic carditis affects the valvular endothelium, resulting in destruction of the valve leaflets. Eventually scar formation occurs, resulting in valves that are either stenotic or insufficient. Valvular dysfunction may be complicated by rheumatic involvement of the chordae tendineae.

Infective endocarditis is an inflammation of the heart, particularly the heart valves. Individuals at risk are those with underlying cardiac anatomic lesions (including rheumatic heart disease, congenital heart disease, and mitral valve prolapse) and IV-drug abusers. The organisms responsible for infective endocarditis are most often streptococci in individuals with underlying cardiac lesions and staphylococci in IV-drug abusers. A variety of other infectious organisms, including fungi and rickettsia, may also cause infective endocarditis.

The most common valvular lesions caused by rheumatic heart disease or infective endocarditis are mitral stenosis, mitral insufficiency, aortic stenosis, and aortic insufficiency. In IV-drug abusers with infective endocarditis, tricuspid insufficiency may occur. In valvular stenosis, there is a reduction in the size of the valve orifice, resulting in decreased flow across the valve and increased pressure upstream from the valve. In **mitral stenosis,** there is increased RAP and PAWP; in **aortic stenosis,** there is increased left ventricular pressure, eventually resulting in left ventricular hypertrophy and even later, left atrial enlargement. The CO may be decreased.

In contrast, in valvular insufficiency, the valve cannot competently close and the chamber upstream from the valve has to pump an increased stroke volume to accommodate the backflow of blood. In **mitral insufficiency,** the blood backs up into the left atrium during ventricular systole, whereas in **aortic insufficiency,** blood backs up into the left ventricle during diastole. Insufficiency and stenosis may affect the same valve.

Clinical picture

The clinical picture seen in the individual with valvular heart disease depends on the specific type and location of valvular damage. In addition, certain manifestations occur rapidly, whereas it may take $\geq$30 yr for others to become clinically apparent.

In **mitral stenosis,** there is pulmonary vasocongestion, resulting in shortness of breath, orthopnea, cough, and hemoptysis. Left atrial enlargement from mitral stenosis commonly results in atrial arrhythmias and palpitations. Other signs and symptoms include an enlarged liver and peripheral edema, consistent with increased systemic venous pressure. On auscultation, there may be an accentuated S_1, an opening snap, and a diastolic rumble. On chest x-ray, enlargement of the left atrium, right ventricle, and pulmonary arteries may be seen, as well as calcification of the valve. The diagnosis of mitral stenosis is confirmed most commonly by echocardiogram.

In **mitral insufficiency,** the prominent alteration is a decrease in the CO, resulting in signs and symptoms such as fatigue and a decreased exercise tolerance. With worsening insufficiency, pulmonary vasocongestion may occur, resulting in shortness of breath, orthopnea, cough, and hemoptysis. On auscultation, a holosystolic murmur may be heard, loudest at the apex. In addition, an S_3 is usually present. On chest x-ray, left atrial and left ventricular enlargement may be seen. The diagnosis of mitral insufficiency usually requires cardiac catheterization.

In **aortic stenosis,** the obstruction to left ventricular ejection of blood results in increased left ventricular work, manifested clinically as angina pectoris and CHF. Syncope, particularly on exertion, is common in aortic stenosis. On auscultation, an S_4 may be heard, as well as an ejection click, paradoxic splitting of S_2, and a harsh, high-pitched crescendo-decrescendo murmur. The diagnosis of aortic stenosis is usually confirmed by cardiac catheterization.

In **aortic insufficiency,** the increased work imposed on the left ventricle to pump an increased volume may result in angina pectoris and CHF. Peripheral pulses may display a characteristic water-hammer pulse, that is, a pulse with a rapid upstroke. BP measurement may reveal a wide pulse pressure. On auscultation, a high-pitched diastolic decrescendo murmur and S_3 and S_4 may be heard. On chest x-ray, aortic valve calcification may be seen.

In tricuspid insufficiency, signs and symptoms of right-sided vasocongestion may be seen, including pleuritic pain, dyspnea, and a productive cough.

Medical interventions

Conservative medical management of valvular heart disease consists of preserving cardiac function and symptom alleviation. When conservative management is no longer effective, valvular surgery is required.

Atrial fibrillation, common with mitral insufficiency, may be treated by cardioversion and with drugs such as quinidine. If the atrial fibrillation cannot be converted to normal sinus rhythm, the ventricular rate may be slowed with digitalis. The possibility of embolization from the fibrillating atria may be reduced by anticoagulation.

In valvular heart disease resulting in CHF, digitalis may be given to improve left ventricular function. Pulmonary congestion may be alleviated by the use of diuretics and adherence to a low-sodium diet.

Valvular surgery may involve valvulotomy or valve replacement. Valvulotomy, also referred to as a commissurotomy, is sometimes performed to repair stenotic valves. Advantages of valvulotomy are a low perioperative mortality and a low incidence of postoperative complications. A significant disadvantage, however, is that the stenosis may recur, requiring further surgery.

Valve replacement surgery involves removal of the diseased valve and placement of a synthetic or tissue valve. Disadvantages of most synthetic valves are that they disrupt laminar flow across the valve orifice and thus increase the postoperative risk of embolic complications. Tissue valves, most commonly porcine valves, do not disrupt laminar flow to any significant degree, but their long-term durability is somewhat less than for synthetic valves.

Valvular surgery is accomplished via a midline sternotomy. For valve replacement surgery, the heart is then arrested and extracorporeal circulation is established. The incidence of postoperative complications is correlated with the duration of extracorporeal circulation time, with longer times resulting in increased complications.

Early postoperative complications include altered mentation ("post-pericardiotomy syndrome"), arrhythmias, infections (including infective endocarditis), respiratory insufficiency ("pump lung"), as well as the complications that may be seen following any type of major surgery. Later postoperative complications include thromboembolism, infective endocarditis, and valve dysfunction. Thromboembolism prophylaxis is usually accomplished by anticoagulation with agents such as dicumarol. Infective endocarditis prophylaxis involves the administration of antibiotics during those times when bacteria may be introduced into the bloodstream, e.g., following minor GU and dental procedures.

Nursing interventions

Nursing interventions for the individual undergoing valvular heart surgery are briefly described below.

Anxiety. (1) Provide information about sensory experiences common during perioperative period (ICU environment, presence of lines, tubes, drains). (2) Prepare family for probable physical appearance of patient immediately postsurgery. (3) Instruct patient in respiratory hygiene techniques. (4) Allow patient to verbalize fears and encourage realistic expectations for recovery.

Possible postsurgical complications. (1) Monitor continuously for arrhythmias. (2) Obtain frequent 12-lead ECGs. (3) Monitor hemodynamic status (MABP, LAP, RAP, CO, physical assessment). (4) Monitor pulmonary status (physical assessment, arterial and venous blood gases, chest x-rays). (5) Monitor renal status (urine output, urine specific gravity, serum creatinine, BUN). (6) Monitor GI status (physical assessment, testing of stool and nasogastric aspirate for occult blood). (7) Monitor hematologic status (measurement of clotting parameters, CBC, physical assessment). (8) Institute vigorous pulmonary hygiene. (9) Provide frequent wound care. (10) Reduce environmental stressors in ICU (lights, noise, awareness of other acutely ill patients). (11) Prepare patient emotionally for transfer to regular nursing unit and eventual discharge home.

CHAPTER 3

THE RESPIRATORY SYSTEM

Mary Jane Densmore and Linda Frigon

ANATOMY AND PHYSIOLOGY REVIEW

To sustain life, the human body must inspire O_2 and expire CO_2—the process of respiration. The primary purpose of the respiratory tract is to conduct air from the atmosphere to the alveoli in the lung, where it comes in contact with pulmonary capillary blood. The entire process of respiration includes every phase of O_2 and CO_2 transport in the airways, blood, and tissues.

THE UPPER AIRWAYS

The upper airways consist of the nose, the mouth, the pharynx, and larynx. The **nose** is a mucous-membrane lined cavity, which is well supplied with blood vessels, serous glands, and hair follicles, and whose main function is filtration, heating, and humidification. The anatomy of the nose makes breathing through the **mouth** necessary when large volumes of air are moved in and out of the lungs. In oral breathing, air is not heated, humidified, or filtered.

The **pharynx** is the area behind the oral and nasal cavities and is divided into the nasopharynx, the oropharynx, and the laryngopharynx. The primary purpose of the pharyngeal musculature is to close the glottis, so as to separate liquids and solids from air, while initiating the act of swallowing.

The **larynx** is the area connecting the upper and lower airways. The opening to the larynx is called the glottis. The functions of the larynx are to act as a gas-conducting channel; to protect the lower airways from foreign substances; to participate in the cough mechanism; and to participate in speech.

The upper airways do not participate in gas exchange and therefore constitute a major portion of what is called anatomical dead space. A part of each breath remains within the upper airways and the tracheobronchial tree and does not reach the gas-exchanging surfaces in the alveoli; therefore, it does not contribute to the exchange of O_2 and CO_2. This anatomical dead space is commonly designated V/D and is approximately equal to 1 ml/lb of ideal body weight.

THE LOWER AIRWAYS

The lower airways consist of the tracheobronchial tree and the lung parenchyma. The **tracheobronchial tree** is a system of bifurcating tubes consisting of muscular, cartilaginous, and elastic tissue. These tubes—the trachea, the two main bronchi, the lobar and segmental bronchi, and the bronchioles—exist for the purpose of conducting air to and from the **lung parenchyma,** where gas exchange takes place between the capillaries and the alveoli (Fig 3–1).

As the tracheobronchial tree progresses from its beginning at the trachea to its termination at the respiratory bronchioles, the size of the airways decrease, whereas the number of airways and the cross-sectional area of the

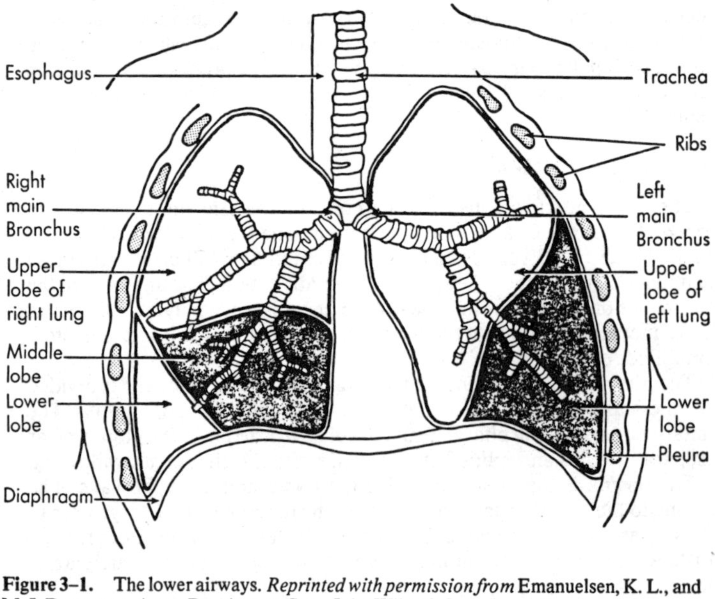

Figure 3–1. The lower airways. *Reprinted with permission from* Emanuelsen, K. L., and M. J. Densmore. Acute Respiratory Care. John Wiley & Sons, Inc., New York. 1981. p. 6.

system increase. The remaining portion of the respiratory tract is primarily concerned with gas exchange. Respiratory bronchioles, alveolar ducts, alveolar sacs, and alveoli make up this portion of the lung and together are often referred to as the acinus.

The respiratory bronchioles are succeeded by a single order of alveolar ducts, whose wall is composed of a musculo-elastic mesh through which alveoli protrude outward. Alveolar ducts give rise to the terminal spray of alveolar sacs, which are the blind ends of the respiratory tract; their walls are alveoli. There are ~300 million in the average adult lung.

Three distinct types of cells are found in alveoli. Type I alveolar cells are the basic structural cells of the alveoli and are called alveolar epithelial cells. Type II alveolar cells are larger than type I and produce pulmonary surfactant. Surfactant is a surface-tension-reducing lipoprotein whose function is to keep alveoli from collapsing as a result of their own elastic recoil. By reducing alveolar surface tension, surfactant equalizes pressure within each alveolus during expansion or contraction on inspiration and expiration. The tendency for alveoli to collapse is not entirely eliminated by surfactant; it is merely controlled, for alveoli must be kept inflated with a certain volume of air. Type III alveolar cells are the alveolar macrophages, which are important cells in the defense against pulmonary infection. The macrophage cells float throughout the alveoli by ameboid movement and phagocytize particles.

Pulmonary circulation

Blood travels from the right ventricle into the pulmonary artery and then branches into the arterioles. The arterioles continue to branch into capillaries that surround the respiratory bronchioles and alveolar sacs (Fig. 3–2). Its main function is to carry mixed venous blood through the alveolar capillaries so that a proper amount of O_2 can be added and a proper amount of CO_2 can be removed.

The pulmonary circulation is a low-resistance, high-flow system. This means that although huge amounts of blood are pumped through it, the pulmonary capillary pressure remains low because the right ventricle is much less muscular than the left and does not pump with nearly so much force. The right ventricular systolic pressure is ~22 mmHg, and the diastolic pressure is ~1 mmHg. The right ventricle is pumping against a system that offers only one-tenth the resistance of systemic circulation. Thus, with less pressure being developed in the right ventricle and less resistance being offered by the pulmonary vascular bed, the pulmonary arterial presure is about 22/8 mmHg. With increased cardiac output and increased blood flow to the lungs, the pressure in the pulmonary circulation does not rise markedly. Because of the great capacity of the pulmonary arterioles and capillaries to dilate and accept more blood, the cardiac output must rise to at least three times that of the resting level before the pulmonary artery pressure is significantly elevated. Although the lungs normally

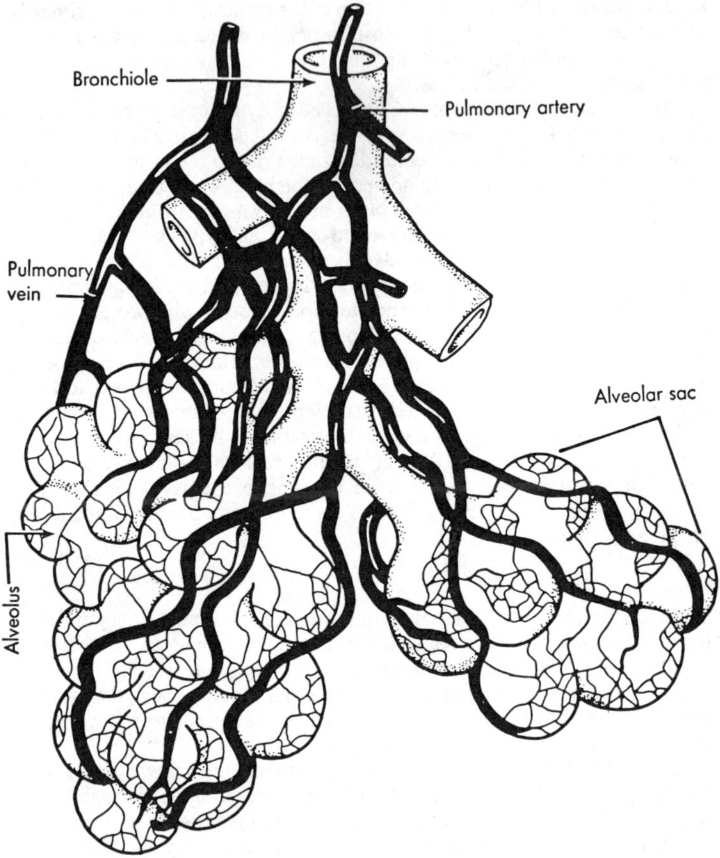

Figure 3–2. Alveoli with pulmonary blood supply. *Reprinted with permission from* Emanuelsen, K. L., and M. J. Densmore. Acute Respiratory Care. John Wiley & Sons, Inc., New York. 1981. p. 9.

contain only 12% of the total blood volume, they can increase their capacity up to 200% of their normal volume during exercise.

The pulmonary vessels, in one way, are very different from those in the systemic circulation—instead of dilating in the presence of low O_2 levels, they constrict. The concept of autoregulation of blood flow that applies to all nonpulmonary capillaries in the body is reversed in the lung. If it were not, the highest blood flow in the lungs would be where the least amount of O_2

was available, and little circulation would occur in those areas where the most O_2 was available. The result would be that the blood in the pulmonary system would pick up the least O_2 available to deliver to the tissues.

The distribution of the capillary circulation is not uniform. Blood flow is greatest in the dependent position of the lungs because of the effects of gravity. The bases of the lungs in the upright position and the posterior part of the lungs in the supine position receive the greatest amount of blood perfusion. Consequently, the lower part of the lungs is relatively overperfused and the upper part of the lungs is relatively underperfused in the upright position. In the apices of the lungs, blood flows only during systole and, therefore, blood is not uniformly distributed through the pulmonary bed.

Bronchial circulation is not accomplished by pulmonary circulation. Blood is delivered to the structural portions of the lungs—the lower trachea, bronchi, visceral pleura, etc.—by the bronchial arteries. Bronchial circulation is part of the systemic circulatory system. The right lung has one bronchial artery, and the left has two. Each artery follows a course along the bronchial tree, subdividing with it. Part of the venous return of bronchial circulation is through the pulmonary veins, which comprise one-fourth of the total arteriovenous shunt in a healthy person. Because bronchial circulation is not part of the pulmonary circulation, it operates under a much higher pressure.

Pulmonary mechanics

The lungs are enclosed in the thorax, a structure composed of bone and muscle. The construction of the thoracic cage is such that it has sufficient rigidity to protect the vital organs, yet it is pliable enough to function as a bellows during the ventilatory cycle. Expansion of the chest cage takes place as a result of upward and outward movement of the ribs and flattening of the diaphragm. Atmospheric air is pulled into the lungs when the movement of the diaphragm causes the development of negative pressure in the airways. The diaphragm, the major muscle of inspiration, is dome-shaped and composed of two hemidiaphragms that are attached to the lower ribs. In its relaxed position, the diaphragm occupies an area in the thorax. When it contracts, the diaphragm moves downward, thereby enlarging the volume of the thorax and stretching the lungs, which move with the thoracic walls. The contraction of the diaphragm is stimulated by the phrenic nerve.

The intercostal muscles also play a role in normal inspiration by pulling the ribs upward and forward, which further increases the size of the thorax and lungs.

The pleural space is a potential space between the layers of pleura that is normally occupied by a small amount of fluid. This pleural fluid acts as a lubricant to decrease friction as the pleural layers slide along one another. The pleura is a continuous membrane that encloses the pleural spaces. The parietal pleura is attached to the interior wall of the thorax and moves with the chest wall. The visceral pleura (lining the lung) is carried along with the thoracic wall because of its adherence to the parietal pleura. This "hugging" of the chest wall can only occur because of the negative pressure in the intrapleural space. Atmospheric pressure is 760 mmHg at sea level and intrapleural pressure is 755 mmHg. This negative pressure is a result of the force moving the chest wall away from the lungs or the lungs away from the chest wall.

Because the two pleural layers normally do not separate, the increased volume of the thorax leads to expansion of the lung. Pressures within the lung that were previously atmospheric are now subatmospheric, creating a pressure gradient between the lungs and the atmosphere. Air then flows into the lungs until a pressure equilibrium is reached. At the end of inspiration, the elastic forces in the lung and the chest dominate and cause higher-than-atmospheric pressure (positive pressure) in the lungs—and air flows out of the lungs.

When the lungs are inflated maximally, the elastic forces of the respiratory system are balanced by the maximum inspiratory muscle forces. Similarly, there is a limit to the amount of air that can be expelled from the lungs and, after a maximal expiration, the elastic forces (mainly the chest wall) tending to expand the lungs are balanced by the maximum expiratory muscle forces. Between these two extremes, the relationship between the elastic forces of the lung and the chest wall is related to the lung volume.

Breathing takes place within the framework established by the boundaries of the maximum excursions of the respiratory apparatus. Changes in lung volumes produced by the action of the respiratory muscles can be studied. The various components of the lung volumes are illustrated in Figure 3–3 and the definitions of each are given in Table 3–1.

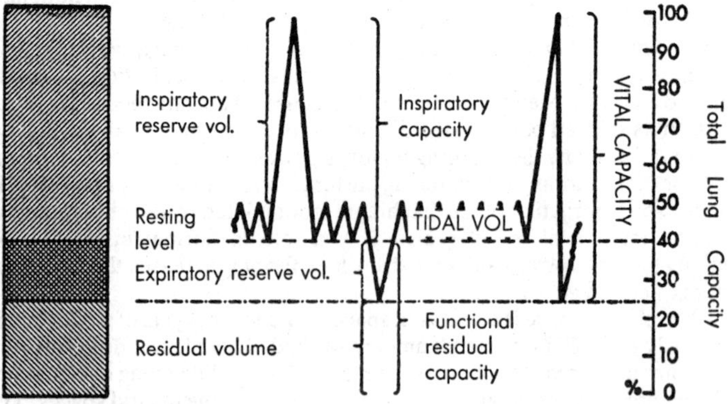

Figure 3–3. The subdivisions of lung volume shown as a proportion of total capacity.

TABLE 3–1

Basic Definitions of Lung Function Measurements

Test	Definition
Vital capacity (VC)	Largest volume that can be measured on complete expiration after taking the deepest possible inspiration without force or effort.
Inspiratory capacity (IC)	Largest volume of gas that can be inspired from the resting expiratory level.
Expiratory reserve volume (ERV)	Largest volume of gas that can be expired from the end-expiratory level.
Functional residual capacity (FRC)	Volume of gas remaining in the lungs at the end of a normal expiration.
Residual volume (RV)	Volume of gas remaining in the lungs at the end of a maximal expiration.
Inspiratory reserve volume (IRV)	The maximal volume of air that can be inhaled to total lung capacity over and above the tidal volume.
Total lung capacity (TLC)	Amount of gas remaining in the lungs at the end of a maximal inspiration.
Tidal volume (V_T)	Volume of gas inspired or expired during each respiratory cycle.
Minute volume (MV)	Total volume of gas either inspired or expired in 1 min.
Forced vital capacity (FVC)	Volume of gas that can be expired as forcefully and rapidly as possible after maximum inspiration.
Compliance (C)	The change in transpulmonary pressure required to effect a given change in the volume of air in the lungs.

Compliance

The change in transpulmonary pressure required to effect a given change in the volume of air in the lungs is a measure of the distensibility, or compliance, of the lungs. When the lung is easy to distend (elastic resistance is low) it has a high compliance; if it is difficult to distend (elastic resistance is high) it has a low compliance. Lungs that have decreased compliance will not expand properly and the vital capacity will be reduced. A stiff lung or a fixed thoracic cage would result in decreased compliance. The distensibility can also be expressed as the change in pressure per unit of volume change, in which case it is called the elastic resistance and is the reciprocal of the compliance.

NEUROANATOMY

There is no single center that controls the power of breathing; several centers and receptors are involved. The primary respiratory center is located in the medulla oblongata of the brainstem. Intermittent bursts of activity in the neurons of the respiratory center initiate nerve impulses that travel down the phrenic and other motor nerves to cause muscular contraction for each inspiration. Increases in alveolar ventilation are the result of an increase in the role of impulses—which determine respiratory frequency—and an increase in the amplitude of the impulses, causing an increase in the tidal volume.

Other parts of the respiratory center include the inspiratory and expiratory centers, which overlap anatomically in the posterior medulla; chemoreceptor areas, which lie on the anterior side of the medulla; and the apneustic and pneumotaxic centers in the pons. Inspiration is normally ended by inhibition, both from the pneumotaxic center and from the vagal efferent impulses. The inhibitory action of the pneumotaxic center is reinforced by stretch receptors in the bronchi and the bronchioles that are activated by inflation to inhibit further lung expansion. Thus, the normal volume of air inspired is in part governed by this reflex, which is called the Hering-Breuer inspiratory reflex.

Changes in PCO_2, pH, and PO_2 levels are sensed by chemosensitive areas in the brainstem and by peripheral chemoreceptors that send impulses by afferent nerves to the respiratory center. The anterior medullary chemosensitive areas are primarily sensitive to CSF pH levels. CSF pH levels change very rapidly with the changes in $PaCO_2$. Thus, a fall in alveolar ventilation will very quickly result in a rise in CSF hydrogen ion concentration and increased stimulation of the respiratory center.

RESPIRATION

Alveolar ventilation

The most important function of the lung and of pulmonary ventilation is to supply tissue cells with enough O_2 and to remove excess CO_2. To accomplish this, pulmonary ventilation must increase the PAO_2 to well above the PO_2 in the venous blood flowing through the alveolar capillaries; thus loading the blood destined for tissue cells with O_2. It must also lower the $PACO_2$ to be below the PCO_2 of the venous blood: this unloads excess CO_2 from the blood destined for tissue cells. The amount of air per minute that a healthy man at sea level should breathe (minute volume or minute ventilation) is the amount needed to keep his PAO_2 ~100 mmHg and his $PACO_2$ ~40 mmHg. This amount varies with the rate and depth of breathing and the volume of anatomic dead space. It also varies with uneven metabolic requirements. Patients with uneven alveolar ventilation, uneven pulmonary blood flow, or impairment of alveolocapillary diffusion require more ventilation to oxygenate their arterial blood supply.

Diffusion

Both internal and external respiration operate by diffusion, the process by which a gas expands because of molecular motion to fill the available volume. CO_2 is 20 times more diffusible across alveolocapillary membranes than is O_2; for this reason, if the membrane is damaged, its decreased capacity for transporting O_2 into the blood is almost always more of a problem than its decreased capacity for transporting CO_2 out.

Transport of gases

Because PO_2 is high in the alveoli and low in mixed venous blood, O_2 diffuses from the alveoli into the pulmonary capillary blood. It is carried in the blood in two ways: as dissolved O_2 in physical solution in the plasma and combined with the Hb in the RBCs. The amount of O_2 dissolved and the amount of O_2 combined with Hb depends upon the PaO_2. Most of the O_2 in the blood is carried in the RBCs in combination with the Hb as oxyhemoglobin (HbO_2). Hb that is not combined with O_2 is called reduced Hb. The extent to which Hb combines with O_2 is usually expressed as the percent of saturation and is illustrated in the following formula:

$$\text{Percent saturated} = \frac{O_2 \text{ content } (HbO_2)}{O_2 \text{ capacity } (HbO_2 + \text{reduced Hb})}$$

The O_2 saturation of the arterial blood in a normal person breathing room air is ~97%. The saturation of Hb depends upon the PO_2 in the plasma. When the PO_2 is high, most or all of the Hb combines with O_2. When the PO_2 is low, as in respiratory disease, only a small amount of the Hb combines with the O_2.

The relationship between the PO_2 and the saturation of the Hb is expressed by the HbO_2 dissociation curve. The characteristic S-shape of this curve illustrates that the Hb clings to O_2 over a fairly wide range of O_2 tensions at the upper end of the scale and gives up O_2 readily at the lower O_2 tensions (Fig. 3–4).

O_2 is brought to the tissues by the arterial blood. The O_2 that is directly available to the tissues is the O_2 in physical solution in the plasma. As it is taken up by the tissue cells, the PO_2 in the plasma falls so that the HbO_2 begins to dissociate.

In this way, O_2 is freed from the RBCs into the plasma and then into the tissues. The HbO_2 dissociation curve shows that the Hb readily gives up O_2 when the O_2 tension drops below 60 mmHg.

Because the O_2 tension of the tissue cells is low (<10 mmHg), the O_2 diffuses rapidly from the blood into the tissue cells.

The HbO_2 dissociation curve shows that the top of the graph becomes nearly flat at a PO_2 level of ~75 mmHg. Therefore, at a PO_2 level of 75 to 100 mmHg, Hb is nearly saturated. At a PO_2 level of 100 mmHg, Hb is 97.4% saturated, and a PO_2 level of over 250 mmHg would be required to increase the saturation another 2.6% to a saturation of 100%.

The significance of these ranges of PO_2 that produce high saturation is that even when the alveolar PO_2 level is reduced below its normal of 100

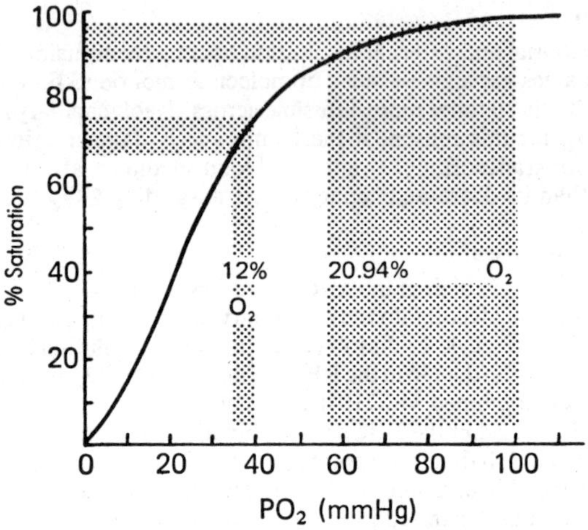

Figure 3–4. The oxyhemoglobin dissociation curve. *Reprinted with permission from* Emanuelsen, K. L., and M. J. Densmore. Acute Respiratory Care. John Wiley & Sons, Inc., New York. 1981. p. 19.

mmHg, Hb saturation remains high until the reduction of the PO_2 level is quite large—nearly 25%. The curve also shows that once the PO_2 level begins to drop, it drops very rapidly.

Hb has a certain affinity for O_2, allowing blood to oxygenate readily in the pulmonary bed. Extreme changes in this affinity can make the Hb less capable of releasing O_2 to the tissues. Various factors—such as the pH, body temperature, and PCO_2 levels—alter this affinity and, in so doing, change the normal relationship between Hb saturation and O_2 tension. A change in the Hb affinity for O_2 changes the position of the HbO_2 dissociation curve. This is known as shifting the curve (Fig. 3–5).

Decreasing O_2 affinity results in a shift to the right: for any given PO_2, there is a lower percentage of HbO_2. The O_2 transport capability of the blood is decreased because O_2 content is decreased. A shift to the right means that Hb affinity for O_2 is less than normal, but the O_2 is also more readily released to the cells. A shift to the right can be a result of acidemia, hyperthermia, hypercapnia, or chronic hypoxemia.

Increasing O_2 affinity results in a shift to the left: for any given O_2 tension, there is a higher percentage of saturated Hb. The effect of increased affinity on tissue oxygenation may be profound. Hb may be thought of as an "oxygen magnet" in the blood; the stronger the magnet, the less susceptible O_2 is to the tissue-pressure gradient in the transfer of O_2 to tissues. A shift to the left can be a result of alkalemia, hypothermia, or hypocapnia.

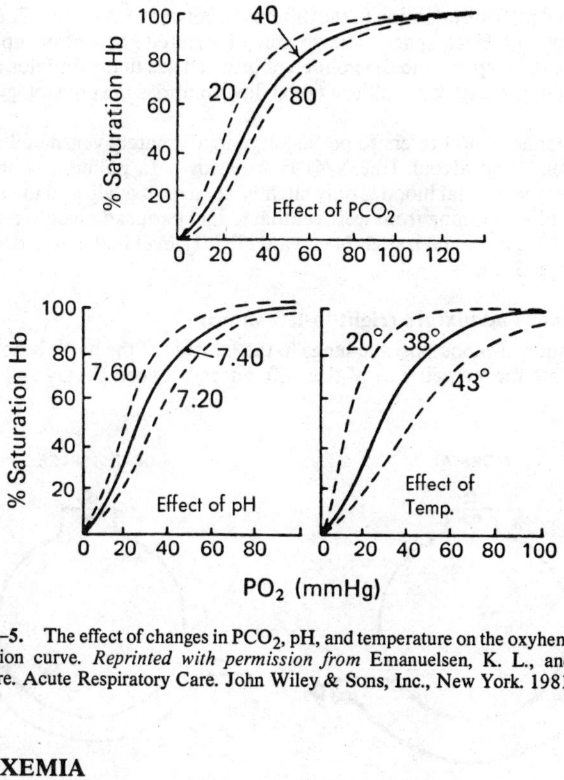

Figure 3–5. The effect of changes in PCO_2, pH, and temperature on the oxyhemoglobin dissociation curve. *Reprinted with permission from* Emanuelsen, K. L., and M. J. Densmore. Acute Respiratory Care. John Wiley & Sons, Inc., New York. 1981. p. 21.

HYPOXEMIA

Disorders that lead to hypoxemia do so through one or more of the following processes.

Ventilation-perfusion imbalance

Uneven distribution of ventilation with respect to perfusion is the most common clinical phenomenon responsible for hypoxemia. If O_2 and CO_2 are to be exchanged, pulmonary blood flow and alveolar gases must come into contact with one another. Interference with normal gas exchange will result if either perfusion (Q) or ventilation (V) is altered. Nonuniformity of V/Q ratios in the lung accounts for a large portion of differences between PAO_2 and PaO_2. When the alveolus is ventilated but not perfused (a dead-space unit), the V/Q ratio is high. Blood that leaves poorly perfused or unperfused alveoli is fully oxygenated so that arterial blood gas (ABG) tensions may be relatively normal. This abnormality can, however, be uncovered by determination of the difference between PAO_2 and PaO_2 and the physiologic dead space. The volume of inspired gas that occupies the anatomic dead space and the volume of inspired gas that ventilates alveoli that are not perfused by capillary blood flow comprise the physiologic dead space.

Pulmonary shunt refers to perfusion of inadequately ventilated alveoli or nonventilated alveoli (the V/Q ratio is low). In pulmonary shunt, a portion of the arterial blood is only slightly aerated, if at all, and then mixes with the blood coming from well-ventilated and perfused alveoli, resulting in a low PO_2 level and a slightly elevated PCO_2 level in the mixed arterial blood (Fig. 3–6).

True venous admixture (right-to-left shunt)

Shunting of blood past the lungs to the left side of the heart is normally responsible for a small part of the differences between PAO_2 and PaO_2.

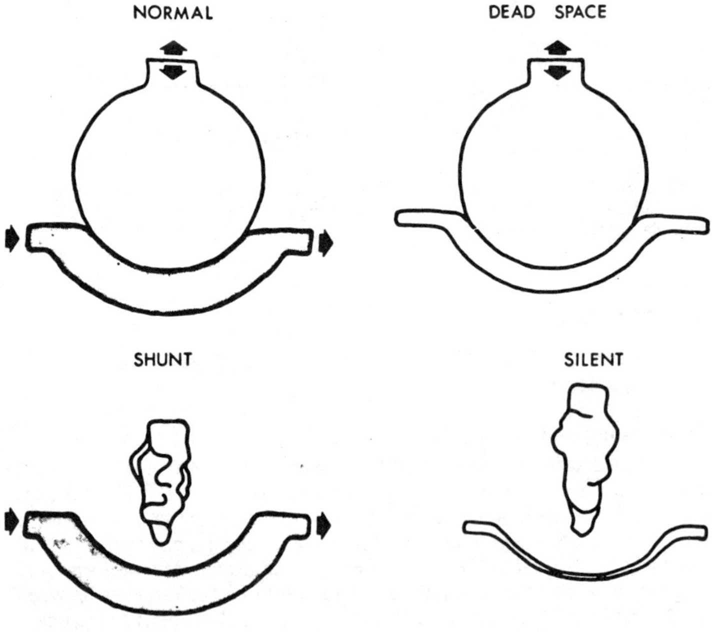

Figure 3–6. Diagram of alveoli and capillaries showing ventilation-perfusion relationships. *Reprinted with permission from* Emanuelsen, K. L., and M. J. Densmore. Acute Respiratory Care. John Wiley & Sons, Inc., New York. 1981. p 28.

Significant degrees of O_2 desaturation, caused by the admixture of unaerated blood, can occur in congenital heart disease, polycythemia, liver disease, and abnormal pulmonary arteriovenous communications.

A qualitative estimate of the shunt can be obtained by allowing the patient to breathe 100% O_2 and then measuring the PaO_2. If there is a greater-than-normal amount of unaerated blood being added to aerated blood, the PaO_2 will not reach the expected value of >500 mmHg. To determine the amount of blood being shunted, one can use the following equation:

$$\text{Percent shunt} = \frac{\text{difference in } O_2 \text{ content between end pulmonary capillary and arterial blood}}{\text{difference in } O_2 \text{ content between end pulmonary capillary and mixed venous blood}}$$

Although an increase in calculated venous admixture is caused by a defect in the heart, it may also occur if there is perfusion of regions of the lung that are not ventilated because of obstruction, collapse, consolidation, or pulmonary edema.

Impairment of gas diffusion (diffusion defect)

The diffusion capacity of O_2 and CO_2 may be decreased when the path for diffusion becomes longer. This occurs when the alveolar membrane is thickened or these membranes are separated by transudate, exudate, or abnormal tissue, or when the surface area of contact between ventilated alveoli and functioning pulmonary capillaries is reduced. A pure diffusion defect is relatively uncommon and is usually associated with a ventilation-perfusion imbalance.

The process of diffusion can be measured quantitatively in man by determining the pulmonary diffusing capacity for O_2 and carbon monoxide. To do so, it is necessary to know the amount of O_2 and carbon monoxide/min that is diffusing across the blood-gas barrier as well as the mean gradient of its partial pressures between the alveolus and the pulmonary capillary.

ASSESSMENT OF THE PATIENT

In the ICU setting, the patient with impending respiratory problems demands immediate evaluation. This should include history—including medical history and pertinent pulmonary history—and physical assessment. After immediate assessment and evaluation occur, further diagnostic studies may be indicated.

Health history

It is very important when recording a medical history to have a careful, organized approach. Initially the symptom that brought the patient into the hospital should be identified, and a determination as to the onset and duration of this symptom should be made. This allows the examiner to classify the problem as an acute, subacute, or chronic one. The history of the present illness should detail the development of the symptoms identified in the chief complaint and related symptoms. Elements of the personal, occupational, or social history may be incorporated (if pertinent), and a list of medications that the patient is currently taking is also important. The patient's previous illness and operations should be recorded in chronologic order. Occupational history is especially important in patients with pulmonary problems because the lungs are constantly exposed to the environment. The patient's social history, including his smoking and drinking habits, should be investigated. The illnesses occurring in family members are important because several pulmonary diseases are hereditary (e.g., asthma and cystic fibrosis). Also, family members may have similar exposures (e.g., TB or other infections).

The pulmonary history should focus on cardinal pulmonary symptoms, which include dyspnea, cough, sputum evaluation, hemoptysis, and chest pain.

Dyspnea. Breathlessness, shortness of breath, or dyspnea is a sensation of difficulty inspiring air into the lungs and is one of the most common complaints of a patient with chest illnesses. Dyspnea may occur slowly and progressively, as seen in chronic emphysema, or can be acute and intermittent, as seen in asthma. Orthopnea is common in left heart failure but may also be seen in COPD.

Cough. Coughing is not a normal symptom in patients who do not smoke, although everyone coughs on occasion. A change in the character or frequency of coughing is one of the most common chief complaints in patients with pulmonary disease. The frequency and severity of the cough, its character and pitch, and its timing, both daily and seasonally, should be determined. The amount and character of sputum produced from the cough should also be noted.

Sputum evaluation. Sputum production may be difficult to assess either because of the patient's lack of awareness or personal distaste in discussing it. It is, however, important to define carefully the duration of sputum production, volume, and character, and presence or absence of blood. The important issue is whether or not these signs and symptoms represent a change from normal.

Hemoptysis. If hemoptysis is present, it is important to note its duration and to specify whether there is gross blood, blood-tinged sputum, or blood-streaked sputum. Most episodes of hemoptysis are caused by bronchitis or bronchiectasis and usually present as blood-streaked sputum, rather than gross hemoptysis. Another common cause of hemoptysis is bronchial carcinoma which, too, is associated with blood streaking.

Grossly bloody sputum is often seen in patients with TB, pulmonary infarction, or bronchial adenoma.

Chest pain. Chest pain is another common symptom in patients with pulmonary problems and warrants careful documentation. There are two types of chest pain: one that arises in the chest wall and is conducted through the intercostal muscles and phrenic nerve; and one that is visceral in origin and is conducted through the afferent fibers of the ANS. Chest-wall pain is sharp and well localized and is increased by deep breathing or coughing (pleuritic pain). Visceral pain is poorly localized and is generally described as central or substernal. This pain occurs with neoplasms of the major bronchi, tumors of the mediastinum, and abnormalities of the heart and pericardium.

Physical examination

Examination of the chest is one of the most important aspects of respiratory nursing care. The methods used in physical assessment of the chest are inspection and observation, palpation, percussion, and auscultation.

Inspection and observation. To obtain an accurate picture of the thorax and its movements, have the patient sitting in an upright position, if possible, with anterior and posterior chest exposed. The symmetry of the chest should be observed, as well as skin color and structural alterations, such as bony deformities. Important diagnostic clues to a patient's pulmonary problem can be obtained by bedside observation of his respiratory pattern. The most important factors to note are the rate, rhythm, depth, and degree of effort involved. Table 3–2 lists the most commonly seen abnormal breathing patterns.

Palpation. Palpation is begun by feeling both sides of the trachea to discover any masses, deviations, or asymmetry. The nurse should then locate the manubrial (sternal) notch, which is situated at the point where the manubrium of the sternum joins the body of the sternum, and note whether the position is in the midline.

Anteriorly, the ribs can be numbered by identifying the second rib and its costal cartilage. The second rib is adjacent to the sternal angle. Posteriorly, the ribs can be numbered in relation to the scapulae (Fig. 3–7).

The chest is palpated to identify areas of tenderness, assess observed abnormalities, assess tone of the chest muscles, confirm the adequacy or inadequacy of respiratory excursion, and examine for tactile fremitus. Tactile fremitus is felt when the vibrations produced by the patient's voice are transmitted through open airways to the periphery of the lungs. To test for tactile fremitus, the patient is asked to repeat words such as *ninety-nine* or *one, two, three,* while maintaining the same pitch and intensity of voice each time; at the same time, the examiner places the palmar base of the fingers against the apices of the posterior chest to the lung bases. The procedure is then repeated over the lateral and anterior areas of the chest.

TABLE 3–2
Abnormal Breathing Patterns

Type of breathing pattern	Characteristics	Disease process
Kussmaul respirations	Regular pattern; moderate-to-rapid rate; large tidal volume; little apparent effort; absent end-expiration pause.	Metabolic acidosis.
Obstructed breathing	Slow rate; increased tidal volume; little apparent effort in inspiration or expiration; may be prolonged and labored; audible wheezing or stridor may be present. If a chronic condition: use of accessory muscles while leaning forward on inspiration; expiration through pursed lips. Low, flat diaphram.	Tumor; mucus plugs; consolidation.
Restricted breathing	Rapid rate at rest; inordinately high respiratory rate with exercise; small tidal volume; little apparent effort.	Kyphoscoliosis; collagen-vascular pulmonary disease, e.g., interstitial fibrosis, LE, scleroderma, rheumatoid arthritis.
Gasping respirations	Irregular pattern; short inspiratory phase associated with extension of the neck; long expiratory phase.	Cerebral hypoxia caused by neurologic insult, shock, cardiac failure.
Cheyne-Stokes respirations	Alternating periods of tachypnea and bradypnea; apneic phase (lasts from 15 to 60 sec) followed by a phase where tidal volume increases with each breath to a peak level, then decreases to the apneic phase.	Increased intracranial pressure, uremia, coma. (Normal in infants and healthy elderly normal adults, individuals at very high altitudes.)
Flail	Paradoxical movement of chest wall at fracture site; affected area drawn in on inspiration, pushed out on expiration.	Multiple rib fractures and disruption of costosternal cartilage.

Normally, there is increased fremitus of the right chest because there is a little more lung tissue on the right.

Fluid, air, or solid tissue in the pleural space slows the transmission of sound waves from the larynx to the chest wall and results in decreased

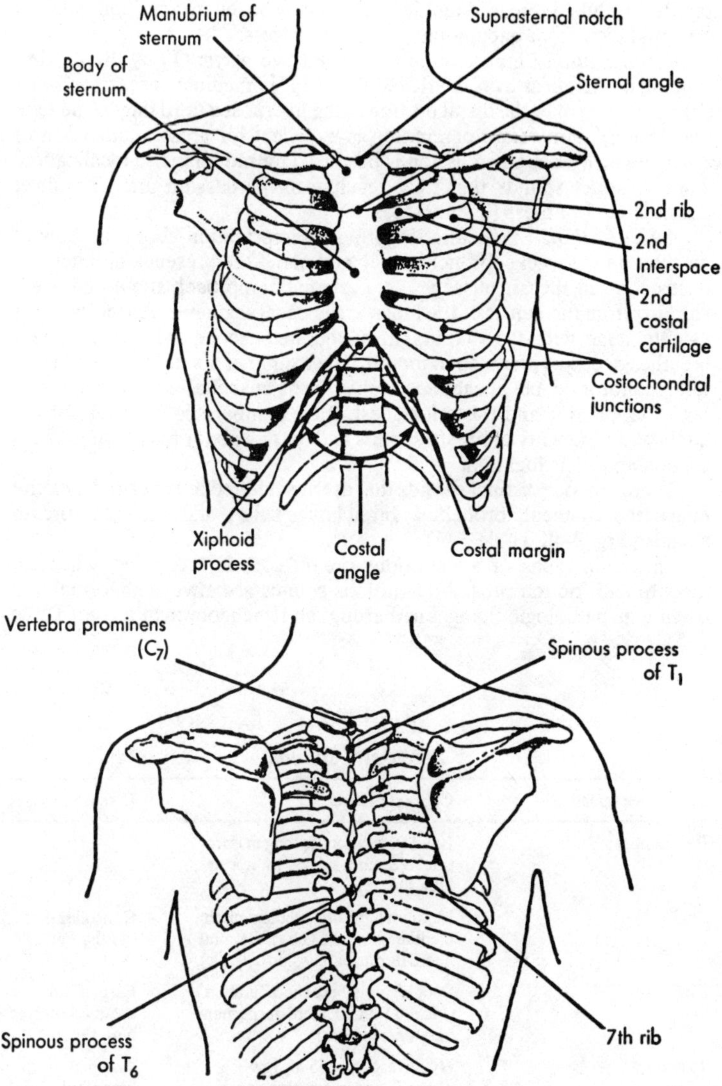

Figure 3–7. The rib cage. (A) anterior view; (B) posterior view.

tactile fremitus. Increased tactile fremitus may be felt in conditions such as consolidation from pneumonia or a lung abscess.

Percussion. Percussion is performed two ways: (1) by direct, firm tapping of the chest with the flexed fingertip (immediate percussion), and (2) by tapping over the distal portion of the interposed third finger (mediate percussion). Immediate percussion is excellent for gross localization of normalities. Mediate percussion is best used for more precise localization. Three distinct sounds that may result from percussion are resonance, dullness, and flatness (Table 3–3).

Auscultation. Auscultation provides information about the flow of air through the tracheobronchial tree and about the presence of mucus or obstruction in the air passages. A systematic approach should be used, working from the apices of the lungs to the basal segments. Auscultation is usually done with the diaphragm of the stethoscope, while the patient breathes deeply with an open mouth. The examiner should then listen to a full respiratory cycle at each location. During auscultation of the lungs on both the anterior and posterior chest, the examiner should listen for the quality and intensity of breath sounds and for any abnormal (adventitious) sounds and their location.

There are four distinct sounds that are auscultated over normal, healthy lungs: the tracheal, bronchial, bronchovesicular, and vesicular breath sounds (Fig. 3–8, Table 3–4).

The main types of adventitious breath sounds are: rales, wheezes, rhonchi and friction rubs. Adventitious sounds are always abnormal and occur with pathologic changes in the lungs and tracheobronchial tree (Table 3–5).

TABLE 3–3

Percussive sounds

Percussive sound	Characteristics	Disease process
Resonant	Loud, low-pitched, long in duration. (Sound heard in normal lung tissue.)	
Dull	Medium intensity, medium pitch, medium duration. (Normal sound heard during percussion of liver.)	Consolidation in lung field.
Flat	Soft, high-pitched, short duration. (Normal sound heard during percussion of thigh.)	Large fluid accumulation in lung field.
Tympany	Hyperresonant, loud, low-pitched, long in duration, musical quality.	Trapped air in lung field.

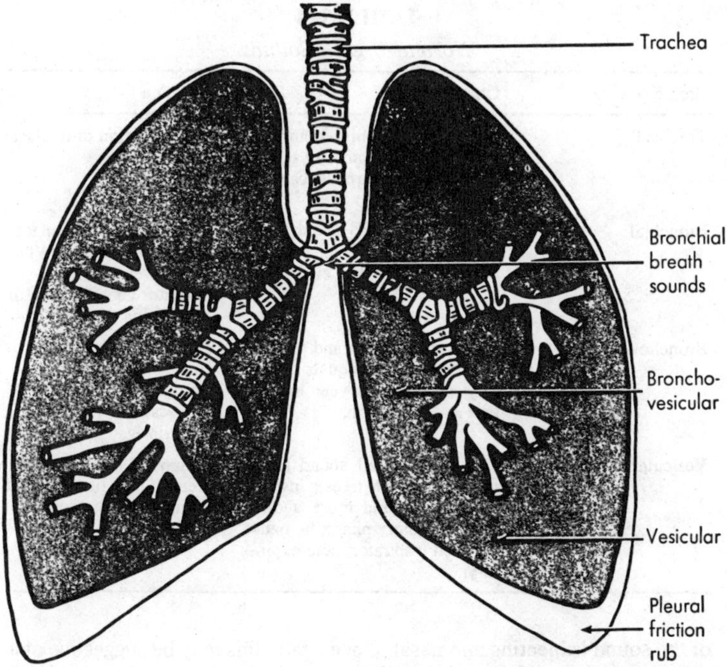

Figure 3–8. Anatomic location of various breath sounds. *Reprinted with permission from* Emanuelsen, K. L., and M. J. Densmore. Acute Respiratory Care. John Wiley & Sons, Inc., New York. 1981. p. 43.

Voice sounds set up vibrations that are transmitted through the bronchial tree. Patients are given words, such as *one, two, three,* to repeat, and the chest is auscultated to hear how the sounds are transmitted. If the words are whispered, the normal transmission of the sound will be faint and the whispered syllables will not be distinct during auscultation. The hearing of whispered words as loud sounds is known as whispering pectoriloquy. Whispering pectoriloquy is extremely useful in the early detection of pneumonia and atelectasis.

Bronchophony is a term given to the spoken syllable that is heard with exaggerated distinctness through the stethoscope. The presence of bronchophony is also associated with pulmonary consolidation.

Egophony is the term used when the *E* sound, spoken by the patient, comes out as an *A* sound when heard through the stethoscope. The quality

TABLE 3–4
Normal Breath Sounds

Breath sounds	Characteristics	Location
Tracheal	Loud, harsh tubular sound; inspiratory and expiratory phases equal in length. No pause between two phases.	Upper portion of trachea.
Bronchial	Loud, high-pitched sound; wind-in-tunnel quality; inspiratory phase is shorter than expiratory.	Second intercostal space on side of sternum. (When heard over lung fields indicates consolidation or obstruction.)
Bronchovesicular	Moderate intensity and pitch; inspiratory phase equals expiratory; no pause between inspiration and expiration.	First and second intercostal space next to sternum anteriorly and intrascapular region posteriorly.
Vesicular	Soft, low-pitched sound (wind rustling through trees); inspiratory; longer and more audible than expiratory phase; no pause between inspiratory and expiratory.	Peripheral lung tissue; all areas of lung tissue except where large airways are present.

of the sound is bleating and nasal. Once again, this may be suggestive of a pulmonary consolidation. Upon listening through the stethoscope, the *A* sound is so distinct over the area of consolidation that the examiner may wish to listen to the spoken word with one ear and auscultate the lungs with the other in order to hear the *E* to *A* change.

The development of skill in chest assessment requires discipline and practice. By using a systematic evaluation of the chest and lungs along with a knowledge of the patient's history the critical care practitioner can develop an appropriate plan of care.

Diagnostic tests

Chest x-ray. After obtaining a complete history from the patient and performing a thorough physical examination, the examiner should be able to arrive at a tentative diagnosis. An x-ray of the patient's chest can give more information and lead to a more definitive diagnosis and is therefore an integral part of the assessment of the patient.

In the ICU, chest x-rays are taken to look for lung pathology, to assess changes in lung pathology, to check for the correct placement of an endotracheal tube, or to look for the presence of pleural fluid or pneumothorax. The routine chest x-ray is usually taken with the patient facing and

TABLE 3–5
*Adventitious Sounds**

Breath sounds	Characteristics	Disease process/location
Crackles (Rales, from the French meaning "to rattle")	Discontinuous sounds, series of popping or crackling sounds, heard usually on inspiration.	Interstitial diseases, such as pneumonia, pulmonary edema, purulent bronchitis, and pulmonary fibrosis.
Fine		Associated with small airway pathology.
Coarse		Associated with large airway pathology, e.g., bronchitis, bronchopneumonia.
Wheezes	High-pitched continuous sounds (usually lasting >250 msec); expiratory wheezes indicate mild asthma; inspiratory and expiratory wheezes indicate more severe asthma.	Arise in small airways.
Rhonchi (meaning snore)	Continuous, low-pitched, turbulent, rumbling, snoring sound; may disappear following a cough (if caused by mucus blockage).	Large airway disease involving either stricture, foreign body, tumor, or mucus secretions.
Pleural friction rub	Loud, grating sound heard primarily at end of inspiration and beginning of expiration; often accompanied by pain or discomfort; best heard anteriorly.	Pleural space; visceral and parietal pleura rubbing together without pleural fluid to serve as a lubricant.
Pericardial friction rub	Similar to pleural friction rub, heard during atrial and ventricular systole; best heard at left sternal border, third intercostal space.	Pericardial space; inflammation caused by pericarditis.

*Terminology of adventitious breath sounds is based on the recommendations of a special committee of the American Thoracic Society and the American College of Chest Physicians.

touching the photographic film, and the x-rays penetrate the chest from the posterior to the anterior (PA view); it gives the sharpest and smallest cardiac shadow because the heart is situated close to the anterior wall of the chest. In the ICU, most x-rays are taken portably, with the patient's posterior chest lying on the photographic plate and the x-rays penetrating from the anterior side. This gives a larger cardiac shadow.

When chest x-ray films are interpreted, the degrees of blackness on the film are compared either with each other or against a film taken earlier. There are four types of densities (blackness) seen on an x-ray. These are gas, or air, water, fat, and metal. Gas is the least dense and absorbs minimal x-rays. Therefore, air-filled structures, such as the lungs, appear to be the blackest on the film.

Water density is seen with soft tissue, muscle, and blood. The heart appears as water density, which is lighter in color than gas density. Fat density is even lighter in color than water density. The lightest of all is metal density, which is seen in bony structures, such as the ribs, because they absorb the most x-rays.

The simple chest x-ray is one of the most fundamental diagnostic tools in the assessment and evaluation of pulmonary diseases. All other radiographic procedures, such as fluoroscopy, tomography, and special contrast studies, are strictly ancillary.

Arterial blood gas analysis. The evaluation of oxygenation and acid-base status is crucial in the management of critically ill patients. *See* Chapter 12 for an in-depth discussion of ABG analysis.

Pulmonary function tests. Pulmonary function testing consists of the performance of a set of maneuvers to detect and quantitate disorders of pulmonary ventilation and gas exchange. In the critically ill patient, this testing will be deferred until the patient's condition permits, as good patient effort is required. These tests provide objective evidence of the presence, type, and degree of pulmonary abnormality and thus allow for assessment of the course of the disease state over time, evaluation of the effectiveness of drug therapy, and determination of the risk of pulmonary complications of surgical procedures. Testing of the pulmonary system requires relatively little invasiveness or risk but does require complete patient cooperation and effort.

MAJOR DISORDERS

ACUTE RESPIRATORY FAILURE

Respiratory failure is the inability of the pulmonary system to provide the adequate exchange of O_2 and CO_2 necessary to fulfill its role of meeting the metabolic demands of the tissues. When the lungs are unable to maintain adequate arterial oxygenation, with or without the impairment of CO_2 elimination, the condition is known as acute respiratory failure.

There are four basic mechanisms that contribute to respiratory insufficiency and failure: hypoventilation, ventilation-perfusion inequality, diffusion impairment, and right-to-left shunt (Table 3–6).

Hypoventilation is the reduction of the alveolar minute ventilation. The ABG picture for alevolar hypoventilation is a decreased PO_2 level, a decrease in oxygenation saturation, and an increase in the PCO_2 level. Any condition that depresses the CNS, restricts the expansion of the lungs or alveoli, blocks the airflow to large numbers of alveoli, or hampers the

TABLE 3–6

Causes of Hypoxemia

Alveolar hypoventilation	Ventilation-perfusion defects	Diffusion defects	Right-to-left shunting
CNS depression: overdose of sedatives or narcotics; anesthesia. Neuromuscular diseases: myasthenia gravis, Guillain-Barré syndrome, poliomyelitis, multiple sclerosis, amyotrophic lateral sclerosis. Spinal cord injuries. Pulmonary diseases: Restrictive (those that impede thoracic or lung expansion): pulmonary fibrosis, pulmonary edema, pleural effusion, pneumothorax, TB, lung cancer. Obstructive (those that block normal ventilatory pathways): emphysema, chronic bronchitis, asthma, cystic fibrosis. Obesity. Deformity: kyphoscoliosis. Pain: surgery, trauma, fatigue. Upper airway obstruction	Atelectasis. Lung cancer. Obstructive pulmonary disease. Pulmonary emboli. Pulmonary artery ligation. Decreased CO.	Pulmonary edema. Pulmonary fibrosis. Pulmonary cysts. Sarcoidosis. Emphysematous bullae. Polycythemia.	O_2 toxicity. Atelectasis Pneumonia. Pulmonary emboli. Pulmonary edema. Shock.

Reprinted with permission from Emanuelsen, K. L., and M. J. Densmore. Acute Respiratory Care. John Wiley & Sons, Inc., New York. 1981. p 169.

movement of the diaphragm and chest wall can cause hypoventilation and consequently hypoxemia.

Ventilation-perfusion inequality is the single most common cause of hypoxemia. An A/a PO_2 difference between $PACO_2$ and $PaCO_2$ that is >10 mmHg indicates a defect in blood gas equilbration between the alveoli and the pulmonary capillaries. This may be caused by one or more of these physiologic disturbances: ventilation of alveoli that are perfused poorly or not at all or perfusion of alveoli that are ventilated inadequately or not at all. Regardless of whether there is too little ventilation matched with normal blood flow or too little blood flow matched with normal ventilation in a large number of alveoli, the result will be an overall reduction in the level of arterial oxygenation. Clinical abnormalities, such as pulmonary emboli or atelectasis, interfere with the balance of ventilation and perfusion in a specific region of the lung.

Diffusion defects are the result of an increase in the anatomic distance gas must travel from the alveolar space to the lumen of the pulmonary capillary. The most common causes of impaired diffusion are pulmonary fibrosis and pulmonary edema.

Right-to-left shunting can result from untreated alveolar hypoventilation, ventilation-perfusion defects, or diffusion defects. When large numbers of alveoli fail to function, a large amount of blood passes from the right to the left side of the heart without being ventilated. There are several clinical situations that may lead to shunting, such as atelectasis, consolidation, and interstitial edema.

Pathophysiology

Decreased intake of O_2 produces a state of hypoxemia, an insufficient amount of O_2 in the blood, leading to a state of hypoxia, an insufficient amount of O_2 at the tissue level. Hypoxia will stimulate the sympathetic nervous system to produce selective tissue vasoconstriction, increase peripheral resistance, and increase heart rate. If the hypoxia is caused by hypoventilation or circulatory deficiencies, hypercapnia will occur. Hypercapnia, a state of excess CO_2 in the body fluids and at the cellular level, causes a local depressant effect on the cellular and tissue function that results in cerebral depression, hypotension, and circulatory failure. The excess of CO_2 also stimulates the sympathetic nervous system to increase the heart rate and the cardiac output. The excess CO_2 in the blood combines with water to form carbonic acid, causing a state of acute respiratory acidosis.

Clinical picture

The diagnosis of respiratory failure is usually made from data compiled from three sources: (1) a history of a condition that may predispose the patient to respiratory failure; (2) clinical manifestations that are associated with respiratory failure; (3) ABG measurements that indicate respiratory failure. Occasionally, pulmonary function tests may be used to make the diagnosis of respiratory failure.

Early clinical manifestations of respiratory failure are subtle in nature. Table 3–7 illustrates the early-to-late progression of symptoms that are related to hypoxemia. It is important to remember that these signs and symptoms may occur simultaneously and may occur at a very rapid rate of progression.

Medical intervention

Acute respiratory failure is often a medical emergency. Therefore, priorities of treatment must be established. The first treatment priority is hypoxemia, because a PO_2 level of 20 mmHg or less causes death within a few minutes and a PO_2 level of 30 mmHg for more than several minutes may cause death or permanent brain damage. The second priority is the treatment of a life-threatening abnormal pH level. Abnormally low pH levels (indicating an acidotic state) can severely depress cellular and metabolic functioning and can precipitate fatal ventricular arrhythmias.

Nursing interventions

Nursing management of a patient with respiratory failure must be based on sound medical knowledge of the syndrome and the problems that can arise.

TABLE 3–7

Signs and Symptoms of Hypoxemia and Hypercapnia

	Hypoxemia	Hypercapnia
Early	Tachycardia Restlessness Increased BP Anxiety Headache Fatigue Cool, dry skin Arrhythmia	Hyperventilation Vasodilation that leads to a decreased BP Warm, diaphoretic skin
Middle	Air hunger Increased respiratory rate Vasodilation that leads to decreased BP Arrhythmia Confusion that leads to lethargy	Headache Hallucinations Drowsiness Asterixis
Late	Cyanosis Diaphoresis Coma that leads to death	Cyanosis Lethargy that leads to coma or death

Reprinted with permission from Emanuelsen, K. L., and M. J. Densmore. Acute Respiratory Care. John Wiley & Sons, Inc., New York. 1981. p 170.

Maintenance of a patent airway. (1) Instruct conscious patient to sit upright and lean forward. (2) Insert oral artificial airway and hyperextend neck in unconscious patient. (3) If endotracheal intubation is necessary, maintain airway patency by frequent suctioning.

Hypoxemia. (1) Assess level of hypoxemia through ABG interpretation. (2) Administer O_2 at level appropriate to maintain adequate arterial O_2 saturation.

Hypercapnia. (1) Assess level of hypercapnia through frequent ABG analysis. (2) Be prepared to assist with endotracheal intubation.

Infection. (1) Administer antibiotic therapy to treat respiratory and systematic infections. (2) Prevent infections from occurring; employ aggressive broncheal hygiene, position changes, and airway suctioning.

Support of ventilation. (1) *See* Chapter 13.

Electrolyte disturbances. (1) Monitor ABGs, serum and urine electrolytes and osmolarity.

Neurologic status. (1) Monitor blood chemistries frequently. (2) Check neurologic status, check level of consciousness, hand grasps, pupils.

Cardiac status. (1) Monitor vital signs frequently. (2) Maintain continuous cardiac monitoring. (3) Obtain ECG's as ordered.

ADULT RESPIRATORY DISTRESS SYNDROME

Adult respiratory distress syndrome (ARDS) is characterized by sudden and overwhelming respiratory failure and may occur in a wide range of previously healthy people who sustain a pulmonary insult. Regardless of the initial cause, the clinical and pathologic features follow uniform patterns, and these patterns define the syndrome.

Pathophysiology

The initial lung injury is to the alveolar capillary membrane. The first manifestation of this injury is an increase in pulmonary capillary permeability. Leaky capillaries permit exudation of fluid into the interstitial space, which causes a decrease in pulmonary compliance. As the leakage of fluid progresses into alveolar spaces, the resultant loss of surfactant causes patchy atelectasis, whereas other alveoli are edematous. Perfusion of these nonventilated areas continues and results in a profound right-to-left pulmonary shunt. This severe O_2 transport problem explains why the PaO_2 can be only partially corrected by high concentrations of inspired O_2.

Clinical picture

The types of lung insults that result in ARDS are multiple and varied and are classed as direct or indirect. Direct insults that result in damage to the alveolar capillary membrane include inhalation of toxic irritants, diffuse alveolar infection or inflammation, fat embolism, and direct chest trauma. Indirect causes that have been reported include traumatic or surgical shock, sepsis, disseminated intravascular coagulation (DIC), pulmonary edema, cerebral trauma, and acute hemorrhagic pancreatitis.

The clinical presentation of ARDS includes marked respiratory distress, diffuse pulmonary infiltration on chest x-ray, decreased pulmonary compliance, marked hypoxemia despite ventilatory assistance, and pulmonary congestion. A reduction in functional residual capacity (FRC) has been a consistant finding in patients with ARDS and has been considered by some to be one of the features that defines the syndrome. An early accumulation of fluid in the peribronchovascular interstitial space directly results in airway closing, distal atelectasis, and loss of lung volume. As accumulation of fluid proceeds and lung volume decreases because alveoli are flooded, there is a reduction of lung compliance. A decrease in the compliance of the lung is another defining feature of ARDS. This means that higher-than-normal ventilator pressures are required to deliver an adequate tidal volume. The loss of lung compliance stems from a decrease in tissue elasticity that is associated with lung congestion. Prolonged courses of ARDS have been associated with the development of pulmonary fibrosis, which causes further reductions in lung compliance. Just before death, it is common for the lung to be so stiff that ventilation is almost impossible.

Hypoxia is an outstanding feature of ARDS and is the result of a combination of factors. Because of alveolar collapse and flooding, a large number of gas-exchange units do not participate in the uptake of O_2 and elimination of CO_2. Capillary blood flow continues to these collapsed alveoli, and this blood returns unoxygenated to the left side of the heart. Thus, intrapulmonary shunting is one factor that contributes to hypoxia. Alveoli with reduced but finite ventilation will contribute to hypoxia because of differences in the matching of ventilation and perfusion; thus, a marked ventilation-perfusion imbalance is another contributing factor.

Medical intervention

Early intubation with controlled ventilation constitutes one of the most important aspects in the prevention and treatment of ARDS. Although mechanical ventilation is traditionally used only as a supportive measure to maintain life while other therapeutic measures are undertaken, considerable evidence exists suggesting that the maintenance of lung volumes improves small-airway function and prevents the development of congestive atelectasis.

The use of positive end-expiratory pressure (PEEP) is an accepted form of therapy in patients with ARDS. PEEP produces a constant, positive, distending pressure across the walls of airways and alveoli. This reestablishes their patency and increases FRC. The patency of newly opened airways and alveoli, maintained by PEEP, reduces the amount of shunting, thereby alleviating the potential for the development of O_2 toxicity. The maintenance of airways and alveoli in an open position cannot be achieved with conventional intermittent positive-pressure breathing (IPPB) because reclosure is permitted as intra-airway pressure returns to atmospheric levels at the end of each inspiration.

Although PEEP is extremely important in the management of patients with ARDS, there are potentially dangerous side effects of which the nurse should be aware. One of the potential complications is a reduction in cardiac output caused by impaired venous return to the heart, which results from pressure on the intrathoracic great veins and on pulmonary capillaries. The magnitude of the effect of PEEP on cardiac output is the result of a balance of several factors: the status of the circulatory and intravascular volumes, the level of end-expiratory pressure applied, the compliance of the lung, and the FRC at the time of the application of PEEP.

Other complications of PEEP are the development of spontaneous pneumothorax or pneumomediastinum, presumably resulting from overdistension and rupture of less diseased and/or more distensible alveoli.

Supplemental O_2 is invariably necessary in patients with ARDS. Because of the potential for O_2 toxicity, it is essential that the lowest possible inspired O_2 concentration be provided to deliver adequate oxygenation at tissue level. The adequacy of tissue oxygenation is difficult to measure precisely, but measurement of ABGs is probably the most assessable measure and, therefore, the most frequently used. The use of arterial lines for the facilitation of drawing ABGs is strongly recommended because of the frequency of drawing arterial blood during the acute stage of the syndrome.

Fluid management is one of the most essential considerations in ARDS. One of the major determinants of fluid fluctuation in the lung is the hydrostatic pressure in the pulmonary capillaries. Because the prevailing pressure assumes even greater-than-normal importance in the presence of increased permeability of the alveolar capillary membrane, increased elevation of capillary hydrostatic pressure caused by overvigorous administration of fluid increases the amount of water in the lung markedly. On the other hand, restoration of adequate pulmonary and systemic perfusion may also be important factors in the prevention of lung damage. For these reasons, it is crucial that volume replacement be carried out judiciously and monitored carefully. Information relating to fluid management obtained from measurements of central venous pressure (CVP) is often inadequate, for it does not provide a reliable indication of the pulmonary capillary hydrostatic pressure, especially in patients with either cardiac or pulmonary abnormalities. The discrepancies between CVP and pulmonary artery wedge pressures (PAWP) are attributable, in part, to the changes in pulmonary vascular resistance that may occur in patients with acute and chronic pulmonary diseases and to differences between right and left ventricular compliance. The positioning of a Swan-Ganz catheter in the pulmonary artery will provide much more valuable information by measurements of PAWPs. It also allows for a sampling of mixed venous blood, which indicates the status of peripheral oxygenation. Fluid should be administered in sufficient amounts to reinstitute and maintain perfusion of critical organs but carefully enough to ensure that PAWP is affected as little as possible.

The indications for corticosteroid treatment of ARDS are not absolute. A number of mechanisms have been suggested as reasons why corticosteroids should be useful in treating the syndrome. These include maintenance of capillary and cell membrane structure, stabilization of lysomal membranes, modification or prevention of platelet aggregation, and enhancement of surfactant production. In the absence of any substantial data regarding complications from short-term, high-dose corticosteroid usage, it is recommended that dosages as high as 30 mg/kg of body weight be used q 8 hr for 24 to 48 hr in patients critically ill with ARDS.

Nursing interventions

With the increased technological sophistication in acute cardiopulmonary care, many patients are maintained with a degree of respiratory failure and elevated airway pressure not previously encountered. The ICU nurse must, therefore, have a complete understanding of the pathophysiology of this syndrome and its treatment in order to provide the quality of care necessary to affect the patient's ultimate prognosis.

Alteration in gas exchange. (1) Ventilate mechanically. *See* Chapter 13. (2) Maintain PEEP. (3) Monitor ABGs (correcting hypoxemia and acidosis) frequently. (4) Monitor mixed venous PO_2. (5) Suction only as absolutely necessary in order to maintian PEEP. (When suctioning is needed, preoxygenate and use PEEP adapter or PEEP bag.) (6) Assess breath sounds routinely. (7) Sedate as ordered and prn to decrease work of breathing.

Alterations in fluid and electrolyte status. (1) Check intake and output hourly. (2) Measure weights daily. (3) Monitor electrolytes. (4) Administer colloids as ordered. (5) Monitor PAWP for worsening of pulmonary edema. (6) Maintain careful hydration.

Underlying disease process. (1) Identify and treat underlying disease process (i.e., shock, trauma, sepsis, aspiration, pulmonary contusion, emboli, etc.).

Immobility. (1) Use air mattress. (2) Turn frequently and provide back care. (3) Institute passive range of motion exercises (only if tolerated and if they do not increase work of breathing or compromise oxygenation—activity of any kind may need to be severely restricted).

Nutritional deficiency. (1) Maintain adequate nutritional support with enteral or parenteral feedings. (2) Check and monitor bowel sounds. (3) Measure weights daily. (4) Monitor nutritional serum and urine laboratory values (i.e., albumen and liver function tests).

Psychological trauma. (1) Provide emotional support to patient and family. (2) Provide hope but prepare family for possible complications and death (ARDS carries an extremely high mortality rate). (3) Establish a means of communication with patient. (4) Sedate as ordered and prn. (5)

Allow time for patient and family to visit. (6) Keep call bell within reach. (7) Explain all procedures to patient and family.

PULMONARY EMBOLISM

Pulmonary embolism (PE) is a major cause of sudden and unexpected death and is responsible for >50,000 deaths in the USA every year. Available data indicate that >95% of all pulmonary emboli arise from thrombi in the deep venous system of the lower extremities. Thrombi occurring in the right cardiac chamber or in other veins account for the remainder. Thus, PE should be viewed as a complication of deep venous thrombosis (DVT), which leads to three important observations: (1) prevention of DVT is the most effective approach to prevention of PE; (2) prompt treatment of DVT may limit frequency of PE; and (3) techniques that allow the diagnosis of DVT in the leg veins will allow identification of a large percentage of patients at high risk of PE.

Pathophysiology

Emboli are usually thrombi that originate in the leg and dislodge, traveling through the venous system into the right side of the heart and into the pulmonary artery, where they lodge in one or both of the branches. Acute obstruction of the pulmonary artery circulation leads to right heart failure, with a resultant decrease in cardiac output. Persons suffering from massive PE often experience associated hemodynamic compromise.

Contributing factors or causes may include venous stasis, hypercoagulability, and venous injury. Venous stasis is a significant complication of prolonged confinement to bed and/or relative immobility. Dilation of the leg veins and pooling of blood creates a situation of decreased venous return and possible clot formation. Hypercoagulable states may be in part the result of or related to the use of oral contraceptives. Other causes include certain blood dyscrasias such as polycythemia vera or sickle cell anemia. Malignancies may also alter the coagulation process.

Massive PE can occlude >50% of the pulmonary circulation. The obstruction of blood flow creates a region of alveolar dead space, and hypoxia results from a decreased ventilation/perfusion ratio.

Clinical picture

The clinical presentation of a patient suffering from PE often varies, depending on size and location of the embolism, and often mimics the signs and symptoms of other disease processes. Symptoms are often vague and nonspecific. They include tachypnea and tachycardia; pleuritic chest pain or chest discomfort might be experienced along with hemoptysis, anxiety, restlessness, dyspnea, and cough. In cases of massive PE, sudden and profound shock can occur; acute respiratory distress, anxiety, tachypnea, and a feeling of impending doom are also likely.

Medical intervention

The diagnosis of PE is often difficult to make because the signs and symptoms vary depending on size and location of the embolism and often mimic other disease processes. Many of the studies used at present do not allow a definitive diagnosis to be made but rather assist in ruling out other possibilities. Definitive diagnosis requires invasive studies that carry with them significant risks; for this reason, noninvasive studies are performed first.

The following tests may aid in the differential diagnosis but are not specific for PE: (1) ECG (alteration of the ST segment and T-wave inversion may be seen); (2) chest x-ray (occasional elevation of the diaphragm); (3) CBC (may indicate an increased sedimentation rate and WBCs may be slightly elevated); (4) ABGs (PaO_2 <80 mmHg with a PCO_2<35 mmHg may be significant); (5) Doppler studies. If these tests do not demonstrate a reason for symptomatology, then studies more specific for PE should be performed.

The V/Q scan is a useful tool in eliminating the possibility of PE; therefore it should be performed prior to angiography. Perfusion scanning is performed first. A radioisotope is injected IV and eight images, or views, are obtained. A positive defect is presumed when there is a persistent absence of flow on several views. A negative study essentially eliminates the possibility of PE, but an abnormal or positive scan is of less value because of its lack of specificity.

Following a positive perfusion study, a ventilation scan is performed to provide additional information. The ventilation scan is done by having the patient inhale radioactive xenon and recording the distribution of radioactivity in the airways. A combination of well-ventilated areas that coresond with poorly perfused lung in a segmental or lobar distribution is indicative of PE, but not specific for it.

Pulmonary angiography is the definitive clinical test for PE. Possible complications of this invasive procedure include arrythmias with the passage of the catheter through the right ventricle as well as adverse reactions to the dye. A positive angiogram is essentially conclusive for PE.

Medical management relies on anticoagulation therapy and bed rest. Table 3–8 provides a summary of anticoagulants currently in use.

Surgical intervention, consisting of ligation or clipping of the inferior vena cava, may be necessary if there are recurrent thromboemboli despite adequate anticoagulation, if anticoagulation is contraindicated, or if there are septic pulmonary emboli from the lower extremities. Partial caval interruption can be achieved by using an external clip, suturing or by means of an intraluminal filter, which entraps pulmonary emboli and prevents swelling of the lower extremities. Pulmonary embolectomy may be indicated if there is marked hemodynamic compromise and medical management is not possible. This procedure carries high risk and therefore is considered only as a last resort.

TABLE 3–8

Anticoagulants Used in Treatment of Pulmonary Embolism

Drug	Usage	Dosage and administration	Nursing implications	Side effects and contraindications
Heparin	Prevent further clot formation	5,000–10,000 U IV bolus, followed by a continuous infusion at 1,000 U/hr. PTT should be maintained in a therapeutic range of 75–90%. If PTT is less than therapeutic, increase heparin by 250 U/hr and recheck PTT in 6 hr. Continue to increase by 250 U/hr until PTT is in therapeutic range. Heparin should be continued for 7–14 days before switching to oral agents.	Obtain base-line coagulation studies prior to initiating therapy and then monitor PTT after any change in dosage; monitor daily coagulation studies as well. Assess systems fully prior to initiating therapy to establish a base line and reassess each shift for any symptom of bleeding. Hold all venipunctures or arterial sticks with firm pressure to prevent bleeding. Have patient use electric razor for shaving.	Contraindications: active bleeding; recent surgery; stroke.
Streptokinase	Massive pulmonary embolism, with hemodynamic compromise and/or pulmonary vascular obstruction of ≥ 50%. Causes active clot lysis, accelerating time of fresh thrombi removal.	Initial dose of 250,000 U IV over 20–30 min followed by a continuous infusion of 100,000 U/hr. Check TT 3–4 hr after initiating therapy to document that the lysis process is taking place. This is demonstrated by an increase in TT. There is no need for further monitoring or change in dosage unless there is no change in TT. Continue infusion for 24–72 hr. (There is no documentation of effectiveness after 24 hr.)	Assess systems fully prior to initiating therapy and reassess each shift for any symptoms of bleeding. If possible, have a line for blood-sample access inserted before starting therapy to prevent or decrease venipunctures after initiating therapy. Have patient use electric razor for shaving. No IM injections. Decrease or eliminate venipunctures.	Contraindications: hypertension (systolic BP 200); active bleeding; recent surgery (≤7 days); stroke (≤2 mo); recent needle puncture of noncompressible veins. Side effects: fever, leukocytosis, allergic reactions, anaphylaxis, bleeding.

		Heparin therapy should be initiated once streptokinase therapy has been completed.	Obtain base-line studies prior to initiation of therapy and check TT after therapy has started.	
Urokinase	Massive pulmonary embolism with hemodynamic compromise. (Used when streptokinase therapy is ineffective: patient is not sensitive to streptokinase or has an allergic reaction. Cost of urokinase is substantial.)	Initial dose of 4,400 U/kg followed by 4,400 U/kg/hr. Effectiveness of treatment and clot lysis is documented by an increase in TT 3–4 hr after initiating therapy. Heparin therapy should be initiated once urokinase therapy has been completed.	Same as streptokinase.	Contraindications: same as for streptokinase. Side effects: less likely to occur with urokinase.
Warfarin (Coumadin)	Prevent formation of thromboembolism.	Initial dose of 10 mg, then 5–10 mg/day to maintain PT 2–2½ times normal. Continue therapy for 3–6 mo.	Observe for signs and symptoms of bleeding. Monitor PT. Initiate discharge planning and patient education.	Side effects: bleeding.

PT, prothrombin time; PTT, partial thromboplastin time; TT, thrombin time.

Nursing interventions

The nurse caring for the hospitalized elderly and/or chronically ill patient plays a very significant and important role in decreasing instances of PE through prevention. A few measures that can be life saving include: (1) identification of those patients considered to be at high risk; (2) encouragement of early ambulation whenever possible; (3) encouragement of pulmonary exercises; (4) use of antiembolism stockings or inflatable boots; (5) encouragement of leg exercises or assistance with passive range of motion exercises regularly; (6) prevention of sudden movement or trauma if venous thrombosis has already occurred; (7) maintenance of appropriate hydration; (8) recognition of signs and symptoms of PE.

Specific problems in the care of the patient with PE are listed below.

Alteration in gas exchange. (1) Supplement O_2 as ordered. (2) Maintain semi-Fowler's position. (3) Institute mechanical ventilation when necessary. (4) Monitor ABGs. (5) Assess and monitor breath sounds q 2 to 4 hr.

Hemodynamic compromise. (1) Maintain hydration as ordered. (2) Administer vasopressors as required. (3) Administer afterload reduction as ordered. (4) Administer digoxin for increased heart rate and right-sided failure as ordered. (5) Observe for signs of decreased CO including decreased BP, CVP, and urine output, changes in level of consciousness, restlessness, diminished peripheral pulses, and slow capillary refill.

Alterations in comfort (chest pain). (1) Administer narcotics as ordered and as needed to reduce splinting.

Anxiety. (1) Explain all procedures to patient. (2) Sedate patient as ordered. (3) Provide emotional support to patient and family. (4) Provide calm, quiet environment.

Immobility. (1) Assist with passive range of motion exercises q 4 to 6 hr. (2) Provide special back care and reposition q 2 to 4 hr.

CHRONIC OBSTRUCTIVE PULMONARY DISEASE

COPD is a functional category of respiratory disorders characterized by obstruction of airflow within the lungs. In addition to asthma, the principal diseases include chronic obstructive bronchitis and emphysema. Synonyms include chronic obstructive lung disease (COLD), chronic airway obstruction (CAO), chronic obstructive pulmonary emphysema (COPE), and chronic bronchitis.

Chronic bronchitis

Chronic bronchitis is a clinical disorder characterized by excessive mucus secretions in the bronchial tree, demonstrated by a chronic, recurring, productive cough. The symptoms are a result of chronic bronchial irritation often caused by environmental factors such as smoking, air pollutants, and infection.

There is no real answer to the question of why some individuals develop chronic bronchitis. Genetic susceptibility seems to have a role in determining the degree to which any individual's respiratory system reacts to toxic substances. The **major cause** of chronic bronchitis is cigarette smoking.

One of the earliest changes in chronic bronchitis appears in the secretory glands of the large airways. Both goblet cells and cells in the mucosal glands increase in size and number, and the normal gland:wall-thickness ratio increases. Epithelial squamous metaplasia also occurs, and goblet cells appear distally in terminal bronchioles, where they are not normally found. Because the chronic inflammation causes an increase in bronchial wall thickness, small airways are particularly likely to become obstructed when their luminal diameter reaches a critical point. The net result is an increased quantity of sputum with decreased clearance. As the disease progresses, the normally sterile lower respiratory tract becomes colonized by bacteria and an increased number of polymorphonuclear leukocytes are found in the secretions. They participate in the stimulation of further bronchial and bronchiolar inflammation and eventual destruction.

Patients with simple chronic bronchitis are afflicted with daily cough and sputum production on most days for ≥3 mo/yr. The diagnosis of chronic bronchitis is made clinically, with confirmation obtained by pulmonary function testing. In the very early stages, an individual may be free of **symptoms** except for cough following respiratory tract infections. The cough may persist for increasing lengths of time, and the infections may be associated with intermittent wheezing. In the more severe form of the disease known as chronic obstructive bronchitis, there is a chronic reduction in forced expiratory volume (FEV), with at least partial reversibility following bronchodialator administration.

In the most severe form, constant wheezing, sputum production, dyspnea, and episodes of respiratory failure occur. The severe bronchitic has often been described by the term "blue bloater" because he is frequently obese, cyanotic, plethoric, and somnolent. Bronchitics have a depressed CO_2 ventilatory response, and hypoxia assumes the role of stimulation for ventilation.

Because respiration is normally stimulated far more efficiently by hypercapnia than by hypoxia, the reduction of sensitivity to CO_2 leads to chronic hypoventilation and hypoxia. As a result of this chronic hypoxia, polycythemia may develop, causing further cyanosis.

Emphysema

Emphysema is a pathologic entity whose diagnosis is made by a combination of clinical signs and symptoms, chest radiographic findings, and pulmonary function deficits.

Emphysema is characterized by an increase in size of the air spaces distal to the terminal bronchioles, with destructive changes in the alveolar wall. The **primary defect underlying emphysema** is the derangement of lung elastin by neutral proteases, which directly results in diminished elastic recoil of the lung and limited expiratory airflow. The end result is the reduction of gas exchange at the respiratory bronchiolar, alveolar ductal, and alveolar septal levels. Two consequences result: (1) air is trapped in increased volume because of the loss of elastic recoil and (2) total gas exchanging surface is diminished.

In the early stages of emphysema mild dyspnea on exertion may be the only symptom. In a more advanced state of the disease, the patient may be described as a "pink puffer." He is frequently underweight and barrel-chested. His supraclavicular fossae are hollowed and his accessory muscles of respiration are hypertrophied. No matter how dyspneic he may be, he remains pink until the terminal stages of his illness. Cough is not a predominant feature, and if it is present is generally nonproductive. The chest is hyperresonant on percussion and upon auscultation breath sounds may be barely audible.

As work of breathing continues to increase and hypoxemia develops, the patient becomes progressively more dyspneic with exertion and eventually is short of breath at rest. Cor pulmonale and polycythemia develop as a result of prolonged hypoxemia and pulmonary artery hypertension, with the greatest reduction of O_2 content occurring during sleep. Most patients with severe emphysema die of respiratory failure and/or cardiac arrythmia secondary to severe hypoxemic episodes.

Medical intervention

Acute respiratory failure in patients suffering from advanced COPD is a relatively common complication. It may also occur in less advanced stages of the disease when a major precipitating event such as viral pneumonia or bronchitis occurs. Muscle weakness and/or fatigue and hemodynamic compromise can also be significant contributing factors. Precipitating factors are the major cause of acute respiratory failure, and treatment must be geared to controlling and/or resolving the cause of the acute insult to effectively manage these patients.

The patient with COPD often lives with some degree of respiratory failure and has preexisting low arterial oxygenation and elevated $PaCO_2$; in these patients, acute respiratory failure is distinguished by worsening of the preexisting hypoxemia and hypercapnia. The impairment of gas exchange can be life-threatening; therefore the goal of therapy is to assure that hypoxemia, hypercapnia, and acidosis do not reach hazardous levels. It is generally accepted that in COPD patients PaO_2 <40 mmHg is life-threatening. Sustained hypoxemia causes impaired cardiac and cerebral function as well as cardiac arrythmias. Acidosis with an arterial pH of <7.2 is considered potentially dangerous and needs prompt attention. Hypercapnia, especially when the $PaCO_2$ exceeds 70 mmHg, is manifested by mental status changes, including confusion and coma.

Supplemental O_2 is one of the most basic and most crucial parts of treatment in the patient with COPD. Hypoxemia, the main source of ventilatory stimulation in the patient with chronic airway obstruction, requires low-flow O_2 delivered by nasal canula or Venturi mask. High concentrations of O_2 may correct hypoxemia but may in turn decrease the ventilatory drive and increase the $PaCO_2$ to dangerous levels, leading to confusion or unconsciousness. O_2 must be administered cautiously, with inspired O_2 concentrations of 24 to 28% by Venturi mask or 1 to 3 liters/min by nasal cannula. (*See* Chapter 13.) Frequent ABG measurements are necessary to guide the nurse, physician, and respiratory therapist in regulating and maintaining adequate O_2 levels and keeping CO_2 retention at a minimum.

A fundamental problem in COPD is the compromise of conducting airways, which results in acute respiratory insufficiency and failure. Very little can be done to resolve the limitation resulting from the impairment in elastic recoil of the lungs; the goal must be to correct the problem of small- and large-airway secretions, decreasing bronchospasm and edema. This may improve overall ventilation. Techniques used to improve airflow include moisture, physical therapy, mucolytics, bronchodilators, and steroids.

Moisture assists in the mobilization of secretions by thinning them so that they can be coughed up with greater ease. Several relatively easy techniques may be employed in delivering moisture, including aerosolized water or saline and nebulizers and humidifiers. An ultrasonic nebulizer may also be used; it delivers high-density water, but these nebulizers are often poorly tolerated and may actually increase airway resistance in some patients.

Physical therapy techniques such as posturing, vibrating, and shaking have demonstrated some effectiveness, especially when used in conjunction with moisture. Vibrating, pummeling, and shaking applied to the chest often create coughing that is productive, especially when used for conditions such as lobar pneumonia.

Mucolytic therapy is used to aid in decreasing the viscosity of pulmonary secretions. Acetylcysteine (Mucomyst) is the only true mucolytic available. Acetylcysteine is often too irritating alone because it can cause bronchospasm; this is usually avoided with concomitant use of bronchodilators.

IPPB is often used to assist the patient in clearing secretions. The effectiveness of IPPB is currently a subject of controversy. The cough, often expulsive, following IPPB is effective in the clearance of secretions. IPPB is often utilized as a method for delivering bronchodilators.

Bronchodilators improve airflow by decreasing bronchospasm in the patient with COPD. The most commonly used bronchodilators include aminophylline and terbutaline. Theophylline levels should be followed closely to ensure that toxicity does not occur, especially in the patients with liver dysfunction or in the elderly. Symptoms of toxicity include GI upset, cardiac arrythmias, and convulsions. Inhaled beta-adrenergic agonists that rapidly improve airflow include isoetharine (Bronkosol), metaproterenol

(Alupent), and terbutaline (Brethine); these can be delivered by IPPB or aerosol.

The use of **corticosteroids** in acute respiratory failure from COPD may improve airflow. The dosage is usually 0.5 mg/kg of body weight of sodium methylprednisolone succinate q 6 hr. More severely ill patients often receive much higher doses.

Management and treatment of the precipitating events or condition that led to the acute respiratory failure must also occur. Acute purulent bronchitis is a common precipitating factor in the patient suffering from COPD. Organisms commonly involved include *Haemophilus influenzae* and *Streptococcus pneumoniae.* The treatment revolves around prompt antibiotic therapy. Antibiotics are continued for 5 to 7 days or until purulent sputum has lessened and leukocytosis and fever are reduced. Bacterial pneumonias are also fairly common in patients with COPD, and again the most likely organisms are *Haemophilus influenzae* and *Streptococcus pneumoniae.*

Acute respiratory failure that cannot be managed by traditional noninvasive means may require intubation and mechanical ventilation, especially when the patient begins to experience fatigue, muscle weakness, and/or cardiac embarrassment. The objective of mechanical ventilation is to allow the patient a period of rest and to treat the condition that precipitated the acute event. After a sufficient period of rest and appropriate medical therapy, attempts at weaning from mechanical ventilation should begin (*see* Chapter 13).

Nursing interventions

Inadequate gas exchange. (1) Monitor ABGs closely, observing for a decreasing PaO_2 and pH, and an increase in $PaCO_2$. (2) Manipulate low-flow supplemental O_2 on physician's order to prevent further worsening of hypoxemia, hypercapnia, and acidosis. (3) Maintain mechanical ventilation as required (*see* Chapter 13). (4) Assess neurologic signs especially with impending respiratory failure.

Airway malfunction. (1) Monitor quality, quantity, and color of secretions; notify physician and document any change. (2) Assess secretions for need of mucolytic therapy or additional moisture. (3) Auscultate breath sounds frequently. (4) Suction patient prn; instill saline down endotracheal tube and bag patient with ambu or anesthesia bag; if tenacious secretions are a problem, this will help to liquify them and removal by suctioning will be easier. (5) Monitor for signs and symptoms of toxicity of bronchodilators, especially theophylline. (6) Apply physical therapy techniques to the chest for specific problems, e.g., lobar pneumonia.

Alterations in fluid and electrolyte balance. (1) Maintain careful hydration prn. (2) Monitor intake and output. (3) Measure weights daily. (4) Examine skin turgor and check for edema. (5) Monitor electrolytes and ABGs.

Immobility and loss of respiratory muscle tone. (1) Turn and reposition frequently. (2) Provide special back care q 2 hr. (3) Assist with passive or active range of motion at least q 4 hr while awake. (4) Begin to get patient out of bed as soon as possible. (5) Encourage patient to cough up secretions if possible.

Nutritional deficiency. (1) Maintain adequate nutrition with enteral or parenteral feedings. (2) Check bowel sounds regularly. (3) Monitor weight and intake and output. (4) Initiate bowel regimen as appropriate.

Psychological trauma. (1) Sedate as ordered and prn, being careful because of tenuous respiratory status. (2) Explain all procedures to patient. (3) Allow time for patient and family to visit and participate in care. (4) Provide undisturbed rest periods. (5) Provide stimulation during waking times. (6) Provide method of communication if necessary. (7) Keep call bell within reach. (8) Assist patient in maintaining independence; allow patient to make some decisions.

ASTHMA

Asthma is a common disorder that affects all age groups. The American Thoracic Society defines asthma as "a disease characterized by increased airway responsiveness to various stimuli and manifested by widespread narrowing of the airways that changes in severity either spontaneously or as a result of therapy." The symptoms may be so mild that the patient is troubled only by a slight cough or so severe that respiratory failure may ensue. The primary characteristics of asthma are prolonged expiration, wheezing, cough, and thick, sticky sputum. Symptoms may be intermittent, with normal pulmonary function between attacks, or they may be chronic and cause severe debilitation from compromised pulmonary function.

All patients with asthma are at risk of developing status asthmaticus. Usually, however, status asthmaticus develops in a patient in whom asthma is poorly controlled and/or is preceded by days or weeks of worsening symptoms.

Pathophysiology

The site of obstruction is in both large and small airways. Although the primary source of increased airway resistance is from disease in large airways, small-airway obstruction occurs and may persist even in the stable phase of the disease. Pathologic examination of the lungs in status asthmaticus suggests three principal mechanisms that increase airway resistance: bronchospasm, mucosal edema, and accumulation of secretions. The airway walls are thickened from an increase in bronchial smooth muscle, enlarged bronchial mucous glands, an increased number of goblet cells, as well as mucosal and submucosal edema.

In status asthmaticus, abnormalities in pulmonary mechanics result in abnormal distribution of ventilation and low ventilation/perfusion ratios in many respiratory units. The result is abnormal gas exchange, causing hypoxemia. Impaired O_2 transfer across the lung is manifested by a widened alveolar-arterial difference in PO_2, while the PCO_2 is usually below normal, indicating alveolar hyperventilation. As the attack worsens and overall ventilation decreases, total gas exchange is impaired and hypoxia and hypercapnia result.

The mechanism for the initiation of bronchospasm is unclear. A common precipitant of asthma in children and young adults is exercise. After episodes of vigorous, steady exercise stop, bronchospasm occurs. Mechanisms for exercise-induced asthma are not clear. Emotional upsets, too, can precipitate bronchoconstriction. An emotional upset can lead to hyperventilation, which in turn causes hypocapnia, which then results in bronchoconstriction. Many of the most serious asthma attacks that lead to hospitalization are precipitated by infection, either bacterial or viral. Asthma induced by viral infections may be due to an allergic response to the virus, a decreased threshhold for stimulation of the irritant receptors of the airways by the respiratory mucosal infection, or an alteration of ANS responses of the airways.

Many patients develop bronchoconstriction when exposed to cold air, dust, air pollution, or cigarette smoke. The same irritants may cause bronchoconstriction in normal persons, but in asthmatics the reaction occurs with a much shorter exposure.

Clinical picture

Status asthmaticus is the term applied to asthmatic episodes that fail to respond to bronchodilators and hydration and are of life-threatening severity. An asthmatic's response to bronchodilators is an important basis for differentiating between a bout of severe asthma and status asthmaticus.

Clinically, patients with status asthmaticus cannot be immediately distinguished from those with severe but easily reversible asthma. Typically, the patients are too short of breath to speak in full sentences and are extremely restless and anxious. Accessory muscles of respiration are in use, and the chest shows little movement with expiration but appears to be in a fixed, distended position. Wheezing is usually audible without the use of the stethoscope. A decrease in systolic BP on inspiration (pulsus paradoxus) is often present and is caused by the combined effects of an increase in airway resistance and an increase in the FRC. Clinical evidence, such as altered ABG levels, cyanosis, and mental confusion, is usually not seen until the patient is critically ill. The continued effects of low airflow and failing respiratory effort because of patient exhaustion may result in absence of wheezing and disappearance of breath sounds. This situation is life-threatening and necessitates immediate assisted ventilatory support.

Medical intervention

The medical management of status asthmaticus should be aimed at three major problems: (1) abnormal gas exchange, (2) airway secretions, and (3) bronchospasm.

Abnormal gas exchange. Because arterial hypoxemia is a regular feature of status asthmaticus, O_2 should be administered routinely, aiming toward reaching a PaO_2 of 60 to 80 torr. It can be administered through a Venturi-type mask or by a double-prong nasal cannula. For any patient who has had a change in mental status or who appears exhausted or whose arterial blood reflects a rising PCO_2, prompt endotracheal intubation and mechanical ventilation is required. It must be kept in mind, however, that invasion of the airway with an endotracheal tube may invoke further bronchospasm and should only be considered after all other measures have failed.

To reach adequate tidal volumes, high driving pressures from the ventilator are needed, achieved through the use of a volume-cycled ventilator with high pressure limits. The need for high pressure limits increases the risk of pneumothorax or pneumomediastinum so that careful observation and assessment must continue while the patient is maintained on assisted ventilatory support.

Airway secretions. IV administration of fluids is used early in the treatment of status asthmaticus to improve the effectiveness of the cough reflex by thinning secretions. A very careful check should be kept on fluid balance and body weight because of the threat of overhydration, especially in elderly patients or those with compromised cardiac function. Removal of bronchial secretions can also be facilitated by postural drainage and good chest physiotherapy, whose frequency and duration should be gauged according to the patient's tolerance. The therapeutic value of aerosol therapy varies from patient to patient, but it can sometimes be helpful in loosening secretions. Use of aerosols should be preceded or accompanied by the administration of a bronchodilator by nebulizer.

Bronchospasm. Although by definition status asthmaticus does not respond to treatment with bronchodilators, these remain an important part of the treatment regimen. They are administered in anticipation of the return of bronchosensitivity and in an attempt to achieve maximal bronchodilation.

The initial pharmocologic agent of choice is SC epinephrine 1:1,000; 0.3 ml is the standard dose. An equivalent dose of terbutaline would be equally effective and should be repeated in 30 to 60 min if no response has occurred.

IV aminophylline is generally the second drug to be given. If the patient has not been receiving therapy po, a standard loading dose of 5 to 6 mg/kg is generally infused within the first 15 to 30 min. This dose is adjusted downward if patients have been receiving therapy po and if they have liver or cardiac disease. Frequent monitoring of serum theophylline levels is necessary to ensure therapeutic and nontoxic dosages.

Although the exact mode of action remains unclear, emerging evidence supports IV administration of corticosteroids in large doses. A typical initial dose is 1,000 mg of methylprednisolone or the comparable dose of an equivalent steroid, followed by 4 mg/kg q 4 hr for the first few days.

Aerosolized bronchodilators have been widely used for the treatment of status asthmaticus, but their effectiveness is somewhat questionable, probably because of ineffective distribution of the drug, resulting from severe airway obstruction and air-trapping.

Nursing interventions

The nursing care of the patient in status asthmaticus is of critical importance. A nurse who works quickly, efficiently, and confidently will be necessary to effectively deal with this critically ill patient. The following nursing care plan is designed to outline the nursing intervention.

Respiratory distress (due to bronchospasm). (1) Loosen constrictive clothing around patient's chest. (2) Sit patient in semi-Fowler's position. (3) Check breath sounds frequently (note if diminished). (4) Administer appropriate bronchodilator drugs as ordered. (5) Administer O_2 as ordered. (6) Monitor ABGs.

Exhaustion. (1) Discourage talking. (2) Keep room quiet. (3) Limit visitors. (4) Check level of consciousness q 1 to 2 hr and report changes.

Dehydration. (1) Administer IV fluids as ordered. (2) Record accurate intake and output. (3) Offer small amounts of ice chips as ordered.

Apprehension. (1) Stay with patient as much as possible. (2) Give verbal reassurance and encouragement. (3) Appear calm.

Adverse reaction to medication. (1) Monitor vital signs and report increases in pulse or BP or repeated emesis. (2) Monitor theophylline level as ordered. (3) Reassure patient that muscle tremors, shakiness, and "hyper" feeling are expected side effects of bronchodilators.

Environmental irritants. (1) Keep environment free from flowers, smoke, dust.

Respiratory failure. (1) *See* nursing interventions for acute respiratory failure *above*.

PNEUMOTHORAX AND HEMOTHORAX

Collection of air, gas, or blood in the pleural space causes the lung to collapse either partially or totally; the degree of collapse and the patient's previous clinical state will determine the significance of the event.

Pathophysiology

Spontaneous pneumothorax often occurs in the absence of trauma and is usually caused by subpleural blebs or bullae through the visceral pleura. There are two categories of individuals most commonly affected by spontaneous pneumothorax, the young and otherwise healthy person and the older person with underlying COPD. In the younger individual the cause is usually a ruptured congenital bleb, whereas in the older individual the blebs or bullae are usually caused by changes in the lung seen with COPD. Other possible causes of spontaneous pneumothorax include mechanical ventilation, fungal diseases, tracheostomy, subclavian venipunctures, cancer, and TB.

Clinical signs and symptoms are often minimal unless the collapse is >40%. If significant underlying pulmonary disease is present, signs and symptoms may occur with <40% collapse. If the pneumothorax is large and there is marked increase in intrapleural pressure, there will be a shift of mediastinal structures, an associated decrease in chest wall motion, and tracheal deviation.

Hemopneumothorax results from air leaking through the visceral pleura, usually because of chest trauma and usually associated with blood loss into the pleural space, thus differing from spontaneous pneumothorax.

Tension pneumothorax may result from any chest injury in which air is allowed to enter the pleural space during inspiration but is unable to escape on expiration. The amount of air in the pleural space progressively increases, and the injured lung collapses. Eventually the increase in pressure pushes against the mediastinum, toward the opposite lung. Any pneumothorax, regardless of size, may potentially become a tension pneumothorax if and/or when volume or positive ventilation is instituted.

Hemothorax may present with or without pneumothorax and is frequently the result of chest trauma. Hemorrhagic shock may occur because of the massive blood loss into the pleural space, and the shock state may be compounded by mediastinal shift, with resultant decrease in venous return.

Clinical picture

The clinical presentation associated with pneumothorax depends on the patient's previous clinical state of health and the degree of lung collapse involved. The signs and symptoms include chest pain, diminished breath sounds over the affected area, and dyspnea; shock may occur if the affected area is significant or the patient's previous clinical state was borderline.

If a tension pneumothorax exists, there will be a mediastinal shift toward the unaffected side, increased respiratory distress, and cyanosis. Distant or absent breath sounds and a widening of the intercostal spaces will occur on the affected side. There will be a tracheal deviation and shift toward the unaffected side.

A patient suffering from a hemothorax may demonstrate signs and symptoms of respiratory embarrassment as well as a dullness to percussion and absent or distant breath sounds on the affected side. If blood loss is significant, shock may occur.

Medical intervention

Management of spontaneous pneumothorax will depend on the size and cause. If the penumothorax is small (10 to 15%) and there are few or minimal symptoms, and there are no signs of increase in size over the next few hours of observation, no treatment is necessary. A larger pneumothorax with significant shortness of breath may be treated by closed thoracotomy and chest tube insertion. If a tension pneumothorax is present, a needle may be inserted to let trapped air escape, especially if the situation appears life-threatening. This procedure is usually followed by closed thoracotomy and chest tube insertion. If there is a continuous air leak after several days or the lung cannot be reexpanded, an open thoracotomy with resection and closure may be required.

Treatment of hemopneumothorax usually requires a large, posteriorly placed chest tube for evacuation of blood and air. If persistent and/or large air leaks occur, suspicion of injury of the more proximal tracheobronchial tree should be investigated by bronchoscopy and, if necessary, surgical repair performed.

In cases of hemothorax, hemorrhagic shock may occur; excessive blood loss must be estimated and replaced. Treatment requires a thoracotomy with chest tube drainage. Continued blood loss may require surgical repair.

Nursing interventions

Pneumothorax. (1) Assess breath sounds q 2 to 4 hr; notify physician of change in quality. (2) Maintain chest tube function; check for air leak in water seal chamber of chest drainage system q 2 to 4 hr; monitor for signs of crepitus or extension of existing crepitus; check and record amount of any drainage q 8 hr. (3) Change dressing as ordered. (4) Explain procedure to patient and offer reassurance.

Hemothorax. (1) Monitor amount of blood loss. (2) Milk chest tubes q 1 to 2 hr. Notify physician of excessive blood loss. (3) Monitor vital signs frequently if excessive blood loss noted. (4) Assess breath sounds q 2 to 4 hr. (5) Measure chest tube drainage. (6) Replace blood as ordered.

Inadequate ventilation. (1) Place the patient in semi-Fowler's position. (2) Administer supplemental O_2 as ordered. (3) Encourage the patient to cough and deep breathe.

Immobility. (1) Assist with passive or active range-of-motion exercises q 4 to 6 hr. (2) Turn and reposition frequently. (3) Provide special back care q 2 to 4 hr. (4) Ambulate as soon as possible.

Pain. (1) Medicate as ordered and prn. (2) Assess the effectiveness of pain control management.

PLEURAL EFFUSION

Pathophysiology

The pleural space normally contains a small amount of fluid that serves to lubricate the surfaces of the parietal and visceral pleura and allows them freedom to slide past each other in normal respiration. Collections of fluid in the pleural space are abnormal. They may be the result of an inflammatory process or malignant disease, but fluid occurs most frequently as a result of cardiac, hepatic, or renal disease. Treatment should be aimed at the underlying disease process, and aspiration of pleural fluid should be used therapeutically for the relief of dyspnea.

Clinical picture

Pleural effusions are usually indicative and/or associated with significant underlying disorders. Symptoms of pleural effusion often include pleural pain and shortness of breath, and sometimes an irritating dry cough may be present. Pleural inflammation begins early in the process and may be indicated by a pleural friction rub heard over the involved area. As fluid in the pleural space increases, the rub disappears and the pain lessens. Dullness to percussion and decreased breath sounds on auscultation are noted. Pleural effusions often result from underlying disorders, which need to be investigated if unknown.

Medical intervention

Chest x-rays may be helpful for diagnosing the effusion, although it may not be apparent even in the case of significant accumulation. Aspiration and examination of the pleural fluid of those patients for whom the diagnosis is not completely clear is essential, and specimens should be sent for cytology, chemical, and bacterial analysis. Treatment for pleural effusions is dependent on the underlying disease state. Closed thoracotomy tube drainage may be necessary to evacuate the accumulation of fluid. If drug therapy (antibiotic or chemotherapy) is necessary, it may be administered directly into the pleural space.

Nursing interventions

Thoracentesis or chest tube insertion for the removal of pleural fluid. (1) If thoracentesis is performed: measure and record amount of fluid withdrawn; include documentation of color and quality; assess breath sounds q 2 hr; check dressing; monitor vital signs q 15 min for the first hour. (2) If chest tube inserted: monitor and record the amount, color, and character of the drainage; report excessive amounts of drainage to the physician; milk chest tubes q 2 to 4 hr; assess breath sounds q 2 to 4 hr; notify physician of changes in quality; change dressing as ordered. (3) Explain procedure and purpose to patient and family.

Inadequate ventilation. (1) Supply supplemental O_2 as ordered. (2) Monitor ABGs. (3) Control pain to prevent splinting.

Pain control. (1) Medicate for pain as ordered and prn. (2) Assess the effectiveness of pain control.

Immobility. (1) Assist with passive or active range-of-motion exercises q 2 to 4 hr. (2) Ambulate as soon as able. (3) Turn and reposition frequently. (4) Provide skin care q 2 hr.

Underlying disease process. (1) Appropriate nursing intervention should be aimed at the specific disease process, i.e. systemic edema, pulmonary edema, CHF, infection, or cancer.

DROWNING

Approximately 8,000 people die from drowning in the USA annually; this figure represents ~10% of all accidental deaths. The greatest percentage of drowning and near-drowning victims are from 10 to 19 years of age and in previous good health. More than half of all drowning occurs in swimming pools and is usually due to the lack of swimming skills, tiring, or an acute medical event while in the water.

Pathophysiology

Of all drowning victims, 10% do not actually aspirate water. Rather, asphyxiation occurs from breath-holding or severe bronchospasm, which prevents water from entering the lungs. These dry drowning victims demonstrate the best chance for survival. The remaining 90% are considered to have suffered from wet drowning. In wet drowning, the victim often makes violent respiratory efforts, and water fills the lungs. When drowning occurs in cold water of $\leq 20°C$, severe bradycardia and hypothermia ensue, delaying irreversible brain damage and decreasing O_2-consumption requirements, thereby prolonging the amount of time hypoxia can be tolerated.

Although submersion in cold water may actually increase chances of survival, possible fatal arrythmias (e.g., ventricular fibrillation) may occur with excessive cooling. It has been demonstrated that survival is possible in warm water for 10 min and in cold water up to 40 min. The type of water (salt water or fresh) in which the drowning has occurred is not as significant as was once believed. Drowning in salt water, a hypertonic solution, causes fluid to be drawn from the plasma into the alveoli, causing a large intrapulmonary shunt. Fresh water alters pulmonary surfactant so that alveoli are unventilated but perfused, causing increased intrapulmonary shunting and hypoxia. Both fresh-water and saltwater drowning causes a V/Q mismatch. Victims who survive near-drowning may develop a secondary near-drowning event, which occurs anywhere from 1 to 72 hr after the initial insult. Demonstrated by a respiratory distress syndrome because of the influx of fluid and protein into the alveoli, this is thought to be caused by the loss of surfactant and a leaky pulmonary membrane secondary to acidosis and hypoxia.

Most near-drowning victims aspirate insufficient amounts of water to create significant disturbances in fluid and electrolyte balance. The values may be altered initially by homeostasis but are usually rapidly restored and not life-threatening. Changes in cardiovascular function are proportionate to the changes in PaO_2 and acid-base balance. Renal function is not usually impaired, although acute tubular necrosis (ATN) may occur secondary to lactic acidosis, hypoxia, or change in renal blood flow.

Clinical picture

The clinical presentation of the victim of near-drowning will vary, depending on several factors: (1) length of time submerged, (2) temperature of the water, (3) state of consciousness, and (4) presence of pulses and respiration at the scene.

At the scene, cardiopulmonary resuscitation (CPR) should be initiated if the victim is pulseless. If the victim has pulses and is breathing spontaneously, supplemental O_2 should be administered, even if the victim is conscious. The signs and symptoms presented may include apnea to mild respiratory distress, frothy pulmonary-edema type secretions, cyanosis, and respiratory acidosis. The stomach may contain large amounts of aspirated water, and the airway needs to be protected from possible regurgitation and aspiration of stomach contents. The victim may demonstrate signs and symptoms of shock, depending on length of time submerged and temperature of the water. Level of consciousness will vary from unconsciousness to fully awake and responsive. The body temperature will depend on the temperature of the water and whether or not cardiac arrest ensued.

Medical intervention

Significant complications of near-drowning are related to decreased PaO_2 and acid-base disturbances, making it imperative to restore both to normal as rapidly as possible. The victim should be removed from the water and basic CPR initiated as early as possible. If the victim has not aspirated water and effective ventilation and circulation are established before circulatory collapse and neurologic damage ensues, the prognosis is excellent. If water has been aspirated, alterations in pulmonary function exist. Initiating effective artificial ventilation is more important than clearing or draining water from the lungs; fresh water is usually absorbed within minutes. It is important to recognize that swallowed water may be significant and that the airway needs to be protected from possible regurgitation and aspiration of stomach contents. If the victim is able to breathe on his own, he may still have a decreased PaO_2 and/or pH, and supplemental O_2 should be provided until specific determination of degree of oxygenation can be made.

Once the victim has been transported to an appropriate facility, the initial emphasis should be on pulmonary care. Intrapulmonary shunting can exceed 70% of cardiac output. Initiating PEEP can dramatically improve V/Q ratios. If the victim is breathing effectively (able to eliminate CO_2 and maintain adequate PaO_2 through adequate ventilation), this can be accomplished with the use of a continuous positive airway pressure (CPAP) mask. If the CPAP mask cannot provide adequate assistance, endotracheal intubation will be required for mechanical ventilation and PEEP. Occasionally bronchospasm is a problem, and the use of aerosolized bronchodilators and/or aminophylline can be effective. It is important to recognize that PEEP is one of the most important ways of medically managing the pulmonary function of the victim of near-drowning, and any interruption of that therapy may cause reflux pulmonary edema with an increase in pulmonary shunting and a corresponding decrease in PaO_2. Metabolic acidosis can be significant and the use of IV sodium bicarbonate may be required. The prophylactic use of antibiotics and corticosteroids in near-drowning victims is an issue under debate.

The prognosis for victims of near-drowning varies. If the individual presents to a medical facility awake or in a semiconscious state, the prognosis is excellent, providing he gets intensive pulmonary support and cardiovascular care. The victim who presents with coma has a much more guarded prognosis. With the comatose patient, it is essential to prevent any further neurologic damage. This may improve the prognosis in many cases of near-drowning. Deliberate hyperventilation will decrease the PCO_2 and reduce the intracerebral pressure in cases of cerebral edema when the PCO_2 is kept at ~30 torrs. The use of corticosteroids may also be effective in decreasing cerebral edema. Other therapy to prevent or reverse increased intracranial pressure includes high-dose barbiturates, muscle relaxants or paralytic agents, and hypothermia, reducing body temperature to 30°C. Intracranial pressure (ICP) monitoring may be necessary with treatment for ICPs >20 torr. Possible treatment includes fluid restriction and/or osmotic diuretics.

Nursing interventions

Alteration in gas exchange. (1) Monitor ABGs frequently for adequate oxygenation and pH. (2) Use CPAP mask or mechanical ventilation with PEEP (*see* Chapter 13). (3) Suction infrequently to maintain PEEP. If suctioning is necessary: preoxygenate before suctioning, use PEEP adapter or PEEP bag. (4) Interrupt PEEP only if absolutely necessary. (5) Assess breath sounds q 2 to 4 hr.

Alteration in acid-base balance. (1) Monitor electrolytes. (2) Monitor pH; treatment of acidosis may be necessary.

Alterations in cardiovascular status. (1) Monitor vital signs closely including CVP and pulmonary artery pressure. (2) Monitor intake and output hourly.

Alterations in renal status. (1) Monitor intake and output hourly. (2) Measure weights daily. (3) Observe changes in electrolytes, BUN, creatinine, urine electrolytes and osmolarity.

Alterations in neurologic status. (1) Monitor neurologic signs for increasing ICP; maintain ICP <20 torr. (2) Maintain head of bed at 30 degrees.

CHAPTER 4

THE HEMATOLOGIC SYSTEM

Mary Alice Higgins Donius

ANATOMY AND PHYSIOLOGY REVIEW

The hematopoietic system is derived from connective tissue and is composed of cellular components and plasma. The cellular components are RBCs, WBCs—including the nongranulocytes (lymphocytes and monocytes) and the granulocytes (neutrophils, eosinophils, basophils)—platelets, and chylomicrons, or fat droplets. The plasma is a liquid intracellular material that contains a fluid or ground substance, a fibrous component that appears at clotting, proteins, and other solids.

The functions of the blood include the distribution of heat; the transportation of respiratory gases, nutrients, and waste products; selective reaction to factors present in specific tissues, such as osmotic tension, pH, temperature, and hormonal levels; the transportation of cellular components among hematopoietic tissues, connective tissues, and other tissues and organs; and control of the effects of infection and tumors.

Normally, hematopoiesis occurs in the bone marrow. Rarely, it may occur in the lymph nodes, liver, or spleen. The stem cells, which are multipotential in their primitive stage, are the precursors of all blood elements. These cells are capable of self-replication and cell differentiation, and they ultimately produce the cellular components of the blood. Figure 4–1 depicts the various committed cells and their developmental stages.

Functions of cellular components

The primary function of the RBC is the transportation of O_2 to the tissues via the protein-and-iron molecule, Hb. A sequence of events controls the production of RBCs. First, hypoxia occurs as a result of

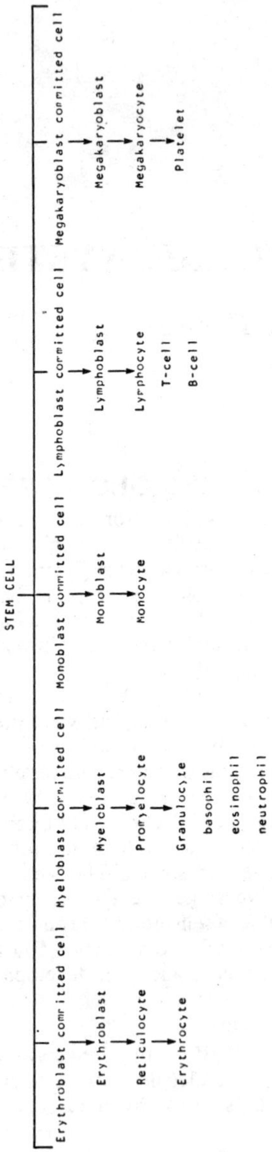

Figure 4–1. Hematopoiesis.

decreased O_2 supply to tissues, causing the kidneys to secrete erythropoietin. Ultimately the erythropoietin circulates through the bloodstream to the bone marrow, where it stimulates RBC production.

The primary functions of the WBC are many and vary, based on the type of cell. Defense against bacterial infection is provided by monocytes, neutrophils, eosinophils, and basophils. B-cell lymphocytes provide defense against viral as well as bacterial infection. T-cell lymphocytes provide defense against viral, fungal, and parasitic infection, cancer cells, and foreign bodies. The WBC also functions in anticoagulation by the production of heparin from basophils.

The primary function of platelets is to assist in clot formation, thereby maintaining homeostasis. Platelet functioning includes the following process: (1) The adhesion and aggregation of platelets to form a plug at the site of the injured vessel; (2) the release of serotonin and epinephrine to cause vasoconstriction; (3) the release of phospholipid to stimulate the cofactor necessary for coagulation; (4) the formation of a fibrin and clot retraction.

Functions of plasma and plasma proteins

The proteins contained in the plasma are essential to homeostasis. Albumin contributes to the maintenance of the osmotic pressure of the blood. Globulins—alpha, beta, gamma—act as transporters for various substances in the blood. Gamma globulin is necessary for antibody production. Fibrinogen, when catalyzed by thrombin, forms the fibrin necessary for clot formation.

The other significant components of plasma are nonprotein substances. Nonprotein nitrogen helps to maintain protein balance in the blood. Glucose supplies energy to the cells, and electrolytes maintain fluid and acid-base balance.

Function of the lymphatic system

The part of the circulatory system that transports fluids and solutes from interstitial spaces into the blood is the lymphatic system. The components of the lymphatic system are: (1) the lymphatic vessels, i.e., capillaries, collecting vessels, and trunks; (2) the lymphatic tissue, which contains lymphocytes and is contained in lymph nodes, mucous membranes, the thymus, spleen, and the bone marrow; and (3) the lymph. The primary functions of the lymphatic system are the return of fluid and proteins from interstitial fluid to the blood, filtration and phagocytosis, and the formation of nongranular WBCs in the lymph nodes.

ASSESSMENT OF THE PATIENT

To make a complete and accurate assessment of the patient, it is necessary to obtain a health history, including a complete review of systems, and a physical examination.

Health history

The assessment of current health status should include a brief nutritional assessment, including iron, vitamin B_{12}, and folate intake. The past health history should consider previous bleeding tendencies or hematopoietic dysfunctions or disorders, immune diseases, and tumors. A family history of these conditions should also be ascertained. The social history should identify exposure to radiation, toxic chemicals, or drugs.

The general health status considered in the review of systems may reveal chronic fatigue, weight loss, and increased bruising and bleeding. Systems and noteworthy symptoms are as follows:

Integumentary. Complaints of increased bruising and bleeding.

Head and neck. Sores on mouth and tongue.

Respiratory. Shortness of breath, dyspnea, orthopnea, dyspnea on exertion.

Cardiovascular. Increased pulse rate.

GI. Anorexia, indigestion, weight loss.

Musculoskeletal. Bone pain, intermittent claudication.

Neurologic. Paresthesia and weakness.

Immunologic. Increased infections, unexplained fever and fatigue.

Mental status. Depression, inability to concentrate, irritability, and malaise.

Physical examination

The significant findings on physical examination of each system is presented in Table 4–1.

Diagnostic studies

RBCs. Diagnostic studies to determine the structure and function of RBCs include: (1) CBC (Table 4–2); (2) bone marrow biopsy examination to determine the number, size, shape, and maturational progress of RBCs; (3) erythrocyte indicies, in which RBC mean cell volume (MCV) is 80 to 100 cu μg; the mean cell Hb (MCH) is 27 to 31 pg; and the mean cell Hb concentration (MCHC) is 31 to 37% of the volume of the RBC; (4) measurement of the life-span of the erythrocyte by isotopic methods; (5) measurement of total iron-binding capacity (TIBC), with the normal value being enough transferrin in 100 ml of serum to bind 250 to 450 μg of iron.

WBCs. Diagnostic studies include: (1) WBC differential — the normal being 4,500 to 11,000 WBCs/μl, which is broken down into mean percentages as follows: segmented neutrophils, 56.0%, bands, 3.0%, eosinophils, 2.7%, basophils, 0.3%, lymphocytes, 34.0%, monocytes, 4.0%; (2) bone marrow biopsy examination to determine the number, size, shape, and maturational progress of WBCs.

Platelets. Diagnostic studies include: (1) CBC, in which the normal is 200,000 to 350,000 platelets/mm; (2) bone marrow biopsy examination to determine the number, size, shape, and maturational progress of platelets; (3) bleeding time, with normal being 1 to 6 min (Ivy) or 1 to 3 min

TABLE 4–1
Physical Examination

System	Symptoms
Integumentary	Color and condition: pallor, icterus, hemolytic jaundice, erythema, temperature, varicosities, edema.
Head and neck	Eyes: scleral icterus, retinal hemorrhages. Ears: evidence of bleeding from the orifice. Mouth: bleeding, pallor, or cyanosis of the mucous membranes. Lymph nodes: enlargement (with or without pain).
Respiratory	Nose: pallor or cyanosis of the mucous membranes, epitaxis. Lungs: rate and rhythm may be increased and shallow, hemoptysis.
Cardiovascular	Pulse: rate and rhythm may be increasing, thready, and irregular. BP: decreasing, postural hypotension. Heart sounds: systolic murmurs. Peripheral pulses: diminishing and irregular.
GI/GU	Hematemesis, melena, hematuria, menorrhagea, ascites, splenomegaly, hepatomegly.
Musculoskeletal	Limited range of motion, hemarthrosis.
Neurologic	Changes in sensory level, coordination.
Immunologic	Evidence of infection.
Mental status	Changes orientation and memory, alteration of mood and affect.

TABLE 4–2
Values for Complete Blood Count of Red Blood Cells

Diagnostic study	Male	Female
Hb level	13.5–18.0 g/dl	12.0–16.0 g/dl
Hct	40–54%	38–47%
RBC count	4.6–6.2 million/mm^3	4.2–5.5 million/mm^3
ESR	0–15 mm/hr	0–20 mm/hr

ESR, erythrocyte sedimentation rate.

(Duke); (4) partial prothrombin time, with normal values from 40 to 100 sec; (5) prothrombin time (PT), with normal being 12 to 14 sec; (6) venous clotting time of 5 to 15 min; (7) thrombin time of $\leq$20 sec; (8) fibrinogen level of 200 to 400 mg/100 ml; (9) clot retraction, which normally begins within 1 hr and is completed within 24 hr.

MAJOR DISORDERS OF RED BLOOD CELLS

ANEMIAS

Pathophysiology

Anemia is the reduction in the concentration of circulating Hb or RBCs. It may result from a variety of causes, including the reduced production of RBCs, the reduced synthesis of Hb by the RBC precursors, the increased destruction of RBCs, and the loss of RBCs from the circulatory system. Anemias are characterized as iron deficiency, megaloblastic macrocytic, and hemolytic (for specific discussion, *see below*).

Clinical picture

The symptoms of anemia result from the reduced capacity of the blood to carry O_2, the change in the total blood volume, and the rate at which these occur. Other symptoms include those associated with the underlying disorder and decreased cardiovascular and pulmonary compensation capacity. Therefore, the nonspecific symptoms include fatigue, irritability, and a vague sense of loss of wellness. The specific symptoms will reflect system involvement including pallor of skin and mucous membranes, tachycardia, systolic flow murmurs, dyspnea, peripheral edema, anorexia, nausea, vomiting, flatulence, abdominal discomfort, constipation, diarrhea, weight loss, headache, vertigo, tinnitus, faintness, chills, feeling of cold, inability to concentrate, drowsiness, restlessness, increased BMR, proteinuria, mild fever (with marked anemia), increased susceptibility to bruising and bleeding (petechiae, purpura, ecchymosis, retinal hemorrhage), scleral icterus, pancytopenia, and symptoms related to underlying pathology.

Complications of anemia include myocardial ischemia, angina, congestive heart failure, renal failure, shock, and complications related to underlying pathology.

Diagnosis is based on health history, physical examination, CBC, blood smears for specific morphology, and complications.

Medical interventions

Medical interventions include iron supplements, blood transfusions, a well-balanced diet, vitamins, O_2 therapy, and treatment of underlying pathology and complications.

Nursing interventions

Hypoxia. (1) Administer O_2 therapy prn. (2) Administer blood transfusions as ordered, assessing for reactions. (3) Administer iron and vitamin supplements as ordered. (4) Monitor laboratory data (CBC, MCHC, MCV, MCH, arterial blood gases [ABGs]). (5) Restrict activity level by assisting with activities of daily living; providing periods of rest following activity; planning for progressive ambulation and activity. (6) Assess for respiratory rate and rhythm. (7) Place in semi-Fowler's position to maintain adequate lung expansion and ease of breathing. (8) Assess skin and mucous membranes. (9) Protect patient from becoming chilled. (10) Assess for signs of confusion and/or irritability. (11) Instruct patient in clear and concise manner, allowing for time to process information.

Tachycardia. (1) Monitor ECG for pulse rate and arrhythmias. (2) Auscultate for systolic murmur.

Anorexia. (1) Provide small, frequent feedings. (2) Provide high caloric supplements as ordered.

Increased susceptibility to infection and bleeding. (1) Maintain strict asepsis in management of wound, IV, and injection sites. (2) Provide proper oral care. (3) Assess for signs of infection both generalized and specific. (4) Provide pulmonary hygiene, including coughing and deep-breathing exercises and change of position while in bed. (5) Assess for signs of bleeding (monitor BP; observe for blood from body orifices and secretions; assess for heme and occult blood in urine, feces, and emesis; assess for petechiae, purpura, and ecchymosis).

Potential for ischemia of vital organs. (1) Assess for signs and symptoms of: angina, MI, left-sided heart failure, renal failure, shock.

Anxiety. (1) Provide emotional support to patient and family regarding critical episode, debilitating effects of anemia, and chronicity of the disorder. (2) Provide instruction related to medical regimen and underlying pathology.

IRON DEFICIENCY ANEMIA

Pathophysiology

The most common form of nutritional deficiency and the most common cause of anemia is iron deficiency. It is the depletion of the total body iron content. It is most frequently seen in children under two years of age and in postmenopausal women. It may be caused by inadequate dietary intake, impaired iron absorption, increased iron loss through bleeding (acute, chronic, or persistent hemorrhage), and by increased requirements for iron.

Clinical picture

Symptoms include fatigue, irritability, palpitations, dizziness, breathlessness, headache, epithelial abnormalities of the nails, tongue, hypopharynx (associated with dysphagia), stomach (associated with gastritis), and nose, and pica. Other symptoms may include menorrhagia, neuralgic pains, vasomotor disturbances, numbness, and tingling.

Diagnosis is based on the health history, physical examination, and laboratory data. Important laboratory findings include decreased serum levels of Hb, MCH, MCV, and MCHC; normal or decreased levels of reticuloctyes and WBCs; an increased platelet count and possibly an increased TIBC. A blood smear shows decreased Hb in each RBC, with central pallor. The degree of change and the number of RBCs affected will increase with the severity of the disease. Erythroid hyperplasia will be noted on bone marrow examination.

Medical interventions

Medical and surgical interventions include treatment of underlying pathology. Iron supplements from dietary requirements may be prescribed.

Nursing interventions

Nursing interventions are the same as for anemia (*see above*).

MEGALOBLASTIC MACROCYTIC ANEMIA

This is a disorder in which the RBC is increased in size and the macrocyte is thicker than normal. The etiologic factors include: (1) defective DNA synthesis, (2) vitamin B_{12} deficiency, and (3) folate deficiency. Table 4–3 compares the etiology, therapeutic interventions, and nursing interventions for these three types of megaloblastic macrocytic anemia.

HEMOLYTIC ANEMIA

Pathophysiology

Hemolytic anemia is the result of an increase in the rate of RBC destruction, with the concomitant inability of the bone marrow to increase the generation rate of RBCs to compensate sufficiently. This condition may result from either an inherited or an acquired disorder.

Clinical picture

The symptoms and complications of *chronic* congenital hemolytic anemia are jaundice, "crisis" periods of asymptomatic disease with episodic symptomatic disease, splenomegaly, cholelithiasis, leg ulcers, severe skeletal abnormalities during growth and development, and symptoms associated with underlying pathology. Symptoms and complications for *acquired* hemolytic anemia are rapid onset, aching pains of the back, abdomen, and limbs, headache, malaise, vomiting, fever, chills, and other symptoms of generalized anemia, underlying pathology, and shock.

Diagnosis is based on the health history, physical examination, and laboratory data including decreased RBC survival rate, increased serum bilirubin (unconjugated), increased lactic dehydrogenase (LDH), hemoglobinuria, leukocytosis, thrombocytosis, and specific morphologic abnormalities. Bone marrow aspiration reveals hyperplasia.

Medical interventions

Treatment depends on the specific diagnosis of the underlying pathology. But in general, medical interventions include making a differential diagnosis, relieving shock, and administering blood transfusions. Surgical treatment includes splenectomy.

Nursing interventions

Nursing interventions are the same as provided for anemia (*see above*) as well as care for the underlying pathology, pre- and postoperative care for splenectomy, and genetic counseling if indicated.

Pain. (1) Assess pain for location, duration, onset, and severity. (2) Administer analgesics as ordered. (3) Position carefully in proper body alignment. (4) Protect from injury and trauma. (5) Provide as calm and quiet an atmosphere as possible.

SICKLE CELL ANEMIA

Pathophysiology

Sickle cell anemia is an inherited condition of abnormal Hb synthesis. It occurs almost exclusively in blacks and is due to the homozygous inheritance of Hb S, which substitutes valine for glutamic acid in position six of the beta chain. The sickling phenomenon occurs when the altered Hb molecules, after prolonged deoxygenation, aggregate into rigid, liquid crystals and distort the cell into the characteristic sickle shape. This results in increased RBC fragility and permeability. Reversal to the normal shape occurs after oxygenation, but cells with the highest concentration of Hb S sickle irreversibly. Repeated sickling and unsickling decrease the cell's ability to return to normal. Hemolysis takes place both intra- and extravascularly, causing occlusion in the microcirculation.

Clinical picture

The clinical picture reflects a history of chronic hemolytic anemia with jaundice, which usually begins in childhood. Other symptoms include recurrent abdominal and limb pain, recurrent pneumonialike symptoms from infections and vascular occlusive episodes, possible delayed skeletal and sexual maturation, cardiomegaly, heart murmurs, dyspnea on exertion, palpitations, pleurisy, episodic abdominal pain, hepatomegaly without tenderness, altered splenic functioning, the inability to concentrate urine, hematuria, conjunctival vessel changes, repeated vitreous hemorrhages, susceptibility to infections, and leg ulcers.

Diagnosis is based on the health history, physical examination, and specific laboratory findings. Blood studies usually reveal a normal RBC, increased or reduced MCV, decreased erythrocyte sedimentation rate (ESR), morphologic distortions (i.e., poikilocytosis, anisocytosis, and the presence of target cells and Heinz bodies), elevated plasma proteins, and possible elevation of WBC and platelet count. Bone marrow aspiration reveals an increased erythroid mass. Sickling tests induce the sickling phenomenon, identify Hb S, and screen the trait.

Medical interventions

Medical treatment for an acute episode includes blood transfusion with normal RBCs, O_2 therapy, analgesics, antibiotics, fluid replacement,

TABLE 4–3

Comparison of the Three Types of Megaloblastic Macrocytic Anemia

Parameter	Defective DNA synthesis	Vitamin B_{12} deficiency	Folate deficiency
Etiology	Inherited Drug-induced	Decreased dietary intake of vitamin B_{12} (rare) Pernicious anemia Gastrectomy Obstruction of gastric mucosa Small-bowel bacterial overgrowth Disease affecting the ileum Chronic pancreatic disease Congenital malabsorption Fish tapeworm	Decreased dietary intake of folates Alcoholic cirrhosis Pregnancy Infancy Hematologic illness characterized by rapid cellular proliferation of RBCs or other marrow components Congenital or drug-induced deficiencies Malabsorption Tropical sprue Celiac disease Regional jejunitis Small-bowel resection
Clinical picture			
Symptoms	Relate to anemia in general	Paresthesia, weakness, incoordination, unsteady gait, inability to perform fine motor skills, personality changes, confusion and psychosis. Other symptoms include those that relate to anemia and underlying pathology.	Glossitis, anorexia, dyspepsia, flatulence, and diarrhea. Other symptoms include those that relate to anemia and underlying pathology.

Diagnosis	1. Health history and physical examination. 2. Laboratory data including: normal MCHC; increased MCV in proportion to the severity of disease; decreased RBC, Hb, Hct; normal-to-low WBC; decreased platelet count; prolonged bleeding time; erythropoiesis of macrocytic RBCs of distinctly oval shape; cellular and hyperplastic bone marrow with megaloblasts.	1. Same as for defective DNA synthesis. 2. Schilling test normal in pernicious anemia and abnormal in B_{12} malabsorption. 3. Evidence of underlying pathology.	1. Same as for defective DNA synthesis. 2. Evidence of underlying pathology.
Medical interventions	Treatment of underlying pathology and of anemia.	Vitamin B_{12} therapy and treatment of underlying pathology and of anemia.	Folate therapy and treatment of underlying pathology.
Nursing interventions	*See* nursing interventions related to anemia and underlying pathology.	*See* nursing interventions related to anemia and underlying pathology.	*See* nursing interventions related to anemia and underlying pathology.

hydration, management of acidosis, treatment and control of complications, and administration of urea.

Nursing interventions

Anemia. *See* nursing interventions related to anemia.

Dehydration. (1) Assess for signs and symptoms of dehydration including: intake and output; oliguria to anuria; condition of skin and mucous membranes. (2) Monitor BP and respiratory rate. (3) Monitor heart rate for tachycardia and murmurs. (4) Maintain IV hydration as ordered as well as oral fluids. (5) Maintain blood transfusions as ordered.

Pain. (1) Assess pain for location, duration, onset, and severity. (2) Administer analgesics as ordered. (3) Maintain on bed rest and position carefully in proper body alignment. (4) Assess for and prevent pathologic fractures. (5) Protect from injury and trauma. (6) Maintain patient safety.

Potential for respiratory infection. (1) Assess for signs of decreasing respiratory function including: increased shallow respiratons; abnormal ABGs; restlessness and irritability; dyspnea, shortness of breath, and orthopnea. (2) Assess for signs of infection including: increased temperature; abnormal breath sounds; coughing and sputum production. (3) Provide pulmonary hygiene (reposition frequently; coughing and deep-breathing exercises). (4) Administer O_2 therapy as ordered. (5) Administer antibiotics as ordered.

Leg ulcers. (1) Cleanse the ulcer as ordered and apply dressing. (2) Elevate legs when sitting. (3) Avoid using knee gatch. (4) Protect from injury and trauma.

Anxiety. (1) Provide emotional support to patient and family regarding chronic illness, genetic disease, and crisis episodes. (2) Obtain genetic counseling for patient and family. (3) Have family members screened for the sickle trait. (4) Teach patient and family how to deal with the crisis episode and how to prevent complications of the disease.

POLYCYTHEMIA VERA

Pathophysiology

Polycythemia vera is an increased production of RBCs, with a resultant expansion of blood volume. Its etiology is unknown but it is comparatively common in Jews and it is more common in males.

Clinical picture

Symptoms occur insidiously and include polycythemia rubra vera, headache, dizziness, tinnitus, visual disturbances, dyspnea, weakness, ascites, and pruritus. Complications include hypertension, CHF, increased potential for respiratory infections, decreased peripheral vascular circulation, bleeding into the skin and mucous membranes, GI and GU bleeding, spleno- and hepatomegaly. Also, thrombus formation may occur with occlusion of vessels in the heart (MI), lower extremities (gangrene), lungs (pulmonary embolism), and brain (cerebrovascular accident [CVA]).

Diagnosis is based on the health history, physical examination, blood and diagnostic studies. The bone marrow aspiration is performed. The fluid appears dark red and there is hyperplasia of all elements. The blood studies will show increased RBCs, Hb, WBCs, platelets, and total blood volume. The MCV, MCH, and MCHC will be decreased. The urinalysis will reveal albuminuria.

Medical interventions

Medical treatment and management includes venesection, or phlebotomy, irradiation of the bones, chemotherapy, and specific treatment of symptoms and complications.

Nursing interventions

Localized hemorrhage. (1) Assess for signs of bleeding including: petechiae and ecchymosis on skin; frank blood from body orifices and in secretions; heme and occult blood in urine, feces, and emesis. (2) Protect from injury and trauma. (3) Prevent shock.

Potential respiratory infection. (1) Assess for signs of infection including: increased temperature; increased WBCs and ESR; increased and shallow respirations; coughing and sputum production. (2) Maintain IV hydration. (3) Administer antibiotics as ordered. (4) Provide pulmonary hygiene (reposition patient frequently; assist with coughing and deep-breathing exercises).

Systemic complications from thrombus formation. (1) Monitor for systemic signs of emboli including: CVA, angina and MI, pulmonary emboli, and gangrene of lower extremeties.

Complication related to medical treatment. (1) Phlebotomy: Instruct patient about procedure; prepare patient for procedure; monitor patient during and following procedure, especially for signs of shock. (2) Chemotherapy and radiation: Monitor for signs and symptoms of the side effects of the treatment and provide appropriate nursing care; provide emotional support related to the treatment and its side effects.

Anxiety. (1) Provide emotional support related to crisis, diagnosis, and prognosis. (2) Provide information related to the disease process and its management. (3) Teach patient to avoid trauma, injury, and elective surgery. (4) Teach patient to advise physicians, dentists, and nurses of the disease. (5) Provide Medic Alert identification.

DISORDERS OF WHITE BLOOD CELLS

LEUKEMIAS

Leukemia is the proliferation of abnormal WBCs. There are two types of acute leukemia and two types of chronic leukemia. Potential causes include genetic predisposition, radiation, drugs, exposure to toxic chemicals, viruses, and bone marrow hypoplasia. The pathophysiology, clinical picture, and medical and surgical interventions for these leukemias are described in Tables 4–4 and 4–5.

The types of treatments used for leukemia follow the progression of the disease. The initial treatment is remission induction therapy, followed by consolidation therapy, which is therapy that is continued or modified once the initial therapy is completed, and maintenance therapy, which reflects decreasing treatment.

Nursing interventions

Anemia. *See* nursing interventions related to anemia.

Pain. (1) Assess pain for location, duration, onset, and severity. (2) Administer analgesics as ordered. (3) Position carefully in proper body alignment. (4) Protect from injury and trauma. (5) Provide adequate rest in as calm and quiet an environment as possible.

Infection. (1) Administer IV antibiotics as ordered. (2) Monitor laboratory data (CBC, blood cultures, sputum culture, BUN, urinalysis, culture of any drainage). (3) Maintain reverse isolation and/or precautions. (4) Reduce fever through hypothermia and antipyretics as ordered. (5) Prevent infection by maintaining asepsis in management of wounds, IVs, Foley catheter, etc. (6) Provide adequate fluids and nutrition.

Potential for hemorrhage. (1) Maintain IV hydration as ordered. (2) Administer blood transfusions as ordered. (3) Administer O_2 therapy as needed. (4) Monitor ECG for heart rate, especially ventricular tachycardia and arrhythmias. (5) Monitor BP. (6) Monitor laboratory data (CBC, ABGs, electrolytes). (7) Monitor intake and output accurately. (8) Assess for signs of bleeding including: petechiae and ecchymosis on skin, frank blood from body orifices and in secretions; heme and occult blood in urine, feces, and emesis. (9) Protect from injury and trauma. (10) Prevent shock.

TABLE 4–4

Acute Lymphoblastic Leukemia (ALL) and Acute Myelogenous Leukemia (AML)

Parameter	ALL	AML
Definition	The proliferation of primarily abnormal lymphoblasts.	The proliferation of primarily abnormal myeloblasts.
Classification	L_1: small and homogenous lymphoblasts. L_2: heterogeneous lymphoblasts. L_3: homogeneous lymphoblasts appear like Burkitt's lymphoma cells.	M_1: no maturation of myeloblasts. M_2: maturation to or beyond promyelocyte stage. M_3: variant, with hypergranular promyelocytes and Auer bodies.

Parameter	ALL	AML
Clinical picture		
Symptoms	Subtle onset (pallor, anorexia, irritability, and malaise). Low-grade fever with intermittent marked temperature elevations, with or without infection. Bleeding tendencies (petechiae, ecchymosis, and mucous membranes) and anemia.	Subtle onset of generalized symptoms over longer period of time. Preceded by a hematologic defect, most often anemia ("preleukemia"). Mild bleeding tendencies (petechiae and mucous membranes).
Complications	Thrombocytopenia, lymph node enlargement, spleno- and hepatomegaly, bone and joint pain, increased susceptibility to infection, meningeal leukemia (headache, nausea, and intracranial pressure), GU manifestations (hematuria, cystitis, and pyelonephritis), and death.	Severe bleeding (GI and GU tracts, and CNS hemorrhage). Thrombocytopenia, lymph node enlargement, spleno- and hepatomegaly, bone and joint pain, increased susceptibility to infection, meningeal leukemia (headache, nausea, and intracranial pressure), GU manifestations (hematuria, cystitis, and pyelonephritis), and death.
Diagnosis	Health history and physical examination. Blood studies: anemia, granulo- and thrombocytopenia, elevated WBC with leukemic lymphoblast cells or leukopenia, increased uric acid, BUN, and LDH. Bone marrow: leukemic lymphoblast cells.	Health history and physical examination. Blood studies: anemia, Auer bodies, macrocytic anemia, thrombocytopenia, leukopenia, hypergammaglobulinemia, and increased uric acid. Bone marrow: leukemic myeloblast cells.
Medical interventions	Chemo-, radio-, and immunotherapy, treatment and prevention of infection, and supportive care therapy.	Same as for ALL
Surgical interventions	Bone marrow transplant	Same as for ALL

LDH, lactic dehydrogenase. *Adapted from* Mahoney, E.A., and Flynn, J.P., editors. *Handbook of Medical-Surgical Nursing.* John Wiley & Sons, Inc., New York. 1983. p. 691.

Anxiety. (1) Provide emotional support to patient and family during the critical episode as well as regarding terminal illness. (2) Provide emotional and physical support to patient and family regarding the side effects of radiation and/or chemotherapy. (3) Instruct patient and family about proper medical regimen and preventing complications.

TABLE 4–5

A Comparison of Chronic Lymphocytic Leukemia (CLL) and Chronic Myelocytic Leukemia (CML)

Parameter	CLL	CML
Definition	A possible clonal disorder that allows for the production of an excessive number of small lymphocytes.	A clonal disorder of the stem cell, which is allowed to proliferate in preference to normal stem cells.
Incidence	Uncommon in people <30 yr; increases as age increases. More common in males and whites; rare in Orientals.	Occurs at any age but most commonly in young or middle-aged adults. More common in males.
Etiology	Unknown. Same causative factors as ALL, except radiation.	Unknown. Same causative factors as AML.
Clinical picture		
Symptoms	Slow onset, anemia, enlarged lymph nodes, spleno- and hepatomegaly, and fever.	Insidious onset, anemia, abdominal fullness, easy bruising and bleeding, massive spleen, fever, very little enlargement of the lymph nodes, and diaphoresis.
Complications	Infection, hemolytic anemia, and hypogammaglobulinemia.	Infection, thrombocytopenia, anemia, thromboembolism, and hemorrhage.
Diagnosis	Health history and physical examination. Blood studies: normal WBCs, decreased RBCs, normal platelet count, and blood smears. Bone marrow examination.	Health history and physical examination. Blood studies: increased WBCs, decreased RBCs, increased platelet count, LAP, and blood smears. Bone marrow examination.
Medical interventions	Chemotherapy (alkylating agents), immunotherapy, radiation therapy, treatment of anemia and thrombocytopenia, and treatment and prevention of infection.	Chemotherapy, radiation therapy, radioisotope therapy, treatment of symptoms, and treatment and prevention of infection.
Surgical intervention	Splenectomy.	None

ALL, acute lymphoblastic leukemia; AML, acute myelogenous leukemia; LAP, leukoycte alkaline phosphatase. *Adapted from* Mahoney, E.A., and Flynn, J.P., editors. *Handbook of Medical-Surgical Nursing.* John Wiley & Sons, Inc., New York. 1983. p. 693.

CLOTTING DISORDERS

DISSEMINATED INTRAVASCULAR COAGULATION

Pathophysiology

Disseminated intravascular coagulation (DIC) is a syndrome that produces an accelerated turnover of various coagulation factors in the blood, resulting in diffuse coagulation within the arterioles and capillaries. Etiologic factors include obstetric conditions, infections, neoplasms, hematopoietic dysfunction, vascular disorders, and massive tissue injury.

Very simply, the intrinsic or extrinsic factors activate the formation of thromboses composed largely of fibrin and aggregated platelets, thus causing widespread occlusions throughout the microcirculation. Ultimately, as a compensatory mechanism, the fibrinolytic system is activated, with the subsequent inhibition of the clotting mechanism, and increases the tendency toward bleeding.

Clinical picture

Thus, this syndrome is characterized by diffusion of fibrin deposits within the arterioles and capillaries and symptoms that reflect (1) the effects of the resultant occlusions in the microcirculation, such as shock, acute respiratory distress, CNS depression, cardiac failure, and renal failure and (2) the effects of the compensatory mechanisms, such as hemorrhage from the vital organs, especially kidneys, brain, adrenals, and heart. Acute symptoms include abrupt, severe bleeding and thromboembolitic manifestations. Chronic symptoms are superficial but extensive ecchymosis, recurrent episodes of bleeding, thrombophlebitis at unusual sites, and the symptoms of the underlying pathology. Complications include hypovolemia with decreased perfusion to vital organs, acute renal failure, and shock.

Diagnosis is based on health history, physical examination and laboratory data, including plasma fibrinogen level, thrombin time, low platelet count, and high increase in fibrinolysis, possible increase in fibrinogen degradation products (FDP) and prolonged PT and partial thromboplastin time (PTT).

Medical interventions

Medical treatment includes anticoagulation therapy and replacement of platelets and coagulation factors. Anticoagulation therapy is a controversial medical treatment, however. Its efficacy in treatment of DIC is difficult to provc and dosage regulation is difficult. Its use is aimed at inhibiting the formation of thrombi in the microcirculation as a result of one of the intrinsic or extrinsic factors of DIC.

Nursing interventions

Occlusion of the microcirculation of vital organs. (1) Assess for complications that may occur in the brain, lungs, heart, and kidneys as a result of occlusion and decreased perfusion.

Hypovolemia. (1) Monitor intake and output accurately. (2) Monitor vital signs carefully for decreasing BP; postural hypotension; increasing pulse rate; increasing respiratory rate. (3) Monitor laboratory data: Hct, BUN, sodium. (4) Maintain IV hydration and oral fluids. (5) Provide proper care of the skin and mucous membranes. (6) Prevent dehydration and shock.

Impaired coagulation. (1) Maintain IV hydration as ordered. (2) Administer blood transfusions as ordered. (3) Monitor ECG for heart rate, especially ventricular tachycardia and arrhythmias. (4) Monitor BP. (5) Monitor laboratory data for PT, PTT, thrombin time, fibrinogen level, and factor assays for II, V, and VII. (6) Assess for signs of bleeding including: petechiae and ecchymosis on skin; painful swollen joints; frank blood from body orifices and secretions; heme and occult blood in urine, feces, and emesis. (7) Administer anticoagulation therapy if ordered and assess for side effects. (8) Instruct patient and family in the proper administration and necessary precautions of anticoagulant therapy. (9) Administer vitamin K as ordered. (10) Provide Medic Alert identification.

Pain. (1) Assess pain for location, duration, onset, and severity. (2) Administer analgesics as ordered (preferably PO). (3) Position carefully in proper body alignment. (4) Apply cold and/or hot compresses to involved joint and immobilize the area.

Anxiety. (1) Provide emotional support to patient and family during the crisis period. (2) Allow and encourage the patient and family to express their concerns and fears about the disease and its prognosis and management. (3) Provide and discuss information related to the disease and its prognosis. (4) Instruct patient and family in the best ways to manage the disease and prevent its complications.

HEMOPHILIA

Pathophysiology

Hemophilia is a genetic clotting disorder that causes severe hemorrhagic diathesis. Type A is the most common coagulation disorder and it affects males with a genetic aberration. Type B is less common and improves with increasing age. Both types of hemophilia are caused by an X-linked recessive trait that produces a deficiency of factor VIII in type A and of factor IX in type B. Both types are classified in the same manner. Subhemophilia is identified as 25 to 50% of the factor present, with moderate bleeding following trauma or surgery. Mild stage is noted as 5 to 25% of the factor present, with unsuspected or serious bleeding following trauma or surgery. The moderate stage is evidenced by 2 to 5% of the factor present; infrequent spontaneous bleeding; and serious bleeding from insignificant injuries. The severe stage is reached when there is <2% of the factor present, prompting severe and frequent spontaneous bleeding, hemarthrosis, and crippling.

Clinical picture

The symptoms of hemarthrosis include pain, limited range of motion of the affected joint, muscle spasm, thickening of the synovia, and crippling.

Complications include subcutaneous and intramuscular hematomas, with resultant increased pressure on vital organs and nerves (e.g., retroperitoneal hemorrhage), acute or chronic GI or GU bleeding, delayed bleeding, hemophilic cysts, poor wound healing, and exsanguination.

The diagnosis of type A and type B hemophilia depends upon an accurate health history and physical examination. Significant laboratory data include prolonged coagulation time in severe stages but normal in all other stages; prolonged PTT in the severe and moderate stages, variable in the mild stage, and usually normal in subhemophilia; normal PT. Thrombocytosis occurs in acute or chronic hemorrhage. Specific diagnostic tests for each type include factor VIII assay for type A and factor IX assay for type B.

Medical interventions

Medical interventions include replacement therapy for type A hemophilia of IV administration of factor VIII in the form of blood or blood products, such as cryoprecipitate and purified or fresh-frozen citrated plasma. For type B, replacement therapy involves the IV administration of factor IX in the form of blood or blood products, including citrated plasma and purified prothrombin complex. Additional interventions for both types are the treatment and prevention of hemarthrosis and bleeding.

Nursing interventions

Hemorrhage. (1) Maintain IV hydration as ordered. (2) Administer replacement therapy as ordered. (3) Administer topical thrombin or other medications to stop superficial bleeding from or under skin. (4) Apply ice and pressure to stop superficial bleeding from or under the skin. (5) Monitor BP and respiratory rate. (6) Monitor ECG for heart rate, especially ventricular tachycardia and arrhythmias. (7) Monitor laboratory data: CBC, ABGs, PT, PTT, and thrombin time. (8) Monitor intake and output accurately. (9) Assess for signs of bleeding. (10) Protect from injury and trauma. (11) Prevent shock.

Pain. (1) Assess pain for location, duration, onset, and severity. (2) Administer analgesics and steroids as ordered. (3) Encourage bed rest but maintain movements of joints.

Anxiety. (1) Provide emotional support to the patient and family during episodes of bleeding. (2) Provide emotional support related to genetic disease, chronic illness, and debilitating disease process. (3) Identify and discuss with patient and family necessary adaptations in life style to prevent complications. (4) Provide Medic Alert identification. (5) Teach measures to avoid the causes and sources of bleeding and complications, especially trauma and elective surgery. (6) Instruct patient to inform physicians and dentists about the condition. (7) Teach patient and family to recognize signs of bleeding. (8) Obtain genetic counseling for the patient and his family. (9) Have family members screened for the genetic trait.

IDIOPATHIC THROMBOCYTOPENIA PURPURA

Pathophysiology

Idiopathic thrombocytopenia purpura (ITP) is a condition that produces thrombocytopenia without apparent exogenous etiologic factors. It occurs most frequently in children and young adults and is the most common form of thrombocytopenia. Its etiology is unknown, but immunologic factors are suspected.

Acute ITP occurs in children two to six years of age and is preceded by an infection 1 to 3 wk prior to the onset of symptoms. It is marked by the abrupt onset of bleeding and a low platelet count. Symptoms last 4 to 6 wk with spontaneous remission.

Chronic ITP, which occurs in young adults of 20 to 40 yr of age, is also marked by insidious onset of bleeding and a decreased platelet count. Its course fluctuates, however, and may last months or even years.

Clinical picture

Symptoms include fever, signs of mild to moderate bleeding (such as petechiae of the skin and mucous membranes, superficial ecchymosis, bleeding from superficial cuts, excessive bleeding after trauma, vesicles or bullae of the mouth, epitaxis, and GI and GU bleeding), intracranial hemorrhage, aplastic anemia, and mild splenomegaly.

The diagnosis is based on the health history, physical examination, and laboratory data. Platelets may be found to be totally absent or only slightly decreased in number. However, they are abnormal in size, morphology, and functioning. Blood coagulation tests reveal a prolonged bleeding time, absent or abnormal clot retraction, and an abnormal prothrombin consumption time (PCT). Anemia is proportional to the amount of blood lost, and bone marrow aspiration reveals megakaryocytes and hyperplasia if blood loss is great.

Medical Interventions

Medical management includes steroid therapy and the symptomatic treatment of bleeding and its complications. Surgical treatment is splenectomy.

Nursing interventions

Localized hemorrhage. (1) Assess for signs of bleeding including: petechiae and ecchymosis on skin, mucous membranes; frank blood from body orifices and in secretions; heme and occult blood in urine, feces, and emesis. (2) Observe for signs of intracranial bleeding. (3) Maintain IV hydration. (4) Protect from injury and trauma. (5) Prevent shock.

Anemia. *See* nursing interventions related to anemia.

Anxiety. (1) Provide emotional support for acute phase of chronic illness. (2) Provide information related to the disease process, its complications, and medical management.

DISORDERS OF THE LYMPHATIC SYSTEM

NON-HODGKIN'S LYMPHOMAS

Pathophysiology

Malignancies of the lymphoid tissues other than Hodgkin's disease are identified as non-Hodgkin's lymphomas (NHL). These are more common in males and are estimated to constitute 2.5% of all malignancies (excluding nonmelanotic skin cancer and cervical carcinoma in situ). Causes include RNA viruses, genetic factors, immunodeficiencies and immunostimulation, immunosuppressive agents, and high-dose radiation exposure.

The Rappaport classification is often used to identify NHL. It was proposed by Rappaport and associates to classify those tumors according to their nodular architecture (i.e., either nodular or diffuse) and also to differentiate according to cellular histology or type (i.e., well-differentiated, lymphocytic nodes; histiocytic nodes; mixed nodes composed of histiocytic and lymphocytic cells; and undifferentiated nodes).

Clinical picture

Symptoms include enlarged, painless lymph nodes, usually in the primary sites of the cervical or supracervical areas, lymphadenopathy at another primary site, and fatigue, malaise, GI symptoms, weight loss, fever, infection, bone pain, and possible splenomegaly. Complications are related to associated organ involvement (liver, spleen, the parenchyma of the lungs, and the kidneys). Infection is also a complication.

Diagnosis is based on health history, physical examination, chest x-ray (mediastinal and hilar nodes), skeletal x-ray (bone nodes), CT scan, and laboratory findings. The CBC is usually normal at diagnosis, uric acid may be increased, calcium may be increased if bone is involved, and albumin may be decreased as the disease advances.

Medical interventions

Medical treatment is radiation therapy to the involved areas, radioisotopes, and chemotherapy.

Nursing interventions

Infection. (1) Assess for generalized symptoms of infection including: increased temperature; increased WBCs and ESR. (2) Assess for systemic signs of infection, especially in the lungs and kidneys. (3) Administer antibiotics as ordered. (4) Maintain asepsis when caring for wounds, IV, or injection sites. (5) Maintain reverse precautions if necessary. (6) Reduce fever if present by means of antipyretics. (7) Maintain IV hydration.

Weakness and fatigue. (1) Maintain O_2 therapy. (2) Provide periods of rest following activity. (3) Assist with activities of daily living.

Bone pain. (1) Assess pain for location, duration, onset, and severity. (2) Administer analgesics as ordered. (3) Position carefully in proper body alignment. (4) Provide warm compresses to affected area and keep area immobilized.

Complications involving affected organs. (1) *See* nursing measures for anemia, pulmonary edema, renal, and liver dysfunction.

Anxiety. (1) Provide emotional support to deal with diagnostic procedures, disease process, and complications. (2) Provide emotional and physical support for radiation and/or chemotherapy. (3) Teach the health care related to the medical regimen and control and prevention of complications.

HODGKIN'S DISEASE

Pathophysiology

Hodgkin's disease is a chronic and progressive tumor of the lymphatic system. It is most common between the ages of 20 to 40 and is more common in males. Causes include viral infections, immunologic dysfunction, and tumor. Histologic classification is based on the presence of the Reed-Sternberg cell, which is a distinctive, giant, tumor cell that is present in Hodgkin's disease and is diagnostic of it. Diagnosis may also be based on lymph nodes with diffuse and mixed infiltration of lymphocytes.

Stage I Hodgkin's disease is noted by single node involvement and single extralymphatic organ or site involvement. Two or more lymph node areas on the same side of the diaphragm involved or an extralymphatic organ or site and the involvement of one or more lymph node areas on the same side of the diaphragm are classified in stage II. In stage III, the lymph node areas on both sides of the diaphragm are involved. This stage may or may not be accompanied by extralymphatic organ or site involvement, spleen involvement, or both. Stage IV is marked by diffuse involvement of one or more extralymphatic organs or tissues with or without associated lymph node involvement. Subclassifications include patients with or without generalized symptoms.

Medical interventions

Medical treatment is radiation therapy, chemotherapy, or a combination of the two. Surgical treatment includes the removal of tumors that may be pressing on a nerve or an organ and splenectomy.

Nursing interventions

Nursing interventions are the same as for NHL and include nursing care for appropriate diagnostic procedures as well as appropriate pre-and postoperative nursing care.

ADMINISTRATION OF BLOOD PRODUCTS

A common medical intervention is the IV administration of blood or blood components including serum, plasma, RBCs, and platelets for replacement and therapeutic purposes. Blood transfusions are used to restore blood volume, prevent shock, or to treat severe chronic anemia.

Nursing interventions

The label and identification form should be checked for corresponding information: the patient's name, room number, hospital number, package number, the patient's blood group and Rh status, and the donor's blood group and Rh status. If the information does not correspond, transfusions should *not* be administered. Blood should be removed from the refrigerator 1 hr before administration. The patient should be identified.

The patient's arm is stabilized on an arm board and the transfusion administered with filter and normal saline, very slowly for the first 15 min. The patient's vital signs are then assessed. If there is no reaction, the rate of flow can be increased. The transfusion should be administered rapidly if patient is suffering from shock or hemorrhage. The patient should be assessed for signs of transfusion reactions (Table 4–6).

If there is a reaction, blood must be discontinued immediately, a physician notified, and blood and a sample of patient's blood sent to the blood bank; fluids and medications are administered as ordered. The patient should be taught to tell health professionals, on future hospitalizations or when donating blood, about the transfusion reaction and the presence or absence of complications.

Nursing interventions in the event of transfusion reactions are listed below.

Hemolytic transfusion reaction. (1) Discontinue transfusion. (2) Administer fluid and medications as ordered. (3) Administer O_2 therapy. (4) Monitor vital signs q 15 to 30 min. (5) Assess and prevent hypotension and shock. (6) Record intake and output accurately. (7) Assess for side effects of medications. (8) Provide emotional support during and after the emergency. (9) Advise the patient of the reaction and the importance of reporting it before future transfusions or before donating blood.

Bacterial transfusion reaction. (1) Same as for hemolytic reaction, except O_2 therapy is not usually needed. (2) Reduce fever.

Allergic reaction. (1) Discontinue transfusion if reaction is severe. (2) Slow down transfusion if reaction is mild. (3) Same as for hemolytic reaction.

Circulatory overload. (1) Discontinue transfusion. (2) Administer digitalis preparation as ordered. (3) Assess for side and toxic effects. (4) Prepare for phlebotomy procedure. (5) Same as for hemolytic reaction.

TABLE 4–6
Transfusion Reactions

Parameter	Hemolytic transfusion reaction	Bacterial transfusion reaction	Allergic reaction	Circulatory overload
Etiology	The hemolysis of RBCs due to an ABO or Rh incompatability. This is the most severe reaction and occurs in one out of 5,000 transfusions.	A rare reaction caused by the administration of blood contaminated by pathogenic organisms. Gram-negative bacteria cause the most severe and even fatal reactions.	Hypersensitivity to the blood received, due to an unknown cause.	Excessive fluid volume in the blood vessels caused by infusion of fluid in too great a quantity or at too rapid a rate.
Symptoms	Chills, fever, hematuria, oliguria, jaundice, headache, backache, dyspnea, cyanosis, chest pain.	Chills, fever, lumbar pain, headache, malaise, hematemesis, diarrhea, warm, dry, pinkish skin.	Mild reactions include mild edema, hives, bronchial wheezing, itching, fever; severe reactions include bronchospasm and severe dyspnea.	Cough, dyspnea, edema, tachycardia, hemoptysis, frothy, pink-tinged sputum.
Complications	Renal failure and shock.	Shock and death.	Anaphylactic shock and death.	Pulmonary edema, congestive heart failure.
Diagnosis	Based on etiology and symptoms.	Based on etiology and symptoms.	Based on etiology and symptoms.	Based on etiology and symptoms.
Medical interventions	Discontinuation of transfusion, administration of IV fluids, O_2 therapy, sedation, prevention and treatment of shock.	Discontinuation of transfusion, administration of IV fluids, medications (vasopressors, corticosteroids, antibiotics), prevention and treatment of shock.	Mild reaction is treated with antibiotics and antihistamins. With severe reaction, the transfusion is discontinued and epinephrine is administered IM.	Discontinuation of transfusion, digitalization.
Surgical intervention	None	None	None	Phlebotomy.

CHAPTER 5

THE NERVOUS SYSTEM

Celeste B. Williams

ANATOMY AND PHYSIOLOGY REVIEW

The **neuron** is the functional unit of the nervous system. Its components are the cell body; axons, which carry the nerve impulses away from the cell body; and dendrites, which carry impulses toward the cell body. Some axons are covered with a myelin sheath, which functions to speed the conduction of impulses. Myelin fibers constitute the white matter of the CNS for the most part; the gray matter consists mainly of nonmyelinated fibers.

Specialized, non-nervous connective tissue cells, the **neuroglia, or glial cells,** support and protect the neurons and act as a selective barrier to the brain. Neuroglia, which outnumber the neurons, are of differing sizes and shapes.

Impulse transmission occurs by both chemical and electrical processes. Impulse conduction along nerve fibers is *electrical.* When the neuron is stimulated, its resting potential is altered to evoke an action potential. Each nerve cell has a membrane potential maintained by ionic concentrations inside and outside the cell. These ionic concentrations create an electrical potential difference across the cell membrane. When the cell's specific threshold is reached, an action potential, or discharge of a nerve impulse, is produced. The transmission of impulse across a synapse—a junction of two nerves—is *chemical.* Synaptic junctions occur in the gray matter and are true anatomic gaps. When an impulse traveling along a neuron reaches a synapse, the excitatory hormone acetylcholine acts on the impulse-receiving cell membrane to increase its permeability to sodium ions. A leakage of sodium ions into the cell causes electric currents to flow along the surface in a wave of depolarization. In a fraction of a second, acetylcholine is destroyed by the enzyme cholinesterase, thus reestablishing the membrane potential of the cell. The most common chemical transmitters are acetylcholine and norepinephrine; however, there are some 30 different substances known or suspected to be transmitters in the brain.

The nervous system is classified into three major systems: (1) the central, (2) the peripheral, and (3) the autonomic.

THE CENTRAL NERVOUS SYSTEM

The CNS consists of the brain and the spinal cord. Cranial bones, vertebrae, and the meninges cover and protect them. The meninges consist of (1) the dura mater, a tough, fibrous white layer, (2) the arachnoid membrane, a delicate membrane with villi projections into the dura, and (3) the pia mater, a transparent meninx lying closest to the brain and containing most of the brain's blood supply.

The divisions, structures, and functions of the brain are described in Table 5–1. Throughout the brainstem are numerous large and small neurons intertwined by small processes. These fibrous neurons constitute the reticular formation, an important part of the extrapyramidal pathway. The **reticular activating system** receives stimuli from the hypothalamus, cranial nerves, and ascending tracts between the spinal cord and the thalamus or cerebellum and motor neurons. It is responsible for cortical activities, such as initiating and maintaining wakefulness. When it is stimulated, it causes diffuse activation of the entire brain. Arterial **blood** from the internal carotid and vertebral arteries supplies the intracranial contents. The vertebral arteries supply the posterior portion of the cranial cavity (brainstem, caudal part of diencephalon, cerebellum, occipital lobes, and parts of the temporal lobes). The internal carotid supplies the anterior and middle brain (including the cerebral hemispheres and most of the diencephalon) and the eye. The vertebral and internal carotid arteries join with communicating arteries at the base of the brain to form the circle of Willis, a frequent site of aneurysm formation. Venous drainage is by way of the cerebral veins and dural venous sinuses, which ultimately drain the venous blood of the brain into the jugular vein. The **ventricles** are cavities within the brain. There are two lateral ventricles, which communicate with the third ventricle through the foramen of Monro. The third ventricle communicates with the fourth ventricle through the aqueduct of Sylvius. The major structures surrounding the third and fourth ventricles include the nuclei of the thalamus, hypothalamus, basal ganglia, and the brainstem. CSF is formed from the blood in the choroid plexuses in both lateral and the third and fourth ventricles by a process of secretion and diffusion. It leaves the ventricular system via the foramens of Magendie and of Luschka to enter the subarachnoid space. It circulates over the brain and down the spinal cord and is absorbed into the subarachnoid space through villi into the large central vein.

TABLE 5–1

Structures and Functions of the Brain

Divisions	Structure	Function
Cerebrum	Largest portion of brain. Divided into two hemispheres by the longitudinal fissure and joined by a band of nerve fibers (corpus callosum), composed of white matter. Hemispheres are mirror images of one another and associated with one side of the body in contralateral control. Cerebral cortex (gray matter) is divided into lobes.	Governs reason, memory, intelligence, sensory-motor functions.
	Frontal	Anterior portion controls personality, behavior; area where values learned; role in memory; exercises some control of BP, heart rate, respiration. Posterior portion controls motor activity of lower extremities.
	Parietal	Receives and interprets sensory stimuli from skin, muscles, joints on opposite sides of body; interprets sensory data, including pain, heat, cold, pressure, size, shape, texture recognition, and body-part identification.
	Occipital	Receives sensory information for sight.
	Temporal	Receives auditory information primarily; also involved in visual reception.
	Insula: located deep within the lateral fissure.	Involved in visceral sensibility and motor activity.
	Limbic system: consisting of a group of structures, including hippocampus, amygdala, gyrus fornicatus, and connections with septal area, hypothalamus, and mesencephalon.	Thought to link higher functioning area with more primitive areas and to house reticular activating system. Affects sexual behavior, emotional response, and motivation.
Cerebellum	Occupies posterior cranial fossa; separated from cerebral hemisphere by the tentorium cerebelli, an extension of dura mater.	Acts to coordinate gross voluntary movement and maintain equilibrium.
Diencephalon	Continuous caudally with midbrain.	

Divisions	Structure	Function
Thalamus	Composed of gray matter and located in medioposterior aspect of each hemisphere. Forms roof of diencephalon.	Serves as relay station for sensory impulses from cord and brainstem on their way to cerebral cortex.
Hypothalamus	Lies below thalamus and above midbrain; contains the stalk of the pituitary gland, linking the nervous system to the endocrine system.	Major center for controlling ANS; also involved in regulation of body temperature, appetite, water balance, and wakefulness.
Brainstem		
Midbrain	Located between pons and diencephalon. Contains important afferent and efferent pathways. Aqueduct of Sylvius passes through lengthwise to connect third and fourth ventricles.	Motor coordination, visual and hearing reflexes.
Pons	Located between midbrain and medulla and serves as relay station between medulla and higher cortical centers. Includes nuclei of 5th to 8th cranial nerves.	Conductive pathway; contains portion of respiratory control mechanism.
Medulla	Lies below pons and is continuous with pons on one end and spinal cord on the other. Includes nuclei for the 9th to 12th cranial nerves.	Functions as connection between spinal cord and brain; contains cardiac, vasoconstrictor, and respiratory centers and mechanisms for controlling reflex activities.

Cerebrospinal fluid

CSF protects the brain and spinal cord against injury and carries nutrients to and removes metabolites from the brain. It is a clear, colorless fluid, with a sp gr of 1.007. Because the sp gr of CSF and water are nearly the same, pressure of CSF is expressed in mmH_2O. The normal pressure range is 60 to 180 mmH_2O in the lateral recumbent position. The quantity of CSF averages from 100 to 150 ml, at one given moment, and is produced at the rate of 18 ml/hr. CSF is composed of traces of minerals and organic materials of the blood (of which protein is the most significant), water, sodium, glucose (65 mg/dl), chloride (120 to 130 mEq/liter), and potassium.

Brain physiology

The brain uses glucose as its source of energy in the production of ATP, necessary in cellular processes. The brain consumes O_2 at a rate of ~49 ml/min, or ~20% of the total resting body O_2 consumption. If the flow of O_2 to the brain is decreased, cytotoxic cerebral edema results in seconds. Total cerebral blood flow (CBF) alters with changes in cerebral perfusion pressure (CPP). CBF is equal to the difference between the mean arterial pressure (MAP) and the intracranial pressure (ICP). Autoregulation assists in keeping CBF constant. Receptors in the brain constantly analyze blood gases, more specifically $PaCO_2$ and PaO_2 and the level of lactic acid. If the $PaCO_2$ rises >45 mmHg, increased CBF will result. Hypoxia (PaO_2 <50 mmHg) leads to arteriolar dilation and increased CBF. CPP must be maintained at 60 to 90 mmHg for adequate CBF. If MAP increases, the cerebral vessels constrict in an effort to limit the amount of blood to the brain. If the MAP falls, the cerebral vessels dilate. Increased lactic acid levels also cause vasodilation.

Intracranial pressure

The volume of blood, CSF, and brain tissue enclosed within the skull are all determinants of the level of ICP. When the volume of one compartment increases, the total pressure will increase, unless there is a reciprocal change in another compartment. CSF is usually the compensating factor because (1) the dura mater of the spinal cord is loosely attached and can accommodate CSF leaving the cranial subarachnoid space, and (2) CSF absorption by the arachnoid villi is partially dependent on CSF pressure. The skull, although nondistensible, has openings for the spinal cord, cranial nerves, and blood vessels, which can allow for some escape of cranial contents.

THE PERIPHERAL NERVOUS SYSTEM

The 12 pairs of cranial nerves, symmetrically arranged and attached to the brain, and the 31 pairs of spinal nerves make up the peripheral nervous system. Each pair of cranial nerves leaves the skull through a foramen at its base. The cranial nerves and their functions are listed in Table 5–2.

The spinal nerves exit from successive levels of the spinal cord. They are designated as 8 pairs of cervical nerves, 12 pairs of thoracic nerves, 5 pairs of lumbar nerves, and 1 pair of coccygeal nerves. The cord itself usually terminates at the level of the second lumbar vertebra. Each spinal nerve begins as a series of fibers from the dorsal root of the cord (sensory) and the ventral root (motor). The sensory, or afferent, fibers transmit impulses from the sensory receptors in the body to receptors in the spinal cord. The motor, or efferent, fibers transmit impulses from the cord to the muscles and glands of the body.

The strip of skin supplied by one pair of spinal nerves is called a dermatome. The general function of the spinal nerves is to convey impulses to and from the brain and its periphery. Many conduction pathways, or tracts, run through the CNS transmitting impulses.

Clusters of nerve cell bodies are grouped as the ganglia. Networks of spinal nerve roots form plexuses. The plexuses of the spinal cord are the cervical, brachial, lumbar, and sacral.

TABLE 5–2
Cranial Nerves and Their Functions

Nerve	Type	Origin	Function
1st Olfactory	Sensory	Cells of nasal mucosa	Smell
2nd Optic	Sensory	Ganglion cells in retina	Vision
3rd Oculomotor	Motor	Midbrain	Movement of eyes
4th Trochlear	Motor	Roof of midbrain	Movement of eyes
5th Trigeminal	Motor, sensory	Lateral aspect of pons	Chewing motions; sensations of cornea, nasal mucosa, face, oral cavity, two thirds tongue, teeth
6th Abducens	Motor	Lower portion of pons	Movement of eyes
7th Facial	Motor, sensory	Lower portion of pons	Muscles of facial expressions; taste, anterior two-thirds of tongue
8th Acoustic	Sensory	Lower border of pons	Equilibrium
9th Glossopharyngeal	Motor, sensory	Medulla oblongata	Secretion of saliva; swallowing motions; taste, posterior one-third of tongue; sensation of pharynx
10th Vagus	Motor, sensory	Medulla oblongata	Swallowing, voice production
11th Spinal accessory	Motor	Medulla oblongata	Shoulder movements, neck rotation
12th Hypoglossal	Motor	Anterior lateral sulcus	Movement of tongue

AUTONOMIC NERVOUS SYSTEM

The ANS is anatomically divided into the sympathetic and parasympathetic systems. Table 5–3 shows their effects on the various organ systems.

ASSESSMENT OF THE PATIENT

Health history

The history of a patient with a neurologic disorder may be extensive. When obtaining a history, focus should be on information that is relevant to

TABLE 5–3
Autonomic Function

Organ	Effect of sympathetic stimulation	Effect of parasympathetic stimulation
Heart muscle	Increases rate, force of beat	Slows rate, decreases force of atrial beat
Lungs, bronchi	Dilates	Constricts
GI tract	Decreases motility, contracts sphincters, inhibits secretions	Increases motility, relaxes sphincters, stimulates secretions
Bladder muscle	Relaxes	Constricts
Eye (pupil)	Dilates	Constricts
Adrenal gland	Stimulates secretion of epinephrine, norepinephrine	No significant effect
Blood vessels		
Coronary	Dilates	No significant effect
Skeletal muscle	Constricts	Dilates
Skin and most others	Constricts	No significant effect

the patient's present condition and the implications for nursing care. Current and significant past medical history should include any traumatic injury, childhood diseases, and pertinent family history (e.g., diabetes mellitus and hypertension). Current medication history should include tranquilizers, sedatives, anticoagulants, aspirin, anticonvulsants, alcohol, or drug dependencies or abuse.

Physical examination

Level of consciousness (LOC). LOC is assessed by asking questions designed to test orientation to person, place, and time, including recent and remote memory. Suggested descriptions of levels of consciousness are: (1) alert and oriented to person, place, and time (patient displays insight into his condition, recent and remote memory, talks willingly and coherently); (2) confused (patient may be quiet and cooperative or restless and irritable, is not oriented to time or place, and may begin to display delusions or hallucinations); (3) stupor (patient lethargic and difficult to arouse, responds only if tactile stimulus applied, does not respond purposefully to pressure or moderate pain); (4) coma (patient is unarousable, with no purposeful response to pressure or pain).

The Glasgow Coma Scale: Used to evaluate LOC, the Glasgow Coma Scale consists of three sections:

Section I, Eye Response:
- Grade 4, opens eyes spontaneously.
- Grade 3, opens eyes to speech.
- Grade 2, opens eyes to pain.
- Grade 1, does not open eyes.

Section II, Motor Response (score in relation to the affected side):
- Grade 6, obeys command.
- Grade 5, localizes pain.
- Grade 4, flexes and withdraws to pain.
- Grade 3, abnormal flexion to pain (decorticate posturing).
- Grade 2, abnormal extension to pain (decerebrate posturing).
- Grade 1, no response to pain (flaccid).

Section III, Verbal Response:
- Grade 5, oriented.
- Grade 4, disoriented but coherent.
- Grade 3, inappropriate.
- Grade 2, incoherent words or sounds.
- Grade 1, no verbal response.

The best score that can be obtained is 15, describing the patient who is awake, alert, oriented, and obeys commands. The scale is used to categorize patients and serves as the basis for therapy.

Movement and sensation. Voluntary motor activity in the upper extremities is assessed by asking the patient to grip the second and third fingers of the examiner's hands and noting whether the grip is of equal strength bilaterally. Voluntary motor activity in the legs is assessed by asking the patient to push his feet against the examiner's hands. If the patient does not respond to simple commands, motor reflex activity is tested with pressure or painful stimuli. Most voluntary activity originates in the motor cortex fibers, which are located in each posterior frontal lobe. Because the fibers cross in the medulla, voluntary movement initiated by the motor cortex is seen on the opposite side of the body. Therefore, loss of voluntary movement on one side of the body could result from damage to the motor cortex, internal capsule, or medulla on the opposite side of the body; or to the crossed pyramidal tract, ventral roots, spinal nerves, peripheral nerves, neuromuscular junctions, or muscles on the same side of the body. An appropriate response to painful stimulus in an unconscious patient is for the ipsilateral side to reach up toward the stimulus or to resist active movement. Painful stimulus to elicit a response is achieved by applying light-to-moderate thumb pressure to the bony ridge under the eyebrow, the supraorbital notch (Fig. 5–1). Caution must be observed to avoid eye injury. The patient with acute cerebral dysfunction will demonstrate **decorticate** posturing (*see* Fig. 5–1) in response to noxious stimulation. The patient lies with one or both arms in full flexion on the chest. Legs may be stiffly extended. Decorticate posturing indicates deep cerebral hemispheric lesions that are starting to press upon the upper brainstem. The

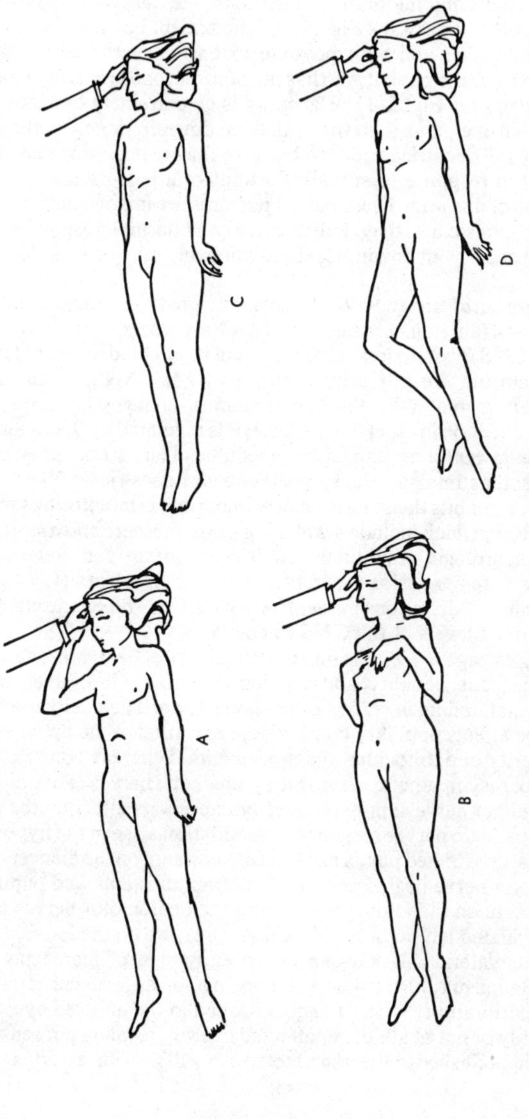

Figure 5–1. Postural responses of the unconscious patient. (A) Response to a noxious stimulus; (B) decorticate posturing; (C) decerebrate posturing; (D) flaccid posturing.

patient with an injury destroying the entire brainstem above the middle of the pons or with massive cerebral hemorrhages destroying or compressing the lower thalamus and midbrain will demonstrate **decerebrate** posturing on both sides of the body (*see* Fig. 5–1). The patient lies with one or both arms stiffly extended and with possible extension of the legs. **Flaccid** posturing describes the patient who has no motor response in any extremity when stimulated (*see* Fig. 5–1). Flaccidity is an extremely ominous sign, indicating extensive damage to the brainstem down to or across the pons. Very often the full decorticate, decerebrate, or flaccid posturing may not be demonstrated in response to stimuli. Portions of a posture may be seen, such as flexion of one arm. These partial postures are important to note and report to the physician; they indicate early abnormal responses. The postures may occur with or without stimulation and may be intermittent or continuous.

Neurologic vital signs. Vital signs can provide valuable clues to nervous system function. Changes in LOC are earlier, more sensitive indicators of CNS dysfunction. Vital signs can be affected by the voluntary nervous system but are primarily controlled by the ANS. Even though **temperature** is regulated by the hypothalamus, changes in temperature may indicate infection in other body sites. **BP** is regulated by the vasomotor center in the lower pons and upper medulla. The lateral area of the vasomotor center stimulates the sympathetic vasoconstrictor fibers, while the medial area inhibits them. Particularly important is monitoring for signs of increased ICP, which include a widening **pulse** pressure and a slow pulse rate. Other neurologic conditions requiring accurate and frequent BP readings are: vascular lesions, cerebral vascular accidents (CVA), and spinal cord injury. Alterations in **respiratory patterns** often correlate with lesions at various levels of the CNS (Table 5–4).

Pupillary changes. Pupils must be checked frequently in a darkened room for size, shape, equality, and reaction to light. Pupils of unequal size may be a normal finding in ~25% of the population. The oculomotor (3rd cranial) nerve affects pupillary constriction, elevation of the upper eyelid, and the majority of extraocular eye movements. Whereas constriction is caused by a parasympathetic nerve, the sympathetic nerves cause dilation. Pressure on either nerve supply reduces or cancels its effect on the pupil; e.g., the sympathetic nerves responsible for dilation arise in the hypothalamus, and thus, constricted pupils can indicate pressure on the diencephalon. The oculomotor nerve begins near the midbrain; thus enlarged pupils can indicate pressure on the midbrain. Because the oculomotor nerves do not decussate, a dilated left pupil could indicate pressure on the left midbrain. Bilateral or unilateral dilation can be an early sign of increasing ICP. Unilateral dilation may also indicate cerebral hemorrhage, uncal herniation, and rapid deterioration. When a light is flashed in the affected eye, it will react sluggishly or not at all; the unaffected eye will respond consensually. Similarly, a light flashed in the nonaffected eye will provide a normal reflex

TABLE 5–4

Respiratory Pattern Variations with CNS Injury

Pattern	Characteristics	Area involved
Cheyne-Stokes	Rhythms altered, hyperpnea to apnea.	May indicate deep cerebral or cerebullar lesions. May occur with upper brainstem injury.
Central neurogenic hyperventilation.	Sustained, rapid, forced inspiration and expiration.	May indicate a lesion of the midbrain. May indicate upper pons areas of the brainstem.
Apneustic	An end inspiratory pause, often followed by expiratory pause.	May indicate a lesion of the mid- or lower pons.
Cluster breathing	Irregular respirations alternating with periods of apnea.	May indicate a lesion of the lower pons or upper medulla.
Ataxic breathing	Irregular respirations with deep and shallow respirations; pauses may occur.	May indicate a lesion of the medulla.

but in the affected eye, it will produce a sluggish or absent consensual response. Increasing ICP next affects the fibers in the center of the oculomotor nerve that control eye movement; increased ICP causes diplopia and ptosis, and the eye looks downward and outward because of the unopposed abducens (6th cranial) nerve.

Reflexes. In an unconscious patient with cervical spinal injury, brainstem function can be quickly assessed by testing the **oculocephalic** reflex, also called "doll's eye" reflex or motion. The eyelids are held open and the head turned quickly, first to one side, then the other. A normal response is for the eyes to move in the opposite direction from the side to which the head is turned, i.e., if the head turns to the right, normal reflex would be for the eyes to move to the left. With severe brainstem involvement, the oculocephalic reflex disappears. Abnormal variations, such as nystagmus (constant cyclical movement of the eyeball), movement of both eyes in the direction the head is turned, or conjugate deviation (deviation of both eyes to either side), may also be seen. To elicit **Babinski's reflex** in the adult is abnormal. The normal response to stroking the lateral aspect of the sole of the foot is flexion of the toes. With a positive Babinski response, the great toe will dorsiflex and the other toes will spread apart, which may indicate an upper motor neuron lesion.

ICP monitoring. The generalized signs and symptoms of increased ICP are a nonspecific headache, blurred vision, decreased LOC, personality changes, nausea, vomiting, papilledema, and Cushing response (bradycardia and systemic hypertension). These signs may appear and indicate increased ICP, but only after pathologic changes have occurred; they do not reflect the degree of pressure elevation.

The three techniques for measuring ICP—intraventricular, epidural, and subarachnoid (subdural)—are described and compared in Table 5–5. Normal range of ICP is 4 to 14 mmHg, with some patients having excursions >100 mmHg.

ICP wave forms: Pulsations from the choroid plexus are transmitted to the CSF in the ventricular and subarachnoid space and produce a mechanical wave form that the transducer electronically converts to an electrical wave form. Normal and abnormal wave forms can be observed. The three types of abnormal wave forms are A waves, B waves, and C waves. On the graph paper the horizontal axis measures time in minutes and the vertical axis measures ICP in mmHg. The **normal** ICP wave form consists of a steep upward systolic slope. The normal range is 4 to 14 mmHg, or 5 to 20 mmH_2O. **Plateau,** or **A** waves, vary in intensity and amplitude and range from 50 to 100 mmHg from 5 to 20 min. These sustained pressure elevations occur on an already elevated mean ICP base line >15 to 20 mmHg. Plateau waves may indicate reduced cerebral perfusion pressure and brain cell hypoxia. **B** waves are sharp, rhythmic oscillations with a sawtooth pattern that may correspond to changes in respirations. B waves occur every half to two minutes and may elevate as high as 50 mmHg but are not sustained. **C** waves are smaller rhythmic oscillations that correspond to changes in BP. They may reach abnormal levels but are not sustained elevations. The significance of B and C waves is not certain; therefore, they are not clinically important.

A carpenter's level should be used to verify that the transducer is level with the patient's third ventricle (outer canthus of the eye). If the wave form morphology on the oscilloscope is damped (meaning depressed wave form), the physician should be consulted. If institutional standards permit flushing, the ICP catheter may be flushed slowly with the ordered amount and type of solution. (Standard saline vials should not be used; they contain alcohol, which can cause cortical necrosis). Aspiration is contraindicated; this technique may aspirate brain tissue into the screw. Neither flush devices nor heparin should be used because of the risk of causing small vessels to bleed. ICP should be measured when the patient is quiet. Activities such as coughing, turning head to one side, or using abdominal muscles to inspire will cause temporary increases in ICP. The transducer should be balanced and calibrated. Trends should be observed, rather than an isolated reading and the readings compared to the patient's base line rather than a standard.

Diagnostic tests

There are numerous procedures available to aid in assessing the location and extent of neurologic damage and prognosis for recovery. The following procedures are the ones most commonly performed on the critically ill patient.

TABLE 5–5

Comparison of Procedures for Measuring Intracranial Pressure

Technique	Procedure	Advantages	Disadvantages
Intraventricular	Catheter introduced into lateral ventricle and connected via pressure tubing and stopcock to pressure transducer. NS or lactated Ringer's solution is the fluid column between CSF and diaphragm of transducer dome.	Direct measure of pressure generated from CSF; provides access for determining volume challenge response; provides avenue for CSF drainage or sampling.	Risk of infection from invasive procedure; insertion of catheter difficult in case of shifting or collapse of ventricle; catheter may become occluded; necessary to recalibrate often.
Epidural	Placement of radio transmitter or fiber optic transducer between skull and dura.	Less invasive; sensor is easily placed; sensor not subject to occlusion; no need to recalibrate.	Accuracy of reflected CSF pressure questionable; no direct route for CSF drainage and sampling; not possible to obtain volume challenge response.
Subarachnoid	Insertion of a screw device through a hole into subdural or subarachnoid space. Transducer may be attached to screw or connected via pressure tubing.	Direct measure of pressure generated from CSF; cerebrum is not penetrated; provides access for determining volume challenge response; provides avenue for CSF drainage or sampling.	Risk of infection from invasive procedure; screw can become occluded; necessary to recalibrate often.

NS, normal saline.

Lumbar puncture. A lumbar puncture is performed to measure CSF pressure, to sample CSF for chemical analysis and for the presence of blood, to lower ICP, or to inject contrast media or medication. Bloody spinal fluid may indicate cerebral contusion, laceration, or subarachnoid hemorrhage. Samples of CSF can be obtained from the lumbar subarachnoid space of the spinal canal, the cisterna magna, and the lateral ventricles.

Queckenstedt test. This test is made when a spinal subarachnoid block from tumor or vertebral fracture is suspected. Normally there is a rapid rise in pressure of CSF in response to jugular compression, with rapid return to normal upon release of compression. Compression to the jugular veins manually or with BP cuff inflated to 20 mmHg for 10 sec during the lumbar puncture with the manometer attached will demonstrate a rise in pressure with compression and a *slow* drop in pressure during release of compression, if there is a block caused by a lesion compressing the spinal subarachnoid pathways. This test is not done if an intracranial lesion is suspected.

EEG. Electrodes applied to the scalp record the electrical activity of the brain, enabling the assessment of cerebral activity. It is useful to diagnose disorders that alter electrical patterns (seizure disorders, indication of brain death, coma, or organic brain syndrome).

Skull x-ray. The skull series reveals configuration, intracranial calcification, density vascular markings, and presence and size of tumors.

Brain scan. Brain scans can detect and evaluate neoplasm and stroke or follow up surgical or radiation therapy to the brain. A radioactive substance is administered either IV or PO, transmitted through the skull, and scanned either with a scanner, which prints out a picture based on the number of counts from the brain as it scans, or a gamma camera, which prints out an image without scanning.

CAT. The head is scanned in successive layers by a narrow x-ray beam. A computer analyzes the data to provide a cross-sectional view of the brain, distinguishing densities in the brain. Lesions appear as variations in tissue density, differing from normal brain tissue. CAT may identify tumor masses, ventricular collapse, brain infarction, hydrocephalus, or hemorrhage in the hemispheres, ventricles, cerebellum, or brainstem that cannot be detected by other procedures. IV contrast medium may be used to define lesion boundries more accurately.

Cerebral arteriography. X-ray study of the vascular system of the brain is made possible by injection of contrast media into the cerebral circulation. Cerebral arteriograms are useful in detecting aneurysms, occlusions, hematomas, tumors, or other lesions sizable enough to block or distort cerebral vessels.

Myelography. The injection of contrast medium or gas into the spinal subarachnoid space via spinal puncture for x-ray examination reveals distortion of the spinal cord, dural sac, or disk. Myelography is used to detect tumors or cysts or herniated intervetebral disks or other lesions.

MAJOR DISORDERS

CEREBRAL VASCULAR ACCIDENT

Pathophysiology

A CVA is the consequence of severe derangement in the blood supply to a portion of the brain. Events in the cerebral circulation that can impair brain function include thrombosis, hemorrhage, embolism, arterial spasm, and compression of cerebral vessels from an external clot, tumor, or swollen brain tissue. Stroke is a term used to describe pathologic events that involve brain tissue and result in neurologic deficits. CVA and stroke are terms used interchangeably.

Thrombosis is the most common cause of CVA. Occlusion of a cerebral vessel may be secondary to an inflammatory reaction in the vessel wall. Thrombosis causes ischemia of brain tissue and therefore edema and congestion in the surrounding areas. As the edema subsides, the brain may regain some functions that were impaired by the edema. Thrombosis may occur during MI or following surgery. It does not usually cause death unless it is massive.

Cerebral **embolism** is produced by such substances as fragments of clotted blood, fat, and bacterial vegetation released from the walls of the heart or valves, which lodge in the cerebral arterial system. Emboli cause necrosis and edema. If the embolus contains bacteria, the infection may extend beyond the walls of the vessel, and encephalitis may develop. If the infection remains contained within the occluded vessel, there may develop an aneurysm, which may rupture. Emboli frequently lodge in the middle cerebral artery.

Hemorrhage may occur outside the dura (extradural), beneath the dura (subdural), in the subarachnoid space (subarachnoid) or within the brain tissue (intracerebral). Intracerebral hemorrhage results from rupture of a cerebral vessel, usually an artery. Extravasations may come from veins and capillaries. Intracerebral hemorrhages usually cause the most extensive permanent functional deficits and the slowest recovery. Rupture of the cerebral artery leaks blood into or around the brain, which results not only in decreased blood supply to the part of the brain normally supplied by that artery, but compression of the surrounding arteries and damage to cells from accumulated blood. Hemorrhage may occur secondary to trauma, aneurysms, occasionally from neoplasms, during periods of anticoagulation therapy, or from disseminated intravascular coagulopathy (DIC). The most common cause of intracerebral hemorrhage is rupture of an arteriosclerotic vessel in the presence of hypertension. Intracerebral hemorrhage is massive and is the most common cause of death in the cerebrovascular disease groups.

Predisposing factors for CVA include hypertension, atherosclerotic plaque, cardiovascular diseases that contribute to emboli formation (coronary artery disease, mitral stenosis, arrhythmias, such as atrial fibrillation, infective endocarditis, rheumatic heart disease, cardiac enlargement, CHF), diabetes mellitus, family history of CVA, oral contraceptives, and cigarette smoking.

Clinical picture

CVAs produce a variety of neurologic symptoms. The patient may experience transient symptoms (e.g., headache or visual disturbances) or they may last indefinitely. The more severe CVA may have a sudden onset in which the patient falls unconscious. Flaccid and generalized or focal seizures may occur.

Warning symptoms include confusion, drowsiness, dizziness, and headache. Occasionally, secondary to a focal spasm or thrombosis of a vessel, symptoms such as transient loss of speech, hemiplegia, or paresthesia of one side of the body may precede the onset of a severe paralysis by a few hours or days.

Symptoms vary with the areas of the hemispheres involved. Hemorrhage compressing nerves on the left side of the brain causes right-sided hemiplegia and vice versa. The speech center in a right-handed person is on the brain's left side (the dominant hemisphere); therefore, hemorrhage in the left hemisphere often produces alterations in speech as well as right-sided hemiplegia. If the CVA involves the region of the thalamus, the symptoms will be manifested by a burning or aching dysesthesia in one half of the body and emotional lability with inappropriate crying or laughing. **Extensive cerebral involvement** often produces conjugate deviation of the eyes or head and eyes toward the side of the lesion. Generally, as the patient's condition improves, these symptoms resolve. Pupillary changes vary after CVA. Frequently, the pupils are unequal in size. Typically, the larger pupil is on the side opposite the cerebral lesion. Changes in reflexes, plantar responses, and other symptoms of focal brain damage are related to the lesion's site.

Except with ruptured aneurysms, CVAs do not cause sudden death. Intracerebral hemorrhage that ruptures into the ventricles is fatal and symptoms of increased ICP may develop. In patients with such fatal complications, there is a rise in temperature and an increase in respiratory and pulse rate before death as a result of damage to vital cerebral centers. The patient may lapse into coma.

Diagnosis makes use of evaluation tools such as skull x-ray, blood work, examination of CSF, EEG, brain scan, ventriculogram, cerebral angiography, or digital subtraction angiography.

Medical interventions

Medical management during the acute phase is aimed at keeping the patient alive and minimizing the extent of cerebral damage. Medications that may routinely be prescribed are: anticonvulsants, such as phenytoin or phenobarbital to prevent or treat seizures; steroids to treat cerebral edema;

antihypertensives if CVA is associated with hypertension; analgesics to treat headache associated with hemorrhagic CVA (aspirin is contraindicated in these patients because it can prolong bleeding time); antifibrinolytics such as aminocaproic acid (Amicar) to prevent rebleeding after the initial aneurysm rupture; stool softeners to maintain regular elimination; and anticoagulants for occlusive CVA.

Surgery may be performed to prevent further strokes in patients with transient ischemic attack (TIAs) or with a moderate completed CVA. Procedures include:

1. Carotid endarterectomy, which removes atherosclerotic plaques from the inner arterial wall.
2. Microvascular bypass. Candidates for this procedure include those with inaccessible carotid stenosis, basilar stenosis, middle cerebral artery stenosis, and/or occlusion. An extracranial vessel is anastomosed with an intracranial vessel, thus bypassing the stenosis or occlusion and creating collateral circulation.
3. Application of a clip to the neck of the cerebral aneurysm, allowing circulation to bypass the defective area.
4. Reinforcement of an inoperable cerebral aneurysm by wrapping the aneurysm with such material as muscle, fascia, muslin, or acrylic resins or other types of plastic.
5. Application of a carotid artery clamp that will reduce BP and flow within the aneurysm. The clamp is gradually tightened over several days to allow growth of collateral circulation to assist with compensating for the reduced blood flow.

Nursing interventions

Risk of aspiration. (1) Turn to the affected side (patient may demonstrate ballooning of the cheek on the affected side with expiration). (2) Suction mouth frequently.

Respiratory insufficiency caused by hypoxia and hypercapnia. (1) Monitor arterial blood gases (ABGs) (hypoxia and hypercapnia may cause increased CBF and ICP). (2) Insert artificial airway if stertorous respirations occur. (3) Suction frequently. Observe for increased ICP with endotracheal suctioning. (4) Assess for need for endotracheal intubation or tracheostomy.

Fluctuating neurologic vital signs. (1) Assess LOC. (2) Check pupil size, reaction to light, and ocular position to detect brainstem involvement from bleeding or infection. (3) Monitor motor function. Note the presence or absence of voluntary or involuntary movements of the extremities, muscle tone, body posture, position of the head, stiffness or flaccidity of the neck. (4) Monitor quality and rates of pulse, respirations, and BP. Elevated BP can reflect increased ICP or rebleeding. (5) Monitor temperature. Elevated temperature will increase CBF, and thus ICP.

Urine retention. (1) Monitor intake and output. (2) Insert Foley catheter prn. (3) Observe for renal calculi.

Arrhythmias. (1) Monitor for evidence of MI; for bradycardia, which may indicate increased ICP.

Disorientation when conscious. (1) Reorient the patient. (2) If patient aphasic, reassure that communication assistance will be given through speech therapist and staff.

Nutritional deficit. (1) Blend or strain food. (2) Provide supplemental vitamins. (3) Provide assistance with meals as needed. (4) Provide meticulous mouth care.

Electrolyte imbalance. (1) Monitor electrolyte balance. (2) Monitor arrhythmias that may result from electrolyte imbalance.

Pulmonary complications. Auscultate lung sounds for signs of pulmonary complications.

Potential skin breakdown. (1) Alternate patient's position frequently. (2) Utilize supportive aids such as eggshell or air mattress.

HEAD INJURY

Trauma to the head may cause fractures of the skull and injuries to the soft tissue such as contusions, edema, hemorrhage, or lacerations. Skull fractures (Table 5–6) become significant when brain tissue is depressed or lacerated or CSF leaks. The most significant effect of head injury is loss of consciousness. The duration of unconsciousness usually indicates the gravity of the injury. The resultant cerebral edema, cellular hypoxia, and prolonged periods of increased ICP may cause more damage than the initial injury.

A **cerebral concussion** is marked by momentary loss of consciousness; posttraumatic retrograde amnesia may occur.

TABLE 5–6

Skull fracture and clinical presentations

Location/type	Clinical picture
Linear	Swollen, ecchymotic, tender area of scalp.
Depressed	
Closed	Contusion, edema of scalp without a laceration.
Open	Scalp laceration; altered level of consciousness dependent on amount of brain damage.
Basal	
Anterior fossa	CSF rhinorrhea if dura is torn; bilateral ecchymotic eyes secondary to blood oozing into the sinuses (referred to as "raccoon's eyes"); injury to 1st cranial (olfactory) nerve.
Posterior fossa	Ecchymosis over the mastoid bone (referred to as Battle's sign); CSF otorrhea if dura is torn and tympanic membrane is ruptured; difficulty in hearing; cranial nerve injuries.

Actual bruising of the brain associated with temporary or permanent structural damage is described as **cerebral contusion.** Coup is the bruising of the brain tissue below the point of injury; countercoup is the rebound propulsion of the brain to the side opposite the injury. Coup-countercoup phenomenon is the consequence of an acceleration-deceleration injury. The opposing forces stress nerve fibers and blood vessels in the brainstem.

The skull encloses the brain in a nearly inexpansible container. When hemorrhage occurs after injury, there is little room to accommodate this increase in volume. Three common hematomas arise from hemorrhage.

Subdural hematoma

Subdural hematoma results from the accumulation of blood below the dura mater, usually from a tear in a cortical vein. It is thought that the venous bleeding stops by tamponade compression and a clot develops in the space between the dura and the arachnoidea and continues to enlarge by extracting fluid from surrounding tissues. A subdural clot is not confined and may spread over an entire hemisphere. An **acute subdural hematoma** develops more slowly than an epidural hematoma and is associated with cerebral contusions and lacerations. Symptoms of deterioration from a subdural hematoma begin within a few hours after injury. **Chronic subdural hematomas** may develop weeks after a injury by imbibing fluid into a small subdural hematoma. Any combination of lateralizing signs such as decorticate posturing and hemiparesis or cranial nerve palsies may be evidenced. There is usually a drastic change in the patient's LOC. Acute subdural hematomas may mimic or occur in conjunction with an epidural hematoma. The mortality rate for patients with an acute subdural hematoma is ~80%. The patient with chronic subdural hematomas with retrograde amnesia may not recall the injury. The bleeding progresses slowly. The hematoma begins as a small clot, comprised of protein and decomposed blood. The dura and arachnoidea encase the mass, which eventually will calcify or slow bleeding from small vessels within the lining of the clot will continue. Symptoms depend upon (1) the size of the clot, (2) the rate of blood accumulation, and (3) how much brain mass is displaced by the clot. Symptoms are present one moment, not the next. The patient may have a headache over the affected region or behind the eye and may experience subtle changes in personality. Certain symptoms, such as clumsiness in one hand or mild hemiparesis, may go unnoticed. As the clot exerts pressure against the brain mass, the brain begins to shift, causing a downward compression of diencephalic and midbrain structures. Eventually, tentorial herniation may result in fatality unless the clot is evacuated. If the clot is evacuated through trephinations (burr holes), the prognosis for recovery is good.

Epidural hematoma

Epidural hematomas present as rapidly expanding mass lesions, which lie in the epidural space between the skull and dura mater. They may be caused by trauma to the middle meningeal artery or the dural sinus. Temporoparietal skull fractures often cause epidural hematomas. Classically an epidural hematoma is associated with a history of a brief loss of consciousness. A lucid period follows, after which the patient lapses into unresponsiveness. Lateralized symptoms such as unilateral or bilateral hemiparesis, ipsilateral dilating pupils, focal seizures, or positive Babinski's sign are typical results of an epidural hematoma. Incipient tentorial herniation may occur. Pulse is slow and bounding, respirations are slow, BP elevates (Cushing phenomenon), indicating increased ICP. This clinical picture is not always present, however, and the most important sign presented will be deterioration in the LOC.

Intracerebral hematoma

Multiple small hematomas may accompany a head injury. A single subcortical hematoma may form in the area of the contusion or lacerated brain or at a distance from the initial injury. The symptoms of an intracerebral hematoma are indistinguishable from those of epidural and subdural hematomas. Diagnostic procedures are similar. Generally, increased ICP and focal symptoms develop a few hours or days after the injury. Surgical interventions offer poor results because of damage to the brain caused by the hemorrhage.

Medical interventions

The initial medical objectives are to determine the precise location of the lesion, distinguish between epidural and subdural hematomas, and then intervene to sustain life and minimize brain damage. Medical management may consist of medications such as steroids (dexamethasone) and osmotic diuretics (mannitol) to reduce cerebral edema. Research suggests that dexamethasone is able to stabilize the endothelial cell membrane to support the junction between these cells, thus preventing loss of serum protein and fluid into the extracellular brain spaces. Mannitol, urea, and hypertonic solutions increase osmolality, resulting in a transfer of fluid from extracellular brain spaces into the blood. This diuretic effect is limited to one or two dosages, however, because solutes from the edematous tissue will pull fluid back into the brain tissue (rebound effect).

Barbiturates are used to induce coma by depressing the reticular activating system. Barbiturate therapy causes a decreased rate of cerebral metabolism, which results in decreased glucose utilization and O_2 demand, which in turn may improve neuronal survival in ischemic brain tissue. Indications for barbiturate therapy are ICP levels >20 mmHg for >30 min and unresponsive to the usual therapeutic modalities. The decrease in ICP during barbiturate therapy may be a consequence of cerebral vasoconstriction, decreased blood volume, and decreased rate of CSF production and secretion. A base-line EEG and brainstem-evoked responses should be done before administering barbiturate therapy and a further series done during barbiturate therapy to assess brainstem functioning.

Surgical interventions include: (1) craniotomy (surgical opening of the skull to remove a tumor, relieve ICP, evacuate a blood clot, or stop hemorrhage); (2)craniectomy (excision of a portion of the skull); and (3) cranioplasty (repair of a cranial defect).

Nursing interventions

Ineffective respirations. (1) Suction endotracheal tube to maintain a clear airway. (2) Observe for elevations of ICP. (3) Monitor ABGs; keep PCO_2 between 25 and 30 mmHg to restrict cerebral blood vessels, reducing CBF, and thus reducing ICP. (4) Maintain mechanical ventilatory assistance.

Hypovolemic shock secondary to multiple injuries. (1) Avoid Trendelenburg's position, which will elevate ICP. (2) Elevate legs; keep the head of bed elevated 15 to 30 degrees.

Infection. (1) Administer antibiotics, tetanus toxoid per physician's order with scalp lacerations or open skull fractures. (2) Observe meticulous aseptic technique during dressing changes.

Decreased LOC. (1) Assess responsiveness. (2) Assess focal motor ability. (3) Assess pupillary reactions and size. (4) Assess vital signs.

Suppressed LOC during barbiturate therapy. (1) Monitor ICP levels; if the BP remains <90 mmHg, initiate vasopressors per physician's order. (2) Monitor CPP. (3) Maintain CPP between 60 and 70 mmHg. (4) Monitor serum barbiturate levels. (5) Monitor all available parameters (e.g., pulmonary artery measurements).

Fluid and electrolyte imbalance. (1) Monitor serum osmolality, electrolytes, BUN, creatinine, output and intake.

Nutritional deficit. (1) Maintain nutritional status. (2) Administer parenteral hyperalimination per physician's order. (3) Maintain nasogastric tube feedings when barbiturate therapy has been discontinued; bowel sounds and function will return slowly.

Potential for skin breakdown, contractures, thrombi. (1) Reposition frequently. (2) Use devices to prevent skin breakdown.

Family anxiety. (1) Provide opportunities for expression. (2) Assist in understanding and coping with patient's comprehensive care.

SEIZURES

A seizure is a paroxysmal, episodal event that causes a disruption in the patient's ongoing mental or behavioral activities. The transient impairment of cerebral function may be manifested by motor, sensory, or psychic phenomena. The common factor in all seizure types is the occurrence of dysrhythmic electrical disturbances of characteristic form and voltage as seen on the EEG. Seizure activity is classified using the characteristic configuration and spikes and waves. A patient has **epilepsy** if there are recurring seizures caused by a primary defect in the brain and not by an extracerebral defect or complication of a transient insult. Most seizures are self-limiting, lasting from 3 to 5 min; in **status epilepticus,** however, seizures are prolonged or occurring at such frequency that the patient does not recover from one episode to the next. Seizures have been classified into two main types: partial and generalized. **Partial,** or focal, seizures result from local disturbances in the brain; there may or may not be loss of consciousness associated. **Generalized** seizures result from a diffuse discharge from the CNS. The etiology of epilepsy includes trauma, birth injuries, infectious disease (e.g., encephalitis), structural lesions, cerebrovascular disease, degenerative diseases (e.g., multiple sclerosis), metabolic disorders, and hereditary factors.

Pathophysiology

Seizure activity is generated by electrical disturbances in the brain. Nerve cells that discharge multiple rapid impulses regardless of the message received are called epileptic cells. Some cells are more susceptible to abnormal electrical activity than others, e.g., hippocampal cells found in the temporal lobe. The resting potential for the hippocampal cells is close to the threshold potential; also, hippocampal potentials are long and decrease slowly to the resting state, which allows for minute external discharges to cause the cell to fire repeatedly.

Clinical picture

Seizures can be described by their clinical signs.

Grand mal (major motor). These seizures produce loss of consciousness, opisthotonos (arched back), and tonic and clonic movements of all extremities. Tonic convulsion refers to the persistent, nonatrophic contraction of a muscle or set of muscles. Clonic convulsion refers to alternating contraction and relaxation of opposing muscle groups producing a jerky, convulsive movement. Many patients experience an aura while conscious: A personalized warning—consisting of a temporary visual, olfactory, or auditory sensation—may precede the seizure. Bladder and bowel incontinence may occur during the seizure. The patient may remain unconscious for several minutes, awakening in a confused, drowsy state followed by sleep. Todd's paralysis, a temporary paresis or paralysis of the extremities, may occur after the clonic phase. The patient may have no recall of the event upon awakening.

Petit mal (absence attacks). These seizures may be inherited and usually occur in childhood. Petit mal seizures have no aura and are shorter in duration (5 to 30 sec). A blank stare indicative of transient clouding of consciousness may be the only symptom. This type of seizure may occur several times a day and may go unnoticed.

Psychomotor (temporal lobe). These usually occur in the adult and produce automatisms (the repetition of inappropriate acts, such as lip smacking, disrobing, hand wringing). These episodes are sometimes confused with psychic equivalents such as déjà vu and hysteria. Post-seizure amnesia follows.

Jacksonian seizures (focal). These seizures result from focal irritation of a part of the motor cortex and may remain localized in the appropriate peripheral area, such as a hand or foot, and progress to other muscle groups and may progress to a grand mal seizure. Consciousness maybe retained in focal seizures, along with transient postictal weakness in the affected muscle group.

Laboratory findings. CSF change is the only abnormality to be found, with a slight increase in CSF protein and WBC count. Skull x-rays may reveal abnormal calcifications, pineal shift, or signs of increased ICP.

Radioactive isotope brain scanning and CAT will locate the site of focal lesions. The EEG remains the most valuable diagnostic tool.

Medical interventions

Nonemergent seizures are controlled with medications such as phenytoin (Dilantin), diazepam (Valium), primidone (Mysline), carbamazepine (Tegretol), ethosuximide (Zarontin), and barbiturates. Status epilepticus, or sustained grand mal activity, is an emergency situation with potential lethal outcome, requiring immediate intervention. The goal of medical management for status epilepticus is to prevent the development of hypovolemia. A variety of pharmacologic regimens to abort the seizure produce response in ~75% of patients within several hours; however, ~25% may require three or four days to respond to any regimen. Complications that may develop during the status epilepticus episode include respiratory depression, cardiac arrest, prolonged coma, hypotension, and aspiration pneumonia.

Diazepam is the drug of choice to suppress seizure activity rapidly. It is given IV in doses ≤10 mg over 3 min. The initial IV dose may be repeated in 20 min, because the patient may begin to seize after the initial effect has dissipated. Diazepam is supplemented with phenytoin. An appropriate alternative to phenytoin is phenobarbital.

Blood samples are screened for toxicology, barbiturates, phenothiazines, narcotics, alcohol, and phenytoin.

If the above regimens are unsuccessful over a 12-to-24-hr period, general anesthesia, which will require intubation, is suggested.

If seizures cause brain damage, surgical procedures may be performed to control them. The neurosurgeon may implant electrodes through burr holes, usually over the temporal or frontal lobes. The implanted electrodes are left in place for 1 to 3 wk. During that period the patient is observed for signs of infection or neurologic deficit. An area of abnormal discharge may be removed surgically. This procedure is limited to those patients with intractable seizures after an intensive medical regimen. These patients are often those with focal motor or psychomotor seizures.

Nursing interventions

Inadequate ventilation. (1) Place an oral airway prior to tonic, clonic movements. (2) Monitor patient's cardiopulmonary status.

Injury during seizure. (1) Maintain a safe environment during seizure activity. (2) Pad the side rails and headboard.

Seizure activity not controlled by therapeutics. (1) Observe and report seizure activities, noting type of aura, duration of the seizure, time, type of tonic, clonic, flaccid movement, LOC. (2) Observe reflexes: bilateral Babinski's signs are common after grand mal seizures; unilateral Babinski's reflexes may indicate a contralateral hemisphere lesion. (3) Note pupillary changes: pupils may constrict, then dilate and remain nonreactive to light. Eyes will deviate away from the hemisphere with the focal leison. (4) Administer medications prescribed. (5) Assess for adverse effects.

Psychological implications. (1) Reinforce education about the disease and its symptoms. (2) Assist the family and patient to understand the importance of the benefit to adapting to normal settings.

MENINGITIS

Pathophysiology

Meningitis is an acute inflammation of the pia-arachnoid membrane in the spinal cord or brain. Meningitis can be caused by almost any pathogenic bacteria, but commonly it is caused by the gram-negative diplococcus *Neisseria meningitidis.* Multiplication of the organisms in the blood produces a fulminating septicemia. Pathogenic microorganisms gain access to the meninges and subarachnoid space. Possible causes of meningitis are infections of the head and face, such as otitis media, mastoiditis, ruptured brain abscess, sinusitis, or tonsillitis, infections in the bones, skin, lungs, or heart valves that are transmitted to the meninges by the vascular system, and trauma or surgery. *Haemophilus influenzae* may cause a viral meningitis.

Clinical picture

Symptoms of meningitis include temperature elevation, rash, malaise and lethargy, headache, stiff neck, and pain while moving the neck. Kernig's and Brudzinski's signs are two classic signs of meningitis. Signs of sepsis usually occur with the rash, including shaking chills, low BP, rapid, shallow respirations, and overwhelming bacteremia. Increasing ICP may lead to headache, generalized convulsions, nausea, vomiting, dilated or irregular pupils, papilledema, elevated BP, and Cheyne-Stokes respirations.

CSF may be clear to purulent. A gram stain reveals diplococci, and the WBC is elevated. Total protein is increased and sugar decreased.

Medical interventions

Antibiotic therapy is the chief treatment modality. Sulfonamides, penicillins, and aminoglycosides in massive doses are the primary drugs of choice. Reduction of increased ICP and/or hyperthermia are also goals.

Nursing interventions

Infectious process. (1) Enforce isolation precautions as necessary. (2) Administer prescribed antibiotics. (3) Monitor the side effects of these potent antibiotics. (4) Monitor patient's temperature. (5) Use tepid sponge baths, prescribed antipyretic drugs, and hypothermia for elevated temperatures. (6) Minimize light and noise, because the patient's sensitivity to external stimuli is increased.

Complications. (1) Monitor neurologic vital signs. (2) Assess patient for vasoconstriction, which may indicate impending coma. (3) Observe for seizure activity.

Anxiety of patient and family. (1) Answer questions. (2) Offer support. (3) Explain to the family about the disease and its treatment.

SPINAL CORD INJURY

Pathophysiology

Trauma to the vertebral column may include concurrent injuries to the head, thorax, and extremities. It is of great concern because of the possibility that an incomplete injury may extend to a complete one. Injury to nerves, soft tissue, and intervertebral disks can lead to laceration and contusion of delicate tissues, fractures, dislocation, paralysis, paresthesia, spinal shock, and motor dysfunction.

During spinal injury, displaced bone may encroach on the spinal canal and compress the cord, interrupting its blood supply. The spinal cord's arterial system does not have extensive collateral circulation. Trauma to the spinal column may completely sever or partially damage the cord. When the cord is transected, it is, in effect, separated from the brain; afferent impulses cannot ascend from below the level of the lesion to the brain, and efferent impulses cannot descend to body areas innervated below the break in the cord's continuity. During the early stages of cord injury, it may be impossible to determine if the cord has actually been transected or traumatized. Complete transection may produce loss of all sensation, spastic paralysis, impaired sexual functioning, and vasomotor instability.

Clinical picture

Cervical injury may cause quadriplegia. Respiratory failure may occur as a result of injury above C-4, which affects the diaphragm and intercostal muscles. The patient experiences paralysis of bowel and bladder function, is unable to void and has bowel incontinence. There may be temperature elevation initially, because perspiration may not occur in paralyzed regions below the level of the cord injury. At a later stage, excessive perspiration may occur in the unaffected regions. **Thoracic injury** may cause paraplegia. Typically, bowel and bladder functions are paralyzed initially. A flaccid paralysis is usually followed by a spastic paralysis. **Lumbar** and **sacral injury** may cause paralysis of the lower extremities and the bowel and bladder, which remain flaccid.

Fractures of the cervical spinal area commonly result from acute hyperflexion of the neck, crushing the body of one or more cervical vertebrae. C-5 and C-6 and L-1 and L-5 are the most common sites for injury. C-5 and C-6 are enlarged at that area because of the many nerve fibers that feed the upper extremities, and maximum movement of the cervical spine occurs at this level, making C-5 and C-6 susceptible to injury. Likewise L-1 and L-5 are the sites of a great number of nerve fibers that feed the lower extremities.

Spinal shock may occur immediately after spinal cord trauma. Spinal shock, or areflexia, is a sudden neurovascular shutdown response. It is indicated by hypotension, which results from loss of vascular tone below the injury level. Bradycardia is seen, and there is also hypothermia, with no sweating below the injury level, and flaccid paralysis with bowel and bladder atony. Patients with upper motor neuron lesions may experience sacral reflexes and priapism. Patients with lower motor neuron lesions have no reflex activity.

Medical interventions

The objectives of medical management are much the same as for the patient with a head injury and include: (1) preservation of life; (2) prevention of further neurologic deficits; (3) prevention of complications; (4) prevention of deformity.

The patient with cervical injuries may be immobilized with skeletal traction (e.g., skull tongs, such as Crutchfield or Gardner-Wells, or halo device). While in skeletal traction the patient may be cared for on a Stryker frame or CircOlectric bed. The phrenic nerve stimulator may be used for patients with injuries above C-4. Conservative treatments involve injection of a basic polypeptide aprotinin (Prasylol) into the affected intravertebral disk to diminish pressure from swelling and reduce associated nerve-root compression. Or neurosurgical procedures may be undertaken to remove the damaged disk.

Nursing interventions

Potential for increased damage to the spinal cord. (1) Maintain immobilization of the spine to obtain a pull along the axis of the cervical spine while the head is in a neutral position. (2) Observe for symptoms of neurologic damage. (3) Assess patient frequently for motor and sensory changes from cord edema, transection, or postoperative hematoma. (4) Record and report loss of sensation or inability to move extremities. (5) If patient in a Stryker frame or CircOlectric bed, keep position extended, not twisted. (6) Maintain a patent airway; respiratory problems from paralysis of intercostal and abdominal muscles are seen with quadriplegic patients.

Potential for experiencing autonomic dysreflexia, or hyperreflexia. (1) Observe for and report the following symptoms: severe pounding headache; shivering followed by profuse sweating above the injury level;

sudden hypotension; bradycardia; flushed skin above the injury level; fast, pounding pulse followed by a progressively slowing pulse. (Patients with injuries above T-8 are at high risk.) (2) Prevent the most common stimuli from initiating dysreflexia, i.e., bladder distension or fecal impactions. (3) Elevate the head. (4) Relieve the causative factor. (5) Call the physician if persistant. (6) Prevent decubiti, which may develop within 6 hr because of inadequate peripheral circulation. (7) Maintain alignment to prevent contractures.

Nutritional deficit. (1) Encourage a high-calorie, high-protein diet to compensate for increased catabolic activity and lack of appetite.

Alteration in psychological stability. (1) Allow patient to use coping mechanism to adapt. (2) Allow patient to control his environment. (3) Allow family to be included in counseling sessions. (4) Provide sexual counseling when patient is ready.

MYASTHENIA GRAVIS

Myasthenia gravis is a disorder of neuromuscular transmission in the voluntary muscles of the body and is characterized by excessive fatigability of muscle function. It primarily affects young women and older men. It may occur in a transient form in infants born to a mother with myasthenia.

Pathophysiology

Myasthenia gravis is characterized by a deficiency of acetylcholine at the myoneural junction. As a result, the skeletal muscle fails to receive the motor impulse properly and fails to contract well or at all. Possible causes of the pathologic deficiency are: (1) presynaptic deficiency in production of acetylcholine; (2) a disturbance of the endplate (postsynaptic); or (3) an abnormality in the muscle fiber itself.

It has also been suggested that myasthenia gravis is produced by an autoimmune mechanism that destroys or inactivates the sensitive acetylcholine-receptor substance. About 80% of myasthenic patients have an antibody to the receptor that can bind to the motor endplate and functionally interfere with neuromuscular transmission. The thymus gland plays an important role in the immunologic process and is implicated in myasthenia gravis. An infectious or neoplastic inflammatory process within the gland could induce intrinsic lymphocytes to produce an antiacetylcholine-receptor antibody that has the potential for cross-reaction with acetylcholine-receptor protein in peripheral skeletal muscle.

Clinical picture

Symptoms in most patients begin with double vision caused by ocular muscle dysfunction and, often, drooping of one or both eyelids. Dysarthria, dysphagia, or dyspnea may occur; or any striated muscle in the body may be involved. A patient with myasthenia often appears in good health upon examination. The face may appear sleepy because of ptosis. Often the limb weakness is asymmetric. Remissions and exacerbations are common. The distribution of weakness is the key clue to diagnosing myasthenia gravis.

To differentially diagnose myasthenia gravis, an anticholinesterase drug is administered and the patient's strength then recorded. Most commonly used are edrophonium chloride (Tensilon) and neostigmine methylsulfate (Prostigmin). By inhibiting the action of acetylcholinesterase, these drugs effectively increase the concentration of acetylcholine at the postsynaptic membrane. Edrophonium effects last a brief time; neostigmine lasts ≤2 hr. After administration of either drug, there is a quantifiable temporary improvement in maintenance of upward gaze or shoulder flexion, which appears within 15 min, with a peak effect in 30 min.

Medical interventions

Management includes **anticholinesterase therapy.** Pyridostigmine bromide (Mestinon) 180 mg PO tid is the usual initial medication. Excessive pyridostigmine results in supramaximal levels of acetylcholine at the postsynaptic membrane and a functional depolarizing block (cholinergic crisis). Symptoms include nausea, vomiting, abdominal cramps, diarrhea, and bronchial hypersecretion. Other drugs used are neostigmine (Prostigmin) and ambenonium (Mytelase). Certain drugs such as magnesium sulfate, morphine or its derivatives, curare, procainamide, quinine, quinidine, and chlorpromazine have been known to increase the muscular weakness and should not be administered. Smoking, drinking, prolonged exposure to the sun, and cold weather may also increase symptoms.

Corticosteroid therapy has been shown to be of benefit, but the most effective method of administration is debatable. ACTH has been used. Although it is not a corticosteroid, it does stimulate the adrenals to increase the circulating corticosteroid level. Many physicians feel that chronic corticosteroid therapy seems to produce a more profound and lasting improvement in myasthenia patients than ACTH.

Thymectomy is used for the management of patients for whom control with anticholinesterase therapy is inadequate. The procedure results in clinical improvement in majority of patients and remission in a moderate number of patients.

Other treatments include procedures such as immunosuppression, thoracic duct drainage, and plasmapheresis, which prove useful in certain refractory crisis situations. Plasmapheresis may be combined with immunosuppressive drug therapy to bring the propensity to synthesize acetylcholine-receptor antibody under control.

Nursing interventions

Progressive muscle weakness, fatigue. (1) Observe and report changes in appearance, the degree of ptosis or facial muscle drooping, and posture. (2) Provide adequate rest, balanced with moderate activity and exercise. (3) Administer medication precisely on time; a delay may worsen symptoms, especially in those with swallowing problems. (4) Monitor for signs of dysphagia. (5) Time meals to occur when there is peak anticholinesterase effect. (6) Keep suction equipment available.

Potential for respiratory failure. (1) Monitor for signs of dyspnea.

Fear of dependency. (1) Allow patient to control his environment. (2) Make the patient feel that attention is given to his individuality. (3) Discuss hopeful aspects of the disease.

Education. (1) Instruct the patient about the importance, action, and side effects of the medication regimen. (2) Emphasize that concurrent illness should be avoided. (3) Encourage patient to wear the Medic Alert identification bracelet.

MULTIPLE SCLEROSIS

Multiple sclerosis is a chronic, progressive disease of the CNS and is characterized by a patchy loss of myelin in the brain and spinal cord.

Pathophysiology

Hypotheses concerning the etiology of multiple sclerosis include viral infection and autoimmune process. Plaques or patches of demyelination are scattered throughout the CNS, affecting the white matter. Because the lesions of multiple sclerosis are diffuse, the symptoms are highly variable.

Clinical picture

The signs and symptoms reflect the location and areas of demyelinization within the CNS. There are remissions and exacerbations.

The patient may present with: (1) weakness, paresthesia of the extremities; (2) abnormal reflexes; (3) tremor, ataxia, incoordination; (4) impaired sense of position; (5) emotional lability; (6) slurred speech.

Diagnostic measures such as evoked-response measurements help to assess such neuronal disorders as multiple sclerosis where lesions may not be apparent clinically. If lesions are 1.5 cm in diameter or larger, a brain scan may be useful in documenting them. Contrast CAT scans may provide another means of locating new lesions.

Medical interventions

The aims of treatment are to help the patient achieve maximum physical capacity and optimum psychosocial adjustment and increase resistance to infection. No specific treatment or cure is known to alter the course of the disease. ACTH may be effective in lessening the intensity or shortening the duration of an acute exacerbation of symptoms. Corticosteroid use remains controversial. Improved care and the use of chemotherapeutic and antibiotic agents in the treatment of secondary complications have prolonged the lives of many patients.

Considerable research is focusing on finding an effective curative treatment for patients with multiple sclerosis.

Nursing interventions

Muscle spasticity. (1) Instruct patient to avoid muscle fatigue. (2) Administer muscle relaxants (diazepam) as ordered. (3) Encourage the patient to do muscle stretching exercises daily to minimize joint contractures.

Muscular weakness and poor coordination. (1) Assist the patient with physical therapy exercises in overcoming incoordination. (2) Refer the patient to resources such as social service, visiting nurse service, Multiple Sclerosis Society, occupational and physical therapy.

Potential for urinary tract infections. (1) Instruct the patient on intermittant self-catheterization, if directed.

GUILLAIN-BARRÉ SYNDROME

Guillain-Barré syndrome is an acute, rapidly progressive disorder characterized by polyneuritis in the extremities and usually occurring after a viral infection.

Pathophysiology

The etiology of Guillain-Barré syndrome is unknown. One theory suggests enteroneuritis may cause a polyneuropathy. Another theory suggests there is demyelination and degeneration of the myelin sheath of peripheral nerves.

Clinical picture

In the acute phase the patient experiences mild tingling or sensations of hands and feet falling asleep. At first, rest may alleviate the paresthesia, then in 1 to 4 days paresthesia becomes constant. Although ascending paralytic progression is typical, descending paralysis, beginning with the cranial nerves or upper extremities, has also been noted. Sensory loss may occur but is less severe than motor loss. Other symptoms in the acute phase include vague malaise, loss of swallowing and gag reflex, and difficulty breathing.

The patient may present with a history of viral infection 2 to 3 wk prior to the onset of symptoms and progressive, ascending weakness. Physical examination may reveal muscle weakness with symmetric involvement; distal muscles are most severely affected. Cranial nerve involvement is demonstrated by symptoms of dysphagia and facial weakness. There is decreased vital capacity secondary to weakness of respiratory muscles.

The diagnosis of Guillain-Barré syndrome may be confirmed by CSF examination, which may reveal an elevation of protein and no leukocytes.

Medical interventions

Accurate diagnosis and supportive therapy are essential. Medical management begins with diagnosing. Supportive ventilation is usually required. It is difficult to predict the course of the disease, how rapidly, and to what extent it will progress, as well as how long it will take to resolve.

Nursing interventions

Once the diagnosis is made, supportive care is instituted. The patient with Guillain-Barré provides the nursing staff with a challenge because the patient must be maintained throughout the acute phase and encouraged during the rehabilitative phase.

Respiratory failure. (1) Assess respiratory status. (2) Maintain a patent airway with endotracheal intubation or tracheostomy prn. (3) Remove bronchial secretions. (4) Monitor ABGs.

Autonomic dysfunction. (1) Monitor vital signs. Wide fluctuations in BP and pulse rate may indicate autonomic dysfunction.

Cranial nerve dysfunction. (1) Assist patient to communicate by finding an alternative. (2) Reassure patient that you will check on his needs frequently. (3) Update the care plan according to what method of communication works best for the patient. (4) Prevent sensory deprivation by encouraging use of a clock, radio, calendar, television. (5) Talk to patient whenever entering the room.

Discomfort from abnormal sensations. (1) Position the patient comfortably. (2) Administer a mild analgesic as directed.

Potential for skin breakdown and contractures. (1) Avoid vigorous exercise, which may increase demyelination. (2) Instruct patient and family on the implications and necessity for avoidance of vigorous exercise.

Nutritional deficit caused by losing gag and swallowing reflex. (1) Monitor the degree of gag and swallowing reflex, especially prior to meals. (2) Assist patient with meals. (3) Have suction equipment available. (4) Maintain high-caloric, high-protein nasogastric feedings as directed. (5) Administer enteral/parenteral nutrition prn.

Depression owing to sudden dependency. (1) Encourage patient and family to talk of fears. (2) Reassure that this syndrome usually disappears and that normal functioning will return.

CHAPTER 6

THE ENDOCRINE SYSTEM

Anita Rubbo Gorman and Michael Hickey

The function of the "core" systems—the heart, lungs, brain, and kidneys—is wholly dependent upon the maintenance of a stable, hospitable biochemical environment. The endocrine system, that extremely powerful regulator of homeostasis, provides such an environment. Constantly responding to minute changes in the chemical composition of the body and to external stressors, the endocrine glands regulate water and electrolyte balance, acid-base balance, the metabolism of nutrients, and the response to stress. This chapter will discuss the characteristics of the major hormone systems and the effects of derangements in their function.

THE PITUITARY GLAND

ANATOMY AND PHYSIOLOGY REVIEW

The pituitary gland, or hypophysis, lies at the base of the brain, connected to the hypothalamus by a narrow stalk. The pituitary is often called the master gland, because its hormones direct the activity of several other endocrine glands. The pituitary is made up of two distinct portions, the anterior and posterior, each with very different cellular structure and functions.

Anterior pituitary

The anterior pituitary, also called the adenohypophysis, produces two types of hormones. It regulates the ovarian cycle by its production of follicle-stimulating hormone, luteinizing hormone, and luteotropic hormone. More important in critical care practice is its production of **tropic**

hormones, which regulate the size and activity of other glands. The production of these tropic hormones is in turn regulated by **releasing** or **inhibiting** hormones produced in the hypothalamus. The interplay of the hypothalamus, anterior pituitary, and target glands is presented in Figure 6–1.

Negative feedback regulation is an extremely important feature of these hypothalamic-pituitary-peripheral gland systems. In negative feedback, rising levels of the peripheral hormone inhibit release of the appropriate releasing and tropic hormones. For example, as plasma cortisol levels rise, there is inhibition of the release of **corticotropin-releasing factor** (CRF) from the hypothalamus and **adrenocorticotropic hormone** (ACTH) from the pituitary. This negative feedback system provides for precise metabolic control and can provide important diagnostic clues in endocrine disease.

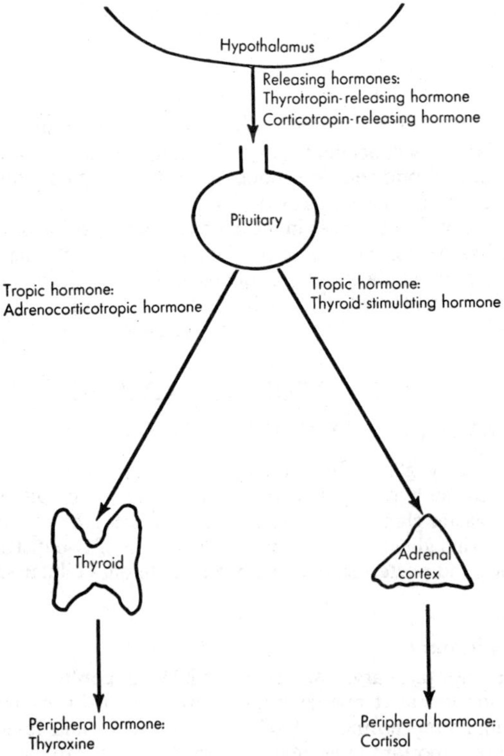

Figure 6–1. Relationship of hypothalamus, anterior pituitary, and target gland.

The role of the anterior pituitary will be discussed further as it relates to specific endocrine glands.

Posterior pituitary

The posterior pituitary, also called the neurohypophysis, is not a true gland, as it does not produce any hormones. Rather, it is a storage area for hypothalamic hormones. The two hormones associated with the posterior pituitary, **oxytocin** and **antidiuretic hormone (ADH)**, are produced in the hypothalamus and then transported via nerve fibers to the neurohypophysis for storage and release. Release of these hormones from the hypothalamus continues even if the pituitary gland is removed. The advantage of such an indirect delivery system is that reserves of the hormones can be available for immediate release when needed.

ADH. ADH acts on the collecting tubules of the kidneys, increasing their permeability to water, which enables free water to pass out of the tubules and back into the circulation, leaving behind it a concentrated urine. In the absence of ADH, water is not reabsorbed from the now nonpermeable collecting ducts, and a dilute urine is excreted. By regulating the absorption or excretion of free water, ADH controls the osmolality of the ECF. Figure 6–2 demonstrates the normal control of serum osmolality by ADH, beginning with an increased osmolality.

It can be seen that if the system is operating properly, concentrated, or hyperosmolal, serum will result in the production of concentrated urine, as free water is retained. Similarly, a dilute serum will result in the excretion of a dilute urine, as free water is excreted in an attempt to normalize serum osmolality.

Serum osmolality, as determined by hypothalamic osmoreceptors, is

Serum osmolality increased

⇩

Raised serum osmolality sensed by hypothalamic osmoreceptors

⇩

Osmoreceptors stimulate ADH release

⇩

ADH causes free water absorption from collecting tubules

⇩

Concentrated urine excreted; retained free water "dilutes" serum, lowering osmolality

⇩

Lowered osmolality sensed by osmoreceptors; ADH production curtailed

Figure 6–2. **Control of serum osmolality by antidiuretic hormone (ADH).**

the major determinant of ADH production. Other factors that increase ADH release include: (1) hypovolemia; (2) pain and stress; (3) hypotension; (4) nausea; (5) manipulation of bowel during surgery; (6) angiotensin II; and (7) hypoxemia. Factors that decrease ADH release include: (1) ethyl alcohol, and (2) cortisol.

While the prime role of ADH is the regulation of osmolality, it may sometimes function as a means of maintaining fluid volume. If the body's homeostatic mechanisms obey any one single overriding principle, it is that adequate fluid volume be maintained at all times. In hypovolemic or hypotensive states, ADH release will proceed even if serum osmolality is normal or low.

DIABETES INSIPIDUS

Pathophysiology

Diabetes insipidus (DI) results from the inability of the hypothalamus to produce ADH or a decrease in the ability of the kidney to respond to ADH. The resultant impermeability of the renal collecting tubules causes a large and ongoing loss of free water via a very dilute urine. As free water leaves the circulation and the serum becomes more concentrated, the failure of the ADH mechanism allows a continued diuresis as long as glomerular filtration is maintained. The hallmark of DI, then, is a diuresis of hypoosmolal urine when the serum is significantly hyperosmolal.

Central DI: Virtually any process capable of damaging the hypothalamus and pituitary is capable of reducing ADH production, resulting in diabetes insipidus. Possible causes include: (1) head trauma and neurosurgical procedures; (2) tumors of the hypothalamic-pituitary region; (3) meningitis; and (4) aneurysms. In as many as half of the cases of this disease, the cause is unknown. It is thought likely, however, that these cases of idiopathic origin are the result of autoimmune processes.

Nephrogenic DI: In nephrogenic DI the production of ADH is normal and appropriate, but the kidney is unable to respond to the chemical message to retain water. Probably the most common etiology of DI that is seen in ICUs is the diuretic phase of acute renal failure, in which the kidney has regained a small portion of its ability to form filtrate but cannot yet respond to ADH and concentrate this filtrate. Other causes of nephrogenic DI are: (1) nephritis, (2) Sjögren's syndrome, (3) hypercalcemia, and (4) drugs.

Clinical picture

Regardless of whether his DI is nephrogenic or central, the patient will present with the same set of symptoms and findings: (1) polyuria, (2) polydipsia if able to drink, (3) increased serum osmolality, (4) urine osmolality within 50 mOsm of serum osmolality, and (5) hypernatremia.

The polyuria seen in DI can be astounding: up to 20 liters/day if ADH production is totally absent; more often, some ADH effect is present and the urine volume is between 3 and 8 liters/day. The onset of the diuresis is often sudden.

The hemoconcentration resulting from this free-water diuresis usually causes a sensation of intense thirst, triggered by a normal osmoreceptor mechanism. The patient will often show a preference for very cold drinks. The thirst is so intense that during administration of the water deprivation test, patients have been known to drink water from any source they can find.

The hemoconcentration is also seen by a rise in serum osmolality and serum sodium (Na), although these increases may be minimal if the person is able to drink enough water to offset his continuous losses. If the person can replace his free-water loss by water ingestion, it is entirely possible for him to live indefinitely without any medical attention; usually, however, the life-style adjustments are too severe to be tolerable. Those who cannot replace their losses, because of impaired consciousness or the unavailability of water (e.g., the typical ICU patient), rapidly become severely dehydrated. This dehydration can lead to hyperosmolality, hypovolemic shock, prerenal azotemia, and death.

The first investigation indicated in a patient with sustained diuresis is to test the urine for sugar. If urinary glucose is high, the patient should be worked up for diabetes mellitus. If urinary glucose is negative, the DI workup should proceed.

The pathognomonic sign of DI is the production of dilute urine when the serum osmolality is high. If the patient has maintained a normal osmolality by water ingestion, the demonstration of this sign will require that serum osmolality be raised and the urinary response to this dehydration studied. The **water deprivation test** consists of withholding fluids until the patient's body weight decreases by 3 to 5% and his serum osmolality rises to >290 mOsm/kg. If the polyuria ceases, DI is almost certainly *not* present. If it continues, urine and serum osmolalities are monitored. Concentration of the urine to >500 mOsm/kg rules out DI; DI is indicated if the urine osmolality does not vary by >50 mOsm/kg from that of the serum. Unless the serum osmolality rises to >290 mOsm/kg, however, there is not a sufficient ADH stimulus to make the test valid.

If the water deprivation test indicates the presence of DI, determining if the disease is central or nephrogenic in origin becomes useful. If the DI is central in origin, the administration of exogenous ADH, as intramuscular vasopressin (Pitressin Tannate in Oil) or, more commonly, as aqueous vasopressin (Pitressin) administered IV will cause a rise in urine concentration as the kidney responds to the AHD. A rise in urine osmolality to >500 mOsm/kg in response to ADH confirms the diagnosis of central DI. Nephrogenic DI is suggested if there is no response to the injected ADH.

Medical interventions

In central DI the administration of exogenous ADH compensates for the deficiency. There are several ADH preparations available, each with its own advantages and difficulties. These are presented in Table 6–1. When some ADH production is present, the hypoglycemic agent chlorpropamide (Diabinese) has been used. This medication acts both to stimulate ADH release and to potentiate its effects on the collecting tubules.

In cases of nephrogenic DI, ADH preparations are of no use, as endogenous ADH levels are already high. The treatment in this instance is the administration of diuretics. Coupled with a Na-restricted diet, these reduce the delivery of Na to the nephronic loop, thus reducing the nephron's ability to dilute the urine.

Nursing interventions

Potential for rapid dehydration. (1) Measure urine output carefully. (2) Pay close attention to weight, a drop of 5% is significant, of 10% is dangerous. Frequent weighing is required during water deprivation test. (3) Monitor serum and urine electrolytes and osmolality.

Intense thirst. (1) Provide adequate iced fluids, except during water deprivation. Understand that until therapy is started, adequate fluid replacement is essential. (2) During the water deprivation test, take whatever measures seem needed to maintain test, while providing encouragement and explanations to patient. Be aware that patients have been known to drink from flowerpots, IV bottles, and urinals during this test.

Potential need for a Na-restricted diet. (1) Assess patient's ability and motivation to learn the diet. Involve family in teaching as needed. (2) Arrange consultation with dietitian.

TABLE 6–1

ADH Preparations

Preparation	Route	Duration of action	Comments
Aqueous vasopressin (Pitressin)	SC, IV	3–6 hr	Short duration a disadvantage long-term but allows precise control in ICU setting.
Vasopressin (Pitressin Tannate in Oil)	Deep IM	6–24 hr	Irritating to tissues; absorption may be erratic; sometimes used in unconscious patient.
Desaminocys^{1}-D-arginine^{8}-vasopressin (Desmopressin acetate)	Nasal	12–24 hr	Drug of choice for maintenance therapy; administration awkward.

SYNDROME OF INAPPROPRIATE ADH SECRETION

The appropriate secretion of ADH occurs when the serum is concentrated and free-water retention is necessary to dilute the serum. In the syndrome of inappropriate ADH secretion (SIADH), there is continued secretion of ADH even when the serum is dilute, or hypoosmolal. The free water retention caused by the ADH further aggravates the hypoosmolal state, and the ADH production is thus deemed inappropriate. The hallmark of this syndrome is the production of a concentrated urine when the serum is dilute.

SIADH is most commonly seen following major surgery. Many of the factors that increase ADH release, such as pain, bowel manipulation during surgery, and emotional stress, may be present, causing the body to activate an ancient response to the anticipated volume loss that accompanies trauma. This response cannot, however, anticipate the several liters of crystalloid fluid that have been administered in the perioperative period. The free water that is retained by the ADH is poured into a system that has been maintained artificially at normal levels, and the result is a diluted serum with a concentrated urine.

Other, more pathologic causes of SIADH include ADH-producing tumors, most commonly oat cell carcinoma, although many other malignancies may also be responsible: pulmonary conditions (e.g., TB and lung abscesses); continuous mechanical ventilation, because of the effects of increased intrathoracic pressure on the left atrial baroreceptors; and drugs (e.g., chlorpropamide, indomethacin, opiates, barbiturates, and nicotine).

Clinical picture

Overloaded with free water—water that is absorbed without accompanying electrolytes—this patient does not exhibit the classic signs of fluid overload (i.e., pitting edema, pulmonary edema, or hypertension) because the retained free water rapidly follows an osmotic gradient into the relatively hyperoosmolal cells. The excess water is thus distributed almost entirely within the cells, and very little remains in the interstitial and intravascular compartments. What is seen clinically are the signs of cellular swelling, particularly in the CNS: anorexia, confusion, disorientation, seizures, and hyperreflexia.

The key laboratory findings are a dilute hyponatremic serum (i.e., plasma osmolality <270 mOsm/kg), coupled with a concentrated urine. If the urine has an osmolality equal to or above that of the serum, it is usually sufficient to suggest SIADH. Volume depletion and chronic CHF may produce a similar laboratory picture, as both will activate ADH and aldosterone secretion. Usually the presence of continued urinary Na excretion (>40 mEq/liter) can be used to rule out these two entities. Hypochloremia and hypokalemia will also be present.

A water-loading test may be used to confirm the diagnosis. The patient is given a large bolus of fluid and the subsequent urine output measured. SIADH is suggested if less than one half of the bolus is excreted; there will usually be an exaggerated loss of Na in the urine as well.

Medical interventions

The approach to SIADH is guided by the severity of the hyponatremia and the accompanying CNS symptomatology. Usually the most effective therapy is strict fluid restriction. As free water is lost naturally via the respiratory tract, electrolyte and osmolal balance will slowly and safely return to normal.

When the serum Na is <115 mEq/liter or the hyponatremia has developed rapidly, however, severe CNS symptoms may be seen. In these cases, more aggressive therapy may be warranted, but the therapy may be as dangerous as the disease itself. The administration of hypertonic (3%) saline will rapidly correct the hyponatremia, but the sudden increase in intravascular tonicity may draw enough fluid into the vascular compartment to precipitate CHF. Furthermore, overly rapid correction of the hyponatremia may cause seizures. Raising the serum Na at a rate >2 mEq/liter/hr is considered excessive. Total correction of the Na level is unnecessary; usually a rise in the serum Na of 10 mEq/liter will relieve the CNS symptoms.

To rapidly treat a hyponatremic crisis without causing intravascular fluid overload, hypertonic saline may be given along with the diuretic furosemide. This results in an unstable electrolyte balance, with rapid losses of potassium and Na. Frequent determinations of serum electrolytes are essential if this therapy is used.

Other approaches to an acute crisis include peritoneal dialysis with hypertonic dialysis fluid or wrapping the patient in blankets to promote fluid loss through perspiration. Drug therapy is limited to the administration of demeclocycline, which blocks the effect of ADH on the collecting tubules.

Nursing interventions

Hyponatremia. (1) Monitor serum electrolytes closely, especially Na level. A rapid rise or fall in this value is dangerous. (2) Observe closely for decreased alertness. (3) Take seizure precautions.

Fluid overload. (1) Weigh the patient daily. (2) Monitor serum Na. (3) Measure intake and output. (4) If hypertonic saline is used, watch closely for signs of CHF: shortness of breath, crackles on listening to lungs, S_3, tachycardia.

Need for fluid restriction. (1) Assess likelihood of patient compliance. (2) Involve family in care. (3) Arrange for continued contact by home health agency if needed.

THE ADRENAL GLANDS

ANATOMY AND PHYSIOLOGY REVIEW

The adrenal glands, located atop the kidneys, are made up of two distinct zones, the **medulla** and **cortex.** The hormones of the cortex are dissimilar in structure, function, and control mechanisms to those of the medulla. The medullary hormones, epinephrine and norepinephrine, are here considered to be a part of the ANS. The cortex, along with its hormones, the corticosteroids, are considered part of the endocrine system. The cortex produces two types of corticosteroids, whose functions overlap slightly but are largely dissimilar. These are the **mineralcorticoids,** typified by the hormone **aldosterone;** and the **glucorticoids,** typified by **cortisol.**

Aldosterone

The major function of aldosterone in homeostasis is the **regulation of ECF volume.** It acts at the distal convoluted tubules of the kidneys, promoting the reabsorption of Na and chloride ions and the excretion of potassium (K). As Na and chloride are reabsorbed, water is drawn out of the tubules with them, and the net result is the reabsorption of isotonic fluid. In this way, fluid can be retained without upsetting the osmotic balance of the ECF. A second function is the **maintenance of normal K levels.** A person lacking the ability to produce aldosterone will die within days if untreated.

Aldosterone production is controlled by multiple factors. Serum electrolyte balance is a major factor, with both hyperkalemia and hyponatremia directly stimulating the adrenal cortex to release aldosterone. When decreased renal perfusion activates the renin-angiotensin system, aldosterone release is stimulated by circulating angiotensin II. Finally, a minor role is played by ACTH, the tropic hormone produced by the anterior pituitary. Aldosterone production is *not* dependent on ACTH, however, and will proceed normally in its absence.

Cortisol

Cortisol affects a wide variety of metabolic processes; indeed, many of its effects are as yet poorly understood. Briefly, the known effects of cortisol are as follows: (1) increases blood sugar by stimulating gluconeogenesis and antagonizing insulin; (2) increases protein breakdown; (3) mobilizes fatty acids from fat stores; (4) decreases thyroid hormone production; (5) exerts a small, aldosteronelike effect on the kidneys; (6) in pharmacologic doses, suppresses inflammation, decreases antibody formation, and stabilizes cell and lysomal membranes; (7) increases gastric acid production; (8) permits normal response to catecholamines (tissue respond poorly to these in its absence); and (9) permits normal function of the cellular Na-K pump.

Not known is the exact usefulness of these effects in helping the body to combat stress. It has been postulated, though not confirmed, that the effects on protein, fat, and carbohydrate metabolism mobilize the basic cellular building blocks, making them available for the maintenance and repair of stressed or damaged cells. It is known that seriously stressed organisms cannot survive without adequate cortisol secretion by the adrenal cortex.

Cortisol production is entirely controlled by ACTH from the anterior pituitary. This ACTH is released both on a normal diurnal cycle and in response to CRF, released from the hypothalamus in response to a wide range of stressors. These stressors include pain, tissue damage, extreme temperatures, hypovolemia, and severe emotional stress. Appropriate cortisol production, therefore, depends upon an intact and functional hypothalamus, anterior pituitary, and adrenal cortex; malfunction of any one of these may result in deranged cortisol production.

ACUTE ADRENAL INSUFFICIENCY

Pathophysiology

Adrenal insufficiency may take one of two forms: (1) **primary,** which is caused by the destruction of the adrenals themselves and results in the loss of both aldosterone and cortisol; and (2) **secondary,** which is caused by a lack of ACTH production and results in the loss of cortisol only. The crisis of acute adrenal insufficiency is the result of the primary form of the disease, and the lack of aldosterone is the cause of the major physiologic derangements seen.

Adrenal damage or destruction is most often caused by poorly understood autoimmune processes but may also result from trauma, infection, or prolonged severe stress. Meningococcal infections, in particular, may lead to adrenal insufficiency.

Although it is possible to survive without cortisol for an indefinite period, a complete lack of aldosterone will lead to death within days. The most striking alteration is the inability to retain Na and water or to excrete K, resulting in dehydration, hyponatremia, and hyperkalemia. Dehydration may lead to prerenal azotemia or even to hypovolemic shock. Hyperkalemia may predispose to cardiac dysrhythmias.

Lack of cortisol is not without harmful effects. The efficiency of the cellular Na-K pump is lessened, furthering electrolyte abnormalities. Absence of cortisol reduces the effectiveness of sympathetic amines, thus reducing cardiac contractility and CO. Hypoglycemia may result from the failure of cortisol to stimulate gluconeogenesis.

Clinical picture

The patient with acute adrenal insufficiency may present with any or all of the following symptoms: thirst, salt craving, progressive fatigue, weakness and weight loss, abdominal pain, and apathy or confusion. Laboratory findings will indicate hyponatremia, hyperkalemia, eosinophilia, elevated BUN and creatinine, decreased plasma cortisol, increased plasma ACTH, and acidosis if shock is present. Physical findings include dehydration and hypoperfusion.

Definitive diagnosis of adrenal insufficiency is established by applying the rapid ACTH test, in which 250 μg of ACTH are administered and plasma checked for cortisol levels at 30 and 60 min. A rise in plasma cortisol of 7 μg/dl indicates a normal pituitary-adrenal axis. An inadequate rise in cortisol levels coupled with a high base-line ACTH indicates primary adrenal disease. If the base-line ACTH level is low, the indication is for secondary disease. In this case, continued ACTH administration over several days will begin to stimulate cortisol production.

Medical interventions

Emergency treatment of acute adrenal insufficiency begins with the administration of IV saline solution to correct the severe dehydration and hyponatremia. Infusions of 5% dextrose in 0.9% NaCl are administered at a rate of 500 ml/hr until there is clinical improvement in the hypovolemic state.

To retain the Na and fluid being administered and to correct metabolic derangements caused by the lack of cortisol, hydrocortisone is administered in dosages of 100 mg IV, followed by 10mg/hr, to a total of 300 to 400 mg. After clinical improvement, the hydrocortisone is decreased by 50%/day to a maintenance dose of 30 to 40 mg/day. Because hydrocortisone in large doses acts like aldosterone to maintain electrolyte balance, no aldosterone replacement is necessary until the hydrocortisone dose drops to <75 mg/day. Below this dosage, an aldosterone replacement, fludrocortisone, may be administered PO. Steroids without any Na-retaining properties, such as dexamethasone (Decadron) and methylprednisolone (Solu-Medrol), *must not* be used in the treatment of acute adrenal insufficiency. These will increase the GFR without increasing Na retention, resulting in a greatly increased Na and fluid loss.

Nursing interventions

Dehydration. (1) Measure intake and output. (2) Monitor electrolytes. (3) Monitor BUN, creatinine, urine osmolality, and urine Na for evidence of acute renal failure.

Hyperkalemia. (1) Monitor ECG for dysrhythmias.

Fatigue, weakness. (1) Institute safety precautions to prevent falls.

Altered state of consciousness. (1) Orient frequently. (2) Allow for family contact.

Inability to respond to stress. (1) Reduce stressors: pain, fear, sleep deprivation, excess noise.

THE PANCREAS

ANATOMY AND PHYSIOLOGY REVIEW

The pancreas is a gland that lies behind and inferior to the stomach and liver. It has both an exocrine and endocrine function. The **exocrine** function is carried out by acinous tissue that secretes digestive enzymes into the duodenum. The **endocrine** function is performed by the islets of Langerhans, which contain two major types of cells, the alpha and beta cells. The alpha cells synthesize **glucagon,** a hormone that acts as a hyperglycemic agent, raising the blood glucose level by promoting the conversion of glycogen to glucose within the liver. Glucagon is secreted in response to a fall in the level of blood sugar.

The beta cells produce the hormone **insulin.** The major action of insulin is to transport glucose into most tissues of the body, including the liver and muscle, where it can be stored as glycogen or burned for energy. Insulin also regulates the rate of cellular conversion of carbohydrate to energy, increases conversion of glucose to glycogen for storage in the liver, and promotes the synthesis of proteins and lipids. The rate of insulin secretion from the pancreas is regulated by the level of sugar in the blood. In the absence of insulin, glucose is unable to enter the cells, resulting in increased glucose concentration in the blood. This condition is called diabetes mellitus.

DIABETIC KETOACIDOSIS

Pathophysiology

Diabetic ketoacidosis (DKA) is a severe complication of diabetes resulting from a relative or absolute lack of effective insulin. DKA may develop over several days or in just a few hours and is characteristic of type I or insulin-dependent diabetes. It may occur as the initial event of undiagnosed diabetes or in uncontrolled diabetes. Other contributing causes of DKA include infection, illness, emotional stress, and rapid growth periods. These stressful events cause increased levels of catabolic anti-insulin hormones, which increase the need for insulin.

With the absence of effective insulin, carbohydrate, fat, and protein metabolism are all affected. Without insulin, glucose is not utilized by most body cells (with the exception of nerve and liver tissue). It therefore accumulates in the blood, resulting in hyperglycemia. The excess blood glucose creates hyperosmosis and water is pulled out of cells into the intravascular compartment. As the blood glucose reaches a level that exceeds the renal threshold, glucose spills into the urine and, acting as an osmotic diuretic, produces polyuria, electrolyte depletion, and eventual dehydration. In response to the dehydration, polydipsia occurs, and thus two of the cardinal symptoms of hyperglycemia are evident: namely, polyuria and polydipsia.

As part of the cycle, fats become mobilized from adipose tissue to be used for energy by the glucose-deprived cells. This shift from carbohydrate to fat metabolism results in ketosis and eventual acidosis. Insulin inhibits the breakdown of fats. Without it, free fatty acids increase in the blood and enter the liver, where many are converted to ketone bodies (acetoacetic acid and beta-hydroxybutyric acid). The ketone bodies are produced faster than they can be metabolized and accumulate in the body, leading to metabolic acidosis.

The body attempts to buffer the mounting acidosis, but the buffering base becomes depleted as the renal mechanism for acid excretion and bicarbonate conservation is overwhelmed. At this point, the lungs attempt to remove carbonic acid by venting CO_2, and the respiratory center is stimulated into the rapid, deep respirations (Kussmaul respirations) characteristic of DKA. The breath acquires a fruity, acetone odor as ketones are blown off. As long as this mechanism can compensate for acid accumulation, the pH will not decline sharply, but when the lungs' alkalosis can no longer offset the metabolic acidosis, symptoms develop quickly.

The body also attempts to provide energy for the cells by breaking down protein, which causes the release of amino acids and electrolytes from muscle tissue. Some of the amino acids are broken down in the liver into glucose and nitrogen, increasing the hyperglycemic and acidotic state and also resulting in further loss of electrolytes.

Unless proper treatment is initiated at this point, the cycle of ketosis, acidosis, and tissue breakdown will end in coma and possibly death.

Clinical picture

The clinical presentations of patients in DKA may vary considerably. Some degree of dehydration resulting from osmotic diuresis and inadequate oral replacement is always evident and is often seen as dry mucous membranes, warm, flushed skin, poor skin turgor, hypotension, tachycardia, and decreased urinary output. GI symptoms are often present, including nausea and vomiting secondary to the acidosis and abdominal pain (often severe) related to electrolyte imbalance.

Altered mental states may range from malaise to frank coma.

Hyperventilation with the characteristic of a deep, sighing respiratory pattern (Kussmaul respirations) is often exhibited, along with the characteristic acetone fruity odor on the breath.

Once the diagnosis of DKA is suspected on the basis of physical findings and patient history, it can quickly be confirmed by laboratory tests.

Initial laboratory tests should include plasma glucose, electrolytes, ketones (serum and urine), creatinine, BUN, CBC, WBC, and pH. Laboratory values for patients experiencing DKA are listed in Table 6–2.

TABLE 6–2

Initial Laboratory Values for Patients Experiencing DKA

Test	Result	Remarks
Glucose	300–800 mg/100 ml	Concentration not related to severity of DKA
Ketone bodies	Strong, at least in undiluted plasma	Measures only acetoacetate, not ß-hydroxybutyrate
HCO_3^-	0–15 mEq/liter	
pH	6.8–7.3	
Na	Low, normal, or high	Concentration dependent on relative H_2O loss
K	Low, normal, or high	Heart responsive to extracellular concentrations
Phosphate	Usually normal or slightly elevated; occasionally slightly low	Associated with phosphaturia; with treatment, marked decrease in levels of both serum and urine phosphates
Creatinine, BUN	Usually mildly increased	May be prerenal
WBC count	Usually increased	Possibility of leukemoid reaction (even in absence of infection)
Amylase	Often increased	Predominant form of salivary gland origin
Hb, Hct, total protein	Often increased	Secondary to contracted plasma volume
SGOT, SGPT, LDH	Can be elevated	Spurious increases due to acetoacetate interference in older colorimetric methods

HCO_3^-, concentration of bicarbonate; K, concentration of potassium; LDH, lactic dehydrogenase; mEq, milliequivalent; Na, concentration of sodium. *Reprinted with permission from* Davidson, M. B. Diabetes Mellitus: Diagnosis and Treatment. John Wiley & Sons, Inc., New York. 1981. p. 203.

Medical interventions

Management of DKA involves a continuous and careful monitoring of the clinical and laboratory status of the patient. The aims of treatment are to reduce the blood sugar and correct dehydration and electrolyte imbalance.

The treatment of the comatose patient must be provided without delay. The risk of pulmonary aspiration is always present, and a nasogastric tube with continuous suction should be inserted until the patient regains consciousness. In alert patients, a nasogastric tube may be necessary only if there are signs of gastric dilation.

Bladder catheterization may be necessary if the patient is not urinating spontaneously.

An ECG is done as soon as feasible and the patient is placed on a cardiac monitor to enable careful assessment and monitoring of K status and replacement.

Other supportive measures may include O_2 administration and, in hypotensive patients, central venous monitoring. The effect of all therapy must be monitored closely, including frequent laboratory determinations for blood glucose levels, electrolytes, and acid-base status.

Insulin. Insulin is the key to therapy in DKA. Only regular short-acting insulin should be used; the longer-acting insulins, such as NPH and Lente, are not effective immediately and therefore are not effective treatment.

The amount of insulin prescribed will vary with the individual patient and is often dependent on the weight of the patient. Typically, an adult will be started with a loading dose of ~10 U bolus IV. This is followed by 5 to 10 U/hr IV (usually 50 U regular insulin to 500 ml of normal saline). The rate of the insulin infusion is titrated in response to blood glucose levels. The continuous IV insulin is continued until the acute phase of ketoacidosis is thought to be over (rarely <6 hr) and the patient's general condition permits administration of fluids PO and insulin SC.

Fluid treatment. IV fluid treatment is started immediately to relieve dehydration. As a rule, the initial fluid administration will be either normal saline (when the intravascular volume depletion is profound) or 0.45% saline (when plasma volume contraction is more moderate). Subsequent fluid replacement again will depend on the state of dehydration.

General guidelines for fluid replacement are as follows: ~1,000 ml of normal saline (or 0.45% saline) the first hour, followed by 200 to 400 ml/hr. The amount of fluid in the first 18 to 24 hr will usually range from 4 to 8 liters.

In the elderly patient and in patients with oliguria, central venous pressure (CVP) monitoring is recommended to avoid overhydration. As blood glucose falls to 250 mg/dl, 5% dextrose is added to IV fluids to prevent hypoglycemia.

Electrolyte replacement. Na is replaced with the initial IV of normal saline.

K treatment usually begins once urinary output is established and/or when serum K is <3.5 mEq/liter. It is important to note that although a patient may have a normal or elevated serum K initially, this value does not reflect intracellular K; the insulin and fluid treatments for DKA cause significant shifts of K back into cells, and unless K replacement is started, hypokalemia may develop rapidly. K is given in the form of potassium chloride or potassium phosphate, 20 to 40 mEq/liter of IV fluid. The rate of flow is adjusted in relation to serum K values and cardiac monitoring (essential in observing for K imbalance).

Bicarbonate replacement in DKA is generally avoided and only indicated for severe acidosis (pH <7.0). The administration of bicarbonate may result in severe hypokalemia and fatal cardiac arrhythmias and when indicated must be used with extreme caution. It is never administered by IV bolus but should be added to IV fluid (0.45% saline) and infused slowly over ≥1 hr.

Nursing interventions

Successful therapy of DKA depends on close, constant professional care of the patient.

Alteration in mental status. (1) Evaluate frequently; may range from normal to deep coma. (2) Have oral suction equipment on hand and suction as necessary. (3) Keep patient turned to prevent aspiration of vomitus. (4) Maintain good body alignment. (5) Observe for changes in patient sensorium carefully.

Alteration in fluid balance. (1) Monitor intake and output carefully. (2) Ensure adequate and prompt rehydration. (3) If possible, avoid catheterization in the noncomatose patient. (4) If the patient has a CVP line, monitor carefully. (5) Assess for fluid overload by checking lung sounds for congestion, observing for neck vein distension, and watching for increasing CVP.

Alteration in electrolyte balance. (1) This therapy will depend on close, regular clinical and laboratory checking. (2) Electrolytes and pH should be checked every 1 to 2 hr until the acute phase is over. (3) Cardiac monitoring is essential to observe for signs of K imbalance. Signs of hyperkalemia include: arrhythmias, peaked T waves, loss of P wave. Signs of hypokalemia include: arrhythmias, inverted T waves, flattened T waves.

Hyperglycemia. (1) Plasma glucose should be checked frequently (q 1 to 2 hr until stable). (2) Urine should be checked for sugar and acetone q 1 to 2 hr initially. (3) Titrate IV insulin carefully. Utilization of infusion pump is essential.

Hypoglycemia. (1) Have glucose testing strips at patient's bedside and test immediately whenever hypoglycemia is suspected. (2) Observe for change in sensorium, restlessness, sweating, complaints of nervousness, tachycardia, increased BP. (3) When plasma glucose is ~250 mg/dl, dextrose should be added to the IV infusion.

Ongoing care. (1) Monitor patient's vital signs and ECG continuously. (2) Maintain a flow sheet with all pertinent clinical and laboratory data. Changes in pH, glucose and K levels, and urine output should be reported immediately. (3) Coexistent problems must be considered and treated along with the ketoacidosis.

Education. For prevention of future episodes of DKA, teach patient the causes, symptoms, and treatment of hyperglycemia. (2) Teach to test urine for glucose and ketones, test blood sugar using one of the home glucose monitoring methods, and to report these results to the physician, especially during illness.

HYPEROSMOLAR HYPERGLYCEMIC NONKETOTIC COMA

Pathophysiology

Hyperosmolar hyperglycemic nonketotic coma (HHNC) is a life-threatening complication of diabetes characterized by marked hyperglycemia, profound dehydration, presence of varying degrees of alteration of mental status, and lack of significant ketosis. It is most commonly seen in patients >60 years of age either with known, mild type II diabetes or with undiagnosed diabetes. Very often these patients have other debilitating diseases, such as renal disease, acute pancreatitis, thyroidtoxicosis, cardiovascular disease, gram-negative pneumonia, or uremia. Other precipitating causes are those that increase carbohydrate load or create hyperadrenocortical states leading to hyperglycemia, such as hyperalimentation, hemodialysis, peritoneal dialysis, extensive burns, pancreatic disease, or a variety of acute stress conditions. Some medications can also precipitate this complication, including control-type steroids, phenytoin, propanol, and diuretics such as thiazides, furosemide, and chlorthalidone. Mechanisms by which hyperglycemia leads to HHNC are similar to those that occur in DKA. The lack of sufficient insulin results in an increase of blood glucose, causing an increase in serum osmolality. In normal osmolar mechanics, large amounts of body water are reabsorbed from the kidneys' distal tubules and collecting ducts. This water, drawn out of urine, is restored to the blood. In the HHNC patient, the plasma osmolarity may go as high as that of water-absorbing tissues. In such a situation, osmosis cannot draw water back from the kidney into the blood because the osmotic gradient is not steep enough. This creates an increase in fluid volume, resulting in the loss of large volumes of water through the kidneys. This osmotic diuresis depletes total body water, Na, and eventually K.

One of the major clinical differences between DKA and HHNC is the lack of significant ketones in the latter. It is thought that in HHNC there is some circulating insulin that prevents lipolysis and eventual ketosis and acidosis. There is not, however, sufficient insulin to prevent the severe hyperglycemia characteristic of HHNC.

HHNC is reported to have a high mortality rate, ~30 to 50%, which reflects the fact that most patients are elderly and have other complicating illnesses. Also, because the signs and symptoms are similar to those of other disorders such as cerebral vascular accidents and organic brain syndrome, HHNC may be misdiagnosed. Misdiagnosis can cause a serious delay in the initiation of treatment, and prompt, appropriate therapy is crucial to the patient's recovery.

Clinical picture

Typically, the onset of HHNC is slow but it moves rapidly to a crisis. There may be a history of days or possibly weeks of polyuria and polydipsia. The presenting neurologic status varies widely, although more than half the HHNC patients present in coma. The other various levels of cerebral dysfunction include drowsiness, confusion, focal or grand mal seizures, and abnormal behavioral manifestations.

Other signs and symptoms correlate with electrolyte and fluid imbalances. Signs such as extreme dehydration (with dry, cracked mucous membranes, poor skin turgor, and soft eyeballs), orthostatic hypotension, shock, tachycardia, and hypothermia are all characteristic of this syndrome. Abdominal symptoms such as nausea and vomiting and pain often occur but are not as frequent as in DKA. Patients may exhibit tachypnea with shallow respirations. Kussmaul respirations and acetone breath, typical of DKA, are not a feature of HHNC.

The diagnosis of HHNC is made on the basis of presenting signs and symptoms, historical data, and laboratory data. Laboratory tests that are most important in making the diagnosis include serum glucose (usually extremely elevated), plasma osmolality (>330 mOsm/kg), and serum ketones (absent or minimal).

Laboratory values that are seen in patients with HHNC are listed in Table 6–3.

Medical interventions

The treatment of HHNC is based on the patient's overall status and directed toward correcting the extreme degree of volume depletion and the

TABLE 6–3

Laboratory Values for Patients Experiencing HHNC

Test	Result	Comments
Plasma glucose	400–2,800 mg/dl	Values are often very high; may exceed 2,800 mg/dl
Osmolality	>350 mOsm/kg	Osmolality levels fall after fluid replacement
Ketones (serum and urine)	minimal or absent	
K	high, low, or normal	Total K is always depleted unless renal failure is severe
NA	low or normal	Serum Na levels usually rise after fluid replacement
Hct	elevated	
WBC	elevated	
BUN	elevated	
Creatinine	elevated	

K, potassium; Na, sodium.

hyperosmolar state and detection and correction of any underlying associated illness.

Fluids. The immediate concern is fluid deficit. The patient is often dehydrated to the extent of 20 to 25% of total body water, averaging ~8- to 12-liter deficit. If hypovolemic shock or hypotension is present, fluid replacement must be started before any other treatment is initiated. The type of fluid replacement is individualized, often according to the preference of the treating physician. Hypotonic saline is often the fluid of choice, although isotonic saline may be used if vascular collapse has occurred.

CVP monitoring is often indicated to monitor fluid replacement, especially in patients with cardiovascular disease. Initial fluids may include either 0.45% hypotonic saline IV or, if hypotension or tachycardia is present, isotonic saline IV until CVP rises. The initial fluid is infused rapidly over a 2-hr period. Hypotonic saline infusions are continued, 1 liter q 2 hr, titrated according to CVP readings. It may be necessary to replace ~6 to 18 liters of fluid, with 5 to 6 liters replaced within the first 12 hr of treatment.

Insulin. Insulin administration is started either with or following adequate fluid replacement as adjunct therapy in lowering blood sugars. Most of the hyperglycemia is corrected with IV fluid replacement because fluid dilutes extracellular glucose and increases renal glucose secretion (if renal blood flow is adequate).

Blood glucose must not be lowered too rapidly in the absence of adequate fluid volume, because of the threat of cardiovascular collapse. Insulin therapy usually consists of low-dose continuous IV regular insulin at ~4 to 10 U/hr. When the blood sugar is lowered to a range of 250 mg/dl, an IV glucose infusion is started to prevent hypoglycemia. Patients in HHNC usually respond quickly to insulin and, as a rule, the total insulin dose required is less than that needed for the treatment of DKA.

Electrolyte replacement. K replacement usually begins as soon as urine output is adequate. Patients may present with K levels that are low, normal, or even high; however, total body K is always depleted, although this may not be evident until volume has been replaced. Potassium chloride may be administered concurrently with insulin and fluid replacement, in amounts of ~20 to 40 mEq/1,000 ml.

Patients may lose calcium, phosphate, and magnesium. These elements must be replaced as needed. Na levels are corrected with fluid replacement.

Additional treatment. Hyperviscosity sometimes occurs in hyperglycemic dehydration, especially in the debilitated patient. Anticoagulant therapy may be indicated for patients at risk.

Because mortality in HHNC is most commonly caused by an associated illness, a search for concurrent illness is an important factor in treating the patient in HHNC.

Patients almost always present with some disturbance in mentation (drowsiness, confusion, and stupor); therefore a nasogastric tube with continuous suction is inserted to prevent pulmonary aspiration. The patient is placed on a cardiac monitor to observe K replacement as well as general cardiac status.

Other supportive measures include bladder catheterization and O_2 as needed.

Nursing interventions

Treatment is directed toward correcting severe dehydration and hyperglycemia and assessing the patient for development of complications that can result from HHNC and its treatment.

Alteration in mental status. (1) Monitor neurologic status by checking pupils, assessing level of consciousness, noting subtle changes in sensorium. (2) Seizure precautions are necessary; 15% of HHNC patients have focal or grand mal seizures. (3) Have oral suction on hand. (4) Record changes and report.

Alteration in fluid balance. (1) Monitor intake and output carefully. (2) Monitor a central venous line for adequate fluid volume. (3) Assess patient for signs of fluid overload: dyspnea, increased CVP, pulmonary rales, congestion, neck vein distension. (4) Check serum osmolality regularly, report any sudden decrease.

Hyperglycemia. (1) Administer regular (short-acting) insulin , IV and/or SC. (2) Control IV insulin by means of infusion pump. (3) Monitor serum glucose frequently (q 1 to 2 hr initially). (4) Have IV glucose at bedside, in case insulin causes sudden drop in blood sugar (plasma glucose at ~250 mg/dl signals need for dextrose to be added to the IV infusion.)

Hypoglycemia. (1) Have glucose strips at patient's bedside. Test whenever hypoglycemia is suspected. (2) Observe for change in sensorium, restlessness, sweating, tachycardia, increased BP. (3) If patient is awake and able to verbalize, respond to complaints of light-headedness, feelings of nervousness, headache.

Electrolyte imbalance. (1) Monitor laboratory results carefully. (2) Obtain electrolytes q 1 to 2 hr until acute phase is over. (3) Observe monitor for K imbalance.

Ongoing care. (1) Monitor vital signs continuously. (2) Keep patient turned to prevent aspiration and maintain good body alignment. (3) Identify and treat other medical illnesses along with the HHNC.

Education. (1) Assess patient's and/or family's understanding of diabetes. (2) Provide information regarding signs and symptoms of hyperglycemia. (3) Teach patients to test their urine for glucose, test their blood using a home monitoring method, and when to contact their physician.

HYPOGLYCEMIA

Pathophysiology

Hypoglycemia is a condition of abnormally low blood glucose levels. It is a common and dangerous complication of insulin therapy and is occasionally caused by oral hypoglycemic agents. Other medical conditions that may cause hypoglycemia include hormonal and metabolic abnormalities and some systemic diseases. The focus of this discussion will be on hypoglycemia in the diabetic patient.

Normal adults usually maintain plasma glucose concentrations of 60 to 150 mg/dl at the extremes of fasting and feeding over a 24-hr period. Plasma glucose must, as a rule, fall <60 mg/dl before symptoms occur; evidence also suggests that a rapidly falling glucose may produce the symptoms of hypoglycemia. In the diabetic, hypoglycemia usually results from an imbalance of insulin, food, and activity—i.e., from skipping or delaying a meal, too much insulin, and/or increased exercise without additional food. Other factors that can complicate metabolic control include: (1) alcoholism (Alcohol may prevent gluconeogenesis within the liver, inhibiting the release of glucose); (2) kidney disease (The kidneys excrete ~7 U of insulin each day. Diseased kidneys retain insulin in the body longer, causing accumulation); (3) medications (Aspirin and other salicylates may contribute to insulin hypoglycemia. Propranolol [Inderal] may block epinephrine from increasing the glucose output from the liver and may also mask the sympathetic nervous system responses to low blood sugar).

Most tissues in the body use fat as a source of energy if glucose is not available. Brain and nervous tissue cannot use any other substance; therefore, many of the signs and symptoms of low blood sugar are caused by the effect of inadequate glucose in brain cells.

The signs and symptoms of hypoglycemia are related both to the glucose deprivation of the CNS and the effects of catecholamine release. Although indications vary among individuals, the physiologic response follows a pattern.

When blood glucose falls <60 mg/dl, the parasympathetic nervous system becomes excited, which may lead to nausea, hunger, and lowered BP. The sympathetic nervous system releases epinephrine to stimulate the breakdown of glycogen into glucose in the liver. This adrenergic effect may cause nervousness, tachycardia, sweating, restlessness, and increased BP. Cerebral function declines, producing lethargy, yawning, blurred and/or double vision, behavior changes, confusion, and uncoordinated movements. Without treatment, the disorder progresses to convulsions, coma, or possible death.

Although most reactions create no permanent adverse effects, severe repeated or prolonged reactions can result in brain damage, impaired intellectual ability, and personality change.

Clinical picture

The clinical presentation may vary depending on the individual's physiologic response and the rate and degree that the blood glucose falls. The conscious, alert patient may identify a variety of symptoms, including feelings of anxiety, nervousness, tingling of the tongue or lips, headache, and palpitations. Other symptoms may include pallor, light-headedness, sweating, and increased BP progressing to the inability to concentrate, slurred speech, personality change, uncoordinated movements (especially when walking), and later, signs of convulsions and coma.

In children, hypoglycemia may be deceptive. Many of the usual signs and symptoms manifested in the adult may not be evident. The child may experience a sudden extreme increase in appetite, headache, drowsiness, and often irritability. If the blood glucose falls during the night, nightmares often occur.

The elderly are especially at risk for low blood sugar because reduced renal and hepatic function, seen more often in older people, have an effect on insulin and oral hypoglycemic agents. Also, elderly people may not readily identify the early signs and symptoms and/or may not respond quickly in treating an episode, increasing the risk for severe and prolonged hypoglycemic attacks.

Any suspicion of low blood sugar in the diabetic patient always requires investigation, even of the most subtle signs and symptoms.

Medical interventions

Management is aimed at normalizing plasma glucose concentration as quickly as possible. A glucose reagent strip is a convenient, fast method of confirming a suspicion of hypoglycemia without the delay of a laboratory report. A blood sample should be drawn for diagnostic testing whenever possible, however, both at the onset of hypoglycemia and after treatment.

The patient who is unconscious or not alert enough to swallow is given IV glucose, usually a 50-ml ampule of 50% glucose, or 1 mg glucagon, IV or SC. Glucagon raises the blood sugar by promoting the reconversion of glycogen reserves within the liver to glucose.

The patient who is conscious, alert, and able to swallow should be given a rapidly absorbed glucose liquid or food.

Nursing interventions

Hypoglycemia. (1) If a patient is unconscious, always check for a Medic Alert tag or other emergency identification to determine if the patient is a known diabetic. (2) Have glucose reagent strips on hand and determine blood glucose immediately if there is any suspicion of low blood sugar. If patient is not alert enough to swallow, IV glucose or glycogen should be given. Liquids absorb faster and should be the treatment of choice when available. Recommended liquids or foods that contain ~10 g of carbohydrate include: 4 oz. of orange juice (or other fruit juice); 4 oz. regular sweetened soda; 2 teaspoons of honey, corn syrup, or jelly; or 2 to 3 teaspoons of sugar. Treatment should be repeated if the symptoms are not relieved within ~10 to 15 min. To prevent a second episode of hypoglycemia, treatment should be followed with a slow-acting carbohydrate or protein food such as milk, bread, or crackers and cheese. (3) Initiate treatment without delay if blood sugar is <60 mg/dl. (4) Observe unconscious patient (DKA or HHNC) for signs of low blood sugar. Check for diaphoresis by feeling the bed clothes for moistness. This may be the only observable symptom of hypoglycemia. (5) Know the time period during which an insulin reaction is likely to occur. The action of insulin (onset, peak, and duration) will depend on the type of insulin administered and may vary according to manufacturer. Determine the differences by reading the manufacturer's information. (6) Observe patient carefully and monitor vital signs after treatment of a reaction.

Education. (1) Teach patient to follow a reasonably constant schedule, spacing meals and snacks to minimize long intervals between food. (2) Teach patient to know the action, duration, and peak actions of the prescribed insulin. (3) Explain need to increase food before engaging in moderate to strenuous exercise. (4) Inform patient of need to wear a medical identification tag and advise on how to obtain it. (5) Teach a member of the family or a friend when and how to inject glucagon. (6) Inform patient of need to carry some form of glucose at all times. (7) Explain need to notify a physician if reactions are frequent, severe, or prolonged. (8) Teach patient to avoid injecting into a site that is to be exercised to prevent rapid absorption. (9) Teach patient to monitor blood sugars carefully using glucose reagent test strip and/or urine testing.

THE THYROID GLAND

ANATOMY AND PHYSIOLOGY REVIEW

The thyroid gland is one of the largest endocrine organs. Located immediately below the larynx and closely affixed to the anterior and lateral aspects of the trachea by loose connective tissue, it consists of two lobes joined by a thin band of tissue, the isthmus. The gland concentrates iodine, which is necessary for the production of the thyroid hormones **thyroxine** (T_4), the most abundant hormone secreted by the thyroid, and **triiodothyronine** (T_3). These hormones are necessary for cell metabolism and energy production and influence utilization of fats, carbohydrates, and protein. They are also essential for normal functioning of the nervous system, for normal growth and development, and for maintaining water and electrolyte balance.

The thyroid gland also produces the hormone **calcitonin,** a noniodinated hormone, which functions to reduce plasma calcium (Ca) by influencing Ca deposits in the bone.

Disorders of the thyroid may be caused by deficient dietary iodine, by the thyroid gland itself, or by abnormal functioning of the hypothalamus or pituitary gland. Conditions arising from these defects include increased output of thyroid hormone (hyperthyroidism, or thyrotoxicosis), insufficient output of thyroid hormone (hypothyroidism), and enlargement of the thyroid gland (goiter).

THYROID CRISIS

Pathophysiology

Thyroid crisis, also referred to as thyroid storm, is a rare acute medical emergency. It occurs in patients with untreated or inadequately treated hyperthyroidism. It often presents with an abrupt onset and requires prompt recognition and treatment.

The pathophysiology of thyroid crisis is not clearly understood. It is known, however, that thyrotoxicosis is caused by increased levels of thyroid hormone and excess adrenergic activity, which results in a hypermetabolic state. Because thyroid hormones act like catecholamines, e.g., epinephrine and norepinephrine, it has been theorized that a sudden increase of these hormones may precipitate the crisis. It is most often brought on by stressful events such as infection, injury, nonthyroid surgery, and thyroidectomy. Other precipitating events include ketoacidosis, toxemia of pregnancy, pulmonary embolism, and discontinuance or decrease of antithyroid medication. In the past, thyroid crisis was most often observed postoperatively in patients with hyperthyroid conditions, but with preoperative measures to control metabolic factors, postoperative thyroid crisis is rare. Most patients who are controlled and maintained in a euthyroid state may undergo the precipitating conditions without ever experiencing a crisis.

Physiologic manifestations of thyroid crisis. Thyroid crisis affects the basal metabolic rate (BMR), and the GI, cardiovascular, nervous, and musculoskeletal systems.

BMR: One of the primary functions of thyroid hormones is to maintain the body's metabolic activities including body temperature. In thyroid crisis, increased quantities of T_4 accelerate the BMR and elevate the body's temperature; the high body temperature together with an increased BMR may cause excessive loss of body fluids, resulting in dehydration. An increased BMR also causes an increased need for insulin. The body is often unable to meet this need and subsequently insulin levels fall, resulting in hyperglycemia.

GI system: Greatly increased T_4 production usually decreases the body's weight. Although the appetite increases, the patient is unable to consume adequate calories to meet the demands of the increased BMR. Gastric motility is also increased, thereby decreasing the absorption of nutrients and vitamins. Often diarrhea results.

Cardiovascular system: Increased metabolism increases the demand of the body's tissues for O_2 and nutrients. The heart compensates by increasing the force of contractions and rate of discharge. T_4 also has a direct effect on the excitability of the heart, increasing the heart rate. The stress of thyroid crisis on the heart is evidenced by tachycardia, atrial fibrillation, and possibly congestive heart failure.

Nervous system: Alterations in nervous system function are very common in thyroid crisis. The physiologic basis for these manifestations is not clearly understood but is thought to be the result of increased adrenergic response, e.g., characteristic changes caused by epinephrine and norepinephrine include nervousness, peripheral tremors, exaggerated reflexes, and delirium.

Musculoskeletal system: It is believed that excessive T_4 increases osteoclastic activity in the bones more than it increases osteoblastic activity. As a result, the bones become porous, and excessive amounts of Ca and phosphorus are lost in urine and stool. This loss of Ca and phosphorus is associated with demineralization of bone and pathologic fractures. The extreme energy expenditure caused by the hypermetabolic state contributes to muscle weakness, fatigue, and weakness.

Clinical picture

The clinical presentation of thyroid crisis is an exaggerated state of hyperthyroidism. Signs and symptoms characteristic of this syndrome include fever ($\leq$104–106°F), cardiovascular changes (tachycardia, atrial fibrillation, and other arrhythmias), and altered mental state (from irritability and restlessness to delirium or coma). Patients are often profusely diaphoretic and may also experience nausea, vomiting, and diarrhea resulting in dehydration and electrolyte disturbances.

Although thyroid crisis is more common as a medical crisis, it may occur following surgical removal of the thyroid gland. In this situation it is thought to be caused by an excessive release of T_4 into the circulatory system and is most likely to occur 12 to 24 hr postoperatively.

Diagnosis is usually made with a careful clinical history and physical examination. There is no laboratory test that aids in the diagnosis of thyroid crisis, but determinations of serum T_4, T_3 and T_3-resin-uptake are valuable in establishing the diagnosis of hyperthyroidism.

Medical interventions

Thyroid crisis is a life-threatening condition and must be treated promptly. Treatment is aimed at decreasing the synthesis and release of thyroid hormones, blocking the adrenergic activity, treating CHF and electrolyte abnormalities, and reducing fever.

The combination of propylthiouracil (PTU), iodide, and dexamethasone is used to restore T_3 concentration to a normal range within ~24 to 28 hr. **PTU**, an antithyroid medication, is administered in dosages of 200 mg PO q 4 hr (900 to 1,200 mg/day). It may be crushed and administered by nasogastric tube if parenteral administration is not available. PTU is usually preferred over methimazole because it inhibits the peripheral generation of T_3 from T_4. If methimazole is used, doses are 1/10 of those for PTU. **Iodides** are administered either as sodium iodide 500 mg to 1 g by slow IV infusion q 8 to 12 hr, or Lugol's solution 30 drops PO daily, in divided doses. **Dexamethasone** 2 mg PO q 6 hr (a large dose) provides glucocorticoid support, inhibits release of hormone from the thyroid and peripheral generation of T_3 from T_4.

ß **Adrenergic blocking drugs**, such as propranolol, are used to decrease heart rate. Dosage is 40 to 160 mg PO/day, in 4 divided doses. If the patient is unable to take medication PO, 1 to 2 mg may be administered IV, not to exceed 6 mg in 24 hr. Cautious titration under close medical supervision and cardiac monitoring is essential. Use of beta-adrenergic blockers is contraindicated in patients with heart block, CHF, asthma, and hypotension.

If the patient fails to respond to these usual medical measures, plasmapheresis may be indicated to remove protein-bound thyroid hormone and lower T_4 and T_3.

In addition, IV fluids and electrolytes may be ordered to correct dehydration and electrolyte imbalance. Diuretics may be indicated for CHF or pulmonary congestion.

Nursing interventions

Alterations in cardiovascular and respiratory status. (1) Monitor vital signs. (2) Place patient on cardiac monitor. (3) Observe for signs of cardiac arrhthymias. (4) Observe for signs of CHF: listen to lung sounds; monitor CVP. (5) Monitor respiratory rate, pattern, and depth. (6) Provide O_2 prn to reduce dyspnea.

Elevated temperature. (1) Monitor temperature frequently. (2) Take measures to reduce fever: hypothermal blanket, ice mattress, cool-water sponging. (3) Administer antipyretics as ordered.

Emotional excitability. (1) Provide quiet, nonstimulating environment. (2) Reassure patient frequently. (3) Provide simple explanations. (4) Allow periods of rest between treatments.

Fluid and electrolyte imbalance. (1) Measure intake and output. (2) Monitor CVP. (3) Monitor laboratory reports for electrolytes. (4) Provide adequate fluid and electrolytes.

Self-care deficit. (1) Be aware of weakness of patient and implement care to conserve strength. (2) Assist with simple activities, such as eating. (3) Turn patient frequently to avoid decubiti.

Potential for poor nutritional status. (1) Offer frequent feedings of nutritious diet. (2) Encourage diet high in vitamins. (3) Administer vitamin supplements as ordered. (4) Assess need for parenteral hyperalimentation.

Education. (1) Explain the rationale for patient's medication schedule and emphasize importance of following it. Aluminum hydroxide gel (Gelusil and Amphojel) may be prescribed to bind phosphate in the intestine. Oral Ca supplementation and vitamin D (dihydrotachysterol) may be also prescribed. (2) Teach patient about the need to follow high-Ca, low-phosphate diet and how to do so. (3) Explain the importance of close medical supervision to future health, particularly eye examinations (may be prone to cataracts, conjunctivitis, and photophobia) and routine checking of serum Ca levels.

THE PARATHYROID GLANDS

ANATOMY AND PHYSIOLOGY REVIEW

Parathyroid glands are very small, pea-shaped bodies situated in or beneath the posterior surfaces of the thyroid gland. These glands secrete parathyroid hormone (PTH), which regulates Ca between blood and bone, maintaining the physiologic levels of Ca and phosphorus in the blood. PTH also increases Ca absorption from the GI tract, increases Ca reabsorption from the kidneys, and causes the kidneys to excrete phosphorus. The activity of the parathyroid glands appears to be controlled by serum levels of Ca.

Calcitonin, the hormone secreted by the thyroid gland, opposes the action of PTH and inhibits the withdrawal of Ca from the bone.

The functions of PTH and calcitonin are closely related to Ca and phosphate metabolism, vitamin D function, and formation of bones and teeth. The role of PTH is to increase Ca concentration in the blood, whereas absorption of Ca from the GI tract and mobilization of Ca from bone is controlled by vitamin D. Ca is necessary in the ECF for cell-membrane permeability, blood coagulation, and neuromuscular activity, as well as being the major component of bones.

HYPOPARATHYROIDISM

Pathophysiology

Hypoparathyroidism is caused by an insufficiency of the PTH. The hormone may be decreased or be biologically ineffective. Removal of or damage to the parathyroid glands during thyroid surgery is the most common cause of hypoparathyroidism. Primary hypoparathyroid conditions are rare and occur as an isolated entity or in association with endocrine deficiencies, such as thyroid disease, diabetes mellitus, adrenal insufficiency, and ovarian disease.

The role of PTH is to increase and control bone resorption, which in turn maintains the proper serum Ca levels. PTH also regulates phosphate clearance by the renal tubules, maintaining the correct balance between serum Ca and serum phosphate. With a lack of or diminished PTH function, bone resorption slows, serum Ca levels decrease, calcifications form in various organs, and severe neuromuscular irritability may develop. Insufficient PTH also decreases the number of phosphorus ions secreted by the distal tubules of the kidney, which decreases the renal excretion of phosphate and causes serum phosphate levels to rise. The condition of hypoparathyroidism is characterized by a decrease in serum Ca concentration (hypocalcemia), an elevation of serum phosphate (hyperphosphatemia), increased bone density, and neuromuscular irritability.

Neuromuscular irritability is related to decreased membrane resting potential and increased excitability of nerve and muscle membranes. The degree of excitability is based on a balanced ratio among Ca, magnesium, and K. Tetany, a general muscular hypertonia, is a common manifestation of neuromuscular irritability. Other manifestations attributed to decreased plasma Ca ions include GI disturbances, cardiovascular changes, personality changes, and ectodermal problems.

Clinical picture

An acute episode of hypoparathyroidism is most likely to occur when parathyroid tissue has become temporarily nonfunctional because of atrophy or accidental removal during thyroid surgery. This condition may cause PTH to decline rapidly, bringing about acute hypocalcemia and hyperphosphatemia.

The patient may initially present with vague symptoms of aches and pains and nausea and vomiting as well as emotional instability (anxiety, irritability, depression, and neurosis). A reduction in the serum concentration of ionized Ca <7.0 mg will cause irritability of the neuromuscular system and contribute to the chief symptom of hypoparathyroidism, tetany. Tetany is characterized by tremors and spasmodic uncoordinated contractions. In overt tetany the signs may include carpopedal spasm, dysphagia, cardiac arrhythmias, decreased CO, bronchospasm, and laryngeal spasms. The patient may experience a constricted feeling in the throat, usually preceded by painful tonic spasms of smooth and skeletal muscles. The face and limbs are usually affected the most by these contractions. Laryngeal spasms are rare, but when they do occur they create a life-threatening situation. The glottis narrows and interferes with respiration. The patient may become cyanotic and develop generalized convulsions. Psychiatric symptoms may range from anxiety, irritability, and depression to frank psychosis and delirium. Latent tetany is suggested by a positive Chvostek's sign (a sharp tapping over the facial nerve in front of the parotid gland causes the mouth, nose, and eye to twitch) and a positive Trousseau's sign (carpal spasm is induced by occluding blood flow to the arm for 3 min).

The diagnosis may be difficult, and laboratory studies are essential. Serum Ca levels are usually low (<9.0 mg/100 ml) and serum phosphate is elevated. X-ray studies of bone show increased density and an ECG may show Q-T interval changes and abnormal T waves.

Medical interventions

Hypocalcemia resulting in tetany has the potential for life-threatening laryngeal spasms and serious cardiac arrhythmias. The goals of treatment are to increase serum Ca levels to normal (9.0 to 10.5 mg/100 ml) and to avoid a recurrence of the condition.

If the patient is awake and responding, a rebreathing bag to produce mild respiratory acidosis may be ordered, because severe tetany increases alkalosis. The patient will be placed on a cardiac monitor.

Ca is administered IV until overt tetany is under control. Calcium gluconate is preferred over other Ca solutions (such as calcium chloride), which are irritants and can cause problems of local inflammation and thrombophlebitis. A suggested dose of calcium gluconate (90 mg of elemental Ca/10 ml ampule) is 200 to 300 mg diluted in 50 to 100 ml 5% DW. This is infused over a period of 5 to 10 min followed by a slower IV infusion over 4 to 6 hr (prn to control symptoms). Ca PO should be instituted as soon as feasible. Patients taking digitalis should be watched carefully for signs of toxic effects (nausea, vomiting, pulse <60) because Ca salts may potentiate the effects of digitalis on the heart.

Magnesium deficiency may accompany hypocalcemia and should be suspected in patients who are hypocalcemic after parathyroid surgery and/or in patients with a history of alcoholism and GI malabsorption. If magnesium levels are low, Ca will not permanently correct hypocalcemia. Suggested for replacement is magnesium sulfate (50%) ~49 mEq in 1 liter of 5% DW infused over first 3 hr (in patients with normal renal function).

Antacids (Aluminum hydroxide gel [Amphojel]) should also be administered (30 to 120 ml/day) to reduce serum phosphorus levels by reducing phosphate absorption.

Chronic hypocalcemia resulting from a deficiency of parathyroid hormone or vitamin D is treated by increasing Ca absorption. Treatment may include Ca supplementation PO, vitamin D (dihydrotachysterol), and if necessary, magnesium supplementation PO. A prescribed diet that is high in Ca and low in phosphorus is also part of the treatment plan.

Nursing interventions

Nursing care of postoperative thyroidectomy patients and patients with known hypoparathyroid conditions demands close observation and careful assessment and should be directed toward anticipating signs of hypocalcemia.

Hypocalcemia. Watch for signs and symptoms of fatigue, weakness, personality change (ranging from irritability to neurosis and frank psychosis), GI disturbances, increased neuromuscular irritability (paresthesias, tetany, dysphagia, and convulsions). (2) Monitor serum Ca concentrations and serum phosphorus concentrations. (3) Have a tracheotomy tray and intubation equipment close by in case of respiratory problems. (4) Monitor vital signs closely. (5) Have calcium gluconate readily available for IV administration in case patient's serum Ca level decreases or signs of tetany are evident.

Tetany. (1) Monitor serum Ca concentrations and serum phosphorus concentrations. (Tetany occurs when serum Ca levels are >9 mg/100 ml). (2) Watch for signs and symptoms of tetany: tingling and numbness of the nose, ears, fingertips, or toes; muscle twitching and spasms (the face and limbs are usually most affected by these contractions, which may cause intense pain); laryngeal spasm may cause a respiratory crowing sound and choking sensation and may progress to respiratory arrest and death; generalized convulsions. (3) Latent tetany may be demonstrated by Chvostek's sign and Trousseau's sign. (4) If tetany is overt, monitor IV administration of calcium gluconate. If calcium salts are used, give with orange juice for quick absorption. (5) Evaluate respirations and observe for possible airway obstruction. Keep tracheotomy tray at bedside. (6) Provide rebreathing bag to reverse alkalosis. (7) Continue to monitor serum Ca and serum phosphorus levels closely.

Altered cardiac status. (1) If patient's serum Ca level is decreased or if signs and symptoms of tetany are observed, place patient on cardiac monitor. (2) Monitor vital signs closely: take radial and apical pulse for 1 full min. Watch for signs of heart failure, lung congestion, and edema; watch for ECG changes: arrhythmias, decreased CO and contractility.

Altered respiratory status. (1) Evaluate respirations and observe for possible airway obstruction. (2) Keep tracheotomy tray at bedside. (3) Provide rebreathing bag to reverse alkalosis.

GI disturbances. (1) Patient may have increased peristalsis, with diarrhea and vomiting. (2) Maintain adequate fluid intake. (3) Measure intake and output carefully. (4) Give oral hygiene frequently.

Alterations in psychological status. (1) Provide emotional support to patient and family. Explain that symptoms of weakness, fatigue, and personality change are caused by hormonal changes. Reassure them that changes will reverse when imbalances are corrected. (2) Provide a quiet, nonstressful environment.

Increased susceptibility to skin problems. (1) Teach patient with chronic hypoparathyroid condition how to deal with problems of dry skin and thin hair: avoidance of frequent bathing; use of lotions and mild soap. (2) Observe skin for breakdown. (3) Turn patient q 2 hr. (4) Assist with passive exercises prn.

HYPERPARATHYROIDISM

Pathophysiology

Hyperparathyroidism is a condition caused by oversecretion of PTH by one or more of the parathyroid glands. **Primary hyperparathyroidism** arises from a disorder of the parathyroid gland(s) and may be caused by an adenoma, carcinoma, or hyperplasia, of which there are two types. One type is characterized by nodule formation and occurs in association with diseases such as peptic ulcer, pancreatitis, tumors of adipose tissue, and diffuse gastric polyps. The second type is rare and involves enlargement of all four parathyroid glands.

Secondary hyperparathyroidism is caused by a compensatory secretion of increased amounts of PTH in conditions where hypocalcemia occurs. These conditons include renal disease, osteomalacia, acromegaly, and intestinal malabsorption syndrome.

PTH functions to control and increase bone resorption, maintaining the proper balance of Ca and phosphorus ions in the blood. Increased amounts of PTH cause excessive osteoclast growth in bones, which increases bone resorption. This in turn causes Ca to leave the bones and enter the blood, causing hypercalcemia.

As serum Ca rises, excessive amounts of both Ca and phosphorus are excreted in urine, and high amounts of calcium phosphate are deposited within the renal tubules.

A myriad of symptoms may result from hyperparathyroidism including renal disorders (renal calculi are common), GI symptoms, bone disorders, and mental changes.

Clinical picture

The patient with hyperparathyroidism may present with a variety of symptoms caused by hypercalcemia, decreased serum phosphate, hyperphosphaturia, hypercalciuria, and decreased neuromuscular irritability. Symptoms range from mild to very severe. In the mildest form there may be no symptoms, and diagnosis may be made through a routine laboratory study of serum Ca. In more severe cases patients may present with the following symptoms:

Renal disturbances. Signs and symptoms may include polydipsia, polyuria, and albuminuria. Renal calculi are common because of mobilization of bone salts resulting from chronic hypercalcemia. Other renal problems may include hematuria, back pain and, in advanced chronic hypercalcemia, nephropathy, and uremia.

GI disturbances. Nausea, anorexia, constipation, ileus, and abdominal pain may be present. Patients may have a history of peptic ulcer or GI bleeding.

Skeletal involvement. Symptoms of bone disease may include joint pain, bone pain, and pathologic fractures of the long bones, ribs, and spine. Bone deformities may be seen in long-standing cases.

Cardiovascular disturbances. Ca imbalance may cause cardiac irregularities. Ionized Ca stimulates heart contractility; therefore, alterations in heart rhythm can occur.

CNS involvement. Patients may have symptoms such as depression, listlessness, personality disturbances, and confusion. In hyperparathyroid crisis, acute psychosis may be present.

Classic laboratory findings include elevated serum Ca (normal 9.0 to 10.5 mg/100 ml) and low phosphorus. The urine will contain elevated amounts of both Ca and phosphorus. Alkaline phosphatase may be elevated in patients with associated bone disease. Other laboratory parameters include radioimmunoassay for PTH, urinary with AMP clearance, determination of GI absorption of Ca, and determination of vitamin D metabolites in plasma. (These tests permit differentiation between nonparathyroid-related hypercalcemia and primary hyperparathyroidism).

X-rays of the bones will usually reveal demineralization of the bone, bone cysts, and sometimes distortion. The ECG may show a shortened Q-T interval.

Medical interventions

The degree of hypercalcemia, the severity of symptoms, and overall status of the patient are factors in deciding treatment.

Dehydration, progressive hypercalcemia, and deterioration of renal function are major problems that can be life-threatening in primary hyperparathyroidism. This condition is often treated by removing the diseased gland(s). If all four of the glands are involved, only three and one-half glands are removed in order to maintain sufficient amounts of circulating PTH.

Before surgery, the general condition of the patient must be stabilized. The goals of preoperative care include reducing hypercalcemia, preventing further renal damage, and correcting or treating other complications such as peptic ulcers, bone fractures, and renal problems. During the preoperative and postoperative periods, the patient is at risk for hyperparathyroid crisis, an emergency condition caused by a rapid increase in serum Ca levels (>20 mg/100 ml). The symptoms of hyperparathyroid crisis include weakness, nausea and vomiting, leg pain, and dyspnea, progressing to mental confusion, dehydration, and coma. Treatment includes administration of IV fluids and phosphorus to promote Ca excretion. Surgery should be delayed until the primary metabolic disorder is treated.

IV saline may be ordered to promote excretion of Ca and hydration to prevent formation of renal calculi. Medications may include: administration of PO and IV phosphate (2 to 4 g/day) to drive Ca back into bone; furosemide (Lasix) to reduce serum Ca levels; and mithramycin to lower Ca by antagonizing bone resorptive effect.

A low-Ca diet may be prescribed to help correct hypercalcemia. Daily serum calcium and BUN determinations may be ordered.

Postoperatively, patients may develop transient hypocalcemia because of removal of the parathyroid glands. Calcium may be administered prn (usually lactate or gluconate) and vitamin D may be ordered to increase absorption of calcium.

The danger of hyperparathyroid crisis remains through the immediate postoperative period because of additional circulating hormone from the parathyroid gland minipulation. To prevent such a crisis, serum calcium levels are monitored carefully and elevations treated promptly.

Nursing interventions

Renal dysfunction. (1) Observe for hematuria. (2) Maintain hydration (diuresis lowers serum Ca). (3) Measure intake and output. (4) Strain all urine if calculi suspected.

GI disturbances. (1) Give small frequent meals. Patient may experience anorexia or nausea and vomiting. (2) Give adequate mouth care. (3) Provide low-Ca diet; eliminate milk and dairy products. (4) Observe for signs of peptic ulcer: heartburn, nausea, blood in stools.

Dehydration and electrolyte imbalance. (1) Maintain hydration.

(2) Monitor intake and output carefully. (3) Check laboratory reports for electrolyte imbalance and report abnormalities.

Potential for respiratory distress. (1) Evaluate respirations. (2) Auscultate lung sounds. (3) Have the patient turn, cough, deep-breathe, (4) Monitor carefully if patient has respiratory condition. Respiratory acidosis can precipitate hyperparathyroid crisis.

Cardiovascular changes. (1) Assess need for placement on a monitor. (2) Observe for cardiac irregularities, i.e., flattened T wave or P-wave changes. (3) Monitor and assess vital signs. (4) Report any irregularities or bradycardia.

Demineralization of bones. (1) Implement safety precautions: side rails, call bell within reach. (2) Observe for pathologic bone fracture. (3) Assist patient with passive/active range-of-motion exercise. (4) Maintain body alignment. (5) Assist with ambulation.

Alteration in mental status. (1) Observe for depression, apathy, paranoia. (2) Inform patient and family about mental changes related to endocrine imbalance. Assure them that these changes will reverse when imbalances are corrected.

Potential for postoperative complication. (1) Observe for neuromuscular irritability; serum calcium ≤7.0 mg/100 ml may lead to tetany. (2) Observe for muscle spasms of feet and hands, muscle twitching, numbness, tingling of nose, ears, fingers, and toes. (3) Observe for laryngeal spasm. (4) Provide calcium gluconate at bedside. (5) Have tracheotomy equipment at bedside.

Hyperparathyroid crisis. (1) Monitor serum Ca levels. Rapid increase >20mg/100ml may induce crisis pre- or postoperatively. (2) Symptoms include nausea, vomiting, leg pain, weakness, mental confusion, dyspnea, dehydration, and coma. (3) Obtain daily serum Ca levels; report any abnormal results.

Potential for bleeding. (1) Check vital signs; watch for increased pulse, decreased BP. (2) Check incision. (3) Monitor drainage. (4) Observe for restlessness, pallor, cool and clammy skin. (5) Check laboratory results: Hct. (6) Observe for edema in operative site. (7) Keep tracheotomy tray at bedside. (8) Support head and neck.

Skeletal complications. (1) Reassure patient experiencing bone pain, cysts, and/or osteoporosis that these conditions will resolve quickly once metabolic condition has been corrected.

Need for medication. (1) If a diuretic is prescribed, furosemide (Lasix) is the drug of choice. Thiazide diuretics should not be administered because they decrease the renal excretion of Ca, thereby causing hypercalcemia.

Education. (1) Teach patient that close medical follow-up is important. (2) Explain need for routine checks of serum Ca levels. (3) Explain why a diet low in Ca may be indicated and assess patient's ability and motivation to follow it. Involve family in teaching as needed. (4) Emphasize need for following the prescribed schedule of medication.

CHAPTER 7

THE RENAL SYSTEM

Lani W. Smith

ANATOMY AND PHYSIOLOGY REVIEW

Adequate kidney functioning is essential for life, a fact that becomes obvious when the multiple functions of the kidneys are considered. These functions include excretion of metabolic waste products, regulation of fluid and electrolyte balance, regulation of acid-base balance, regulation of arterial BP, and regulation of erythropoiesis.

STRUCTURES

Macroscopic anatomy

The kidneys are bean-shaped organs that sit in the abdomen outside of the peritoneal cavity, one on either side of the spine. They lie between approximately the twelfth thoracic and third lumbar vertebrae, with the left kidney lying slightly lower than the right. The kidneys are protected from physical trauma by their fibrous capsules and by the perinephric fat in which they lie. Each weighs ~150 g.

Blood is supplied to the kidneys via the renal arteries, which branch off the aorta and enter the kidneys at the hilum, an indentation on the medial border. At rest, the kidneys receive about one quarter of the CO. Renal vein drainage follows the same general pathway to the inferior vena cava. Renal nerves also enter the kidneys at the hilum.

When sliced open from top to bottom, the kidneys reveal two main areas: the outer cortex and the inner medulla. The medulla contains the renal pyramids, the apices of which are the papillae. The papillae empty into calyces, which in turn coalesce to form the renal pelvis. The renal pelvis is the beginning of the urinary tract. Figure 7–1 depicts the kidney's macroscopic anatomy.

Urine formed in the cortex and outer medulla enters the renal pelvis and then the ureter. The ureters are narrow but distensible conduits between the kidneys and the bladder. Urine flows through the ureters assisted by ureteral peristalsis.

The urinary bladder is essentially a reservoir for urine. It consists mainly of a very flexible muscle, the detrusor, which can be passively stretched when distended by urine and which can forcefully contract during micturition. The normal capacity of the bladder is ~400 ml.

The bladder lies between the symphysis pubis and the rectum and seminal vesicles in men, and between the vagina and uterus in women. It is supported in place by the levator ani muscle.

Urine enters the bladder from the ureters at the trigone. The ureters enter at an oblique angle, which serves to prevent reflux and thus protect the kidney. Urine leaves the bladder via the urethra, whose opening also lies in the trigonal area at the base of the bladder. The opening to the urethra is

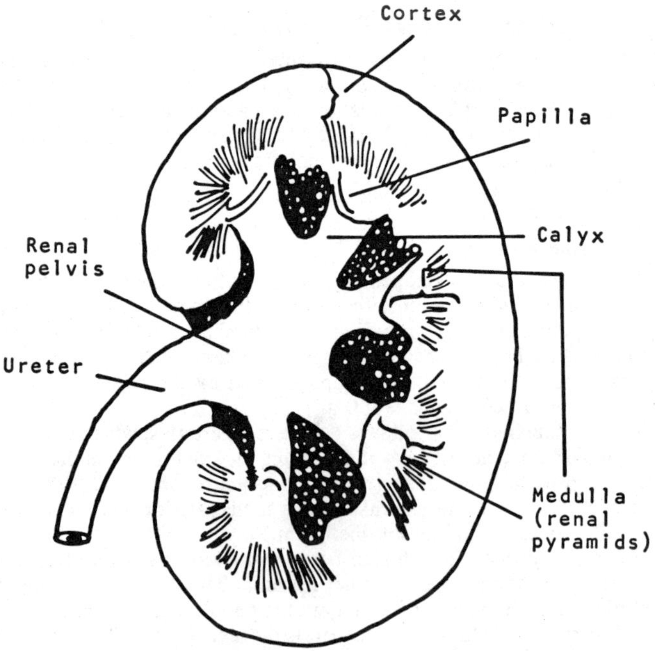

Figure 7–1. Macroscopic anatomy of the kidneys.

surrounded by muscle fibers forming the internal sphincter. The bladder is largely under parasympathetic nervous system control.

The urethra is the conduit from the bladder to the outside. In females, it is ~4 cm in length and lies just in front of the vagina. In males, the urethra is longer because it traverses the length of the penis. Immediately below the bladder, it is surrounded by the prostate gland. In males, the urethra serves not only as a conduit for urine, but also for seminal fluid. Figure 7–2 depicts the macroscopic anatomy of the urinary system.

Microscopic anatomy

Each kidney is composed of about one million functional units called nephrons: ~90% of these nephrons lie solely within the renal cortex; the other 10% extend into the renal medulla and are important in the concentration of urine. Each nephron consists of two parts, the glomerulus,

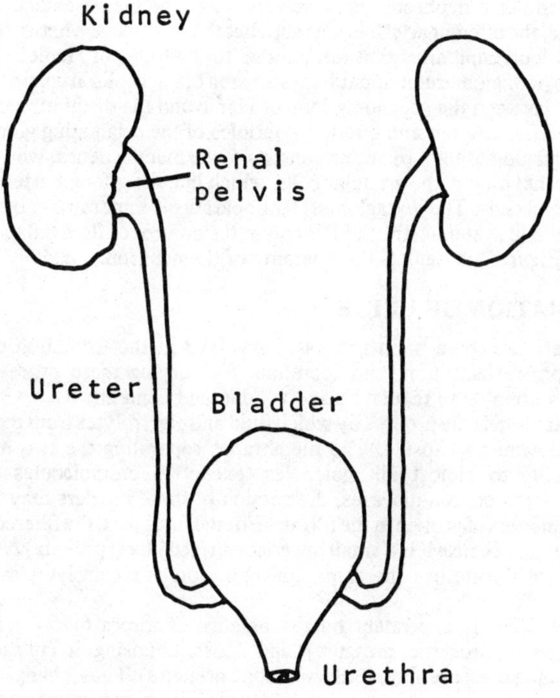

Figure 7–2. Macroscopic anatomy of the urinary system.

where the initial filtration of plasma occurs, and the tubule, where modification of the filtrate occurs and urine is formed.

The glomerulus consists of a tuft of capillaries surrounded by a hollow capsule known as Bowman's capsule. Blood is separated from the capsule by a set of highly permeable membranes that allow filtration of fluid into the capsule. On average, filtrate is formed at the rate of ~125 ml/min; this is expressed as a glomerular filtration rate (GFR) of 125 ml/min. Over the course of the day, ~180 liters of filtrate is formed. Because the average plasma volume is only ~3 liters, the entire plasma volume is filtered ~60 times/day.

Exiting Bowman's capsule is the renal tubule. The filtrate flows first through the proximal convoluted tubule, then through the loop of Henle, and finally to the distal convoluted tubule and medullary collecting ducts. The medullary collecting ducts converge and eventually empty into the renal pelvis.

Blood leaving the glomerular capillaries enters the efferent arterioles, which then branch to form the peritubular capillary system. In the juxtamedullary nephrons, in which the loops of Henle extend into the medulla, the efferent arteriole also supplies the vasa recta, a network of thin, hairpin-loop capillaries that run parallel to the loops of Henle.

The juxtaglomerular apparatus is an area of the nephron where the renal tubule, between the ascending loop of Henle and the distal tubule, passes between the afferent and efferent arterioles of the originating glomerulus. The juxtaglomerular apparatus consists of the macula densa, which is part of the renal tubule, the granular cells, which line the afferent arteriole, and mesangial cells. The juxtaglomerular apparatus is important in the control of renal and systemic arterial BP and in the control of fluid balance in the body. Figure 7–3 depicts the anatomy of the nephron.

FORMATION OF URINE

There are three main processes involved in the formation of urine: filtration, reabsorption, and secretion. By varying these processes, the kidneys are able to regulate urine volume and content.

Filtration is the process by which fluid and electrolytes from the plasma enter Bowman's capsule. The membranes separating the two areas are permeable to almost all molecules, except macromolecules such as proteins. (In certain diseases, destruction of these barriers may result in large amounts of protein in the filtrate. For the most part, the filtered protein is albumin, because it is a small but concentrated blood protein.) Normally, the initial filtrate has the same concentration of electrolytes as plasma water.

The GFR is dependent on the balance of forces favoring filtration (capillary hydrostatic pressure) and those opposing it (intracapsular hydrostatic pressure and capillary oncotic pressure). Thus, changes in renal arterial pressure or plasma protein concentration can change the GFR.

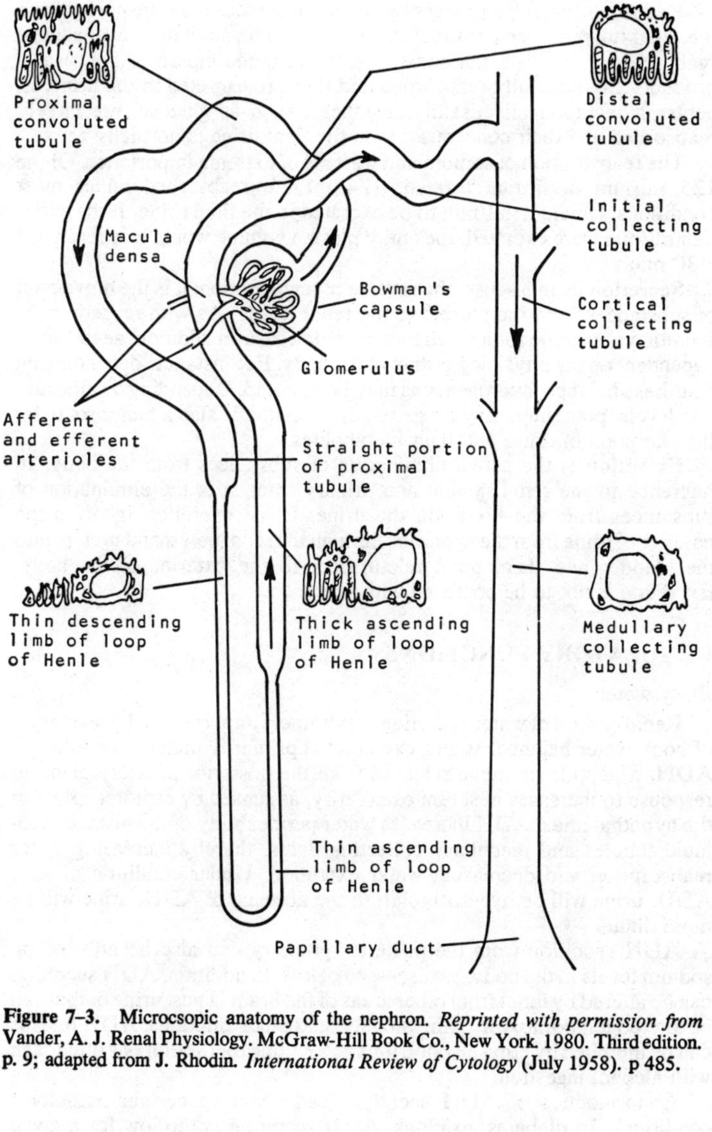

Figure 7–3. Microcsopic anatomy of the nephron. *Reprinted with permission from* Vander, A. J. Renal Physiology. McGraw-Hill Book Co., New York. 1980. Third edition. p. 9; adapted from J. Rhodin. *International Review of Cytology* (July 1958). p 485.

GFR can be estimated clinically by measurement of creatinine clearance.

Reabsorption is the process by which substances are transported from the renal tubule to the peritubular capillaries. The amount of a substance reabsorbed is specific to that substance. For instance, most metabolic waste products are minimally reabsorbed and thus are excreted in the urine. In contrast, metabolically useful substances, such as glucose, are largely reabsorbed and their concentration in the final urine is normally zero.

The reabsorption of sodium and water is of extreme importance. Of the 125 ml/min of filtrate formed, 124 ml are reabsorbed under most conditions, leaving 1 ml/min to be excreted in the final urine. If the entire 125 ml/min were excreted, the entire plasma volume would be excreted in ~30 min.

Secretion is, in a sense, the reverse of reabsorption; it is the movement of substances from the plasma to the renal tubule. As with reabsorption, secretion is specific for a given molecular species. In addition, secretion is dependent on the physiologic state of the body. For instance, depending on acid-base balance, hydrogen ions may be secreted. Depending on aldosterone levels, potassium may be secreted. Secretion is also a major route for the excretion of drugs and their metabolites.

Excretion is the actual elimination of substances from the body. In reference to the renal system and urinary tract, it is the elimination of substances from the body via the urine. Urine excretion involves the passage of urine from the nephrons through the renal pelvis and ureters into the bladder and then, upon micturition, to the exterior of the body. Excretion is not to be confused with secretion.

REGULATORY FUNCTIONS

Body water

Renal control of water excretion is extremely important in the regulation of body water balance. Water excretion is primarily under the control of **ADH,** a peptide hormone released from the posterior pituitary gland in response to increases in serum osmolarity, as sensed by osmoreceptors in the hypothalamus. ADH increases water permeability of the distal convoluted tubules and medullary collecting ducts, thereby increasing water reabsorption and decreasing water excretion. Under condition of high ADH, urine will be hyperosmolar; in the absence of ADH, urine will be more dilute.

ADH secretion from the posterior pituitary can also be affected by sodium levels in the body, as discussed below. In addition, ADH secretion can be altered by input from other areas of the brain. Thus, urine output can be altered temporarily by pain, anxiety, and other emotions. ADH release can be inhibited by ethyl alcohol, thus accounting for the diuresis often seen with alcohol ingestion.

Abnormalities of ADH secretion can occur in certain pathologic conditions. In diabetes insipidus, ADH secretion is too low for a given serum osmolarity, and the result is the excretion of large volumes of very dilute urine. In the syndrome of inappropriate secretion of ADH (SIADH), ADH is secreted from an ectopic site and secretion is not inhibited by low serum osmolarity; the result is water overload and scanty quantities of concentrated urine. SIADH is most commonly seen as a complication of certain types of lung cancer.

Electrolytes

Of all of the electrolytes in the body, sodium, potassium, and calcium are the ones whose levels the kidney regulates most closely. The regulation of **sodium (Na^+)** is important because it is the most abundant extracellular ion. As such, it is the most important determinant of ECF volume and, more importantly, extracellular intravascular (plasma) volume.

Na^+ is freely filtered at the glomerulus: ~65% is actively reabsorbed in the proximal tubule and an additional 25% in the loop of Henle. On average, by the end of the nephron, all but 1% of the filtered Na^+ load has been reabsorbed. It is this active reabsorption of Na^+ that is responsible for the passive reabsorption of water and many other substances across the tubule-capillary boundary. Thus the regulation of Na^+ levels and total body water are closely intertwined.

Na^+ levels in the body are regulated in two main ways: by altering the amount of Na^+ filtered at the glomerulus and by altering the amount of Na^+ reabsorbed. Altering the amount of Na^+ filtered is accomplished by altering the GFR, which in turn can be altered by a variety of factors, including a change in arterial BP or changes in vascular volume. For instance, a drop in arterial BP activates baroreceptors that reflexly activate the sympathetic nervous system. This causes renal vasoconstriction, particularly to the afferent arteriole, thereby decreasing GFR and Na^+ filtration. The reverse happens with an increase in arterial BP. Hypovolemia, e.g., from profuse diaphoresis, emesis, or diarrhea, also can cause a decrease in GFR. This occurs because with a decrease in intravascular volume, there is increased capillary oncotic pressure, which tends to hold fluid in the capillaries and decrease filtration. The reverse happens with hypervolemia.

The reabsorption of Na^+ is under multiple controls: aldosterone, natriuretic hormone, sympathetic stimulation, and the renin-angiotensin system. Aldosterone is a steroid hormone, released from the adrenal cortex, primarily in response to angiotensin and to changes in plasma Na^+ and potassium (K^+). Receptors for plasma Na^+ and K^+ are located in the adrenal cortex itself. Angiotensin is the most important controller of aldosterone levels; it will be discussed in greater detail below. Aldosterone acts on the distal convoluted tubule and medullary collecting ducts to increase Na^+ reabsorption.

Natriuretic hormone is released from the atria of the heart in response to increased atrial stretch, caused by increased plasma volume. Increased levels of natriuretic hormone cause decreased Na^+ reabsorption and thus increase Na^+ excretion.

Sympathetic stimulation has multiple effects resulting in increased Na^+ reabsorption. These effects include direct effects on the renal tubule to increase Na^+ reabsorption and stimulation of renin release, which increases angiotensin formation and thereby stimulates aldosterone release.

Control of **K^+** levels in the body is critical because of the role K^+ plays in the maintenance of resting membrane potential and thus in nerve and muscle excitability. K^+ levels are also primarily regulated by the kidney. Like Na^+, K^+ is freely filtered at the glomerulus. Also like Na^+, 65% is actively reabsorbed in the proximal convoluted tubule and another 25% in the loop of Henle.

Control of K^+ excretion is primarily achieved by altering K^+ secretion in the distal tubule and medullary collecting duct. Altered secretion may result directly from changes in serum K^+ levels that alter the concentration gradient for ion movement. Altered secretion may also result from changes in aldosterone levels. Aldosterone, under the control of factors described above, stimulates K^+ secretion in exchange for Na^+ reabsorption in the distal convoluted tubule and medullary collecting duct.

Acid-base changes can also affect K^+ secretion. Alkalosis stimulates K^+ secretion; acidosis may either stimulate or inhibit K^+ secretion.

Calcium (Ca^{++}) levels in the body are under multiple controls because of the importance of Ca^{++} for muscle contraction. Renal regulation of Ca^{++} levels is primarily under the control of parathyroid hormone (PTH). PTH is a peptide hormone released from the parathyroid gland in response to low serum levels of ionized Ca^{++}. In the kidney, PTH causes increased Ca^{++} reabsorption in the distal tubule, thereby decreasing Ca^{++} excretion. PTH also causes decreased renal **phosphate** excretion.

In addition, the kidney plays an important role in the biochemical activation of **vitamin D.** Vitamin D acts primarily on the intestine to increase Ca^{++} and phosphate absorption.

Acid-base balance

Acid-base balance in the body is under the dual control of the respiratory and renal system. Whereas the respiratory system can respond rapidly to changes in acid-base status, the kidney is more effective over a long period of time in maintaining normal acid-base balance. *See* Chapter 3 for discussion of the respiratory control of acid-base balance and Chapter 12 for specifics of interpretation of arterial blood gases.

There are several buffer systems in the body, the most important being the **bicarbonate system.** Water (H_2O) and carbon dioxide (CO_2) combine to form carbonic acid (H_2CO_3), which then breaks down into hydrogen ion (H^+) and bicarbonate (HCO_3^-). The pH of the body is dependent upon the relative amounts of CO_2 and HCO_3^-. Serum CO_2 levels are primarily under the control of the respiratory system, whereas serum HCO_3^- levels are primarily under the control of the kidneys. HCO_3^- excretion by the kidney can be varied by changing the level of HCO_3^- reabsorption or by adding new HCO_3^- to the plasma flowing through the renal vasculature.

HCO_3^- is freely filtered at the glomerulus. Most of it is actively reabsorbed, with 80 to 90% being reabsorbed in the proximal tubule and the remainder in the loop of Henle and the distal tubule. In acidosis, the kidney can compensate by adding new HCO_3^- to the plasma, coupled to the excretion of an equivalent amount of acid. This is accomplished by secreting a H^+, which is trapped by either phosphate, which was filtered at the glomerulus, or ammonia, which is synthesized in the renal tubule cell and then actively secreted. In alkalosis, the reverse occurs; there is decreased HCO_3^- reabsorption in the distal tubule, resulting in increased HCO_3^- excretion and return of the plasma pH to normal.

BP

The kidneys play an important role in the control of arterial BP because of their ability to stimulate the renin-angiotensin system. The kidneys sense alterations in BP in at least two ways: (1) direct pressure sensing by the granular cells lining the afferent arteriole in the juxtaglomerular apparatus and (2) sensing of sodium chloride delivery to the macula densa. In response to decreased pressure or decreased sodium chloride delivery, the juxtaglomerular apparatus secretes renin. Renal sympathetic nerve stimulation can also stimulate renin production, whereas angiotensin is inhibitory.

Renin catalyses the conversion of angiotensinogen, a plasma protein, to angiotensin I. Angiotensin I is converted to angiotensin II by angiotensin-converting enzyme, which is located primarily in the lungs. Angiotensin II is a potent vasoconstrictor. Angiotension-II-mediated vasoconstriction increases peripheral vascular resistance, and thus arterial BP rises. In addition, this vasoconstriction affects renal arterioles. Angiotension-II-mediated constriction of the afferent arteriole results in decreased GFR. In addition to its vasoconstrictive effects, angiotensin II is the most potent stimulator of aldosterone release from the adrenal cortex. As discussed above, this causes increased Na^+ reabsorption in the distal tubule and medullary collecting duct. Angiotensin II also directly causes increased tubular Na^+ reabsorption. Finally, angiotensin II acts in the CNS to (1) facilitate sympathetic nervous system activity, thereby increasing peripheral vasoconstriction and increasing CO; (2) increase ADH secretion, thereby increasing water reabsorption in the kidney; and (3) increase the sensation of thirst, thereby stimulating the person to increase water intake. In summary, the net effect of angiotensin II formation is increased peripheral vasoconstriction, increased CO, increased Na^+ and water reabsorption, and finally increased arterial BP. Angiotensin II is also converted to angiotensin III, whose physiologic effects are not well understood.

Erythropoiesis

When there is reduced O_2 delivery to the kidneys, renal erythropoietic factor is released. This factor acts to break down a circulating plasma protein into erythropoietin. Erythropoietin acts on the bone marrow to stimulate RBC production. Thus, the kidneys are important in the control of erythropoiesis.

ASSESSMENT OF THE PATIENT

Health history

Relevant areas about which information should be obtained in patients with possible diseases of the kidneys or urinary tract are outlined in Table 7–1.

Physical examination

Inspection. There are few specific manifestations of renal disease that will be apparent on inspection of the patient. Signs of renal failure that may, however, be seen include general malaise, Kussmaul respirations, anorexia, dry and scaly skin, dry and brittle hair, edema, and uremic fetor.

If the patient requires urinary drainage devices, these should be inspected for evidence of proper functioning. Of particular importance is the condition of the penile skin with the use of condom catheters and the condition of the peristomal skin with urinary diversions.

Palpation. The kidneys are mainly inspected by palpation. By placing one hand under a supine patient's abdomen and the other hand above, it is possible to palpate the kidneys. Enlargement may indicate hydronephrosis, tumor, or polycystic kidney disease. Tenderness on palpation may indicate acute inflammation. It is important to assess for tenderness at the costovertebral angle by gently striking over the area.

To assess the amount of urine in the bladder, palpation may be used. This may only be possible, however, if the bladder contains ≥150 ml of urine. Furthermore, even a grossly distended bladder may not be palpable if the bladder wall is flaccid.

Percussion. It is possible to assess the amount of urine in the bladder by percussing the borders of the bladder. As with assessment by palpation, there must be ≥150 ml of urine in the bladder for it to be percussible.

Auscultation. The abdomen should be auscultated for the presence of abdominal or renal bruits. These may indicate the presence of renal artery stenosis.

It is possible to estimate the size of the bladder by placing the stethoscope just above the symphysis pubis. A fingernail is then gently drawn across the patient's abdomen, moving from the stethoscope toward the estimated border of the bladder. A loud sound will be heard to the limits of the bladder; beyond the bladder wall, the sound will be much softer.

Diagnostic tests

Urinalysis is an inexpensive and highly valuable diagnostic test. For it to be most reliable, a clean midstream urine specimen should be obtained and examined as soon as possible after collection. Although laboratory analysis may be desired because of its higher degree of quantitative accuracy, rapid qualitative screening may be performed at the bedside with the use of tablets or dipsticks.

Bacteriologic studies are important in identifying causes of renal or urinary infection. An optimal specimen for culture and sensitivity is not contaminated by organisms from outside the urinary tract; usable specimens are clean-catch midstream-voided or catheterized specimens. A colony count of >100,000/ml is usually considered to be evidence of significant bacteriuria.

Cytologic studies are best performed on morning urine, collected using a clean-catch technique. These studies are useful in the diagnosis of neoplasms.

Although useful information can be obtained from random single specimens of urine, it is sometimes necessary to obtain a 24-hr collection to quantitate the amount of a given substance excreted or to find an average value when there is significant circadian variation. An optimal collection is free of contamination by toilet paper, feces, or menstrual fluid. During the collection period, urine should be preserved either chemically or by refrigeration, depending on the nature of the test.

Analyses of blood specimens may also help to diagnose renal and urinary tract disease, because renal failure causes changes throughout the body.

Measurement of creatinine clearance is often carried out to estimate GFR. Typically, to measure creatinine clearance, a 24-hr urine specimen is obtained for measurement of urine volume and average urine concentration of creatinine. Plasma creatinine concentration can be measured at any time during the 24-hr period of urine collection. The normal creatinine clearance is 125 ml/min; a decrease indicates a decrease in GFR, consistent with deterioration of renal function.

A variety of studies may be carried out to help in the diagnosis of renal or urinary tract disease. The common tests are presented in Table 7–2.

MAJOR DISORDERS

ACUTE RENAL FAILURE

Acute renal failure (ARF) is a rapid decrease in renal function, or more specifically, in the GFR, which may or may not be accompanied by oliguria or anuria. ARF is also commonly referred to as acute tubular necrosis, although necrosis may not always be apparent histologically.

Pathophysiology

Causes of ARF may be broken down into three general categories: prerenal, postrenal, and intrarenal. **Prerenal** failure results from decreased perfusion to the kidneys, leading to ischemia and tubular damage. This hypoperfusion may result from a variety of systemic circulatory abnormali-

TABLE 7-1
Health History

Assessment	Possible abnormality
Usual pattern of micturition	
Frequency	High residual urine volume Inflammation/infection Nervousness
Urgency	Inflammation/infection
Dysuria	Cystitis Prostatis
Nocturia	Primary renal disease CHF with edema Prostate enlargement Drinking fluids late at night
Problems initiating flow, dribbling	Prostate enlargement
Usual urine characteristics	
Color	
Brown, maroon, pink, red	Bleeding secondary to trauma, neoplasms, transfusion reactions, drugs
Nearly colorless	Large fluid intake Interstitial nephritis Diuretics Diabetes insipidus
Orange, amber, brown	Dehydration Bile pigments in urine Drugs (phenazopyridine)
Odor	Infection
Amount	
Decreased	Dehydration Renal failure Obstruction to urinary flow
Increased	Overhydration Diuretics Diabetes insipidus Diabetes mellitus
Pain	
Location Association with voiding	Dull ache at costovertebral angle: renal obstruction, pyelonephritis, ureteral obstruction Ureteral pain radiating from costovertebral angle to scrotum/vulva: stones, clots Bladder pain Constant: urinary retention With voiding: infection

Assessment	Possible abnormality
Medications	
Diuretics	For treatment of CHF, hypertension, renal disease
Parasympathomimetics, parasympatholytics	May affect bladder functioning
Antibiotics	For treatment of various renal/bladder infections
Nephrotoxins	May damage the kidney
Fluid balance	
Weight gain	Fluid retention Renal failure
Weight loss	Diuretics Renal failure
Incontinence Frequency Amount Related to coughing, sneezing	Neurogenic bladder, organic brain syndrome, urinary tract infection, prostate enlargement
Usual diet	
Fluid consumption	Decreased fluid intake can lead to renal failure
Milk, meat consumption	High milk or meat intake predisposes to certain types of renal stones
History of renal or kidney disease	May predispose to further renal or kidney disease
History of other diseases Diabetes mellitus Hypertension SLE	May predispose to renal or kidney diseases
Family history of renal or kidney disease	Polycystic kidney disease

ties, including decreased CO from shock, cardiac failure, or cardiac arrest. Excessive fluid loss (e.g., from profuse diaphoresis, diabetes insipidus, or diarrhea) can cause hypovolemia, which in turn can lead to renal hypoperfusion. Insufficient fluid intake (e.g., from a decreased ability to sense thirst or an inability to obtain adequate fluids) can also cause hypovolemia and renal hypoperfusion. Renal hypoperfusion can also result from the use of nonselective systemic vasoconstrictors, such as levarterenol or high doses of dopamine. Finally, renal hypoperfusion can result from obstructions to renal blood flow, e.g., blood clots or traumatic injuries.

Postrenal causes of ARF are abnormalities that prevent the normal outflow of urine from the kidneys to the bladder and then outward from the

TABLE 7-2
Diagnostic Studies

Name of test	Procedure	Possible findings	Associated care
KUB	Flat plate x-ray of kidneys, ureters, bladder.	Gross malformation of organs Renal calculi	No special care required
IVP	KUB, then injection of radiopaque dye. Serial x-rays before and after voiding.	Altered renal anatomy Renal calculi Postvoiding residual urine	Preprocedure: Check for iodine sensitivity NPO or clear liquids for 12 hr before test Bowel cleanout as ordered Postprocedure: Encourage fluids Watch for delayed dye reaction
Retrograde pyelogram	Injection of radiopaque dye into kidneys via cystoscope. Serial x-rays.	Confirmation of results of IVP	Same as for cystoscopy (*see* below) Check for iodine sensitivity
Renal angiography	Injection of radiopaque dye into renal vasculature. Vascular access is variable; femoral route is common.	Delineation of renal vasculature; stenosis, trauma, neoplasms	Preprocedure: Same as for IVP Postprocedure: Bed rest for several hours Observe puncture site for bleeding Check peripheral pulses and vital signs frequently Watch for delayed dye reaction
Renal biopsy	Visualization of kidney by fluoroscopy or ultrasound, then insertion of biopsy needle percutaneously or via open incision.	Diagnosis of renal parenchymal disease	Preprocedure: NPO for 6–8 hr before test IV line in place Obtain informed consent Sedation as ordered Assess for bleeding disorders, hypertension Postprocedure: Assess for bleeding, vital signs, pain, hematoma, Hct Chest x-ray to check for iatrogenic pneumothorax Bed rest for 24 hr Encourage fluids For open biopsy: general postoperative care
Renal vein catheterization	Catheterization, usually via femoral vein, under fluoroscopy. Collection of blood specimens.	Measurement of renal vein renins, useful in diagnosis of hypertension	Same as for renal angiography

Name of test	Procedure	Possible findings	Associated care
Voiding cystogram	Bladder catheterization; instillation of radiopaque dye, removal of catheter. X-rays before, during, and after voiding.	Ureteral reflux Ureteral stenosis Measurement of postvoiding residual urine volume	Check for iodine sensitivity.
Cystometrogram	Bladder catheterization; instillation of fluid; measurement of intravesicular pressure and correlation with urge to void.	Determination of cause of incontinence	No special care required.
Renal ultrasound	Noninvasive sonography.	Visualization of renal anatomy	No special care required
Cystoscopy	Local or general anesthesia. Passage of rigid or flexible cystoscope into the bladder under strict surgical asepsis. May involve ureteral catheterization.	Removal of calculi	Preprocedure: NPO Bowel cleanout Obtain informed consent Sedation as ordered Antibiotics if at risk of endocarditis Postprocedure: Bed rest. General postoperative care. Encourage fluids Observe for urine retention, bleeding, infection
Renal scan	Injection of radioisotope, usually technetium-99m.	Identification of intrarenal masses, renal anatomy	Handle urine with gloves for 24 hr postprocedure.

IVP, IV pyelogram; KUB, kidneys, ureters, bladder.

body. Such abnormalities include ureteral or urethral strictures, urolithiasis, prostate enlargement, urinary catheter obstruction, and renal or urinary tract trauma. In these conditions, obstruction of urine outflow causes increased backward pressure, resulting in barotrauma and decreased physiologic functioning.

Intrarenal causes of ARF include abnormalities intrinsic to the kidneys themselves. Such causes include renal parenchymal disease (glomerulonephritis, pyelonephritis, etc.), transfusion reactions (resulting in glomerular capillary damage), renal trauma, renal involvement from certain systemic diseases (SLE, etc.), and the nephrotoxic effects of various chemicals (such as the aminoglycoside antibiotics, radiographic contrast materials, heavy metals, and certain organic solvents).

Clinical picture

ARF occurs in four stages: onset, oliguric, diuretic, and recovery. During the **onset stage**, renal damage occurs, but signs and symptoms of renal failure are not apparent. In the **oliguric stage**, which typically lasts 10 to 14 days, urine output is decreased to <400 ml/day. In addition, there is elevation of the BUN and serum creatinine, decreased clearance, fluid retention (resulting in weight gain, pulmonary edema, peripheral edema, hypertension, etc.), electrolyte imbalance (hyperkalemia and hyponatremia), and evidence of the uremic syndrome (anorexia, nausea, vomiting, asterixis, decreased level of consciousness, convulsions, anemia, metabolic acidosis, pruritus, etc.). Oliguria (urine output <400 ml/day) may not be present in as many as 50% of patients in the oliguric stage of ARF; however, these patients still exhibit an inability to concentrate urine and thus exhibit many of the other signs and symptoms apparent during the oliguric stage.

During the **diuretic stage**, urine output increases to >400 ml/day, but the serum creatinine and BUN continue to rise for a few days. Eventually, as renal function improves, serum chemistries plateau and then return to normal. Concurrently, signs and symptoms of ARF improve and disappear. The diuretic stage of ARF typically lasts for two to eight days.

Finally, during the **recovery stage**, renal function returns to normal and signs and symptoms of renal failure disappear. Full clinical recovery may take up to a year, although biochemical studies may reveal permanent minor defects in renal function.

Between 30 and 60% of patients with ARF will die. Mortality rates are higher in older individuals, in individuals with serious underlying diseases, and individuals who develop ARF as a sequela of trauma or surgery. The most frequent cause of death in ARF is infection.

Medical interventions

In ARF, medical intervention is aimed at (1) eliminating, if possible, any causes of renal failure; (2) minimizing demands on the kidney; (3) supplementing renal function artificially to preserve life; and (4) controlling the manifestations of renal failure.

Eliminating causes of renal deterioration involves looking for responsible factors such as renal vascular obstruction, systemic circulatory abnormalities, urine outflow obstruction, and the presence of nephrotoxins. As much as possible, all contributing factors should be corrected.

Minimizing demands on the kidneys involves controlling fluid, solute, and nutrient administration. A high-carbohydrate diet is usually provided to minimize protein breakdown. Fluids are administered IV and PO to a limit of the previous day's urine output plus estimated insensible fluid losses ($\sim$600 ml/day). K^+ and magnesium intake is limited.

Supplementing renal function artificially to preserve life involves peritoneal dialysis or hemodialysis. These treatment modalities will be discussed below.

Controlling the manifestations of renal failure involves (1) treating cardiovascular complications of volume overload with digitalis and judicious fluid administration; (2) correcting hyperkalemia with IV Ca^{++} and HCO_3^-, IV glucose and insulin, or PO or rectal administration of K^+ binding ion exchange resins, such as sodium polystyrene sulfonate (Kayexalate); (3) correcting metabolic acidosis with IV sodium bicarbonate ($NaHCO_3$); and (4) preventing or controlling GI blood loss with antacids, histamine receptor antagonists (cimetidine, ranitidine, etc.), and GI intubation as required. Antacids containing phosphate binders (such as Amphojel) are used in preference to those with high Ca^{++} or magnesium levels.

Nursing interventions

General aspects of nursing management of the patient with ARF are presented here. Dialysis is discussed below.

Alteration in fluid balance. (1) Weigh at same time of day, using same scale each day, subtracting weight of bedclothes. (2) Measure hourly urine output. (3) Monitor serum osmolarity, urine osmolarity, urine specific gravity, sensation of thirst. (4) Make physical assessment for signs and symptoms of volume overload.

Hyperkalemia. (1) Monitor serum K^+. (2) Assess for ECG changes consistent with elevated K^+: peaked T waves, widened QRS complexes, loss of P waves, ventricular dysrhythmias. (3) If blood administration is required, ensure that blood is fresh, not stored.

Anemia. (1) Assist with activities of daily living to reduce O_2 demand. (2) Prevent complications of decreased activity: have patient turn, cough, and deep breathe; perform joint exercises. (3) Minimize bleeding: draw minimal amounts of blood for tests; use stool softeners to prevent lower GI bleeding from irritation.

Altered level of consciousness. (1) Institute seizure precautions in early stages of ARF. (2) Help family understand metabolic causes of altered level of consciousness. (3) Keep bed in low position, with siderails up. (4) Allow time for patient to process information presented to him. (5) Minimize extraneous environmental stimuli.

Increased susceptibility to infection. (1) Practice strict aspesis in management of surgical wounds, drains, urinary and IV catheters. (2) Ensure adequate pulmonary hygiene (coughing and deep-breathing, postural drainage, etc.) (3) Provide skin care to prevent pressure necrosis. (4) Provide mouth care to prevent parotiditis. (5) Monitor temperature and observe for other signs of infection. (6) Ensure adequate nutrition: give mouth care; provide small, appetizing portions; maintain pleasant environment during meals.

Change in body image related to disease and/or therapy. (1) Provide emotional support to patient and family.

Lack of understanding about dietary restrictions. (1) Obtain dietician consultation. (2) Allow self-choice of meals, with supervision, while in hospital. (3) Include family and significant others in diet teaching.

Lack of understanding about medications. (1) Provide written instructions about medications (times to take, side effects to watch for, indications).

Anxiety related to disease. (1) Provide information about sensations patient will experience during planned tests and procedures. (2) Allow as much control over situation as possible.

CHRONIC RENAL FAILURE

Chronic renal failure (CRF) results from a variety of sustained injuries to the kidneys, resulting in the clinical syndrome often referred to as uremia. Unlike ARF, in CRF the damage to the kidneys is irreversible.

Pathophysiology

In CRF, renal function declines over an extended period of time because of any of a number of pathologic processes such as glomerulonephritis, polycystic kidney disease, nephrosclerosis, systemic hypertension, SLE, or diabetes mellitus. The result of this decline in renal function is widespread, involving all of the functions of the kidney: excretion of metabolic wastes, regulation of fluid and electrolyte balance, regulation of acid/base balance, and erythropoiesis.

Because the kidneys cannot excrete nitrogenous end products of protein metabolism (primarily urea), they accumulate in the blood and cause a variety of problems, collectively referred to as the uremic syndrome. Not all of the manifestations of the uremic syndrome are the direct consequence of impaired renal excretion, however, because dialysis to remove accumulated substances does not correct all of the manifestation of the uremic syndrome.

Clinical picture

Signs and symptoms in a given stage of CRF depend largely on the GFR. In early CRF, when the GFR is 40 to 60 ml/min, renal function is adequate to maintain the patient in a symptom-free state. When the GFR decreases further, to between 25 and 40 ml/min, signs of renal failure begin to be evident, including hypertension, anemia, glucose intolerance, increased serum uric acid, polyuria, nocturia, and hypertriglyceridemia. In this stage, patients usually are symptom free, but any additional stress on the kidneys can result in overt manifestations of uremia. When the GFR decreased to <25 ml/min, overt renal failure, the uremic syndrome, is apparent.

The uremic syndrome involves disturbances in all body systems. Neurologic abnormalities include weakness, fatigue, lethargy, decreased level of consciousness, muscular irritability, peripheral neuropathy, and sleep disorders. Cardiovascular abnormalities include hypertension, pericarditis, and accelerated atherogenesis. GI abnormalities include anorexia, nausea, vomiting, peptic ulcer, gastritis, GI bleeding, hepatitis, and ascites. Integumentary abnormalities include altered pigmentation, pruritus, ecchymosis, and uremic frosts. Fluid and electrolyte abnormalities include alterations in body water (overhydration or dehydration), Na^+ (hypernatremia or hyponatremia), hyperkalemia, metabolic acidosis, hyperphosphatemia, and hypocalcemia. Other abnormalities seen in the uremic syndrome include glucose intolerance, hyperuricemia, hypertriglyceridemia, anemia, bleeding abnormalities, increased susceptibility to infection, splenomegaly, leukopenia, and lymphocytopenia.

Medical interventions

Medical management of CRF involves measures to slow the progression of renal deterioration, measures to correct or compensate for signs and symptoms of CRF, and dialysis/transplantation. Measures to slow the progression of CRF primarily involve dietary therapy. Protein intake is generally restricted to <40 g/day, in order to reduce the rate of accumulation of nitrogenous end products while preventing protein catabolism from body stores. In addition, adequate carbohydrate and vitamins are administered.

Medical measures to correct or compensate for the signs and symptoms of CRF are similar to those in ARF. They include management of the cardiovascular complication of volume overload, correcting hyperkalemia, correcting metabolic acidosis, and preventing or controlling GI blood loss.

Dialysis and transplantation are discussed below.

Nursing interventions

Problems common to patients with ARF and CRF are presented in the discussion of ARF. Management of fluid and electrolyte imbalances and nursing management of the patient undergoing dialysis or renal transplantation are discussed below. In addition, however, patients with CRF have problems specific to this disorder as presented here.

Pruritus. (1) Provide starch, vinegar, or oatmeal baths. (2) Keep nails short to prevent skin damage from scratching. (3) Apply lanolin-based skin lotion. (4) Administer ordered antipruritic medications. (5) Use superfatted soaps or bath oils.

Metallic taste in mouth. (1) Provide frequent oral hygiene. (2) Provide candy, gum, cold liquids frequently. (3) Obtain consultation with dietician. (4) Obtain dental consultation if indicated.

Altered skin integrity. (1) Use padded side rails to prevent trauma. (2) Turn patient and change position frequently. (3) Provide air mattress, eggshell mattress, or water bed to prevent decubiti.

Hypertension. (1) Monitor BP accurately: use correct size cuff; if arterial line in place for BP measurement: ensure that the transducer is at heart level; ensure that the system is free of air bubbles, clots. (2) Monitor for signs of complications: fluid overload, signs of increasing intracranial pressure, etc.

Peripheral neuropathy. (1) Obtain physical therapy consultation. (2) Use footboard to prevent foot-drop. (3) Provide daily foot care. (4) Prevent foot trauma: use heel pads, etc.

POTASSIUM IMBALANCES

In the body, K^+ is crucial for maintenance of the resting membrane potential. The normal extracellular K^+ concentration is between 3.5 and 5.0 mEq/liter; the intracellular K^+ concentration is much higher, ~140 mEq/liter. K^+ levels are closely regulated in the body, as discussed above (*see* Anatomy and Physiology Review).

HYPERKALEMIA

Hyperkalemia is an elevation of extracellular (serum) $K^+ > 5.0$ mEq/liter.

Pathophysiology

Hyperkalemia is most often the result of altered renal handling of K^+, as in renal failure. Hyperkalemia can also result from overingestion of K^+ (usually in the setting of somewhat impaired renal function), extensive tissue damage (e.g., following shock, burns, or trauma), metabolic acidosis, adrenal insufficiency, or administration of aldosterone antagonists, such as spironolactone (Aldactone).

Clinical picture

Signs and symptoms in hyperkalemia depend on the degree of elevation of extracellular K^+. At mildly elevated levels, the predominant signs and symptoms are irritability, nausea, vomiting, and diarrhea. Peaked T waves may be seen on the ECG. With increased extracellular K^+, muscle weakness occurs, potentially severe enough to interfere with respiration. On the ECG, severe hyperkalemia may be manifested as loss of P waves, widening of the QRS complex, and ventricular dysrhythmias. Death in hyperkalemia usually results from degeneration of this abnormal cardiac electrical activity to ventricular fibrillation and asystole.

Medical intervention

Emergency medical treatment of hyperkalemia is aimed at driving extracellular K^+ into the cells of the body. This may be accomplished by the IV administration of hypertonic dextrose and insulin or $NaHCO_3$. In addition, Ca^{++} may be administered to protect the heart from the toxic effects of hyperkalemia.

To rid the body of excess K^+, oral or rectal K^+-binding ion exchange resins such as sodium polystyrene sulfonate (Kayexalate) may be administered. In the setting of normal renal function, K^+-wasting diuretics such as furosemide (Lasix) may be given. In patients with diminished renal function, dialysis may be needed to rid the body of excess K^+.

Nursing interventions

The patient with hyperkalemia requires careful monitoring for signs and symptoms. K^+ intake should be limited. Foods high in K^+, such as many fruits and vegetables and most salt substitutes, should be avoided. The use of medications with high K^+ content, such as penicillin G, should be carefully evaluated. K^+-sparing diuretics such as spironolactone (Aldactone) should be discontinued. If blood transfusions are required, fresh rather than stored blood should be used.

To minimize the leakage of intracellular K^+ into the extracellular space and thus further elevation of extracellular K^+ levels, measures to prevent tissue damage should be instituted. These measures include controlling infection, prevention of bedsores, and provision of adequate calories and carbohydrates in the diet to prevent protein catabolism.

HYPOKALEMIA

Hypokalemia is a decrease in extracellular (serum) K^+ to <3.5 mEq/liter.

Pathophysiology

Hypokalemia most often results from excessive K^+ loss from the body, rather than from insufficient intake. Excessive K^+ loss commonly occurs as a result of the administration of K^+-wasting diruetics, such as furosemide (Lasix). Another cause of excessive K^+ loss is the loss of body fluids rich in K^+, through vomiting, diarrhea, or GI suctioning. Hypokalemia can also result from diabetic ketoacidosis, severe burns, metabolic alkalosis, stress, and hyperaldosteronism. Insufficient K^+ intake rarely occurs but may be seen in patients who take little or no nutrition PO. Individuals normally excrete ≥ 40 mEq/day of K^+.

Clinical picture

Hypokalemia affects all excitable tissues of the body, resulting in muscular weakness, fatigue, shallow breathing, decreased GI motility, anorexia, decreased level of consciousness, tetany, and paresthesias. Cardiac arrhythmias are common; flattened T waves and prominent U waves may also be seen on the ECG. Death from hypokalemia usually results from degeneration of these arrhythmias or from respiratory paralysis.

Medical interventions

Medical therapy in hypokalemia is directed toward replacement of the body's K^+ stores, either IV or PO.

Nursing interventions

The patient with hypokalemia should be carefully monitored for signs and symptoms. K^+ intake PO may be augmented by increasing the intake of K^+-rich foods, such as many fruits and vegetables. Most salt substitutes are also high in K^+. If PO K^+ supplementation is ordered by the physician, it should be administered with adequate fluids to prevent mucosal irritation; juices may be mixed with most PO preparations of K^+ to mask the bitter taste.

IV administration of K^+ should be carefully moniotred. No more than 20 mEq/hr should be administered. Local pain at the IV injection site can usually be eliminated only by slowing the rate of infusion.

Patients with hypokalemia are prone to digitalis toxicity. Hypokalemic individuals who are on digitalis should receive adequate K^+ supplementation prior to administration of routine digitalis doses.

SODIUM IMBALANCES

Na^+ is the chief extracellular cation and as such is important in maintenance of extracellular osmotic pressure and ECF volume. In addition, Na^+ plays a critical role in the action potential of excitable cells. Na^+ levels in the body are closely regulated between 136 and 146 mEq/liter, by mechanisms described above (*see* Anatomy and Physiology Review).

HYPERNATREMIA

Hypernatremia is an elevation of extracellular (serum) $Na^+ > 146$ mEq/liter.

Pathophysiology

Increased Na^+ most commonly occurs in the setting of decreased water intake, particularly in those individuals with decreased ability to sense thirst. Alternatively, increased Na^+ may result from excessive loss of hypotonic body fluids, as in diabetes insipidus or the diuresis after high solute loads (such as in hyperglycemia). Finally, increased Na^+ can result from excessive Na^+ intake, e.g., from excessive intake of salty foods, overadministration of salt tablets, or IV administration of hypertonic saline.

Clinical picture

The signs and symptoms of hypernatremia include thirst, flushed skin, dry mucous membranes, and increased tissue tugor. A low-grade fever is often present. Urine output is usually decreased because of the interrelationship between Na^+ and ECF volume. Neurologic findings include restlessness, agitation, convulsions, and decreased deep tendon reflexes.

Medical interventions

Medical therapy for hypernatremia usually consists of the PO administration of water or the IV administration of hypotonic solutions.

Nursing interventions

Nursing management of the patient with hypernatremia involves monitoring fluid balance (daily weights, intake and output recording, measurement of vital signs), maintaining skin integrity (mouth care, frequent position changes, back care), and protection against convulsions (seizure precautions).

HYPONATREMIA

Hyponatremia is a decrease in extracellular (serum) Na^+ to <136 mEq/liter.

Pathophysiology

Hyponatremia can result from excessive Na^+ loss, as in diarrhea or vomiting, excessive use of diuretics such as furosemide (Lasix), or excessive diaphoresis. Alternatively, hyponatremia may result from excessive water intake, resulting in dilution of the extracellular Na^+ stores. This can result from excessive PO ingestion of plain water, particularly after exercising in a hot, humid environment, excessive use of tap-water enemas, excessive administration of hyptonic IV fluids, and excessive GI irrigation with hypotonic solutions.

A less common cause of hyponatremia is SIADH. Increased ADH release will cause inappropriate water retention, resulting in overhydration and hyponatremia. SIADH is a complication of certain malignancies. It can also occur in a variety of other setting including CNS disease.

Clinical picture

The signs and symptoms of hyponatremia depend partly on the etiology of the problem. However, general observations include neurologic changes (such as apprehension, weakness, personality changes), GI symptoms (such as abdominal cramps, nausea), orthostatic hypotension, and cool, clammy skin. Urine output may be decreased.

Medical interventions

Medical intervention depends primarily on the cause of the problem. If the problem is the result of insufficient body Na^+, Na^+ may be administered

PO or IV. If the problem results primarily from excessive body water, the usual therapy is restriction of fluid intake and the judicious use of diuretics.

In SIADH, demeclocycline (Declomycin) may be administered to inhibit the effects of ADH on the renal tubule.

Nursing interventions

As with hypernatremia, nursing management of the patient with hyponatremia involves monitoring fluid balance (daily weights, measurement of intake and output, measurement of vital signs), maintaining skin integrity (back care, frequent position changes), and protection from convulsions (seizure precautions).

If fluid restriction is required, the allotted amount should be carefully allocated over the course of a day; fluids administered as or with medications should be taken into account. Mouth care should be provided frequently to minimize associated discomforts. Visitors should be alerted to the need for restricting the patient's fluid intake. Any IV administration sets should be equipped with microdrip volume-control chambers.

CALCIUM AND PHOSPHATE IMBALANCES

Ca^{++} is the most abundant cation in the body, whereas phosphate (PO_4^-) is a major extracellular anion. Most of the body's Ca^{++} and PO_4^- is deposited in the bones and teeth. The concentrations of extracellular (serum) Ca^{++} and PO_4^- are closely regulated in the body by three hormones: PTH, calcitonin, and vitamin D_3. The normal total serum Ca^{++} concentration is between 9 and 10.5 mg/100 ml; the normal concentration of serum PO_4^- is between 3 and 4.5 mg/100 ml.

The physiologically important form of serum Ca^{++} is the amount that is ionized; that fraction accounts for ~50% of the total Ca^{++} in the blood. The amount that is ionized can be affected by a variety of factors, the most important being serum pH. An increase in the pH (alkalosis) results in a smaller fraction of the available Ca^{++} being in the ionized form; acidosis causes the reverse. Ca^{++} also binds to albumin; changes in the serum albumin levels can affect the amount of free ionized Ca^{++} in the blood.

PTH, released from the parathyroid gland in response to low serum-ionized-Ca^{++} levels, causes increased Ca^{++} and PO_4^- to be mobilized from the bone; it also causes decreased Ca^{++} and increased PO_4^- excretion from the kidneys. Calcitonin, released from the thyroid gland in response to high serum-ionized-Ca^{++} levels, causes Ca^{++} and PO_4^- deposition in the bone. Vitamin D_3, the active form of vitamin D, causes increased GI absorption of Ca^{++}. Increased activation of vitamin D occurs in the setting of low serum-ionized Ca^{++}.

In the body, Ca^{++} serves important physiologic functions in muscle contraction, synaptic transmission, secretion of endocrine and exocrine glands, and blood coagulation. In addition, Ca^{++} is an important regulator of a variety of metabolic pathways in the cell. PO_4^- is a coenzyme in many metabolic pathways and is also an important buffer in the body.

HYPERCALCEMIA

Hypercalcemia is an increase in the concentration of total serum Ca^{++} >10.5 mg/100 ml.

Pathophysiology

Hypercalcemia may result from abnormal regulation of Ca^{++} levels (as in hyperparathyroidism), excessive mobilization of Ca^{++} from the bones (resulting from immobility, fractures, and certain bone tumors), decreased renal Ca^{++} excretion (as in renal failure), excessive Ca^{++} intake, or excessive vitamin D intake.

Clinical picture

Signs and symptoms of hypercalcemia include muscle weakness, bone pain, flank pain, diarrhea or constipation, nausea and vomiting, lethargy, and coma. Peptic ulcers and kidney stones may result as a complication of hypercalcemia.

Medical interventions

To increase Ca^{++} excretion, IV saline (0.9%) may be administered concurrently with a diuretic such as furosemide (Lasix). Glucocorticoids such as prednisone may be administered to decrease Ca^{++} mobilization from bone and to decrease renal Ca^{++} reabsorption. Mithramycin may be administered to patients in whom the increased Ca^{++} levels are associated with certain forms of malignancies. Sodium phosphate may be given PO or rectally to increase Ca^{++} deposition in the bones. Propranolol may be administered to prevent certain cardiovascular effects of hypercalcemia. In some cases, dialysis is used to lower serum Ca^{++}. Patients with hyperparathyroidism may require surgery.

Nursing interventions

Measures to increase Ca^{++} deposition in bone may be useful in hypercalcemia. These measures include active or passive exercises. Because of neuromuscular weakness, patients should be carefully monitored while exercising, and measures should be instituted to prevent injury. Ca^{++} intake PO should be reduced by eliminating milk and other rich sources of Ca^{++} from the diet. The ECG should be monitored carefully for arrhythmias.

HYPOCALCEMIA

Hypocalcemia is a decrease in the concentration of total serum Ca^{++} to <9 mg/100 ml.

Pathophysiology

Hypocalcemia may result from abnormal regulation of serum Ca^{++}, insufficient Ca^{++} intake, or excessive Ca^{++} losses. Abnormal regulation of Ca^{++} most often occurs after thyroid surgery in which all or part of the parathyroid gland is accidentally removed. Insufficient Ca^{++} intake, e.g., in people who ingest few milk products, may cause hypocalcemia; however, it more often results in osteoporosis, with preservation of serum ionized-Ca^{++} levels. Excessive Ca^{++} losses most often occur in the setting of acute pancreatitis, diarrhea, massive burns, and peritonitis. Hypocalcemia can also result from decreases in the fraction of circulating Ca^{++} that is ionized, as in alkalosis. Hypocalcemia is a common complication of renal failure, partly because of abnormal renal handling of Ca^{++} and PO_4^-, and partly because of decreased renal activation of vitamin D.

Clinical picture

Signs and symptoms of hypocalcemia include neuromuscular irritability (muscle cramps, facial grimacing, tingling and numbness of the extremities, increased deep tendon reflexes, tetany, convulsions), positive Trousseau's sign (carpal spasm following brief vascular occlusion), positive Chvostek's sign (lip and cheek spasm following stimulation of the facial nerve) and ECG abnormalities (prolonged Q-T interval and arrhythmias). With prolonged hypocalcemia, osteoporosis may occur.

Medical interventions

Ca^{++} supplements may be administered PO or IV, usually in the form of calcium gluconate or calcium chloride. In chronic cases, supplementing the diet with PO Ca^{++} and vitamin D may be useful.

Nursing interventions

Nursing management of the patient with hypocalcemia involves preventing the complications of neuromuscular irritability and ECG monitoring for arrhythmias.

HYPERPHOSPHATEMIA

Hyperphosphatemia is an increase in the serum PO_4^- concentration to >4.5 mg/100 ml.

Pathophysiology

Hyperphosphatemia results primarily from impaired renal excretion of PO_4^-. It can also result from excessive PO_4^- administration in the therapy of hypercalcemia or hypophosphatemia.

Clinical picture

Patients with hyperphosphatemia are usually asymptomatic, unless their condition is caused by or exacerbates Ca^{++} imbalance in the body. The clinical pictures seen in Ca^{++} imbalances are previously described.

Medical interventions

Medical intervention is usually aimed at correcting any underlying imbalance of Ca^{++} metabolism. Such interventions are previously described.

Nursing interventions

Nursing intervention is also aimed at alleviating problems associated with Ca^{++} imbalance. Such interventions are previously described.

HYPOPHOSPHATEMIA

Hypophosphatemia is a decrease in the serum PO_4^- concentration to <3 mg/100 ml.

Pathophysiology

Hypophosphatemia most commonly occurs as a sequela of liver disease, diabetic ketoacidosis, or excessive HCO_3^- intake. Excessive PTH causes increased PO_4^- excretion of the kidneys; however, this is usually accompanied by increased PO_4^- mobilization from the bones.

Clinical picture

Signs and symptoms of hypophosphatemia include hemolytic anemia, abnormal platelet function, and neurologic changes (encephalopathy, weakness, and fatigue). Demineralization of bone may occur, resulting in bone pain and pathologic fractures. Typically, serum Ca^{++} levels are normal, whereas PTH levels are low or normal.

Medical interventions

Because of the interrelationship of Ca^{++} and PO_4^- levels, medical interventions must take both into account. Sodium phosphate may be administered PO or rectally. IV administration of sodium phosphate carries a risk of renal damage.

Nursing management

The patient should be monitored for the signs and symptoms of hypophosphatemia described above. In addition, measures to prevent pathologic bone fractures should be instituted. The patient with neurologic changes from hypophosphatemia should be carefully protected from overexertion or self-inflicted minor injuries.

RENAL DIALYSIS

Dialysis is a technique used to rid the body of metabolic wastes, toxins, and excess fluids in instances of drug or chemical poisoning and ARF or CRF. Dialysis is based on the principle that solutes will diffuse across a semipermeable membrane in proportion to their concentrations on each side of the membrane and their relative permeability through the membrane. There are two main ways in which dialysis may be accomplished: hemodialysis and peritoneal dialysis. In hemodialysis, an artificial membrane separates blood from the dialysate, whereas in peritoneal dialysis, the peritoneal membrane acts as the dialyser.

HEMODIALYSIS

Hemodialysis is an efficient method for ridding the body of excess fluid and waste products, particularly in the setting of CRF. Although hemodialysis can reverse many of the manifestations of CRF, it is by no means a cure for the disease.

In hemodialysis, the patient's blood is pumped through an external dialysing machine. Inside the machine, the blood passes through a series of channels separated from the dialysate by a semipermeable dialysis membrane. In ARF, access to the patient's bloodstream for hemodialysis is usually via large-bore needles or catheters. In patients with CRF, who will probably require long-term dialysis, access to the bloodstream is more commonly via an arteriovenous (AV) shunt or AV fistula.

An **AV shunt** is an external connection between a large artery and a large vein. During dialysis, the shunt is opened and connected to the dialysis machine. Advantages of an AV shunt are that it can be used immediately and that percutaneous cannulation is not required. Disadvantages are a high rate of malfunction because of clotting or hemorrhage, some degree of interference with patients' activities of daily living, and a risk of local infection. In addition, the average AV shunt has a shorter life span than does an AV fistula.

An **AV fistula** is a surgically created opening between an artery and a vein. During dialysis, large-bore needles are inserted percutaneously into the fistula. The advantages of using an AV fistula are that after the surgical wound heals, it requires almost no maintenance care, interferes minimally with patients' activities of daily living, can be used over a period of years, and is rarely subject to clotting or hemorrhage. Disadvantages are that it cannot be used immediately after formation; several weeks must be allowed for healing of the surgical scar.

Solutions used as dialysates have approximately the same osmolarity as serum but usually contain little or no K^+. Glucose concentrations may vary but are usually in the physiologic range of 100 to 200 mg/100 liters. Most other electrolytes are present in the same concentrations as they would be in normal serum.

Common complications of hemodialysis include dialysis disequilibrium syndrome, hypotension, hemorrhage, transfusion reactions, and hepatitis. Dialysis disequilibrium syndrome is probably the result of too rapid removal of solute from the blood, particularly of urea, resulting in cerebral edema. Signs and symptoms of the dialysis disequilibrium syndrome include headache, blurred vision, confusion, hallucinations, nausea, vomiting, paresthesias, leg cramps, anxiety, hyperventilation, and seizures.

Nursing interventions

Nursing management of the patient who requires hemodialysis is outlined below. The actual dialysis is usually carried out by specially trained personnel; thus, the specifics of dialysis treatments will not be discussed here.

Thrombosis. (1) Check for bruit, thrill. (2) Check for pain. (3) Do not measure BP or draw blood in affected extremity.

Infection. (1) AV shunt: Clean with povidone-iodine at insertion site, apply dry sterile dressing; avoid getting site wet. (2) AV fistula: Immediately postoperatively, apply sterile dressing; clean site daily with povidone-iodine until wound is healed and no dressing is required. Assess for infection or inflammation at dialysis needle insertion site.

Dislodging of AV shunt. (1) Cover with dressing. (2) Keep wrapped with gauze. (3) Keep cannula clamps available at all times.

Risk of hemorrhage postdialysis. (1) Check partial thromboplastin time (PTT) postdialysis. (2) Be prepared to administer protamine to reverse dialysis-associated heparin overdose if PTT is prolonged.

PERITONEAL DIALYSIS

Peritoneal dialysis involves repeated instillation and drainages of dialysate into and from the peritoneal cavity. The large peritoneal membrane functions as a semipermeable dialysis membrane, allowing the diffusion of various substances. Thus, many substances present in the blood that are normally excreted by the kidney can diffuse across the peritoneal membrane into the dialysate solution instilled into the abdomen and then can be removed from the body with the dialysate. Peritoneal dialysis is often preferred over hemodialysis because of its technical simplicity and because it causes gradual rather than sudden fluid and electrolyte shifts.

Access to the peritoneal cavity is achieved by means of a rigid trocar for single-episode dialysis or, more commonly, via a flexible Tenckhoff catheter. Tenckhoff catheters may be left in place over an extended period of time, allowing patients with CRF to be treated with peritoneal dialysis.

The repeated instillations and drainages of dialysate required in peritoneal dialysis may be accomplished manually or with automatic cycling machines. Typically, an acute peritoneal dialysis treatment lasts between 24 and 48 hr. In patients with CRF, continuous ambulatory peritoneal dialysis (CAPD) may be used, with four to five exchanges of dialysate occurring over the course of each day.

Complications of peritoneal dialysis include peritonitis, pain, difficulty in accomplishing drainage of the dialysate from the peritoneum, extravasation of the dialysate into other tissues, and atelectasis.

The dialysis solution is usually close to plasma in terms of electrolyte composition and is slightly hypertonic, to aid in removal of excess fluid. The most commonly used solution contains 1.5% glucose and has an osmolarity of ~370 mOsm/liter. To remove more fluid from the body during the dialysis, solutions containing 4.25% glucose, with an osmolarity of ~525 mOsm/liter, may be used. K^+ may be added to the dialysate, depending upon the patient's serum K^+ concentration. Heparin may be added to the dialysate early in the course of treatment to prevent clotting of the trocar or catheter. Antibiotics may be added to prevent or treat peritonitis.

Dialysis solutions should be kept sterile. They are usually warmed to body temperature prior to instillation. Usually the adult patient can accommodate 2 liters of dialysate at a time.

Nursing interventions

Nursing management of the patient undergoing peritoneal dialysis is outlined below.

Dependence on proper functioning of dialysis catheter. (1) For rigid trocar: ensure that the trocar is securely fastened to the abdomen, allowing little movement; if duration of dialysis <48 hr routine wound care is not indicated. (2) For Tenckhoff catheter: routine wound care postoperatively; before each dialysis treatment, clean carefully with povidone-iodine and sterile water; use strict aseptic technique. (3) If dialysate fails to drain from peritoneal cavity, reposition the patient. (4) Administer heparin as ordered to prevent catheter clotting. (5) Monitor catheter insertion site for signs of inflammation, drainage around catheter.

Risk of infection. (1) Observe strict aseptic technique in handling peritoneal dialysate. (2) Check vital signs frequently. (3) Routinely culture dialysis drainage, usually with first exchange, and then every ten exchanges. With CAPD, culture monthly or prn. (4) Observe for signs and symptoms of peritonitis (fever, elevated WBC, abdominal pain, and cloudy dialysis drainage). (5) Check dialysate for contamination prior to instillation.

Alteration in fluid and electrolyte balance. (1) Record cumulative intake and output during acute dialysis procedure. By convention, if the patient retains dialysis fluid, a positive fluid balance exists. If more fluid drains out than was instilled, then a negative fluid balance exists. (2) Administer proper dialysis solution, depending on fluid balance: 1.5% or 4.25% glucose. (3) Add K^+ to dialysate, as ordered; monitor serum K^+ levels. (4) Weigh patient before beginning dialysis procedure and then $\geq$ q 24 hr during acute or chronic dialysis. Weigh while the abdomen is empty of dialysate. (5) Monitor serum chemistries, BUN, creatinine, glucose.

Discomfort during dialysis procedure. (1) Position patient in semi-

Fowler's position during procedure to decrease pressure of dialysate on diaphragm. (2) With CAPD, little or no activity restriction is required. (3) Provide back care as indicated. (4) Administer analgesics as ordered and prn.

Anxiety related to dialysis procedure. (1) Explain all procedures, taking into account patient's physical and emotional status. (2) Maintain quiet environment; eliminate extraneous noise and unnecessary personnel. (3) Allow uninterrupted rest periods.

RENAL TRANSPLANTATION

Renal transplantation is a major treatment modality for CRF, as an alternative to chronic dialysis. Most donor kidneys are from cadavers; however, use of donor kidneys from histocompatible living donors may reduce the incidence of postoperative kidney rejection.

Individuals who may benefit from renal transplantation usually have irreversible CRF, are relatively young (usually <40 yr of age), have a normal urinary tract, and are free from other major diseases such as coronary artery disease, cancer, COPD, and peptic ulcer. Individuals with uncontrolled hypertension, renal infections, or in whom the diseased kidneys may be pathogenic for the transplanted kidney may undergo ureteronephrectomy prior to transplantation. Psychological stability is an important determinant of postoperative adjustment.

Living kidney donors are usually relatives who are histologically matched on the basis of human lymphocyte antigen tissue typing. Prior to kidney donation, donors undergo extensive psychological and renal evaluations to ensure that the donation procedure will not adversely affect their health.

Perioperative care for living donors is similar to that for any form of major surgery, with particular attention paid to assessment of renal function. Complications specifically related to kidney donation are rare.

Cadaveric kidney donors are individuals who are clinically dead on the basis of an impartial medical evaluation. Individuals with fixed and dilated pupils, who are unresponsive to any external stimuli, who require artificial ventilatory support, are arreflexic, and who have essentially flat EEG recordings are usually considered clinically dead and thus may be suitable kidney donors. Donors should be <65 yr of age, be free from renal disease, diabetes mellitus, hypertension, systemic infections, and cancer. Once suitable donors have been identified and family permission for renal donation has been obtained, renal function in the donor should be maintained, with life support equipment and medications, until harvesting of the kidney can take place. Many medical centers and hospitals have transplant coordinators who can assist with the evaluation and management of prospective donors.

Perioperative care for the kidney transplant recipient is complex. Of primary importance is maintenance of renal function, with prevention or early recognition of complications. Such complications include obstruction of urine outflow (secondary to kinking of the urinary catheter or clots), hypovolemia, renal vascular occlusion, acute tubular necrosis, and ureteral leaks. Because immunosuppressive therapy is required following kidney transplantation, postoperatively recipients are at high risk of infection, locally or systemically.

Long-term complications of transplantation result primarily from immunosuppressive therapy. These complications include Cushing's disease glucose intolerance, cataracts, infections, GI ulceration, leukopenia, aseptic necrosis of the bones, malignancies (particularly lymphoma), and psychosocial instability (with high rates of suicide and divorce posttransplant).

Patients who undergo renal transplantation must be observed for signs and symptoms of rejection. Although rejection most commonly occurs early posttransplant, it may occur at any time postoperatively. Signs and symptoms of rejection include: redness, swelling, and pain at incision; fever; elevated WBC; decreased urine output; weight gain; rising BUN and serum creatinine; edema; elevated BP; anorexia; decreased creatinine clearance; and proteinuria. Patients who are in the early stages of a rejection crisis may be managed with increased doses of immunosuppressives such as corticosteroids, azathioprine, and cyclophosphamide.

CHAPTER 8

THE GASTROINTESTINAL SYSTEM

Marsha Evans Orr

ANATOMY AND PHYSIOLOGY REVIEW

Figure 8–1 illustrates the major and accessory organs and structures of the GI tract.

UPPER GASTROINTESTINAL TRACT

The primary role of upper GI structures is to prepare food substances for the major chemical digestive process that occurs in the lower GI tract.

The cheeks, gums, lips, teeth, tongue, palate, and glands of salivation constitute **the oral cavity,** where the process of digestion begins. Mastication helps to grind food into small particles that can be acted upon by digestive enzymes. Glands near the oral cavity secrete substances that lubricate food particles and begin enzymatic digestion of carbohydrate substances. Because digestive enzymes reach only the outer surfaces of food, chewing is especially important to enhance the rate of digestion. Ptyalin, an amylase in saliva, breaks down starches. The pH of saliva is between 6.0 and 7.4, and a total volume of ~1,200 ml is secreted daily. Salivation is triggered by taste, touch, smell, and reflexes from the stomach and intestines. Mucus secretions in saliva help to lubricate food for passage through upper GI structures.

The pharynx has three divisions—the nasopharynx, the oropharynx, and the laryngeal pharynx—which all participate in deglutination. As food is swallowed, the upper esophageal sphincter relaxes, and food is easily propelled into the esophagus.

The esophagus propels food from the pharynx to the stomach in peristaltic waves, which are controlled by impulses from the vagus nerve. Mucus secretions in the esophagus provide lubrication and prevent

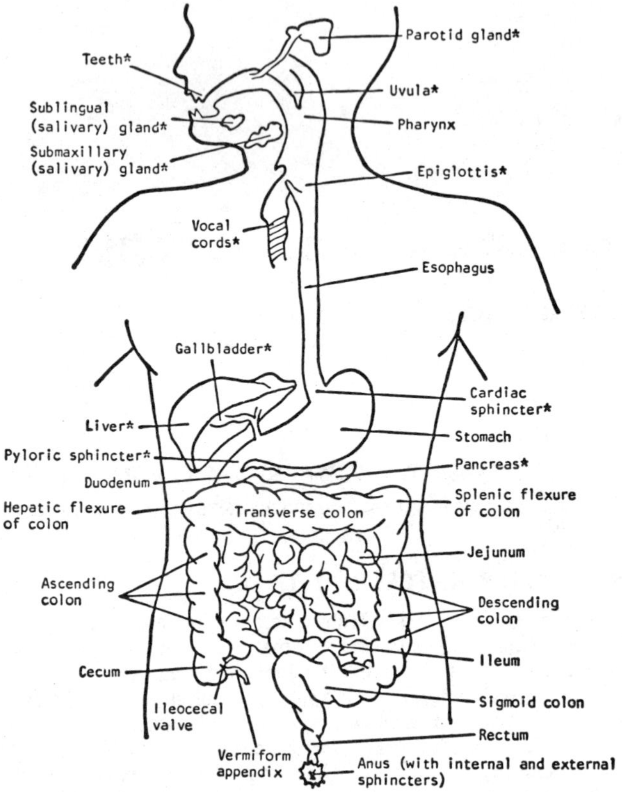

Figure 8–1. Anatomy of the GI tract and associated structures. Asterisks indicate associated structures. *Adapted from* Lewis, C. M., Nutrition: The Basics of Nutrition. Family Nutrition. F. A. Davis Co., Philadelphia. 1977. p. B-75, and Guyton, A. C. Textbook of Medical Physiology. W. B. Saunders Co., Philadelphia. 1981. Sixth edition. p. 784.

irritation of the mucosa. The gastroesophageal sphincter, a ring-shaped muscle at the distal end of the esophagus, helps to prevent reflux of powerful stomach-acid secretions. The sphincter relaxes as a peristaltic wave of swallowing occurs, and food can easily pass into the stomach.

The **stomach** is a muscular pouch having mechanical (food storage, mixing, and propulsion) and secretory (pyloric and gastric glandular) functions. By the time food particles leave the stomach, they have been prepared for digestion by the enzymes within the small intestine. The stomach has two major segments, the corpus and the antrum. The amount of food ejected from the stomach with each contraction is controlled by the pyloric sphincter at the distal antrum.

Food is mixed within the stomach by two types of wavelike motions: weak constrictor waves in the corpus and powerful peristaltic movements in the antrum. These constrictor and peristaltic waves occur about once q 20 sec. As digestive secretions mix with food, a semiliquid substance (chyme) is formed.

Pyloric glands, located in the antrum, secrete mucus to protect the stomach lining from the powerful digestive juices secreted by the gastric glands. Most of the gastric glands are located in the mucosa of the corpus section. They are composed of three types of cells—mucous neck cells, chief cells, and parietal cells—which secrete mucus, enzymes, and hydrochloric acid (HCL) respectively.

The mechanisms for secretion of various digestive juices are rather complex: neurologic, tactile, or chemical stimulation can affect secretory activity. In response to the thought, sight, smell, or taste of food, the hypothalamus or cerebral cortex sends messages to the stomach through the vagus nerve, and gastric secretion is stimulated. Food entering the stomach causes local secretory stimuli, and these messages cause parasympathetic stimulation of the gastric glands; ~2 liters/day of gastric juices are produced in this manner. Food entering the intestine stimulates secretion of gastrin through hormonal and neurologic mechanisms. All these mechanisms occur almost simultaneously.

Secretion of gastric juices can occur in response to negative stimuli, such as stress, as well. Emotional distress can stimulate the secretion of large amounts of pepsin and acid. Without the neutralizing effect of food and mucus, acidic secretions can lead to the development of a peptic ulcer.

HCL and pepsin have a major role in the digestion of carbohydrates and proteins. A very acidic pH is necessary to prevent inactivation of pepsin. The chief cells secrete pepsinogen, a proenzyme that is converted to pepsin in the presence of HCL. Pepsin acts upon aromatic amino acids. HCL also hydrolyzes a small amount of starches and disaccharides.

Other enzymes secreted in the stomach play a minor role in digestion. Gastric lipase hydrolyzes some short- or medium-chain fats, and gastric amylase hydrolyzes starches. Rennin produced in the stomach slows the passage of milk through the GI tract and is an essential substance for the normal digestive process of infants.

LOWER GASTROINTESTINAL TRACT

The small intestine has three major divisions: the duodenum (20 to 30 cm long), the jejunum (~2.5 m long), and the ileum (3.5 m long).

Propulsive and mixing movements occur with the greatest frequency in the duodenum and gradually decrease in frequency in the lower segments of the small intestine. Mixing, or segmental, contractions combine chyme with the intestinal secretions. Peristaltic waves propel chyme along the small intestine toward the ileocecal valve.

The small intestine secretes mucus, ECF, and enzymes. Mucus helps to protect the mucosa of the duodenum from digestion by gastric acid. ECF, in amounts of ~2 liters/day, helps to liquify chyme and enhances the process of absorption. Enzymes secreted in the small intestine include: enterokinase (activates trypsin); amylase (hydrolyzes starches); peptidases (split polypeptides into amino acids); sucrase, maltase, isomaltase, and lactase (split disaccharides into monosaccharides); and lipase (splits lipids into glycerol and fatty acids).

The specialized structures of the lumen of the small intestine promote absorption of nutrients. The lumen wall is composed of: (1) the serosa, or external layer, (2) the muscularis, (3) the submucosa, (4) and the mucosa, or internal layer. The villi also have tiny featherlike projections called microvilli ("brush border"). The villi and microvilli increase the absorptive surface of the intestine several hundred times. Water, ions, and nutrients are absorbed through the small intestine; ≥8 liters/day of water diffuse through the lumen of the small intestine. Water is also transported from the plasma into the lumen to maintain the isotonicity of chyme. Sodium, chloride, calcium, iron, potassium, magnesium, and phosphate are major ions that are absorbed through the mucosa. About one-seventh of all the body's sodium stores (25 to 35 g) are absorbed through the small intestine daily.

The small intestine is a primary site for the absorption of the major nutrients: carbohydrates, proteins, and fats. Carbohydrates are absorbed as monosaccharides; galactose and glucose have the most rapid transport into plasma. Proteins are absorbed as amino acids. Monosaccharides and amino acids are absorbed during—and appear to be dependent upon—sodium transport. Fats are transported by micellular solubilization to the epithelial cells, where monoglycerides and fatty acids diffuse into the cells, leaving bile acid micelles in the chyme. These micelles then transport additional monoglycerides and fatty acids to the surface of epithelial cells. Bile salts are carried in chyme to the distal ileum, where they are absorbed and returned to the liver to be secreted again as bile. Bile salts can be recirculated several times. One to one-half liter of chyme passes through the ileocecal valve into the large intestine each day.

The **large intestine (colon)** is ~150 cm long and has six segments: (1) cecum, (2) ascending colon, (3) transverse colon, (4) descending colon, (5) sigmoid colon, and (6) rectum. The ileocecal sphincter divides the ileum from the cecum and prevents backflow of material into the ileum. Gastrin relaxes the ileocecal sphincter to promote passage of chyme into the colon. Contraction of the sphincter is stimulated by reflexes from a distended cecum.

Propulsive and mixing movements transport contents of the colon to the rectum. During mixing movements, fecal contents are exposed to the surface of the colon by being slowly turned and compressed. Mass movements occur primarily in the transverse colon and are responsible for moving feces into the rectum. Overdistension and irritation can produce powerful mass movements. Usually, the rectum is empty and mass movements propel feces into the rectum to stimulate the process of defecation. Two sphincters control passage of fecal material from the anus: the internal anal sphincter, composed of smooth muscle, and the external anal sphincter, composed of striated voluntary muscle. Movement of feces into the anus causes relaxation of the internal and external sphincters. Parasympathetic impulses from the spinal cord produce the powerful peristaltic waves normally involved in defecation. Feces are composed of bacteria, undigested food fiber, epithelial cells, fat, inorganic matter, and bile pigments, which give feces their characteristic brown color.

Mucus secretions protect the intestinal wall from irritation by acids. Severe irritation of the colon causes large quantities of water, electrolytes, and mucus to be secreted, producing the watery mucoid diarrhea common in diseases such as enteritis.

About one-fifth of the water present in the chyme that enters the colon will be absorbed in the proximal colon. Sodium and chloride ions are also absorbed into the plasma from the colon. Bacterial action in the colon enables vitamin K, vitamin B_{12}, thiamine, and riboflavin to be absorbed.

HORMONES

Gastrin, cholecystokinin, and secretin are three main hormones produced in the GI tract that are extremely important for normal processes of digestion. The action of these hormones is complementary to the digestive process.

Gastrin, composed of amino acids, is secreted in the antral portion of the stomach in response to mechanical (distension of the stomach by food) and chemical (substances such as alcohol, caffeine, and proteins) factors. Gastrin is absorbed into the bloodstream and subsequently stimulates production of HCL in the stomach. Gastrin continues to be secreted until the pH of stomach contents drops <2.0. The feedback mechanism that controls gastrin secretion helps to maintain optimal pH levels for digestion and to prevent hyperacidity of the stomach.

Cholecystokinin-pancreozymin (CCK-PZ), composed of amino acid complexes, is secreted by the small intestine and carried by the bloodstream to the gallbladder. The net effect of CCK-PZ is to produce a flow of bile into the small intestine. Thus, it has an important indirect role in the digestion of lipids. Gastric secretion is moderately inhibited by CCK-PZ.

Secretin is a polypeptide produced in an inactive form (prosecretin) by the mucosa of the small intestine. Chyme, and HCL in particular, trigger the production of prosecretin. Chyme also converts prosecretin to secretin, which causes the production of large amounts of pancreatic fluid containing bicarbonate. This pancreatic fluid neutralizes the acid substances entering the duodenum. Pancreatic enzymes require a neutral pH for digestive activity to occur. In addition, pancreatic fluid protects the duodenum from ulceration by acidic substances.

Other hormones secreted by the intestinal tract are vasoactive hormone, gastric inhibitory hormone, and polypeptides. These affect small-intestinal and gastric secretions.

BLOOD SUPPLY

The GI system is highly vascular and contains a large proportion of the total CO. The liver alone handles approximately one-fourth of the total CO per minute. Blood flow to the intestines, spleen, liver, and portal venous system is called the splanchnic circulation.

The GI organs receive oxygenated blood from major arterial structures branching off from the aorta. The venous system drains blood from GI structures into the central venous circulation (vena cava) and to the portal system.

The portal venous system receives nutrient-rich venous blood from the major intestinal organs: stomach, intestines, spleen, and pancreas. Large venous blood vessels, such as the inferior mesenteric, superior mesenteric, left and right gastroepiploic, splenic, and coronary veins, drain into the portal vein. The portal vein divides into two main branches as it enters the liver and continues to divide until small branches (interlobular veins) become sinusoids, which flow between the hepatocytes. The hepatocytes are drained by central veins that converge to form sublobular veins. The sublobular veins enlarge to form hepatic veins that empty into the inferior vena cava.

Arterial blood also perfuses the liver from the hepatic artery. Tiny branches of the hepatic arterial system empty into the sinusoids, making the liver unique in having a mixed venous and arterial blood flow between hepatic cells. Changes in arterial and venous pressures within the liver's vascular system can produce dramatic changes in hepatic blood flow patterns.

Approximately one-fourth of blood flow to the liver is supplied from the arterial system, and about three-fourths is supplied by the portal system. Various mechanisms control hepatic blood flow. Increased pressure within the right atrium of the heart leads to increased blood volume in the liver. Decreased O_2 concentration in portal blood will induce increased arterial blood flow. Stimulation by the parasympathetic nervous system causes constriction of the large vessels and sinusoids, and increased permeability of the sinusoids allows proteins to diffuse easily into the extravascular spaces.

NEUROLOGIC INNERVATION

The gut is richly supplied with nerve fibers that receive impulses from the ANS via parasympathetic and sympathetic fibers. Because of the nature of smooth muscle, ions can pass easily from one muscle fiber to another. Innervation of the GI system affects three major functions: (1) stimulation of movements of the abdominal structures, especially in the intestines, and subsequent movement of food along the GI tract, (2) alteration in the quantity of GI secretions, and (3) changes in the quantity of blood flowing to and from GI organs.

Smooth muscle fibers

In the GI tract, smooth muscle fibers receive almost constant electrical stimulation and exhibit two major types of contractions; tonic and rhythmic. Tonic contractions are continuous and control the amount of steady pressure upon food substances by bowel segments and by bowel sphincters. Rhythmic contractions vary in rate and intensity and are controlled primarily by a complex structure of neurons called the intramural nerve plexus. The electrical activity in smooth muscle can be described as slow waves and spikes. Slow waves produce no muscle contraction unless affected by stretch, acetylcholine, or parasympathetic impulses. Spikes produce most of the muscle contractions. The slow-wave-and-spike electrical activity is sometimes referred to as the enteric nervous system (ENS) and can be compared to the electrical conduction system within the heart; the ENS and the cardiac electrical systems function independently, but both can be affected by ANS stimulation. The intramural plexus also affects some of the secretory functions of the gut.

Autonomic nervous system

Autonomic control of GI functions is accomplished through parasympathetic and sympathetic nerve fibers. Autonomic stimulation can alter activity throughout the entire length of the GI tract.

Parasympathetic fibers leading to the gut arise from either the cranial or sacral divisions of the spinal cord. The vagus nerves are the major fibers arising from the cranial division. Vagal stimulation has a powerful effect upon the function of the esophagus and stomach; to a lesser extent it also affects the function of the small intestine and colon. Fibers originating in the sacral section of the spinal cord control the anus, sigmoid colon, and rectum and thus, defecation.

Sympathetic fibers leading to the GI tract leave the spinal cord from the lower thoracic vertebrae (T-8 through T-12) and the upper lumbar vertebrae (L-1 through L-3). Unlike the parasympathetic distribution of nerve fibers, sympathetic fibers are very evenly distributed to all parts of the GI tract.

The sympathetic and parasympathetic nervous systems work in opposition to each other. In general, the sympathetic nervous system is inhibitory in nature, but it has excitatory effects upon the ileocecal and anal sphincters and causes slight increases in gastric secretion. Because parasympathetic stimulation has such a powerful effect upon GI activity, destruction of parasympathetic nerve tracts (primarily the vagus and sacral nerves) can have a profound effect upon peristaltic activity and bowel tone. After a time, however, the bowel compensates by increasing its excitability. Destruction of sympathetic nerve tracts causes very little alteration in GI function. The greatest control over motor function in the gut is accomplished via the intramural plexus and the GI tract's intrinsic electrical activity.

ACCESSORY ORGANS OF DIGESTION

The pancreas, gallbladder, and liver are considered accessory organs of digestion (*see* Fig. 8–1). Although these three organs are not an intrinsic part of the GI tract, they have major roles in the process of digestion.

Pancreas

The pancreas is located slightly posterior and caudal to the stomach in the right and left upper quadrants of the abdomen. The **head** of the pancreas lies within the curve of the duodenum and is much wider than the **tail** section near the spleen. The head and tail sections are divided by the midsection, or **body,** of the pancreas.

The pancreas has an extensive ductal system. Small ductules enlarge into major ducts that eventually empty into the duct of Wirsung, which transverses the pancreas and joins the common bile duct in the head. Within the duodenum, at the outflow tract of the common bile duct, the ampulla of Vater is located. A sphincter within the ampulla (sphincter of Oddi) can impede or enhance flow of bile and pancreatic secretions into the duodenum.

The pancreas accomplishes both endocrine and exocrine functions by means of specialized cells. Alpha and beta cells secrete hormones glucagon and insulin (*see* Chapter 6). Acinar cells secrete bicarbonate and the three major digestive enzymes, lipase, amylase, and trypsin. These enzymes are secreted in an inactive form and are converted to an active form within the duodenum. Lipase breaks down triglycerides to fatty acids and glycerol, amylase breaks down polysaccharides to glucose and maltase, and trypsin breaks down the protein bonds of amino acids. The arterial blood supply to the pancreas is from the celiac and superior mesenteric arteries. Venous flow from the pancreas drains into the portal circulation.

Gallbladder

The gallbladder is a pear-shaped organ attached to the inferior surface of the liver. Multiple folds within the epithelium of the gallbladder enable this organ to expand to a maximum volume of ~50 ml of bile.

The major functions of the gallbladder are to collect, concentrate, and store bile. The hepatic ducts carry bile produced by the liver to the gallbladder via the cystic duct. Hepatic bile consists of ~97% water. The gallbladder absorbs the water until bile is four to ten times more concentrated.

Concentrated bile contains bile salts, bile pigments, lecithin, and cholesterol. Bilirubin is the major bile pigment. Bile salts are essential for fat absorption. Upon reaching the small intestine, most of the bile salts are reabsorbed.

Contraction of the gallbladder occurs in response to neurologic (vagal) and hormonal (secretin, CCK-PZ, vasoactive intestinal peptide, and gastrin) stimulation. Contractions cause bile to flow out of the gallbladder, into the common bile duct, through the ampulla of Vater, and into the duodenum.

Arterial blood reaches the gallbladder through the hepatic and cystic arteries. Venous blood drains through the cystic vein and into the portal vein.

Liver

The liver is a large, extremely complex organ, located in the right upper quadrant of the abdomen. It is divided into four main lobes; right, left, caudate, and quadrate. Within each lobe are the liver lobules, which are the functional units of the liver. The lobules may be conceptualized as spokes in a wheel, with each lobule as a spoke and a central vein at the hub (Fig. 8–2).

Arterial and venous blood flows from portal venules and arterioles into sinusoids between plates of hepatic cells. Phagocytic Kupffer cells within the sinusoids remove bacteria from the blood. The Kupffer cells are part of the body's reticuloendothelial system. Channels, called canaliculi, are also located between hepatic plates and carry bile toward the bile ducts. Some fluid diffuses from the sinusoids and collects in the spaces of Disse, also

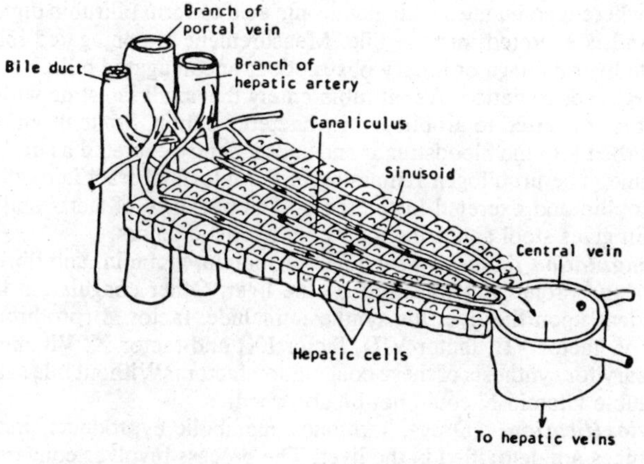

Figure 8–2. Schematic representation of a liver lobule. *Reprinted from* Orr, M. E. Acute Pancreatic and Hepatic Dysfunction. John Wiley & Sons, Inc., New York. 1981. p. 118.

located between the hepatic plates. The spaces of Disse drain into the lymphatic system.

The liver has six major functions: (1) metabolism, (2) bile production and bilirubin metabolism, (3) coagulation factor production, (4) detoxification, (5) blood storage and filtration, and (6) vitamin and mineral storage.

Metabolism. Metabolism of carbohydrates, proteins, and fats is an extremely important hepatic function. The liver regulates blood glucose levels by converting glucose to glycogen (glycogenesis); glycogen back to glucose (glycogenolysis); and by converting deaminated amino acids and glycerol to glucose (gluconeogenesis). The liver functions in protein metabolism by: (1) deamination of amino acid complexes; (2) formation of plasma proteins, such as albumin, globulin, and fibrinogen; (3) transamination of amino acids; and (4) conversion of ammonia to urea. Its specific functions in fat metabolism include: (1) beta oxidation of fatty acids to acetylcoenzyme A (Acetyl Co-A); (2) formation of plasma lipoproteins, phospholipids, and cholesterol; and (3) conversion of large quantities of carbohydrates and proteins to fat.

Bile production and bilirubin metabolism. The hepatic cells form ≤1 liter/day of bile. The bile then flows into the bile canaliculi, which drain into the terminal bile ducts and finally empty into the hepatic ducts. From the hepatic ducts, bile is carried through the cystic duct into the gallbladder, where it is concentrated and stored (*see above*).

The bilirubin excreted in bile represents the byproduct of several metabolic processes. As fragile mature RBCs are phagocytized by the reticuloendothelial system, "free" or unconjugated bilirubin is formed. This free bilirubin is immediately bound with albumin and carried to the liver, where it conjugates with glucuronic acid to form bilirubin diglucuronide and is excreted into the bile. Measurement of conjugated bilirubin reflects liver damage or biliary obstruction; unconjugated bilirubin represents RBC degradation. As bilirubin enters the small intestine within the bile, it is converted to urobilogen by bacterial action. Some urobilogen is reabsorbed into the bloodstream and subsequently excreted as urobilin in the urine. The urobilogen remaining in the intestinal tract is oxidized to sterocobilin and excreted in the feces. The presence of sterocobilin and urobilin gives stool and urine their characteristic colors.

Coagulation factor production. Albumin, globulin, and fibrinogen are plasma proteins synthesized by the liver. Other coagulation factors dependent upon the liver for synthesis include: factor II (prothrombin), factor V, factor VII, factor VIII, factor IX, and factor X. Vitamin K is necessary for synthesis of these coagulation factors. Without bile salts, the fat-soluble vitamin K could not be absorbed.

Detoxification. Drugs, hormones, metabolic byproducts, and other substances are detoxified in the liver. The process involves conversion of these substances to a water-soluble form through oxidation, reduction, hydrolysis, or conjugation so that the toxic substance can be excreted in the urine or bile. During this process, certain substances can cause damage to the hepatocytes.

Blood storage and filtration. The liver is a vast reservoir for blood, having a capacity of $\leq$400 ml. When hemorrhage occurs, large amounts of blood can drain from the liver sinusoids to replace the blood loss. Increased pressure in the venous outflow tract can cause significant increases in portal pressure from the extra blood volume within the liver. Blood filtration occurs within the liver as Kupffer cells remove foreign particles or bacteria from blood flowing within the sinusoids.

Vitamin and mineral storage. Iron is stored in the liver in the form of ferritin and is released when circulating iron levels decrease. Vitamins A, D, and B_{12} are stored in the liver. Vitamin A reserves are extensive and can last from one to two years.

ASSESSMENT OF THE PATIENT

Health history

A history is usually provided in the medical record at the time of a patient's admission to the ICU, unless the admission is an emergency; however, the critical care nurse continues to elicit pertinent information about the patient's current and past medical history, general health, and specific symptoms. Table 8–1 summarizes important areas besides the standard general ones for assessment of the critically ill patient with known

TABLE 8–1

Elicitation of a Health History for the Patient with GI Tract Disease

Current or past illnesses	Signs and symptoms
Diseases of the GI tract	Abdominal pain
GI bleeding	Change in bowel habits
Anemia	Change in appetite
Clotting Disorders	Nausea or vomiting
Trauma	Edema
Surgery	Changes in weight
Exposure to toxins	Dyspnea
Contagious diseases	Fatigue
Alcohol pattern	Dark stools
Allergies	Dark urine
Cancer	Easy bruisability or bleeding
Infections	Indigestion
Chronic illnesses	Hair loss
Medication history (including OTC drugs)	Jaundice
	Change in sleep pattern

OTC, over-the-counter.

or suspected GI tract disease. If the symptoms are present, data about the onset, location, character, duration, pattern, intensity, progression, and relief factors are needed to identify disease and establish disease progression.

General assessment data helps the nurse identify the patient's general state of health, social support network, financial resources, coping skills, and physical resources. Skillful discharge planning and comprehensive care are best achieved when areas of need are identified early in treatment.

Physical examination

In the ICU, physical examination of the patient is an ongoing process performed by the nurse, using the techniques of inspection, auscultation, percussion, and palpation. The critically ill patient is in a dynamic physical state, with an increased risk of multiorgan failure. Physical assessment techniques are among the crucial bedside tools used by the critical care nurse to determine the patient's condition.

Inspection. The abdominal contour is observed for symmetry. The contour can be rounded, flat, or scaphoid (concave) and should be symmetric. Masses, fluid, and hernias cause asymmetric contours. Indications to note include: scars (past surgery or trauma), striae (pregnancy or weight loss), dilated veins (increased vascular pressures), rashes (nutritional problems), and angiomata (liver disease). Sometimes peristaltic waves or pulsations can be observed, particularly when the person is thin. Auscultation and percussion are used to determine whether visible pulsations are normal or abnormal. Skin color should be uniform; hyperpigmentation or jaundice indicates pathology. Changes in the distribution of hair on the abdomen sometimes accompany disease. Pubic hair is often absent in a patient with severe liver disease. The presence, size, location, and appearance of wounds, fistulas, stomas, or ulcerated areas is documented. Base-line data is carefully and thoroughly charted so that changes can be identified and interpreted.

Auscultation. Auscultation is performed before percussion and palpation because the latter techniques can alter bowel sounds. Bowel sounds are auscultated in all four quadrants. Although bowel sounds are normally heard at a rate of 3 to 12/sec, the most frequent sounds are heard over the ileocecal valve. Normal sounds are soft gurglings and clickings. When bowel function becomes abnormal, the character of sounds changes. Hyperperistalsis is accompanied by loud rushing sounds and growls (borborygmi). Infrequent or absent sounds accompany paralytic ileus, peritonitis, or late bowel obstruction. Early bowel obstruction is characterized by high-pitched and loud rushing sounds. The location, intensity, character, and rate of bowel sounds are documented.

Venous hums and bruits may be heard as blood passes through a partially obstructed vessel. Bruits, with a sound similar to cardiac murmurs, usually indicate obstruction or narrowing of an artery, whereas hums occur with venous obstruction.

Friction rubs, heard during inspiration, may occur in the presence of inflammation or tumor. Rubs are generally heard directly over a diseased organ.

Bruits, hums, and friction rubs are abnormal findings and should be reported to the physician if these sounds have not been noted during previous examinations.

Percussion. Percussion is used during examination of the abdomen to estimate the size of the liver and spleen, to detect gastric or abdominal distension, and to determine whether ascites is present.

The liver is percussed as dullness over the right upper quadrant; for a normal-sized liver, the dullness should begin at about the level of the sixth intercostal space and end at the lower margin of the ribs. Enlargement of the liver is determined by measuring the area of dullness; the normal liver size (vertically) is ~7 cm for women and ~10 cm for men.

The spleen is located in the left upper quadrant of the abdomen and is percussed as dullness at the level of the tenth rib. Because it is located more posteriorly than some of the other abdominal organs, the spleen is percussed at the midaxillary line. Enlargement is indicated when dullness to percussion extends toward the midline beyond the midaxillary line.

When empty, the stomach collapses upon itself; however, there is often a gas bubble within the stomach that can be percussed as a tympanic sound. Normally, the stomach is percussed in the left upper quadrant of the abdomen near the left costal margin. A large tympanic area indicates distension of the stomach. During inspiration, an enlarged spleen can obscure the area of tympany over the stomach; the percussed area will change in sound from tympany to dullness.

Percussion can be used to detect fluid within the abdomen. Fluid is suspected in the presence of abdominal distension but can be missed if the patient is obese. Sometimes fluid can be displaced as a wave that travels from one side of the abdomen to the other. The examiner taps one side of the abdomen, and the fluid wave can be felt on the opposite side. Fluid pools over the flank area when the patient is supine and can be percussed as a dull area. The borders of the dull areas on both sides of the abdomen are marked. Then the patient's position is changed and the area is percussed again. Shifting areas of dullness indicate the presence of fluid.

Palpation. Light, deep, and moderate palpation of the abdomen is performed to determine the size and characteristics of organs, to assess for pain, and to identify abnormalities such as masses, distension, or fluid. The patient is assisted to a supine position with knees slightly flexed to promote relaxation of the abdominal muscles. The depth of palpation is gradually increased, beginning with light palpation over the entire abdomen and progressing to deep palpation over specific organs. Masses and distension are generally discovered during light palpation, but deeper palpation is sometimes required to determine the characteristics of a mass. Organs are assessed using moderate to deep palpation. The liver edge is normally palpated at the right lower costal margin during inspiration and feels smooth and sharp. An enlarged liver is palpated a number of fingerbreadths below the rib margin. Liver disease sometimes produces a rough (hobnail) texture, with blunting of the liver edge. The spleen is palpated at the right costal margin during inspiration and usually cannot be located by palpation unless it is enlarged. If tender areas are located during palpation of organs, the areas should be further assessed. Visceral pain is typically dull and difficult to localize, somatic pain is sharp and well localized, and inflammation typically produces rebound tenderness. Palpation is generally performed last in the sequence of physical assessment techniques, with assessment for pain performed last.

MAJOR DISORDERS

GASTROINTESTINAL HEMORRHAGE

GI organs are well supplied with arterial blood, with certain organs, such as the liver and spleen, acting as reservoirs for blood. With each heartbeat, a large proportion of the CO circulates to abdominal structures. Therefore, GI hemorrhage can rapidly become life-threatening. The loss of an O_2-rich blood supply to vital organs, such as the brain, heart, and kidneys, leads to tissue hypoxia. Prolonged tissue hypoxia causes multiple organ failure. GI hemorrhage is a crisis situation that requires skillful medical and nursing interventions. The goals of these interventions are to restore blood volume, to reverse tissue hypoxia, and restore fluid and electrolyte balance.

Two of the most common GI disorders that lead to hemorrhage are esophageal varices and peptic ulcers.

ESOPHAGEAL VARICES

Pathophysiology

Esophageal varices develop as a consequence of portal hypertension; the increased pressure within portal vessels causes collateral circulatory channels to develop in structures such as the esophagus, stomach, and rectum. The distended, fragile, collateral vessels protrude outward into the internal lumen of the esophagus and bleed readily when irritated. Generally, the varices are clustered near the junction of the esophagus and stomach.

Esophageal varices develop most often as a complication of cirrhosis of the liver, and their development is an ominous prognostic sign. The mortality rate associated with bleeding esophageal varices is >50%. Other conditions that can lead to the development of esophageal varices include hepatitis, schistosomiasis, portal vein thrombosis, CHF, and hepatic vein obstruction.

Clinical picture

Hemorrhage from esophageal varices can be sudden and massive with hematemesis, melena, and upper gastric pain as initial symptoms, but a more subtle sign, such as anemia, can sometimes lead to the diagnosis. Bleeding must be distinguished from other types of GI pathology, such as gastritis, peptic ulcers, and Mallory-Weiss syndrome.

Because esophageal varices are most often associated with portal hypertension, other signs and symptoms of liver disease (ascites, muscle wasting, jaundice, spider angiomata, splenomegaly, testicular atrophy, or hepatic encephalopathy) are commonly present.

Laboratory tests usually reflect blood loss and provide confirmation that some degree of hepatic dysfunction is present. The Hct, Hb, RBC, and WBC are decreased. BUN is often elevated, reflecting an increased metabolism of nitrogenous wastes (i.e., blood) from the intestines. Liver function tests (*see* Cirrhosis) are often abnormal. Arterial blood gas samples show decreased oxygenation and acidosis.

Endoscopic evaluation of the esophagus is the most direct method of confirming the presence of esophageal varices; however, the use of endoscopy as an emergency procedure remains controversial. Endoscopy can help to localize the area of hemorrhage when surgical interventions are planned. In addition, endoscopy is indicated when bleeding is not controlled by initial medical treatments. Long-term morbidity and mortality associated with esophageal varices do not, however, appear to decrease when endoscopy is performed on an emergency basis.

Celiac and superior mesenteric angiography is also used to localize the site of esophageal bleeding. Contrast material is injected into the celiac and superior mesenteric arteries and its movement through the splanchnic system observed using radiographic techniques. Extravasation of contrast material indicates a site of bleeding.

Upper GI radiographic films using barium are sometimes ordered; however, these films are relatively insensitive and detect only ~50% of the varices actually present.

Medical interventions

Primary **medical** interventions are: (1) restoration of blood and fluid volume, (2) balloon tamponade with a Sengstaken-Blakemore tube, (3) vasopressin therapy, (4) percutaneous transhepatic embolization (THE), and (5) endoscopic sclerosis of varices. Each of these emergency nonsurgical methods may be used alone or in combination.

Blood volume. Whole blood or blood components are used for restoration of blood and fluid volume. Care must be taken to avoid cardiovascular collapse.

Balloon tamponade. A multiple-lumen tube with esophageal and/or gastric balloons is passed through the esophagus into the stomach. The balloons are carefully inflated to exert pressure directly upon the bleeding vessels. The Sengstaken-Blakemore tube has three lumens: (1) a lumen for inflation of a 45- to 60-ml esophageal balloon; (2) a lumen for inflation of a 300-ml gastric balloon; and (3) a lumen leading to the distal end of the tube that can be used for iced saline lavage and aspiration of stomach contents.

In general, the Sengstaken-Blakemore tube is most effective for esophageal bleeding.

Significant complications are esophageal rupture and pulmonary aspiration. Although tamponade is relatively effective, rebleeding is common.

Vasopressin. This drug has potent vasoconstrictive properties, especially upon the splanchnic arteriolar bed. To lower portal venous pressure, vasopressin infusions are given by either the intra-arterial or IV routes. The intra-arterial route was initially thought to be more effective, but recently IV infusions have been described as being equally effective. The initial dosage of vasopressin is 0.3 U/min, which is maintained for 30 min; this dosage is then advanced by 0.3 U q 30 min until bleeding is controlled or a maximum dose of 0.9 U is achieved. Vasopressin is effective in controlling a discreet bleeding episode ~50% of the time, but rebleeding is common. Complications of vasopressin therapy are water intoxication, myocardial ischemia or infarction, intestinal ischemia, transient ischemic attacks, cardiac arrhythmias, and cerebrovascular accident. Constant cardiac monitoring during vasopressin therapy is essential to detect the presence of cardiac arrhythmias.

Percutaneous THE. This is a technique of cannulating the intrahepatic branch of the portal vein and is performed under fluoroscopic guidance. The intrahepatic catheter is then passed into the coronary vein that leads to the esophagus, and this vein is obliterated using Gel-foam or sclerosing agents. Other collateral vessels leading to the esophagus can also be selectively cannulated and injected. THE is 50 to 90% effective in controlling hemorrhage, but its performance requires a great deal of technical expertise. Complications of THE include portal vein thrombosis, pulmonary emboli, bleeding into the peritoneum, and sepsis. THE cannot be performed if a surgical shunt procedure is anticipated because of the risk of portal vein thrombosis.

Injection sclerotherapy. This technique involves direct visualization of varices through a flexible endoscope and selective injection of sclerosing agents into or around the distended vessels. Sclerosing agents include sodium morrhuate, sodium tetradecyl sulfate, ethanolamine oleate, and, occasionally hypertonic glucose, thrombin, or cephalothin sodium. The protocol followed by most endoscopists uses 2 ml of 5% sodium morrhuate injected over 10-to-15 sec. The patient's condition is first stabilized using techniques such as vasopressin, blood replacement, and balloon tamponade, because the therapy is difficult to perform in the presence of active bleeding. Sclerotherapy is able to control acute variceal hemorrhage in 71 to 96% of patients; its long-term effectiveness in preventing rebleeding episodes is not yet known.

The following complications have been reported: worsening of hemorrhage, esophageal stricture, esophageal ulcer formation with or without perforation, aspiration pneumonia, pleural effusion, tachycardia, and worsening ascites. Complication rates are lower for skilled endoscopists and patients having nonemergent procedures.

Oral propranolol. Propranolol lowers portal venous pressure and has been used in Europe to prevent GI bleeding in cirrhotic patients who have had recurrent esophageal or gastric bleeding. The therapeutic dose is 20 to 180 mg PO bid, a dose that also tends to significantly lower heart rate. Although the overall morbidity associated with variceal bleeding has not changed, the drug does seem to prevent recurrent bleeding ≤1 yr for most patients.

Surgical interventions for bleeding esophageal varices generally involve methods to decompress the portal venous system by shunting blood into a nearby, low-pressure, venous channel. Several types of portal vein shunting procedures have been devised. Portocaval and splenorenal shunts are the most common surgical procedures performed.

Overall, long-term survival following shunting procedures is not impressive; the surgical intervention does not seem to prolong life, and the opinion of some physicians is that the trade-off for surgical intervention is death by hepatic coma rather than death by hemorrhage. If milder hepatocellular dysfunction is present, however, the patient tends to have better results. Child's classification of liver disease (Table 8–2) is often used as a guide in selecting the most suitable patients for surgical shunting procedures. Patients whose liver disease is classified within Child's classes A and B have much better results after portacaval shunts.

Major complications of portacaval shunting procedures are hepatic encephalopathy, ascites, shunt thrombosis, hemorrhage, edema of lower

TABLE 8–2

Child's Classification of Liver Dysfunction

Group	Characteristics
A	Serum bilirubin <2.0 mg/100 ml Serum albumin >3.5 g/100 ml No ascites No neurologic dysfunction Adequate nutrition
B	Serum bilirubin 2.0–3.0 mg/100 ml Serum albumin 3.0–3.5 g/100 ml Ascites, responsive to treatment Minimal neurologic dysfunction Adequate nutrition
C	Serum bilirubin >3.0 mg/100 ml Serum albumin <3.0 g/100 ml Ascites, poorly responsive to treatment Coma Malnutrition

extremities, myelopathy, and paraplegia, with hepatic encephalopathy the most common.

Nursing interventions

Hypovolemia. (1) Carefully replace blood and fluid with colloids, blood products, and fluids. (2) Assess cardiovascular status during fluid replacement (pulse, BP, and intravascular pressures: ([central venous pressure, pulmonary artery wedge pressure, CO]). (3) Monitor respiratory status during fluid replacement (breath sounds, respiratory rate, arterial blood gases, body temperature). (4) Obtain body weight daily.

Hypercalcemia. (1) Assess for signs and symptoms of hypercalcemia (lethargy, confusion, anorexia, constipation, hypertension, ECG changes [shortening of Q-T interval]). (2) Evaluate serum calcium levels. (3) Consider the need to alternate calcium carbonate antacids with another type to reduce calcium intake.

Hypokalemia. (1) Assess for signs and symptoms of hypokalemia (hypotension, weakness, confusion, paresthesia, shallow respirations, and cardiac irritability). (2) Evaluate serum potassium levels. (3) Consider the need to alternate magnesium hydroxide antacids with other types to decrease potassium loss.

Anemia/hypoxia. (1) *See* Hypovolemia, 1, 2, 3. (2) Evaluate Hb and Hct levels; consider fluid status. (3) Ensure that Sengstaken-Blakemore tube is sufficiently inflated and in the correct position. (4) Monitor for complications of vasopressin therapy (cardiac arrhythmias, changes in mental status, decreased urine output, or ECG changes that indicate ischemia). (5) Evaluate clotting studies for abnormalities (lengthened prothrombin time, decreased clotting factors). (6) Evaluate effectiveness of O_2 therapy. (7) Provide for adequate rest to decrease O_2 needs. (8) Assess for signs of massive blood loss (i.e., >1,000 ml): a decrease in BP of 10 mmHg and an increase in pulse of >20 bpm when the patient is upright. (9) Evaluate stool, gastric aspirates, and BUN levels for evidence of continued bleeding.

Acidosis. (1) Assess for signs and symptoms of acidosis (tachypnea, malaise, stupor, Kussmaul respirations). (2) Evaluate serum and arterial pH. (3) Correct hypoxia, anemia, and hypovolemia.

Hyperglycemia. (1) Assess for signs of hyperglycemia (polyuria, elevated serum glucose, glucosuria, and elevated capillary blood glucose).

Discomfort from Sengstaken-Blakemore tube. (1) Carefully release pressure of balloon at intervals. Remove tube after 48 hr. (2) Provide frequent mouth and nose care; provide padding around areas where tube is inserted. (3) Use extreme care in administering analgesics; assess for hypotension.

Confusion. (1) Assess for orientation to time, person, place. (2) Assess for symptoms of encephalopathy (*see* Table 8–6). (3) Reorient frequently. (4) Explain procedures in lay terms. (5) Correct hypoxia, anemia, hypovolemia, ammonia intoxication, drug (cimetidine) dosage, and other etiologies of confusion.

Fear. (1) Enable patient to verbalize fears. (2) Enhance effectiveness of support system. (3) Provide reassurance. (4) Promote appropriate stages of grieving.

PEPTIC ULCERS

Pathophysiology

Peptic ulcers disrupt gastric mucosa; the ulcer crater extends into the muscularis mucosa and causes pain and bleeding. A scar is left when the ulcer heals. Commonly located in the pyloric region of the stomach and in the duodenum, ulcer craters can be single or multiple erosions. Ulcers are symptoms of a chronic disease process (peptic ulcer disease) or occur in association with major trauma, burns, or other types of critical illness (stress ulcerations).

Duodenal ulcers, the most common type of peptic ulcers, occur in males twice as often as females. The incidence of duodenal ulcer disease peaked early in the twentieth century and has been declining ever since. Although an excess of gastric acid and an alteration in the mucous protection of the stomach are primary causal factors, a myriad of other factors—such as heredity, emotion, environment, medications, diet, and physiology—may also have a role. Contrary to popular belief, there is no such thing as an "ulcer personality," but duodenal ulcers perhaps occur more frequently in people who cannot easily express emotion.

Gastric ulcers, usually located in the pyloric region of the stomach, affect men and women with equal incidence and tend to occur in an older population. Aspirin, alcohol, other gastric irritants, anxiety, and depression are possible causes. Gastric ulcers may run in families and are more common in patients with type A blood. Gastritis occurs in association with gastric ulcers more often than with duodenal ulcers. Studies to differentiate gastric ulcer from carcinoma are usually performed.

Stress ulcers are multiple shallow erosions of the gastric mucosa that do not involve the muscularis mucosa and do not leave scars. They are typically found in the fundus of the stomach within 72 hr of a critical illness or episode of trauma, such as sepsis, shock, major trauma, severe hemorrhage, jaundice, renal failure, and respiratory failure. Stress ulcerations are also called Curling's ulcers, when they are associated with burned patients. A decreased blood supply to the gastric mucosa is thought to be a primary factor in stress ulcer development.

Clinical picture

The various types of peptic ulcers have many symptoms in common and, therefore, often require differential diagnosis. Abdominal pain is a cardinal symptom that generally occurs between meals when the stomach is empty. The pain is often described as being a gnawing, burning, pressing, aching or "hunger" pain. It is well localized rather than being diffuse. Certain foods, such as coffee, alcohol, or juices, often produce pain, while milk or antacids afford relief within a few minutes. Gastric ulcer pain can occur closer to mealtime than duodenal ulcer pain; distension of the stomach by a meal may also cause gastric ulcer pain. Weight loss can occur as a result of pain.

Bleeding occurs more often from gastric and stress ulcerations than from duodenal ulcers. Hematemesis or melena can herald the onset of sudden, massive bleeding. When the onset is rapid, faintness, pallor, tachycardia, hypotension, diaphoresis, thirst, and anxiety are common symptoms. Milder bleeding episodes can be accompanied by pallor, fatigue, and postural hypotension.

Diagnostic studies for peptic ulcers include radiographic and endoscopic techniques as well as laboratory tests. Gastric ulcers often appear on x-rays as punched-out, round shapes. Duodenal ulcers are slightly more difficult to elicit by x-rays; flecks of barium that do not move or a change in the outline of the duodenal bulb may indicate ulcers.

Because of the difficulty of x-ray diagnosis, endoscopy has gained in popularity as a diagnostic tool. Flexible, fiberoptic endoscopes enable physicians to (1) directly visualize gastric and duodenal ulcers, (2) determine their exact location, and (3) determine whether single or multiple ulcers are present. Gastric and duodenal ulcers are nearly identical in appearance, as both types have a white base, a sharply punched out crater, and a red rim. Duodenal ulcers are often multiple. Studies such as cytology and biopsy can also be performed during endoscopy. Endoscopy can be done as an emergency procedure to locate an area of bleeding, but massive hemorrhage usually obscures the endoscopist's view.

Stool samples are helpful to determine when mild active bleeding is occurring. Generally, the stool samples are positive for blood as long as active bleeding is taking place but become negative between bleeding episodes. Other causes of blood in the stool, such as hemorrhoids or rectal fissures, must also be considered.

Laboratory tests are helpful to determine the extent of bleeding of an ulcer, but not for diagnosis. The most significant laboratory tests are Hct, WBC, BUN, liver function studies, and serum ammonia levels. The Hct value may not accurately reflect the amount of blood loss for the first 72 hours of a bleeding episode because hemoconcentration has occurred. As the patient's fluid volume is replaced, the Hct falls. The WBC is often elevated $\leq$20,000 cells/mm^3. As bleeding is controlled, the WBC drops to a normal level. Elevations in BUN are common and reflect metabolism of blood from the intestine. Generally, BUN levels decrease within 2 hr after bleeding has stopped. Serum ammonia levels are sometimes elevated and also reflect metabolism of blood from the GI tract.

Medical interventions

Most **medical** interventions are directed toward neutralizing and decreasing production of stomach acid. These measures include nasogastric suction, antacid therapy, and histamine H_2 blockers (Table 8–3). Other

TABLE 8–3

Histamine H_2 Receptor Antagonists

Drug	Major actions	Route of excretion	Therapeutic dosage	Major side effects	Drug interactions
Cimetidine (Tagamet)	Inhibits action of histamine at the H_2 receptor sites of parietal cells. Inhibits gastric acid secretion stimulated by food, histamine, pentagastrin, caffeine, and insulin.	Urine	300 mg PO qid 300 mg IV q 6 hr (reduce with renal or hepatic dysfunction)	Confusion, diarrhea, dizziness, rash, headache, agranulocytosis, and slight increases in serum creatinine.	Warfarin-type anticoagulants, phenytoin, lidocaine, and theophylline. Antacids may interfere with cimetidine absorption if given simultaneously; administer between cimetidine doses.
Ranitidine (Zantac)	Inhibits action of histamine at the H_2 receptor sites of parietal and gastric cells. Decreases hepatic blood flow by $\leq 20\%$. Increases nitrate-producing organisms in the GI tract.	Urine	150 mg PO bid (reduce with renal or hepatic dysfunction)	Headache, malaise, dizziness, constipation, nausea, abdominal pain, rash, decreased WBC and platelet count, slight increase in serum creatinine, some increase in SGOT, and GGT.	Propantheline. (Antacids do not interfere with ranitidine.)

GGT, gamma glutamyltransferase.

drugs, such as sulfated disaccharides and bismuth compounds, form a protective barrier over the ulcer to protect it from acid and pepsin. When moderate to severe bleeding is occurring, however, all these measures take on secondary importance.

In the event of GI bleeding, the major goal of medical therapy is to restore hemodynamic stability by replacing blood, fluid, and electrolyte losses. Initially, whole blood is administered and later blood products, such as packed RBCs, are given to enhance O_2-carrying capacity without adding excess fluid volume. Administration of blood products is guided by hemodynamic monitoring, urine output, laboratory values, and arterial O_2 levels.

Iced saline lavage has been a standard treatment of upper GI bleeding for many years, under the assumption that gastric cooling constricts arterial vessels and subsequently decreases bleeding. Its efficacy has never been proven. On occasion, epinephrine has been added to further constrict vessels. More recent studies suggest that iced lavage, with or without epinephrine, does not decrease—and may actually prolong—bleeding. Feeding when GI bleeding is occurring remains controversial. Most physicians continue to order NPO and use gastric suction to remove blood from the GI tract in hopes of minimizing the amount of ammonia produced as blood is metabolized.

Bland, soft, liberal milk diets after a bleeding episode were once a standard therapy to buffer stomach acid, but histamine H_2 blockers have replaced dietary measures. In addition, milk is as effective as histamine in stimulating the production of gastric acid, and an increased level of calcium in the blood causes even further stimulation of acid production. Rough foods were thought to scrape off tissue around an ulcer, but there is no evidence to support this assumption. Spices such as pepper, chili powder, and Tabasco sauce do cause some inflammation of stomach lining, but other spices and flavorings do not cause irritation and, therefore, foods need not be tasteless. Generally, patients are told to eat the foods that they can tolerate without experiencing pain. Frequent meals are more effective in buffering acid and preventing pain. Milk in small amounts may be helpful to provide relief from ulcer pain.

The patient is sedated during what can be a terrifying experience, with diazepam the sedative of choice. Anxiety and fear cause increased gastric secretion and, therefore, work against efforts to reduce acidity.

Regardless of the type of treatment, 80 to 90% of patients stop bleeding spontaneously. Massive bleeding is not a benign occurrence; the mortality rate is ~10%.

Other complications of ulcers that require medical or surgical interventions are perforation, obstruction, intractable pain, and the milk-alkali syndrome.

Indications for **surgical** treatment of peptic ulcers include massive bleeding, perforation, and recurrent ulcer formation, especially in an elderly person. Surgical approaches include, (1) resection of the segment of the stomach where the majority of acid producing glands are located (antrum), and (2) disruption of the parasympathetic nerve tracts that carry impulses to the stomach and increase acid production (vagotomy). The four most common surgical procedures performed are, (1) partial gastrectomy, (2) vagotomy with pyloroplasty, (3) antrectomy with vagotomy, and (4) selective vagotomies such as parietal cell vagotomy. Complications of surgical interventions include delayed gastric emptying, diarrhea, fat malabsorption, pancreatic insufficiency, lactase insufficiency, and recurrent ulcers. By far the most troublesome and common complication is recurrent ulcers.

Nursing interventions

Nursing interventions are the same as those discussed for esophageal varices.

PANCREATITIS

Pathophysiology

Acute pancreatitis is characterized by a process of inflammation and destruction of pancreatic tissue, ranging from mild to severe. Severe pancreatitis may be accompanied by cyst formation, hemorrhage, and necrosis. Chronic pancreatitis exists when tissue damage persists beyond the removal of the initiating agent. Chronic pancreatitis is characterized by persistant pain, pancreatic endocrine and exocrine insufficiency, and mechanical obstruction of the pancreas and related structures. Acute and chronic pancreatitis can be recurrent.

The release of pancreatic enzymes and vasoactive substances into the peritoneal cavity can cause damage to structures adjacent to the pancreas; proteolytic substances can erode into blood vessels and viscera. Necrotic tissue is an excellent medium for bacterial growth and increases the risk of abscess formation. Alterations in pulmonary, cardiovascular, renal, and GI systems may result.

The most common etiologic agents associated with pancreatitis are alcoholism, biliary tract disease, trauma, hyperlipidemia, and iatrogenic causes, such as medications, operative procedures, and endoscopic retrograde pancreatography (ERCP). Other causes include hereditary factors, peptic ulcer disease, hypercalcemia, vascular diseases, infectious agents, toxins, hypotension, and tumor.

Clinical picture

Abdominal pain, nausea, and vomiting are cardinal features of pancreatitis. The abdominal pain is severe and radiates to the flank areas from the epigastric area, often causing the patient to double over. Upper abdominal tenderness and guarding can also be present. Other physical signs and symptoms are diaphoresis, fever, tachycardia, and hypotension. Because these symptoms are similar to other types of GI pathology, diagnosis involves careful clinical and laboratory evaluation.

Certain physical and laboratory findings have a positive correlation to severe acute pancreatitis. Table 8–4 presents signs that are associated with an increased risk of death, major complications, and prolonged ICU stays. Laboratory tests are helpful in diagnosing pancreatitis, but none are unequivocal. Serum and urine amylase values are elevated early in the disease. These studies are most reliable in the first 24 to 48 hr after the onset of symptoms. The amylase:creatinine clearance ratio compares urine and serum levels of amylase when some renal insufficiency is present. A clearance ratio >6% suggests pancreatitis. Serum lipase levels may also be elevated. Serum calcium, Hb, and albumin may be decreased; blood glucose, lactic acid dehydrogenase (LDH), SGOT, BUN, WBC, serum triglycerides, alkaline phosphatase, and bilirubin may be increased. Electrolyte levels are often abnormal and reflect hydration status.

Pancreatic secretion tests (fecal fat and secretin tests) are rarely used in the acute phase and may be most helpful for the management of chronic pancreatitis. Radiographic tests, such as films of the chest and abdomen and upper-GI contrast studies, can demonstrate findings that suggest pancreatitis. Segmental ileus of the small bowel, dilation of the transverse colon, unclear margins of the psoas muscle, increased density in the epigastric area, pleural effusions, duodenal edema, and pancreatic enlargement are nonspecific findings that suggest pancreatitis and help to rule out other types of GI pathology.

TABLE 8–4

Ranson's Prognostic Signs

Time period	Factor	Value
Admission	Age	>55 yr
	Blood glucose	>200 mg/dl
	WBC count	>16,000/mm^3
	Serum LDH	>700 IU/liter
	Serum SGOT	>250 U/liter
Initial 48 hr	Hct	>10% decrease
	Serum calcium	< 8 mg/dl
	Base deficit	> 4 mEq/liter
	BUN	> 5 mg/dl increase
	Fluid retention	> 6 liters
	Arterial O_2 tension	<60 mmHg

LDH, lactic acid dehydrogenase. *Adapted from* Ranson, J. H. C., K. M. Rifkind, D. J. Roses, S. O. Fink, K. Eng, and F. C. Spencer. Prognostic signs and the role of operative management in acute pancreatitis. *Surgery, Gynecology and Obstetrics* (July 1974). pp 69–81.

Ultrasonography can diagnose a pancreatic mass or pseudocyst but is less helpful for uncomplicated pancreatitis. CAT demonstrates changes in the size and configuration of the pancreas and may be used in conjunction with radiographic contrast material to help delineate structures.

ERCP, performed by a skilled endoscopist, can identify obstruction, dilation, and stenosis of pancreatic ducts and so is most commonly used to diagnose chronic pancreatitis and carcinoma of the pancreas.

Diagnostic paracentesis is occasionally performed to examine the volume, character, amylase content, and WBC count of peritoneal fluid; however, clearly delineated ranges of normal values have not been established.

Medical interventions

Pain control. Meperidine is the drug of choice for pain management and is typically administered in doses of 50 to 100 mg q 4 to 6 hr. Although meperidine produces some constriction of the sphincter of Oddi, morphine is believed to cause more profound constriction and is, therefore, seldom used.

Fluid and electrolyte replacement. Fluid loss with pancreatitis occurs from several sources: vomiting, reduced fluid intake because of pain and nausea, fluid sequestration outside the vascular space because of inflammation, and removal of additional amounts of fluids and electrolytes by nasogastric suction. In severe pancreatitis, ≥6 liters of fluid may be sequestered in extravascular spaces. Crystalloid and electrolyte solutions are often administered to restore and maintain intravascular fluid. Fluid status and response to treatment must be carefully monitored during replacement therapy. Central venous (CVP) or pulmonary pressure (PAWP) recordings help to ensure that fluid replacement does not cause CHF or pulmonary edema.

Electrolyte replacement during an acute episode of pancreatitis is also important. Serum levels of chloride, sodium, potassium, and calcium are likely to be decreased. Levels of serum electrolytes must be carefully monitored during fluid replacement therapy.

Other medications. Medications such as glucagon, cimetidine, insulin, somatostatin, anticholinergics, and corticosteroids have all been used in treatment of pancreatitis. None is of proven value and, in fact, some may mask the occurrence of complications. Antibiotics are often administered during an acute episode of pancreatitis to prevent infection. Studies in groups of patients with mild pancreatitis have failed to demonstrate the benefit of antibiotic therapy.

Preventing pancreatic secretion. Measures such as bed rest, nasogastric suction, sedation, and fasting are used to prevent pancreatic stimulation. Activity and anxiety increase gastric secretion, which can subsequently trigger pancreatic secretion. Nasogastric suction decompresses the stomach but, more importantly, removes stomach acid to help prevent pancreatic stimulation. If PO feeding is begun before pancreatic inflammation has subsided, a dramatic exacerbation of symptoms can occur. Parenteral nutrition may be required for prolonged fasting states. Elemental diets administered via the jejunum are used by some physicians. Close monitoring for signs and symptoms of an exacerbation of pancreatitis is required.

Peritoneal lavage. This treatment for severe acute pancreatitis is relatively new. The rationale is that removal of toxic substances and necrotic material from around the pancreas helps to prevent complications, and lavage does seem to decrease the early mortality rate for severe pancreatitis, but long-term mortality remains unchanged. A peritoneal dialysis catheter is inserted, by cutdown, into the peritoneum. Two liters of an isotonic balanced electrolyte solution are then introduced into the abdomen and allowed to remain for ~30 min before being drained off by gravity. Ampicillin, heparin, and potassium are added to the lavage solution. Peritoneal lavage may begin within 48 hr of the diagnosis of pancreatitis and continue for 2 to 4 days. Major complications of lavage are visceral injury during insertion of the dialysis catheter, respiratory failure, hyperglycemia, and intraperitoneal sepsis.

Surgical interventions include (1) cholecystectomy, performed when biliary obstruction is the known etiologic factor for pancreatitis; (2) pancreatic resection and evacuation of necrotic material, reserved for cases of severe hemorrhagic pancreatitis and often futile, as generally both procedures are complicated by intra-abdominal sepsis and death; and (3) drainage of pseudocysts. Pancreatic pseudocysts sometimes occur as a complication of pancreatitis. The fluid within a pseudocyst contains dissolved tissue and pancreatic enzymes. Pancreatic pseudocysts carry a 10 to 14% mortality rate. Pseudocysts often resolve spontaneously, but large, persistent cysts are troublesome and may become abscesses. Internal and external drainage procedures are used to treat pseudocysts. Internal drainage is accomplished by creating an opening between the cyst and the stomach, jejunum, or duodenum. External drainage involves creation of a drainage tract from the cyst to the abdominal wall.

Nursing interventions

Hypovolemia. (1) Assess patient for decreased urine output, decreased CVP, hypotension, decreased PAWP, decreased CO and cardiac index, increased pulse rate, increased urine sp gr, poor skin turgor, dry mucous membranes. (2) Evaluate cardiovascular and respiratory status during colloid and electrolyte solution replacement. (3) Evaluate renal functions by means of urine sp gr, urine output recordings, serum osmolarity, and laboratory data (creatinine, BUN). (3) Evaluate changes during fluid replacement.

Hyponatremia. (1) Assess patient for the following signs and symptoms: nausea, vomiting, headache, confusion, lethargy, convulsion, coma, acid-base imbalances. (2) Evaluate serum sodium levels.

Hypochloremia. (1) Assess patient for the following signs and symptoms: alkalosis, hypoventilation, hyperexcitability. (2) Evaluate serum chloride levels and pH.

Hypokalemia. Assess patient for the following signs and symptoms: cardiac arrhythmias, hypotension, weakness, lethargy, confusion, paresthesias. (2) Evaluate serum potassium levels.

Hypocalcemia. (1) Assess patient for the following signs and symptoms: tremors, tetany, cardiac arrhythmias, laryngospasm, convulsions, paresthesias, positive Chvostek's or Trousseau's signs. (2) Evaluate serum calcium levels and albumin levels.

Hypomagnesemia. (1) Assess patient for the following signs and symptoms: tetany, tremors, twitching, hallucinations, confusion, hypotension, tachycardia, positive Chvostek's or Trousseau's signs. (2) Evaluate serum magnesium levels.

Hypoxia. (1) Assess patient for the following signs and symptoms: tachypnea, confusion, tachycardia, hypotension, dyspnea, restlessness, cyanosis, cardiac arrhythmias. (2) Evaluate arterial O_2 levels (PO_2, O_2 saturation). (3) Evaluate arterial CO_2 levels and pH. (4) Promote maximum oxygenation: turn, cough, deep breathe; position patient to maximize chest excursion; use postural drainage and suctioning as needed to mobilize and remove secretions.

Hypotension. (1) Monitor pulse and BP. (2) Administer vasopressors as indicated. (3) Evaluate Hb and Hct to assess for intraperitoneal bleeding. (4) Correct fluid and electrolyte imbalances.

Protein calorie malnutrition. (1) Assess for signs and symptoms of malnutrition (muscle wasting; depletion of body fat stores, energy; weight < 80% of ideal, NPO for more than 5 days, depleted albumin levels, depleted lymphocyte count, depleted transferrin, negative nitrogen balance). (2) Safely administer parenteral nutrient solutions, with particular attention to: preventing sepsis; preventing electrolyte, mineral, or vitamin imbalances; evaluating the patient's tolerance of the fluid volume, glucose load and fat load (if applicable); recognizing metabolic complications early. (3) Safely administer enteral nutrient formulas, with particular attention to: evaluating the patient's response (i.e., does feeding exacerbate symptoms of pancreatitis?); preventing aspiration of feeding; preventing or treating diarrhea. (4) Evaluate adequacy of nutritional support (weight gain, positive nitrogen balance, intact immunity). (5) Assess for signs of fat malabsorption; (steatorrhea, bulky, fatty foul-smelling stools).

Hyperglycemia. (1) Assess for signs and symptoms of hyperglycemia (polyuria, elevated serum glucose, glucosuria, and elevated capillary blood glucose). (2) Evaluate serum glucose levels and test urine for glucose and ketones. (3) Administer insulin therapy with special care: assess effectiveness in lowering blood sugar; monitor for signs and symptoms of hypoglycemia at times of insulin peak effect (tremors, diaphoresis, tachycardia, dizziness, loss of consciousness).

Pain. (1) Assess pain (location, character, intensity, duration, timing, precipitating events, comfort measures that work, accompanying symptoms). (2) Administer and assess the effectiveness of analgesics. (3) Use other comfort measures to enhance pain relief (touch, positioning, relaxation, distraction, imagery, and stimulation of the skin). (4) Maintain patency of the nasogastric tube to prevent stimulation of the pancreas; provide mouth and nose care to decrease discomfort from nasogastric tube.

Anxiety. (1) Explain procedures in lay terminology. (2) Provide reassurance. (3) Enhance support system. (4) Enable patient to verbalize concerns. (5) Enable patient to maintain as much control as possible over own care.

Alcoholism/low self-esteem. (1) Assess for signs and symptoms of alcohol withdrawal (tremors, fever, hypertension, tachycardia, diaphoresis, confusion, and hallucinations). (2) Administer sedatives as needed to control withdrawal symptoms. (3) Provide interventions for long-term alcoholism treatment (Alcoholics Anonymous [AA] and other modes of treatment). (4) Provide intervention for family members (Alanon and family counseling services).

HEPATIC FAILURE

Two major complications associated with hepatic failure are cirrhosis and hepatic encephalopathy.

Cirrhosis of the liver

Cirrhosis is characterized by scarring, with fibrosis and areas of tissue regeneration. This process produces nodules, which give the liver a typical hobnailed appearance. The widespread structural changes involve most areas of the liver and subsequently are more destructive than a discreet lesion. Early on, the liver is enlarged, but, as fibrous bands continue to form, it actually shrinks in size. Cirrhosis is characterized as micronodular (fibrous bands thick and uniformly shaped), macronodular (fibrous bands of various shapes and sizes), or mixed (both types of fibrous tissue present.)

Chronic alcohol abuse is the leading cause of cirrhosis in the USA; other causes include: hepatitis (type B), biliary stasis, severe right-sided CHF, industrial compounds, hemochromatosis, Wilson's disease, schistosomiasis, congenital syphilis, alpha-1 antitrypsin deficiency, fibrocystic disease, and galactosemia.

Symptoms. Early symptoms of cirrhosis are weakness, fatigue, anorexia, and weight loss. As the disease becomes more widespread, additional symptoms appear, such as low-grade fever, constipation, abdominal distension, and dyspepsia. Late symptoms characteristic of severe hepatic dysfunction are listed on Table 8–5.

Diagnosis. Laboratory values, liver biopsy, radiographic studies, and ultrasound techniques are used to diagnose cirrhosis. Common **laboratory tests** include: alkaline phosphatase, SGOT, SGPT, gamma glutamyltransferase (GGT), albumin, and bilirubin. Elevated levels of

TABLE 8–5
Signs and Symptoms of Hepatic Dysfunction

Anemia, ascites, ataxia, atrophy of prostate and testes, caput medusae, cardiac myopathy, edema, esophageal varices, fetor hepaticus, gastritis, gynecomastia, hemorrhagic diathesis, jaundice, nodular liver, nystagmus, ophthalmoplegia, palmar erythema, pancreatitis, pectoral alopecia, peripheral neuritis, spider angiomata, splenomegaly, thrombocytopenia.

SGOT, SGPT, and GGT indicate cellular damage, with the GGT being most specific for the liver; none of the enzyme tests suggests the cause of liver damage. The alkaline phosphatase elevates in biliary obstruction but is also elevated in bone disease and other conditions. (Occasionally, the 5′-nucleotidase test is used to distinguish between skeletal or hepatic causes of alkaline phosphatase elevations.) The electrophoretic pattern of serum albumin shows decreased albumin and elevated globin fraction in cirrhosis. If hepatobiliary obstruction is present, the total bilirubin will increase. The serum test for ornithine carbamoyltransferase (OCT) is very sensitive for hepatocellular disease and is increasingly used in diagnosis of liver disease.

Tissue samples obtained by **needle biopsy** of the liver can demonstrate the cellular changes characteristic of cirrhosis. Occasionally, the liver capsule is so tough that the needle cannot pierce it. Complications of liver biopsy are pleurisy, hemorrhage, intrahepatic hematomas, fracture of the biopsy needle, and puncture of nearby viscera.

The **liver-spleen scan,** using technetium-99m, typically shows a patchy uptake of contrast material and splenomegaly.

Ultrasound techniques can be used to determine patency of the portal vein and to demonstrate ascites without exposing the patient to radiation.

CAT is helpful to diagnose the general shape of the liver, abdominal and hepatic tumors, and dilated bile ducts but is limited in diagnosing hepatocellular damage.

Hepatic encephalopathy

A complication of hepatic dysfunction characterized by alterations in neurologic and psychiatric functions, hepatic encephalopathy's exact cause is unknown; the most widely believed theory holds that toxic substances (such as ammonia, mercaptans, fatty acids, and aromatic amino acids), absorbed from the gut and unaltered by the liver, reach the systemic circulation. Alkalosis, hypokalemia, and hypoglycemia often accompany severe liver dysfunction. Ammonia absorbed from the intestines is still considered the most likely cause of hepatic encephalopathy.

Symptoms. Early symptoms are rather vague and nonspecific, such as: forgetfulness, fatigue, drowsiness, irritability, untidiness, frequent yawning, emotional instability, and flattening of affect. As the disorder becomes worse, more dramatic alterations can be observed and assessed.

Table 8–6 illustrates a method of staging based upon neuromuscular and psychogenic alterations.

Diagnosis. Although serum ammonia levels are often elevated in the presence of this disorder, the amount of ammonia does not correlate well with the stage of encephalopathy. Bedside assessment techniques more accurately reflect the alterations that accompany various stages. Common assessment techniques include (1) asking the patient to write his name, construct a star with toothpicks, draw a spiral or star, add a series of numbers, repeat a series of numbers, and—beginning with the number 49—serially subtract 7; (2) checking the patient for fetor hepaticus, asterixis, hyperreflexia, positive Babinski's sign, unsustained clonus, and hyperventilation. Alterations in the plasma amino acid pattern are common in hepatic failure. The level of aromatic amino acids becomes elevated in relationship to the branched chain amino acids. This finding has led to development of specialized enteral and parenteral nutrient formulas for the patient with hepatic failure.

Medical interventions

Major **medical** interventions for hepatic failure are (1) treatment of precipitating causes, (2) reducing production of ammonia, (3) institution of low protein, low sodium, or specialized amino-acid-formula diets, and (4) avoidance of hepatotoxic drugs.

Treatment of causes. A variety of substances and events can cause hepatic failure; however, in the presence of chronic liver dysfunction, the following mechanisms can cause "acute" failure: hemolysis secondary to hypersplenism, GI bleeding, impaired urea production, decreased production of clotting factors, arteriovenous shunting, accumulation of ascites, decreased renal blood flow, altered plasma amino acid patterns, sepsis, and

TABLE 8–6

Stages of Hepatic Encephalopathy

Stage	Neuromuscular alteration	Psychogenic alteration
I (Prodromal)	Slight tremor	Variable mood Variable confusion Slowed mental processes Untidiness
II (Precoma)	Obvious tremor	Enhanced symptoms of stage I Drowsiness Inappropriate behavior
III (Stupor)	Tremor	Stuporous, but arousable Marked confusion
IV (Coma)	Tremor absent	Unresponsive most of the time

drugs. Treatment is primarily supportive; efforts are directed toward preventing failure of other organs such as the heart, lungs, and kidneys. Electrolyte and mineral imbalances are corrected. The patient's intravascular volume is carefully replaced, and antibiotics are used to treat sepsis.

Ammonia reduction. Neomycin sulfate or lactulose is prescribed to supress ammonia production in the gut. By decreasing the number of intestinal bacteria, **neomycin** decreases the amount of ammonia produced by bacterial action. Dosage of neomycin is 4 to 9 g PO/day or a 1 to 2% retention enema. Ototoxicity and nephrotoxicity are the most serious adverse effects. **Lactulose** decreases the pH of the intestine, thus trapping ammonia in the bowel for excretion. The recommended dosage of lactulose syrup is 20 to 30 g PO tid or qid. Lactulose can also be given as a 1-liter retention enema q 4 to 6 hr. Major side effects are abdominal distension, cramping, and diarrhea, although the production of two to three soft stools per day is desirable for successful therapy. Concomitant lactulose and neomycin therapy may decrease the effectiveness of ammonia suppression.

Diet therapy. Diet therapy for hepatic failure consists of salt and water restriction, protein restriction, and replacement of fat-soluble vitamins and minerals. Protein tolerance in hepatic dysfunction varies, but if hepatic encephalopathy occurs, protein intake may need to be restricted to 20 to 60 g/day. Changes in neuromuscular and psychogenic function may indicate an enteral or parenteral nutrition formula. Hepatic-Aid II and Hepat-Amine are, respectively, enteral and parenteral products that provide an increased amount of branched chain amino acids and a decreased amount of aromatic amino acids. If a PO diet is tolerated by the patient, nitrogen-rich foods such as salami, cheese, ham, buttermilk, potatoes, peanut butter, margarine, mayonnaise, onions, gelatin, catsup, and french dressing are avoided.

The fat-soluble vitamins, A, D, E, and K, are typically depleted in hepatic failure. Alcohol abuse causes depletion of folic acid and vitamin B_{12}, as well. Minerals such as calcium, zinc, and magnesium are also often depleted in hepatic failure. Multivitamin preparations that contain these minerals are chosen.

Sodium and fluid restriction are important when ascites and edema are present. Sodium may initially be limited to 2 to 3 g/day, but severe ascites must be managed by more limited sodium intake.

Abstinence from alcohol is essential to prevent rapid deterioration of remaining hepatic function and inadequate nutritional intake.

Drugs. Many drugs are metabolized and excreted as a result of liver processes. Drug dosages must often be reduced in the presence of hepatocellular dysfunction. Any drug addition to the medication regimen requires assessment for hepatic encephalopathy.

Except for transplantation, there are no direct **surgical** interventions for correcting hepatocellular dysfunction (or improving hepatocellular function). Palliative measures are available for complications such as portal hypertension and intractable ascites. Surgical shunting procedures can decompress the portal system, especially in vessels that are most likely to lead to massive hemorrhage. Ascites that does not respond to conventional diuretic therapy is managed by insertion of a peritoneovenous shunt, which allows ascitic fluid to flow from the peritoneal cavity to the jugular vein or superior vena cava by means of a pressure gradient. During inspiration, intrathoracic pressure decreases and ascitic fluid ascends through the shunt to the systemic circulation. Inspiratory exercises and abdominal binders enhance flow through the shunt. The Denver shunt, an adaptation of the LeVeen valve, is fitted with a duckbill or miter valve that, when manually compressed, increases flow through the peritoneovenous shunt. Complications of the peritoneovenous shunts are hemodilution, disseminated intravascular clotting (DIC), CHF, GI bleeding, hyperbilirubinemia, ascitic fluid leak from the incision, wound infection, and device failure from occlusion.

Liver transplantation is performed in a select number of major medical centers and thus is not a widely available surgical intervention. Selection criteria for recipients of liver transplant include age, presence of extrahepatic infection, general health, emotional stability, nature of the liver disease, and presence of complications. Major postoperative complications are rejection, cholestasis, and infection. Recipients have a one in five chance of surviving one year.

Nursing interventions

Providing nursing care for a patient with hepatic failure is a formidable task for the nurse. The actual physical care required is extensive. Some patients will be in the terminal stages of liver disease and, therefore, the nurse will need to assist the patient and family with the process of grieving. If alcohol abuse is the underlying etiology for liver disease, intervention and referral to a counseling program for family members is extremely important.

Excess nitrogenous substances in blood. (1) Administer lactulose/neomycin sulfate to decrease blood ammonia levels. (2) Evaluate serum ammonia levels. (3) Assess dietary protein intake, especially in relationship to neuromuscular and psychogenic status. (4) Assess for side effects of lactulose/neomycin therapy (ototoxicity, decreased renal function, diarrhea, abdominal distension). (5) Provide nutritional support appropriate to patient's ability to tolerate protein.

Hyperbilirubinemia. (1) Assess sclera, mucous membranes, skin of trunk and neck for signs of jaundice. (2) Evaluate bilirubin level.

Hepatorenal syndrome. (1) Record volume, character, color, and sp gr of urine. (2) Evaluate renal function studies: BUN, creatinine. (3) Assess effectiveness of diuretic therapy. (4) Assess effectiveness of peritoneovenous shunt.

Impaired ability to detoxify substances. (1) Check route of excretion of medications. (2) Assess effect of newly prescribed medications upon neuromuscular and psychogenic status.

Alteration in protein, fat, and carbohydrate metabolism. (1) Evaluate tolerance of dietary protein intake (assess for progression of hepatic encephalopathy, evaluate serum ammonia level, evaluate amino acid profile, if available). (2) Evaluate tolerance of dietary fat intake (assess for steatorrhea, evaluate serum triglyceride levels). (3) Evaluate tolerance of dietary carbohydrate intake (evaluate serum glucose levels, assess for signs and symptoms of hyperglycemia). (4) Provide appropriate amounts and types of major nutrients. (5) Safely administer enteral or parenteral nutrient formulas (if indicated).

Alteration in vitamin metabolism and absorption. (1) Supplement fat-soluble vitamin (A, D, E, K) intake. (2) Protect vitamin preparations from heat and light. (3) Evaluate for signs and symptoms of fat soluble vitamin deficiencies (decreased prothrombin time, bone pain, hair loss, scaly skin lesions, and poor wound healing).

Ascites. (1) Measure abdominal girth. (2) Monitor cardiovascular status; pulse, BP, and intravascular pressures (CVP, PAWP, CO). (3) Monitor respiratory status (breath sounds, respiratory rate, lung excursion, and arterial blood gases). (4) Evaluate renal function (urine output, creatinine, BUN). (5) Evaluate effectiveness of diuretic therapy. (6) Evaluate effectiveness of peritoneovenous shunt (decreasing abdominal girth, increased urine output, increased respiratory excursion). (7) Monitor for complications of peritoneovenous shunt (hemodilution, CHF, DIC, GI bleeding, shunt occlusion, sepsis). (8) Enhance flow through peritoneovenous shunt (apply abdominal binder, assist patient to perform inspiratory exercises).

Hepatic encephalopathy. (1) Perform bedside assessment to determine stage of encephalopathy. (2) Evaluate serum ammonia level. (3) Evaluate patient's tolerance of dietary protein intake (*see above*). (4) Provide safety measures to prevent injury from falls, burns, skin breakdown. (5) Assist family to cope with patient's altered mental status.

Decreased immunity. (1) Provide care of invasive lines to prevent sepsis. (2) Mobilize pulmonary secretions to prevent pneumonia. (3) Prevent complications related to parenteral/enteral nutrition. (4) Promote adequate nutritional balance.

Discomfort. (1) Use protective positioning and turning to prevent skin breakdown. (2) Provide mouth and skin care. (3) Carefully administer analgesics, if indicated.

Loss/grieving. (1) Encourage patient and family members to express feelings. (2) Promote a normal process of grieving. (3) Enhance support system.

Alcoholism/low self-esteem. (1) Assess for signs and symptoms of alcohol withdrawal (tremors, fever, hypertension, tachycardia, diaphoresis, confusion, and hallucinations). (2) Administer sedatives as needed to control withdrawal symptoms. (3) Provide intervention for long-term alcoholism treatment (Alcoholics Anonymous [AA] and other modes of treatment). (4) Provide intervention for family members (Al-Anon and family counseling services).

CHAPTER 9

BURN CARE

Margaret A. O'Neill DeVito

FRAMEWORK

THE SKIN

The skin, the largest organ in the body, is the body's natural integument. A severe burn injury disrupts this integument and has the potential of affecting the function of every major body system.

The skin is divided into three main layers: the epidermis, the dermis, and the subcutaneous layer. Each layer plays a major role in protecting the body from injury.

The **epidermis** is a thin layer formed by keratinocytes. The outermost layer, the epidermis is directly exposed to the environment. The keratinocytes synthesize keratin, a flexible, threadlike protein that serves as a protective barrier against the invasion of bacteria and other foreign substances. The epidermal layers originate in deeper layers and migrate to the surface. This is a continuous process that replenishes keratin as it is sloughed off in the course of daily living. The loss of excessive amounts of body fluids is also prevented.

The **dermis** is the middle layer and is composed of a fiberlike structural protein called collagen. The dermal layer nourishes and supports the epidermis. The epidermis and dermis are bound together by the dermal papillae, fingerlike projections that protrude into the epidermis. The dermis contains nerve fibers, which extend through the dermal papillae. These nerves are sensitive to pressure, pain, touch, and temperature. The dermis also contains sweat glands and sebaceous glands. The excreted oil of the sebaceous glands keeps the skin pliable and lubricated. Also found within the dermis are scattered clusters of epidermal cells that contain the roots from which body hair grows.

The **subcutaneous** layer is the innermost skin layer. Composed mainly of fat cells, the subcutis gives support to the outer two skin layers. Within the subcutis are found the largest skin arteries. This layer serves to insulate the body from heat and cold. The subcutis also acts as a protective cushion against mechanical shock.

The epidermis, surrounded by a layer of lipid tissue, provides a water-vapor barrier to the skin, preventing fluid loss and dehydration under normal circumstances; when disrupted by a burn injury, dehydration through evaporation can occur. This further complicates the fluid and electrolyte imbalance that accompanies a burn injury.

The ducts of the sweat glands located in the dermis routinely carry fluids that contain water, salt, and waste products from the blood to the surface of the skin. This fluid (perspiration) helps to regulate the body temperature, cooling the skin as sweat evaporates. Destruction of the skin by a burn injury results in disruption in body temperature regulation.

The body's sensory impulses are carried to the CNS by nerve fibers that extend through the dermis and end in the papillae of the epidermis. With a burn injury, the sensory perceptions are altered as a result of damage to the skin layers. The actual depth of a burn injury is directly related to the amount and intensity of sensory perception that the burn patient has.

The skin reflects a person's outward appearance, which is extremely important to self-concept and body image. Psychological implications associated with a burn injury are as devastating to an individual's sense of identity as the physiologic alterations that occur.

ETIOLOGY OF BURNS

Incidence

Burn injuries are the third leading cause of accidental death in the United States. Each year ~2 million Americans are burned and 12,000 people die annually from severe burns; ~75,000 people suffer severe burns involving ≥30% of the total body surface and are hospitalized in ICUs.

The initiation of the proper plan for treatment of the burn patient is paramount in reducing morbidity and mortality. The initial assessment of the depth of the burn injury and percentage of total body surface area (BSA) involved with the injury generally determine what type of setting is best prepared to care for the burn injury. Robert P. Hummel suggests a measure for choice of treatment location: Minor burns (second-degree, <15% of BSA, and third-degree, <3% of BSA except face, hands, and feet) are treated on an outpatient basis; moderate burns (second-degree, 15 to 25% BSA, and third-degree, <10% BSA except face, hands, and feet) can be treated by a community hospital; major burns (second-degree, >25% BSA; third-degree, >10% BSA; third-degree burns of face, hands, feet; respiratory complication; serious associated injuries; and electrical burns) should be sent to a burn unit or center. When a burn patient is triaged to a treatment facility appropriately, there will be a greater chance that he will recover successfully from the injury.

Types of burns

Generally a burn injury is referred to as a thermal burn, electrical burn, or chemical burn.

Thermal burns. Thermal burns are the most common type of burn experienced. They occur as a result of the transfer of energy from a heat source to the body. Flames, hot surfaces, hot water, the sun, etc., are examples of sources that result in a thermal burn injury. Varying depths of thermal injury can occur, depending upon the length of time of exposure and the intensity of exposure to the source. A thermal burn caused by a flame or fire results in what is called a **dry burn.** This type of burn is often much deeper than what can be seen. Highly concentrated heat comes into direct contact with a localized area and can burn deeply into the soft tissue that is underlying the skin. Damage to the layers of skin and underlying soft tissue can be extensive.

A thermal injury can also be referred to as a **moist burn.** This results from a scald injury caused by exposure to a hot liquid, usually steam or substances such as boiling water. The main difference between a dry burn and a moist burn is in the amount of burn surface area involved. Steam or boiling water can conduct heat to a larger area and frequently injures a more extensive BSA.

Electrical burns. Electrical burns are classified as low-tension or high-tension electrical injuries. A low-tension injury generally results when there is contact with $<$350 volts of electricity, high-tension injury when there is contact with $\geq$350 volts. Low-tension injuries usually occur at home. High-tension injuries are often work-related and represent the largest proportion of electrical injuries admitted to the hospital. Because an electrical burn results in the passage of an electrical current directly through the body, an electrical burn is often difficult to evaluate. The actual tissue damage at the entrance and exit points of the electrical current may appear minor; the passage of an electrical current through the body can, however, cause significant underlying tissue destruction not easily detected upon visual examination. An electrical-burn victim must be carefully assessed for signs and symptoms of shock and internal injury.

Chemical burns. Chemical burns are very common to industry. In this type of work setting there may be frequent exposure to or contact with strong acids or alkalis. Contact with household items such as drain cleaners, paint removers, etc., can also cause this type of injury. Tissue damage from exposure to a chemical is dependent upon the length of time of exposure of the chemical to the skin, the concentration, the amount exposed to the skin surface, extent of penetration into the skin, and the action of the chemical on the skin. The chemical agent present will cause progressive skin and tissue damage until it is inactivated. Therefore, once a chemical burn is sustained, it is important to remove the chemical from the skin surface with water or a chemical neutralizing agent as soon as possible.

PHYSIOLOGIC CHANGES

When a burn injury is sustained, there is a threat to body homeostasis. Considerable disequilibrium can be caused in all the body's systems.

Cardiovascular function

The immediate postburn period is marked by alterations of cardiovascular function. A dramatic **increase in permeability** is caused by heat injury to the capillaries and smaller blood vessels of the circulatory system, the vasculature surrounding the involved area becomes permeable to fluids, electrolytes, and various molecular substances. Plasma and protein escape from the blood vessels. The hypoproteinemia that results decreases vessel pressure and allows fluid to flow into tissue. The increase in capillary permeability is immediate in the area burned, resulting in edema; several hours after the injury edema often occurs in other parts of the body. Fluid is extravasated into the body's interstitial spaces. Capillary permeability gradually returns to normal within 24 to 48 hr postburn. This process is a result of activation of the body's compensatory mechanisms and proper fluid replacement.

Hypovolemia results from the loss of intravascular volume. The undamaged, intact tissues give up fluids to compensate for the loss of readily available circulating plasma. As a result, generalized dehydration often occurs, compounded by the continued escape of fluid from the damaged capillaries. The deficit in plasma and blood volume that results from these hemodynamic changes contributes to the decrease in CO seen in the early postburn period.

Hemodynamic changes, such as hemostasis and hemoconcentration, are often two early responses to disruption of the cardiovascular system. Because fluid shifts from the bloodstream to the tissues, plasma becomes highly concentrated. The blood that remains in the vessels becomes thick and increases in viscosity, resulting in a rise in the Hct level. This increased viscosity of the blood impairs peripheral blood flow, and hypoperfusion to body tissues is the end result.

Generally, on the second to fifth postburn day this process begins to reverse itself. The fluid that has escaped into the interstitial spaces begins to flow back into the vascular and cellular compartments. The capillary walls begin to reestablish their nomral permeability, and edema will begin to resolve. As the fluid is drawn back into the vascular space, extensive diuresis occurs. The circulating blood volume begins to be restored, and CO begins to increase. Close monitoring of the patient is critical at this point to prevent further complications.

Fluid/electrolyte balance

Increased capillary permeability also affects the electrolyte balance of the body. Electrolytes escape through the injured blood vessels, and as a result more sodium than water is drawn into the interstitial space, disrupting the cells' normal sodium/potassium balance. The lymphatic system, which under normal circumstances would work to remove increased tissue fluids, becomes overloaded with this increased fluid volume and functions ineffectively, resulting in edema. The body's normal buffering action is disrupted. With an imbalanced acid:base ratio and imbalanced electrolyte concentrations, a metabolic acidotic state exists.

Fluid-and-electrolyte-replacement therapy must be addressed carefully with each patient, with close attention to the composition of the fluid lost and the rate of loss. The extent and type of burn injury, age of the patient, and cardiovascular status are key factors to consider when initiating fluid replacement. Fluids can be replaced PO or parenterally, depending on how much BSA has been damaged (<15% of the total BSA for adults, <10% for children: PO; larger burns: parenterally). A number of formulas are available for initial fluid resuscitation. Most formulas recommend that 0.5 to 0.6 mEq of sodium/kg of body weight/percent of total BSA burned be replaced. Several of the more popular formulas being used are the Evans, Brooke, and Parkland formulas. In recent years a resuscitative regimen designed by Monafo has been introduced. This formula involves the administration of hypertonic saline and is somewhat different from the standard formulas used. The fluid replacement formulas use a combination of crystalloids and colloids. Colloid preparations generally used are plasma protein fraction, dextran, and human albumin. Crystalloid preparations are generally lactated Ringer's solution and normal saline. Patient response to each formula used must be monitored closely, and alterations made when necessary.

The literature on fluid replacement therapy is extensive. Individual health-care providers are urged to pursue this subject further when caring for the burn patient.

Pulmonary function

Respiratory complications often occur in the burn patient. They can be seen immediately, and if treatment is initiated early, complications that compound the injury can be decreased.

Immediate respiratory complications are usually related to the burn injury itself. These generally occur within two hours of the initial injury. Smoke inhalation injuries are caused by the inhalation of the variety of gases and particles contained in smoke. When smoke inhalation is minimal there may only be an irritating cough with no shortness of breath or hypoxia; however, these irritating effects may eventually cause severe wheezing and bronchospasm in some patients.

Inhalation of carbon monoxide may also occur, causing serious complications for the patient. Carbon monoxide is a colorless, odorless, tasteless, very toxic gas that is a product of the incomplete combustion of carbon. Carbon monoxide readily combines with Hb, displacing O_2 to form carboxyhemoglobin. This loss of O_2 results in tissue hypoxia. The end result of this process has serious ramifications for the burn patient. The more O_2-dependent organs (brain, heart) tend to show the earliest signs of damage. The patient will present with signs of confusion, lethargy, and eventual unconsciousness. This condition can be accompanied by arrhythmias leading to cardiac arrest.

Additional complications are pneumothorax or pulmonary contusion resulting from the trauma associated with a burn injury.

Delayed complications are usually a result of the fluid resuscitative measures taken or occur because of the area involved with the burn injury. Any facial or neck injuries should alert the practitioner to the possibility of concurrent respiratory complications.

Airway obstruction may occur in the first 24 to 48 hr. This is usually associated with edema of or a direct injury to the soft tissue of the upper airway. Patients should be closely assessed for signs and symptoms indicative of an airway obstruction. Complaints of fullness or heaviness in the throat, dysphagia, or increased irritation of the throat, nares, etc. indicate possible interference with the patency of the airway. Placement of an oral or nasal endotracheal tube may be necessary. Once facial edema and further signs of airway obstruction have resolved, the patient can be extubated.

Pulmonary edema commonly accompanies a burn injury. This is directly related to the amount of fluid required for proper fluid replacement during the resuscitative phase of the injury. Signs and symptoms frequently associated with pulmonary edema are the presence of pink-tinged or white frothy sputum, distended and engorged neck veins, dyspnea, perspiration, and cyanosis. Atelectasis often accompanies an inhalation injury. Aggressive pulmonary toilet with inspiratory positive pressure breathing (IPPB) and postural drainage are a few of the treatment measures that must be taken to avoid this complication.

The patient's weakened pulmonary function and exposure to airborn bacteria makes him a prime target for the development of pneumonia, which requires initiation of antibiotic therapy.

Prolonged immobilization with a serious burn injury puts the patient at risk for the development of venous thrombosis and possible pulmonary embolus. Early mobilization and initiation of active and passive range-of-motion exercises can decrease the incidence of this occurrence.

GI function

A patient's GI function is frequently altered with a burn injury. The presence of edema and hyperemia of the mucous membranes of the GI tract often result in gastric dilation and possible paralytic ileus. Gastric acidity may be elevated, reflected by a decrease in the pH of gastric juices. There is evidence of elevated blood histamine levels in stressed and traumatized individuals. Histamine normally stimulates the production of gastric juices; when histamine levels are elevated, there are increased gastric juices. The diminished production of gastric mucus and adrenal hyperactivity also result with a burn injury. Thus, the burn patient is prone to the development of a gastroduodenal ulcer, referred to as Curling's ulcer.

Renal function

The renal function of the burn patient is altered by the impact on this system resulting from impairment of the other major body systems. The kidney damage that occurs is directly related to the fact that other vital organs are being adequately perfused. Cerebral and cardiac perfusion demands often result in the decreased perfusion of the kidneys, which leads to oliguria within the first 48 hr of a burn injury. The tendency for kidney perfusion to increase within the second 48 hr postburn is great because of the dramatic fluid shift back into the circulating bloodstream. The increased volume of circulating blood causes an increase in urine production and urine output.

CLASSIFICATION OF BURNS

Each type of burn sustained—thermal, electrical, or chemical—can cause varying degrees of injury to the involved area. The first 48 hr of a burn injury must be spent stabilizing and managing the burn patient. The actual depth of the burn injury has very little effect on the initial management, but classifying the depth of a burn injury is extremely important. Proper classification will result in successful planning of the course of therapy to be used with the patient.

Burns have been classified as first, second, or third degree, according to the depth of tissue destruction. More recently, burns have come to be referred to as either partial-thickness or full-thickness injuries. The management of the burn wound is dependent upon whether the burn sustained is a superficial, partial-thickness, or full-thickness injury (Fig. 9–1).

Superficial wound. A superficial wound generally results when some agent causes irritation to the epidermal layer of skin. With this wound there is no destruction of tissue. A superficial, or first-degree, burn wound is seen as reddened, slightly inflamed skin. The skin temperature is warm, and minimal discomfort results. This type of wound is similar to the typical sunburn.

Partial-thickness wound. A partial-thickness burn wound results when there is destruction of the local tissue from epidermis into dermis. With this type of wound (formerly known as second-degree), there is some portion of the epidermal or dermal appendages intact. This type of wound

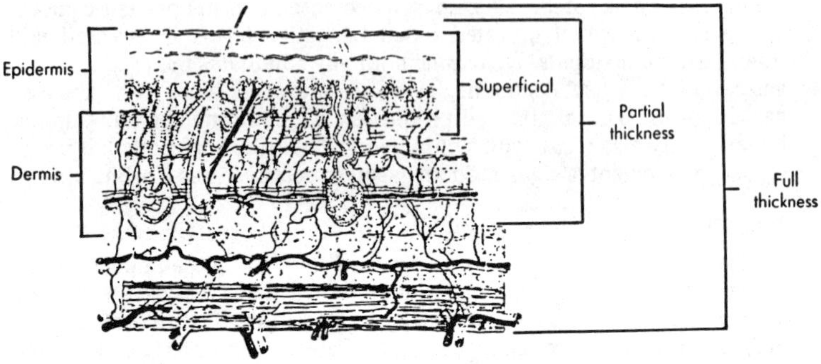

Figure 9–1. Depths of burns.

has the eventual potential to become epithelialized. A partial-thickness injury is often referred to as a superficial-partial-thickness or deep-partial-thickness injury.

Superficial-partial-thickness wound: A superficial-partial-thickness injury involves only the epidermis and extends at times to the outer portion of the dermal papillae. Pain is usually associated with this injury because sensitive nerve endings remain intact. This type of wound is often covered with blisters and once debrided, the epidermis appears shiny, bright pink or red and very weepy.

Deep-partial-thickness wound: A deep-partial-thickness wound involves the entire epidermis along with the dermal papillae. It leaves intact the hair follicles and sweat glands, from which are generated epithelial elements that eventually cover the wound. This type of wound is painful because uninjured nerve endings are irritated. These burns appear from pink or red to dull white or tan and are usually soft and somewhat pliable. In an extensive deep-partial-thickness burn, an eschar or thick, leathery covering may form.

Full-thickness wound. A full-thickness (third-degree) burn wound is characterized by irreversible damage to all of the epidermal and dermal components. Surgical grafting is necessary to promote healing of this injury. This type of injury is usually painless because of the destruction of the nerve endings in the involved area. The wound appears tan in color and is hard and dry. Often, thrombosed blood vessels are visible in the underlying surface of the wound. The degree of skin tissue damage that occurs precipitates a surface dehydration, and an eschar may develop over the wound.

ASSESSMENT OF THE PATIENT

The patient who enters an ICU with a burn injury will need immediate attention. The initial assessment should include a general physical examination, along with a history of how the burn occurred. The major body systems should be assessed.

An adequate airway and breathing pattern is a priority with the burn patient. Physical assessment of the pulmonary status includes inspection of the respiratory pattern. Measurement of oxygenation and arterial blood gases (ABGs) are frequently ordered and need to be monitored closely. Periods of apnea, slow regular or irregular breathing, and tachypnea are documented if found to be present on physical examination. Chest expansion is assessed. Feeling the chest contour will help to assess the degree of expansion. The upper airway and chest wall are palpated. Actual percussion of the chest is important: dull or tympanic sounds can indicate the possibility of an abnormal respiratory pattern. Rales, rhonchi, narrowing of the tracheal lumen, or absence of breath sounds can be detected through auscultation. Frequent chest x-rays are ordered to monitor the pulmonary status.

With fluid replacement therapy, the presence of edema may mask the patient's body weight. If possible, it is helpful to know the patient's most recent preburn weight. One indicator of a positive response to fluid therapy is the subsequent 10 to 20% increase in the patient's weight. By the eighth to tenth postburn day, the patient's weight should begin to return to normal. Weight is taken and recorded on a daily basis in the ICU.

An indwelling Foley catheter is inserted. Close monitoring of urinary output is important when rapid fluid replacement is taking place. A range of urine output of 0.5 to 1 ml/kg of body weight/hr is satisfactory. Urine should be assessed for quantity and character (color, consistency) and the specific gravity measured. A heavy pigmentation in the urine should be recorded and reported because this signals myoglobinuria, which can lead to acute tubular necrosis. Acute renal tubular necrosis occurs as a result of obstructive nephropathy, a condition that occurs when heavy protein pigments precipitate in the renal tubules. In this circumstance, it may be necessary to increase the rate of fluid administration or administer an alkalinizing agent such as sodium bicarbonate ($NaHCO_3$) to resolve the problem. Urine electrolytes must also be closely monitored, particularly sodium. Kidney perfusion is considered normal when 60 to 100 mEq/liter of sodium is excreted from the urine.

The burn patient must be closely assessed for level of consciousness. Sudden changes in mental status, such as disorientation, increased restlessness, or confusion may indicate an inadequate fluid resuscitative effort.

MANAGEMENT

A peripheral IV line is inserted. This is usually positioned in an area in which central venous pressure (CVP) readings may be taken concurrent with fluid replacement. Because cutdowns are a frequent source of sepsis, they are avoided whenever possible. IV lines should be cared for as required by the hospital policy. Fluid replacement therapy will employ the formula of choice of the physician. Resuscitative efforts are based upon the combined amount of partial- and full-thickness injury, the total BSA involved, and the patient's weight. The total BSA involved must be accurately assessed for successful treatment to result. There are a number of methods used to estimate the percentage of total BSA burned; one, the Rule of Nine, is used for a quick estimate (Fig. 9–2).

If a central venous line has been placed, CVP readings are taken concurrently with vital signs. These parameters are measured frequently. Peripheral pulses may need to be heard with a Doppler probe if peripheral edema or an eschar formation hinders the ability to accurately palpate the pulse. An arterial line may be needed to monitor BP accurately if it is difficult to obtain the measurement with a cuff. An elevated temperature is

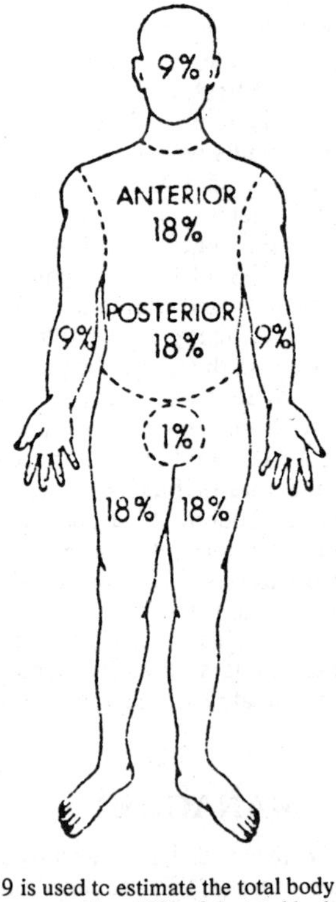

Figure 9-2. The Rule of 9 is used tc estimate the total body surface involved with burn injury. The head and arms are considered 9% of the total body surface; the anterior trunk and posterior trunk and each leg are considered 18% of the total body surface.

common with a burn injury. Administration of an antipyretic may be required. The respiratory rate usually falls within the upper limits of the normal range. A Swan-Ganz catheter may be placed if the area burned involves ≥50% of total BSA or, if a history of previous cardiopulmonary disease exists. When possible, the Swan-Ganz catheter should be removed in ≤72 hr. ECG tracings are monitored regularly. A normal ECG tracing suggests that fluid replacement therapy has been successful.

A Levin tube is usually placed as soon as possible to decompress the bowel. The intestines of the traumatized patient are prone to distension and ileus. Removal of gas via the nasogastric (NG) tube reduces distension and discomfort. Proper care of the NG tube is important to prevent further debilitation of the patient. The nares should be checked for signs of irritation and breakdown. Placement of the NG tube should be checked at regular intervals. To assure patency of the NG tube, irrigations with 10 to 30 ml of normal saline should be done at two hour intervals. The tube is usually attached to intermittent, low-presure wall suction, and proper functioning of this equipment must be maintained. Oral hygiene must be administered regularly to the patient with an NG tube.

The nurse measures and records the amount, color, and consistency of the NG aspirate. The pH of gastric secretions should be checked with pH-sensitive paper every hour and the gastric environment kept alkaline. Antacids are often ordered by the physician to be administered at hourly intervals via the NG tube to maintain the gastric pH at >6.0. Generally 30 to 60 ml of antacid, followed by 10 to 20 ml of water are prescribed. The NG tube is clamped for 15 to 20 min to allow time for alkalinization to occur. Another sample of gastric content is aspirated after clamping and checked for the desired effect. Assessment of bowel sounds, NG aspirate, and stool passage are features of ongoing monitoring of GI function.

Extensive laboratory studies are employed to closely monitor progress. ABGs are measured and O_2 saturation studies are conducted to assess the quality of respiratory function. CBC, BUN, creatinine, glucose levels, serum and urine sodium, potassium, chloride, bicarbonate, and osmolality studies are closely monitored. Additional laboratory studies may be indicated in particular situations. Laboratory studies serve as excellent indices for successful or unsuccessful resuscitative measures.

As hospitalization may be lengthy for the burn patient, measures must be taken to promote proper rest. Rest periods should be planned during the day. Daily hygiene, elimination care, and optimum comfort measures must be provided on a consistent basis.

The initial efforts to stabilize the patient are directed toward stabilization of the patient's physiologic status. But it is also important that initial efforts be directed at promoting patient comfort, cleansing and debridement of the burn wound. It is important to cleanse the wound with an antimicrobial solution such as povidone-iodine to decrease the chance of extensive bacterial invasion at a later stage. The wound should be rinsed thoroughly and dressed with a bulky dressing.

Pain is usually treated initially with low doses of IV analgesics. Oversedation can make assessment of neurologic status difficult. Analgesics work to reduce the pain, which is often accompanied by anxiety and fear. A prophylactic dose of a tetanus toxoid is often administered.

Once the burned individual has begun to respond to the initial efforts toward stabilization of his physiologic state, focus on wound management can begin.

BURN WOUND TREATMENT

There are a wide variety of treatment regimens available for the burn wound. Many depend on the type of wound and the treatment preferred by the medical and nursing staff.

Every effort must be taken to control the patient's endogenous and exogenous environment to prevent wound infection and sepsis. When a burn wound treatment is performed, strict isolation must be enforced. Gown, gloves, and mask are worn during dressing changes or direct patient contact, and strict hand washing is imperative. Isolation techniques vary depending on the design of the treatment facility.

An optimum enviroment for the cultivation, multiplication, and spread of bacteria exists with a burn injury. The presence of necrotic tissue and the loss of the skin's protective function predisposes the patient to infection. Any pathogens present rapidly spread through body tissue and enter the vascular system. It is extremely important to detect the infecting organism as soon as possible. Blood and wound cultures facilitate this identification process. Once the pathogen is identified, proper antibiotic therapy should be initiated, along with application of the chosen topical antibiotic agent to the wound. At periodic intervals, further blood and wound cultures should be taken to assure proper antibiotic coverage. If infection is present and not properly treated, a partial-thickness injury can easily be converted to a full-thickness injury.

The actual burn dressing change often causes intense pain and becomes an added stressor on the already debilitated patient. The appropriate medication must be administered to help alleviate the pain and discomfort. Frequently used are injectable doses of narcotics, such as meperidine hydrochloride in an average dose of 50 to 75 mg for the adult and .5 mg/lb for the child. The patient may often find that listening to a favorite song or tape is helpful in distracting attention during a dressing change. The use of various relaxation response measures may also be beneficial.

The burn wound must be cleansed thoroughly with an antimicrobial agent. The cleansing solution must then be thoroughly rinsed away so not to interfere with the chemical properties of the topical agent used to promote healing. Any excess hair should be removed whenever possible to decrease the chance of bacterial invasion.

Treatment of blisters is controversial. Generally, they are thought to be a natural protective mechanism and therefore should remain intact until spontaneously broken, at which time loose skin must be debrided.

Environment. Dressing changes should be done in a closed environment, such as the patient's room or specially equipped dressing rooms. If possible, patients should be placed in trauma tanks, Hubbard tanks, or tubs for wound cleansing. Hydrotherapy is frequently ordered for wound cleaning and debridement procedures. The nurse must be organized and proceed in a manner that facilitates an extensive, thorough treatment within a time frame tolerable for the patient. Short rest periods should be arranged to promote optimum tolerance.

Wound cleansing. After a sterile field is prepared, the old dressings are removed and discarded in the proper receptacle. The burned area is washed, using a gentle, firm, circular motion. Once cleansed, the wound is rinsed with normal saline and inspected for signs of infection, granulation tissue, and healing. The nurse should observe for the presence of any odiferous smells, unusual drainage, or increased amounts of drainage.

Debridement. Debridement is the actual removal of unhealthy, nonviable tissue from the wound. Burn wounds should be mechanically debrided with each dressing change until the wound becomes free of eschar and necrotic debris. A dressing set equipped with forceps, scissors, and clamps should be used to probe the wound for tissue that should be removed from the wound's surface. Minor bleeding may occur as a result of this procedure and can be controlled by using silver nitrate sticks or by applying firm pressure to the area. Profuse bleeding, not easily controlled, should be reported to the physician. A final cleansing and rinsing of the wound should occur after debridement is completed.

Dressing of the wound. The status of the patient's wound and physician preference indicates the choice of topical agent to be used. Table 9–1 offers a current list of available topical agents. Burn wounds are dressed using an open or closed technique.

When wounds are treated with the **open dressings,** they must be monitored closely for the presence of the topical agent. It is important that the topical agent be reapplied prn in areas where it has been removed by patient activity. A bed cradle can be used to keep bed linens from coming in contact with the skin and causing removal of the topical agent.

A **closed dressing** provides an occlusive wrap to the wound. It is beneficial to impregnate the gauze used for the dressing with the topical agent prior to applying the gauze to the wound, which can be done by using a sterile tongue depressor. If this is not possible, a sterile gloved hand can be used to apply the topical agent to the wound in a thin layer. When silver nitrate solution is the agent of choice, it is important that the gauze dressing remain moist at all times. Precut, perforated red-rubber catheters wrapped into the gauze dressing can be used to maintain moisture. The ends of the catheters should be left exposed for instillation of the silver nitrate solution, providing for easier application of the solution and patient comfort. Closed dressings can be secured in place by using sterile, elasticized net coverings.

TABLE 9–1
Topical Drugs

Topical agent	Advantages	Disadvantages
Silver sulfadiazine (Silvadene) Destroys bacteria by altering DNA and cell metabolism.	Wide spectrum of activity. Long lasting. Works up to 48 hr. Painless and somewhat soothing. Does not cause metabolic derangements or electrolyte imbalance. Not nephrotoxic.	Repeated application directly to the wound may cause buildup of medication that is difficult to remove. May cause a rash in unaffected skin. May be the source of pruritus. Depresses granulocyte formation.
Mafenide acetate (Sulfamylon) Bacteriostatic against gram-negative and gram-positive organisms.	Effective against *Pseudomonas.* Penetrates thick eschar. Relatively nontoxic. Isolation not necessary.	Causes burning pain on application. May cause systemic metabolic acidosis. May cause hyperpnea. May cause rash in unaffected skin. Inhibits epithelial proliferation, and therefore should be discontinued as soon as the wound is clean.
Silver nitrate Bacteriostatic chemical effective in reducing colonization.	Controls surface bacteria. Inexpensive. Easily applied. Does not require isolation. Reduces evaporative water loss from burns.	Caustic substance that stings on application. May cause electrolyte imbalance by drawing sodium, potassium, calcium, chloride, and magnesium from the burn wound. Stains everything it comes in contact with. Does not penetrate eschar.
Nitrofurazone (Furacin) Inhibits enzymes necessary for bacterial metabolism.	Broad spectrum of activity. Effective against *Staphylococcus aureus.* Not absorbed systemically. Low incidence of sensitivity.	May cause contact dermatitis in unaffected skin. A side effect that is not necessarily considered a disadvantage is that this preparation turns urine a reddish color.
Scarlet red Nonantiseptic. Applied in the form of gauze soaked with oil-based red dye.	Applied to donor site during skin grafting. Promotes healing. Protects donor site.	Infection may develop beneath the scarlet-red gauze, which may have systemic effects. Stains and irritates skin. May cause some discomfort.
Bismuth tribromphenate (Xeroform) Nonantiseptic preparation.	Debrides and protects donor site. Protects graft.	Removal may be painful because it sometimes adheres to the wound.

Topical agent	Advantages	Disadvantages
		Neither antiseptic nor antimicrobial.
Povidone-iodine (Betadine) An iodine solution, ointment, or foam.	Effective against gram-positive and gram-negative organisms, fungi, protozoa, and viruses. Microbicidal against many infections not controlled by Silvadene.	May cause metabolic acidosis because of elevated serum iodine levels. Stains clothing and linen. Causes dry, crusting, and scabbing wound. May cause skin rash in unaffected area. May cause an allergic reaction.
Sodium hypochlorite (Dakin's solution) A chlorine-based solution.	Bacteriocidal. Aids in debriding wounds. Aids in cleaning and draining "soupy" wounds.	Dissolves blood clots. May inhibit clotting. May irritate the skin.
Sutilains ointment (Travase) Topical enzymatic agent.	Dissolves necrotic tissue by proteolytic action. Facilitates removal of eschar and purulent exudate.	Mild, transient pain on application. May cause paresthesia, bleeding, or dermatitis. Dressings must be kept moist at all times.

Reprinted with permission from Hills, S.W., and J.J. Birmingham. Burn Care. John Wiley & Sons, Inc., New York. 1981. p. 88–89.

The patient who is severely burned may develop an eschar over the wound, causing pressure to underlying tissue. An **escharotomy** may be necessary to remove this thick, leathery surface. Postescharotomy, warm saline compresses are applied to the skin. Frequent circulation checks and elevation of the affected area are important.

Full-thickness injury will require a surgical grafting procedure. The newly grafted skin and the donor site require meticulous nursing management. Physicians vary in their approach to grafting techniques and the care of the grafted wound and donor site. Specific institutional protocols must be followed. The grafted wound must be immobilized for a period of time to allow for adherence of the newly grafted skin. Dressings should be secured in place. When dressings are removed, the technique must be steady and slow so not to dislodge the graft.

Donor site care must follow strict aseptic technique to prevent infection. Various agents are available to promote healing of the donor site such as scarlet red, Xeroform, and Op-Site, and again physician and nurse preference often indicates the choice of treatment for the donor site.

Once healing of the burn wound has occurred, the patient may experience dryness of the skin, caused by destruction or damage to the sebaceous glands. A natural, nonallergenic lubricant should be applied to the skin to decrease the chance of cracking and pruritus. The lubricant should be lanolin-containing and mild and can be applied as often as necessary. The newly formed skin is very thin and must be protected at all times from further harm.

ADDITIONAL NURSING CONSIDERATIONS

Rehabilitation

The nurse is responsible for proper maintenance of the old as well as new skin. Often immobilized for prolonged periods of time, the patient is at risk for the formation of decubiti and pressure sores. Active and passive range-of-motion exercises are initiated as indicated. Frequent rotation of the patient in bed or use of an air-fluidized bed are measures to be taken.

Proper positioning of the patient is essential throughout the hospital stay (Table 9–2). Proper positioning can greatly decrease the amount of scarring and musculature contractures that result due to the initial injury. Although

TABLE 9–2

Policy for Positioning Burn Patients

Area	Position
Neck	Towel roll or hyperextension mattress to be used. No pillows for anterior neck burns. Patients positioned in neck hyperextension.
Shoulders	Patients with axillary burns positioned in 90-degree abduction and external rotation. Patients may be taken out of braces or slings only for ROM, meals, and dressing changes unless otherwise specified by the treatment program.
Elbows	Full extension. If burns are only on the posterior aspect, some flexion is desirable.
Hands	Safe position of up to 35-degree wrist extension, 70-degree flexion of MPs, extension of the PIP and DIP joints. Thumb in abduction and opposition, avoiding hyperextension of the DIP joint.
Knees	Position in full extension. When burns are only on the anterior aspect, some flexion is desirable.
Hips	15-degree to 30-degree abduction for burns of the medial aspect of the thigh. Extension of the hip.
Feet	Neutral position.

DIP, distal interphalangeal joints; MP, metacarpal phalangeal joints; PIP, proximal interphalangeal joints; ROM, range of motion. *Adapted with permission from* Hummel, R.P., editor. Clinical Burn Therapy, A Management and Prevention Guide. John Wright PSG Inc., Littleton, Mass. p. 281.

scarring and contracture formation are unavoidable with some severe burns, every effort for their prevention must be taken. Early involvement with the physical and occupational therapist is necessary to decrease any potential problems. Supportive clothing, proper positioning, and early physical therapy are suggested for each patient. Efforts such as these will help to decrease the amount of disability and disfigurement that is associated with the burn wound.

A team approach is vital during the patient's rehabilitative phase. Input is needed from all health-care disciplines when planning care to promote wellness and independent functioning for the patient.

Nutrition

The overall metabolic response to a burn injury is characterized by an increased basal metabolic rate (BMR) along with an increased protein metabolism, resulting in depleted stores of protein. The increased BMR is proportional to the degree of injury. The burn wound results in a rapid heat loss for the body. This, along with an increase in adrenergic activity brought on as a stress response to the injury, increases the body's energy expenditure. Protein loss occurs through the burn wound itself and also because of the depletion of glycogen stores and fatty acids. Protein stores are mobilized to meet energy demands and ultimately become further depleted. Eventually, negative nitrogen balance and a catabolic state develop. The process is complicated by the fact that there is an initial weight loss for the patient because of the loss of an excessive amount of fluid via the wound.

An integrated multidisciplinary approach is vital to accurately assess the nutritional requirements of the burn patient. Each patient should have a nutritional assessment and nutritional metabolic profile made early in the hospitalization. Certain parameters, such as the patient's anthropometric (body) measurements, laboratory studies, diet, and nutritional standards are included in this profile, which lays the groundwork for nutritional planning.

With a burn injury, there is often anorexia or an inability to consume food because of the physiologic changes that have occurred. To promote optimal healing, the patient's caloric intake should be four times the normal intake. The protein requirement recommended for an adult to remain in positive nitrogen balance is 0.8 g/kg of body weight; the loss of protein from a burn wound increases this daily requirement by two to four times. Available energy stores also become depleted with this type of injury. Essential vitamin and mineral requirements must also be maintained. Therapeutic doses of vitamins should be prescribed for the patient. Laboratory studies that monitor serum levels of calcium, zinc, phosphate, and iron should be watched closely.

It is important to have the patient begin consumption of food and fluids PO as soon as possible. Once the fluid resuscitative phase is completed, parenteral nutrition will begin. Total parenteral nutrition (TPN), consisting of a 12 to 25% dextrose solution with a 4 to 6% crystalline amino acid solution is administered via a central venous line. If a central line cannot be maintained, a lower dextrose solution may be infused peripherally. A fat solution is administered with TPN to supply fatty acids and calories. Close monitoring of the patient's blood and urine glucose levels is necessary when administering high concentrations of dextrose solutions (*see* Chapter 11).

Once the patient is able to tolerate food and fluid in the GI tract, enteral feedings should begin. Enteral and parenteral feedings can be administered simultaneously to provide for adequate nutritional requirements (*see* Chapter 11). The hypertonicity of tube feeding solution may cause diarrhea, which further depletes the patient's fluid/electrolyte balance. Prescription of an antidiarrheal medication may be needed to resolve this problem.

If the patient is able and willing to take fluids PO, this is strongly encouraged. Dietary supplements, such as burn milkshakes, can be made by the dietary department. Burn shakes are rich in calories and protein and generally well tolerated by the patient. These should be given as between-meal and bedtime snacks. Patient's family members should be encouraged to bring in favorite foods from home. These items can be calculated into the nutritional demands of the patient.

The postburn patient's nutritional requirements may be as great as two-and-one-half times his preinjury requirements. A successful team effort can make this challenge a manageable one.

Psychological impact

The psychological ramifications of a burn injury can be as difficult for a person to recover from as are the physiologic alterations of body state. The emotional needs of the patient cannot be underestimated. Often associated with a burn injury are fears of death, loss of function, and loss of body image, resulting in behaviors associated with denial, avoidance, and withdrawal. The threat of disfigurement and deformity are realistic because of the severe insult to the body caused by the burn injury. The plan of care for psychological support has to be as thoroughly planned, implemented, and evaluated as that initiated for physiologic support.

Nurses working with burn patients must become attuned to their own feelings on death and disfigurement. Coping with personal feelings of anger, despair, and frustration that emerge when working with such a patient population is of paramount importance (*see* Chapter 19). Establishing a sense of trust between the patient and the nurse is essential. A positive approach is especially important when working with burn patients. In daily interactions, discussion must revolve around the realistic goals that the patient can expect to reach, and signs of progress must be pointed out. The lines of communication between the patient and nurse must be kept open, and they must work together at restoring the greatest degree of independence for the patient.

A person who has sustained a burn injury is forced to deal in some way with a new body image, a new self-identity, and often has to adapt to an alternative work style. This is not an easy accomplishment.

When a person is burned, he is removed from the family unit for an extended period of time. Efforts must be made to include the family in the plan of care. The family should be helped to understand many of the feelings and psychological reactions that may be displayed by their injured family member. Guilt often accompanies this type of injury; the family members may view the injury as their fault. This feeling of guilt can be heightened by the anger and hostility shown by the injured family member.

Involvement of the family in the treatment regimen, wound healing process, and physical therapy program can help the family to better understand the injury. It is often helpful to arrange for family meetings, which allow family members to meet with others experiencing a similar traumatic event and are helpful in reducing anxiety. Such meetings serve as excellent support systems for families involved in such a crisis situation. *See* Chapter 19 for further discussion.

CHAPTER 10

MULTIPLE TRAUMA

Linda C. Degutis

FRAMEWORK

Trauma is defined as an injury that is produced by an outside force. It is essentially a disease of the young. Its most frequent victims are males between the ages of 15 and 35. Trauma is the leading cause of death for those under age 40 and accounts for >1,000,000 disabling injuries each year. Trauma is most frequently caused by motor vehicle accidents. Other injuries result from falls, gunshot wounds, stabbings, and assaults.

Although many advances have been made in the care of the injured person, it is estimated that 150,000 to 175,000 people die each year as a result of trauma. Deaths that occur outside the hospital are usually due to hemorrhage or massive head injury, whereas 50% of trauma deaths in the hospital are caused by CNS injury. The majority of other deaths, which generally occur several days to weeks after injury, are caused by sepsis and multiple organ failure (MOF).

As transport times from the scene of the accident to the hospital have decreased, a number of patients who would have died in the past are surviving to be admitted to ICUs for treatment. The main goals of caring for these patients in the ICU are twofold: (1) stabilization of the patient and (2) prevention of complications that are known to result in increased morbidity and mortality. To provide optimal care for these patients and meet these goals, it is important to understand the body's physiologic response to trauma, the nature and severity of injuries these patients suffer, and the factors that place these patients at increased risk for development of complications.

Approximately 10 to 15% of hospitalized trauma victims will require admission to the ICU for care. The decision to admit the patient to the ICU is based on the patient's clinical status in the ED or OR. The conditions that may require care in an ICU are: (1) hemodynamic instability; (2) necessity for mechanical ventilation; (3) prolonged period of hypotension in ED or OR; (4) single life-threatening injury; (5) more than one serious or life-threatening injury; (6) head injury with altered level of consciousness after admission; (7) cervical spine injury with neurologic deficit; and (8) conditions (unrelated to injury) that place patient at increased risk for morbidity and mortality (i.e., age).

Trauma patients in the ICU fall into one of two categories; those who will require a long period of care in the ICU due to the extent of their injuries or complications and those who will need only a brief (generally ≤48 to 72 hr) period of continuous monitoring. Those patients who require prolonged ICU stays are at highest risk for mortality and morbidity.

It should be remembered that frequently the trauma patient is not admitted to the ICU until several hours after arrival at the hospital because of the time required for diagnostic studies as well as surgical intervention, when necessary. During this lag time, however, the patient who is seriously injured requires close monitoring and rapid intervention if problems occur. It is important to be aware of events that have taken place and the patient's progress during this period of time. Therefore, accurate documentation of assessments and interventions in the ED and OR as well as communication between staffs of these units are essential.

When receiving report on a trauma patient, the following information should be obtained: (1) mechanism of injury, (2) condition upon arrival in the ED, (3) injuries sustained, (4) interventions and patient's response to them, (5) diagnostic studies done and results, (6) current status (ventilatory, hemodynamic, neurologic) and (7) whether the patient's family has been notified of admission and extent of injuries.

Mechanism of injury

Knowledge of the mechanism of injury will allow the nurse to understand the extent of injuries the patient has suffered. Whether an injury is penetrating or blunt will have a significant effect on the organs injured. Stab wounds generally cause less tissue destruction than bullet wounds. The extent of injury is based on location of the wound as well as length of the object used to inflict the wound and whether the object was manipulated once the victim was stabbed.

Penetrating injury resulting from a gunshot wound can result in damage to tissues quite distant to the initial point of entry. Factors that affect the extent of tissue injury include velocity, shape, and size of the bullet. The extent of tissue damage is dependent upon the kinetic energy of the projectile and is proportional to the difference between kinetic energy on entry and kinetic energy on exit.

Hollow-point bullets deform on impact, thus increasing the amount of kinetic energy transmitted to the tissue. Other bullets fragment, and these fragments continue to travel through the tissue in several directions. The path of the bullet is also affected by the tissue it comes in contact with. It may be deflected off bone and "bounce" around a body cavity, causing damage to several organs before it exits or loses kinetic energy.

Cavitation is an important principle to understand in relation to gunshot wounds. This is the momentary acceleration of a tissue in a direction that is both forward and laterally away from the missile's track. Acceleration of the bullet creates a temporary, water-filled cavity around the bullet and its track. Foreign objects such as clothing, as well as tissue fragments may be sucked into the track. Cavitation occurs most readily in those tissues with low tensile strength, such as the liver and other parenchymal organs.

In blunt trauma, an important consideration is also the kinetic energy involved in the accident. Horizontal deceleration occurs as one moving object strikes another object (initial impact). An individual in the moving vehicle continues to move until stopped (second impact) by another object (seatbelt, steering wheel, windshield). Internal body structures may continue to move in a horizontal plane after the second impact occurs. These structures are in danger of tearing at points of relative fixation. Other injuries occur as a result of direct contact with immovable objects. The extent of injury in this case is dependent on the force with which an individual strikes or is struck by an object, the size and shape of the object, and the angle at which the object is struck. Although this is a simplification of the process that occurs, it illustrates the forces in play during an accident.

ED management

The condition of the injured patient upon arrival in the ED will provide clues as to the initial blood loss experienced, as well as the severity of injury. In addition, knowledge of injuries actually sustained will alert the nurse to the potential problems that may be encountered as well as to the level of care that will be necessary. Awareness of the necessity for interventions and the patient's response to them is important in determining the patient's current status. A patient who has not responded adequately to blood and fluid resuscitation is likely to have an undiscovered source of bleeding.

Diagnostic studies are important to determine the extent of specific injuries. If the patient has not completed all the studies necessary, the nurse must be aware of what studies will need to be performed after the patient has arrived in the ICU in order to plan the patient's care. Knowing the patient's clinical status prior to transfer to the ICU will allow a more accurate patient assessment and will also allow for preparation prior to the patient's arrival in the ICU.

Families are often the lowest priority during the time of initial assessment and care of the trauma patient. It is, however, important to ascertain whether they are aware of the extent of the patient's injuries and the reasons for the patient's admission to the ICU. The nurse should, whenever possible, provide the family with orientation to the ICU and prepare them for the appearance of the patient prior to their initial visit with him. Frequently, the first contact family members have with their loved one after admission is in the ICU.

THE BODY'S RESPONSE TO TRAUMA

Injury results in both local and systemic physiologic responses. Wound healing or local responses are affected by the body's systemic reaction to trauma. In the individual with minor injury such as a simple laceration, wound healing occurs in several steps. An inflammatory reaction occurs at the site of injury, resulting in removal of damaged tissue. Next, collagen is deposited in the wound and the tensile strength of the area is increased. Finally, the collagen develops into a strong weave, and maximum tensile strength of the healed wound is achieved at some time up to six weeks or more after the initial injury. After major trauma, the ability of this healing process to take place is limited by alterations in blood flow, immune response, and nutritional status.

Hemodynamic response

The most common hemodynamic problem related to trauma is **hypovolemic shock.** This occurs as a result of hemorrhage or, less commonly, the loss of ECF that occurs in patients with abdominal injuries and major crushing injuries. The body's homeostatic mechanisms attempt to compensate for this volume loss through peripheral vasoconstriction, increased CO (by increasing heart rate), and migration of ECF into the vascular compartment. This response is effective as long as blood volume loss is <30% of total blood volume. After 30 to 40% of blood volume is lost, the body is unable to maintain a state of homeostasis for very long. Anaerobic metabolism occurs, resulting in lactic acidosis, which causes myocardial depression as well as depression of other organ functions. If uncorrected early in this phase, hypovolemic shock progresses to an irreversible shock state in which damage to the organs continues, and despite aggressive attempts at fluid volume restoration, organ dysfunction occurs and the patient dies.

Treatment of hypovolemic shock is aimed at restoring adequate blood volume to improve tissue perfusion. Initially, up to three liters of crystalloid solution may be infused. If the patient still remains hypotensive, replacement of volume with blood that has been typed and cross-matched should be initiated. Other treatment measures include use of the military anti-shock trousers (MAST) and autotransfusion using autotransfusion devices.

Cardiogenic shock may occur in the trauma patient who has suffered a major myocardial contusion. This is a result of failure of the heart as a pump caused by extensive damage to the cardiac muscle. Treatment of cardiogenic shock may include inotropic drugs or, in severe cases, use of the intra-aortic balloon pump to support circulation.

Neurogenic shock may also occur in the trauma victim. This is manifested by a decreased BP and peripheral vasodilation. There is a decrease in intravascular volume and so these patients may require fluid volume replacement. In multiply injured patients whose hypotension might be caused by hypovolemia or neurologic injury, it is assumed that shock is caused by blood volume loss, and fluid is given to restore adequate vascular volume. This will also help to maintain cerebral perfusion pressure.

Metabolic response

The basic metabolic response to trauma is an increased energy expenditure. Its extent is dependent upon the severity of injury. Components of this response include changes in metabolism of carbohydrates, fat, and protein.

After trauma, serum glucose rises; at the same time, insulin secretion is unchanged, and the action of insulin is blocked. These conditions are related to the increase in circulating catecholamines following injury. This response is evident for a short period of time in the early posttraumatic state. After the patient is stabilized, the glucose returns to its normal level and circulating catecholamines are decreased. Amino acids, derived from protein, are required for wound healing, liver metabolism, and RBCs and WBCs. If protein is not provided by another source, skeletal muscle is catabolized.

Thus, because of increased energy expenditure related not only to injury but also to therapy such as mechanical ventilation, the trauma patient has greater than normal caloric requirements. Initiation of appropriate feeding early in the hospital course (3 to 4 days postinjury) may prevent consequences of malnutrition. If possible, enteral feeding is initiated. If abdominal injuries make enteral feeding impossible, however, parenteral nutrition is used. Calculation of the number of calories to be provided over 24 hr is based upon the patient's weight and metabolic state. The importance of early nutritional support cannot be overstressed, as it is extremely difficult to reestablish an adequate nutritional state once the patient has become undernourished. (*See* Chapter 11 for a detailed discussion of nutritional support.)

Immunologic response

Host defense mechanisms are altered by injury. Trauma depresses the immune response, thus placing the patient at increased risk for the development of sepsis. Inadequate nutrition also decreases the ability of the body to generate an adequate immune response. Because sepsis is one of the leading causes of late death in the trauma patient, it is important to optimize the function of the host defense mechanisms.

ASSESSMENT

Once the trauma patient arrives in the ICU, the nurse performs an initial assessment. This includes an assessment of ventilatory, hemyodynamic, and neurologic status as well as a thorough appraisal of the patient's injuries. Notation should be made of invasive lines that have been placed and whether they were inserted utilizing appropriate technique. Tubes (Foley catheter, chest tubes, nasogastric tubes, drains) should be checked for proper function. Traction, if applied, should be assessed for proper alignment. A detailed, accurate initial assessment will prove invaluable in setting priorities for care. A format for the initial ICU assessment of the trauma patient is provided in Figure 10–1.

Priority setting in the care of the trauma patient focuses on maintaining adequate ventilation and circulation, prevention of complications, and treatment of life-threatening problems as they occur. Most life-threatening injuries are taken care of prior to the patient's arrival in the ICU. Some of these injuries may not be diagnosed initially, however, and will become apparent during the course of hospitalization.

An awareness of potential complications will allow the nurse to formulate a plan of care that will include measures to prevent these problems. These measures should be integrated into the overall plan of care for any trauma victim. Interventions when complications do occur are based on the nature of the complication and its severity. A more detailed discussion of these problems is presented later in this chapter.

While the patient's psychological function is not one of the initial priorities of care, it should be of concern soon after the patient is stabilized. The nurse should be aware of the patient's unfamiliarity with the environment and need to adjust to the situation. A simple but thorough explanation of what has happened may help orient the patient and decrease initial anxiety. The family is a valuable resource in providing the patient with contact with the outside world.

SPECIFIC INJURIES AND INTERVENTIONS

THORACIC INJURIES

Penetrating trauma

Those patients who experience penetrating injuries to the thorax may have injuries to the abdominal organs as well. Trauma to the great vessels or heart carries a high mortality rate if not treated promptly. Patients with injuries to the cardiovascular system may require thoracotomy immediately upon arrival in the ED to control hemorrhage and allow open cardiac massage. These patients will require massive volume replacement and transfusion, which places them at high risk for developing complications if they survive their initial injuries.

Blunt trauma

Blunt injuries to the chest are usually the result of an unrestrained occupant of a motor vehicle striking the steering column or other parts of the vehicle. Only 10 to 15% of these injuries require surgical intervention; the remainder can be managed with close observation and interventions designed to prevent complications such as pneumonia or respiratory failure.

Injuries to the chest may be divided into three categories: life-threatening, potentially life-threatening, and non-life-threatening injuries. Those injuries that are life-threatening require immediate intervention as do many of the potentially life-threatening injuries. Non-life-threatening injuries require treatment but not immediately.

Life-threatening injuries

Airway obstruction must be corrected to prevent hypoxia leading to cardiac arrest. The airway may be obstructed by malpositioning of the patient, foreign objects (i.e., food, teeth), or injury to the trachea or larynx. A few patients may require emergency cricothyroidotomy in order to provide an adequate airway. A cricothyroidotomy is managed in the same way as a tracheostomy for purposes of ventilation and suctioning.

Tension penumothorax results from an accumulation of air inside the pleural cavity, causing compression of the lung on the affected side and shifting of the mediastinum toward the unaffected lung. This occurs when a one-way valve either from the lung or chest wall allows air to enter the pleural cavity but not escape. This injury necessitates immediate insertion of a large-bore needle into the second intercostal space in the midclavicular line on the affected side. This converts the tension pneumothorax into a simple pneumothorax and allows time for the insertion of a chest tube in order to definitively treat the pneumothorax.

An **open pneumothorax**, or "sucking chest wound," may occur after penetrating chest trauma. This opening in the chest wall causes intrathoracic pressure to equal atmospheric pressure, thus interfering with ventilation. Immediate intervention involves covering the open wound with an occlusive dressing that is taped securely on three sides. Leaving one side open allows air to escape from the thorax during expiration, thus preventing a tension pneumothorax. A chest tube is then inserted through another incision; definitive surgical treatment is then necessary to correct the defect.

Massive hemothorax is a blood loss of 2,000 to 4,000 ml into the thoracic cavity. This is usually the result of injury to the pulmonary vasculature. This injury is usually accompanied by shock resulting from the large blood loss. Volume loss is replaced prior to the insertion of a chest tube. A thoracotomy is usually necessary in order to repair the injured vessel(s) and control hemorrhage. After surgery, these patients must be monitored for increased bleeding as well as respiratory distress. If bleeding continues at a rate of 150 to 250 ml/hr, the patient will probably need to return to the OR for reexploration.

Flail chest is defined as a paradoxical movement of all or a portion of the chest wall. It results when there are fractures of several ribs at more than one site, which causes the flail segment to move independently of the rest of the chest wall and results in impairment of ventilation. If the patient has a large flail segment or bilateral flail segments, intubation and volume ventilation

FIGURE 10–1 *Initial ICU Assessment of the Injured Patient*

Patient name: ________ Age: ________ Sex: ________ Date: ________ Time: ________

Transported from: ________ (OR, ER, Radiology) ________ Family present: ________

Brief history/mechanism of injury: ________

Ventilatory status

airway: patent ________

type of artificial airway:

ET tube: ________

trach tube: ________

none: ________

breathing: rate ________

quality: ________

breath sounds:

right: ________

left: ________

Ventilatory therapy:

O_2: mask ________ cannula ________

% O_2 ________

Ventilator: IMV ________ TV ________

FIO_2 ________ PEEP ________

ABGs: ________

Chest tubes: ________

right: ________ air leak: ________ drainage: ________

left: ________ air leak: ________ drainage: ________

Hemodynamic/circulatory status

pulse: ________ BP: ________

cardiac rhythm: ________

central pressures: CVP ________ PAD ________ PCWP ________

IV therapy:

a. site ________ fluid type ________ infusion rate ________

b. site ________ fluid type ________ infusion rate ________

c. site ________ fluid type ________ infusion rate ________

d. site ________ fluid type ________ infusion rate ________

Urine output: ________ Sp gr: ________

IV Medications (continuous drips):

a. med ________ infusion rate ________

b. med ________ infusion rate ________

c. med ________ infusion rate ________

Neurologic status

Glasgow Coma Scale (GCS)

Eye opening:	spontaneous	4
	to voice	3
	to pain	2
	none	1
Verbal response:	oriented	5
	confused	4
	inappropriate words	3
	incomprehensible words	2
	none	1
Motor response:		
	obeys commands	6
	localizes pain	5
	withdraws (pain)	4
	flexion (pain)	3
	extension (pain)	2
	none	1

Total GCS ______

GI status

Bowel sounds ______

Abdominal tenderness ______

Abdominal distension ______

N/g tube/O/g tube ______

amount/type drainage ______

other drain(s): types ______

location(s) ______

amount/type drainage ______

Musculoskeletal status

Traction: location(s) ______

type ______

External fixation ______

location(s) ______

Casting: location(s) ______

Neck immobilization ______

type ______

Skin

Lacerations/avulsions/abrasions:

location(s): ______

Incision(s); location(s) ______

Diagnostic studies: ______

Operative procedures: ______

Description of injuries: ______

with positive end-expiratory pressure (PEEP) will most likely be necessary to provide internal stabilization of the flail segments and ensure adequate ventilation. In any case, the patient with any degree of this injury must be carefully monitored for increased PCO_2 (indicating inadequate ventilation) as well as other clinical signs of respiratory distress. Overhydration must be avoided to minimize ventilatory compromise that may already be present as a result of the underlying pulmonary contusion that accompanies flail chest.

Cardiac tamponade is the filling of the pericardium with blood, resulting in compression of the heart muscle and decreased filling of the heart. It may result from blunt trauma but is most commonly seen in patients with penetrating injury. Pericardiocentesis is performed initially to decrease the compression of the heart and allow for time to transport the patient to the OR for definitive repair of the injury.

All of these life-threatening injuries must be managed while the patient is in the ED; however, the patients must be closely monitored in the ICU for respiratory distress. Interventions to prevent complications must be carefully planned and the plan closely adhered to.

Potentially life-threatening injuries

Pulmonary contusion is present in a large number of patients with chest injuries. It does not result in an immediate threat to life but is often responsible for the gradual development of respiratory failure. In cases involving extensive contusion, the patient may require intubation and mechanical ventilation until the contusion resolves. Other patients may be observed in the ICU. All patients with this injury must be monitored closely for signs of respiratory distress and inadequate ventilation. Overhydration must be avoided to prevent further respiratory compromise.

Aortic rupture or tear accounts for a number of deaths following trauma. In blunt injury, there are two common sites of rupture or tear of the thoracic aorta. In a horizontal deceleration injury, as in a motor vehicle accident, damage to the vessel occurs at the ligamentum arteriosum (just distal to the take-off of the left subclavian artery), which is a point of relative fixation of the aorta. In falls, or vertical deceleration injuries, the damage occurs at the aortic root. Of patients with injuries to the major vessels in the chest, 80 to 90% die prior to arrival at the hospital. In those patients who survive, prompt repair of the injury is necessary. After operation, the patient must be monitored for signs of hemorrhage, and distal circulation should be checked frequently. Hypertension is to be avoided, which may be done through the use of medications, such as nitroprusside, and avoidance of overhydration.

Associated injuries that may suggest the potential presence of aortic damage include fractures of the first and second ribs, massive hemothorax, and sternal or scapular fractures.

Injuries to the **tracheobronchial tree** are often the result of penetrating trauma. Gunshot wounds cause extensive tissue destruction and require prompt repair to ensure adequate ventilation and to control hemorrhage if damage to neighboring vessels has occurred. Bronchial injuries are uncommon but have a high mortality rate. They must be treated promptly and usually require surgical intervention.

Airway management in patients with injuries to the trachea and larynx may be difficult, because the presence of the injury and concomitant edema may interfere with intubation. Intubation or tracheostomy may be prolonged to ensure an adequate airway while the damaged tissues are healing.

Trauma to the **esophagus** is rare. Infection of the mediastinum may occur, contributing to a high mortality rate. Surgical intervention is necessary to repair the defect, if possible, and provide drainage of the mediastinum and pleural space. Postoperatively, the patient must be carefully observed for signs of infection.

Myocardial contusion usually occurs as a result of blunt trauma to the chest. Patients with this injury are managed like those with MI. They must be closely monitored for dysrhythmias (a right bundle branch block or premature ventricular contractions are commonly seen). Fluid restriction may be necessary but should not take precedence over adequate volume replacement in those patients who have experienced great loss of blood. The contusion resolves within a few days, but if there is concern about myocardial function, diagnostic studies such as technetium scanning or MUGA scanning may be performed.

Non-life-threatening injuries

Rib fractures without displacement or of only a single rib, while not life-threatening in themselves, place the patient at risk for pulmonary complications. The patient experiences pain on motion and has difficulty taking a maximal inspiration and coughing because of pain. Older patients or those with preexisting lung disease are at higher risk for complications.

A **simple pneumothorax** occurs when air escapes from one lung into the pleural space and compresses the lung. The patient develops a ventilation-perfusion defect because the blood that circulates through the nonventilated portion of the lung does not become oxygenated. Treatment consists of placement of a chest tube, with drainage connected to a water-seal system. This allows for evacuation of the air in the thoracic cavity and reexpansion of the collapsed lung.

Laceration of a small vessel in the chest can lead to a **simple hemothorax.** This bleeding is not extensive and does not require operative repair. Intervention consists of placement of a large-bore chest tube to drain the blood. Bleeding through the chest tube must be closely monitored because an increase in drainage to >150 to 200 ml/hr over three to four hours or a total loss of >1,500 ml generally indicates a need for thoracotomy to repair the injury.

All patients with chest injury must be monitored closely for signs of respiratory distress. These patients are also at high risk for development of pulmonary complications, and interventions should be directed at avoiding these complications. Such routine procedures as chest physiotherapy, suctioning at regular intervals, and frequent repositioning will help to minimize the risk of the development of complications.

ABDOMINAL INJURIES

Penetrating trauma

Penetrating injuries to the abdominal organs are most frequently the result of a gonshot wound to the abdomen or thorax. Stab wounds are seen less commonly. The abdominal organ most often injured is the liver. The other organs commonly injured include the small bowel, stomach, colon, major vessels, mesentery, omentum, and spleen.

Mortality resulting from penetrating abdominal injury is related both to the specific organ or organs injured and the number of organs injured. Death shortly after any of these injuries is usually due to hemorrhage, whereas later deaths result from infection and MOF that is often preceded by sepsis.

Treatment of penetrating abdominal injuries is dependent upon the nature and extent of the injury. In some institutions, patients with stab wounds to the abdomen are placed under observation after the wound is cleared and debrided, provided the patient remains hemodynamically stable. As a rule, however, patients with gunshot wounds and extensive stab wounds to the abdomen require surgical exploration.

Diagnostic studies, such as abdominal x-rays, IV pyelogram (IVP), cystogram, and arteriogram, may be done to exploration if the patient's condition permits and the extent of the injury is unclear. These studies do not take priority over definitive treatment in patients who are hemodynamically unstable, however.

Blunt trauma

The majority of blunt injuries to the abdomen are the result of vehicular accidents. The most frequently injured organ in blunt trauma to the abdomen is the spleen. Other organs that are often injured include kidney, intestines, and liver. The mortality rates for these injuries depend not only on the abdominal organ(s) injured but also on injuries to other systems.

Abdominal vessels

The abdominal vessels are rarely injured in blunt trauma; however, no matter what the etiology of the vascular injury is, surgical intervention is necessary to control hemorrhage, repair the injured vessel, and restore circulation. After repair, the patient must be monitored for hemorrhage and adequacy of distal circulation.

Spleen

Most splenic injuries are diagnosed during the initial evaluation of the patient in the ED. Splenic injury usually presents with an abnormal abdominal examination and positive blood on peritoneal lavage. The presence of lower left rib fractures should raise suspicions of splenic injury. It is frequently a cause of hypotension in patients who have sustained blunt abdominal trauma. The extent of splenic injury dictates the intervention necessary. Small lacerations may be repaired; however, multiple or major lacerations or rupture of the spleen generally require splenectomy to control hemorrhage. Postoperatively, patients who have undergone splenectomy are at a high risk for mortality if sepsis occurs, because the spleen serves an important function in the immune response. Care of the patient after splenectomy or splenorrhaphy involves close monitoring for signs of hemorrhage or infection.

Liver

Trauma to the liver is usually diagnosed in the ED. Patients with this injury may also have an abnormal abdominal examination and positive peritoneal lavage. Liver injury should be suspected in patients with fractures of the lower right ribs. Liver injuries can result in massive hemorrhage and require prompt intervention.

The majority of liver injuries can be easily repaired and do not require resection. The goal of operative intervention is to control hemorrhage and remove severely damaged or nonviable tissue. Rarely will a patient suffer a liver injury that is so extensive that repair is impossible. Patients who have sustained liver trauma are at risk for malnutrition, GI bleeding, coagulation abnormalities, abscess formation, and biliomas.

The risk of malnutrition is decreased if the patient begins receiving parenteral nutrition early in the hospital course. Glucose levels should be closely monitored to avoid hypoglycemia. Liver function studies may remain abnormal for as long as a few weeks after resection. Antacids should be started as soon as possible to decrease the risk of GI bleeding. The patient should be monitored carefully for signs and symptoms of hemorrhage and abscess formation.

Pancreas

The pancreas is not frequently injured; however, undiagnosed pancreatic injury carries a high mortality and morbidity. Diagnosis of penetrating injury to the pancreas is easily made at operation, but blunt trauma to this organ is difficult to evaluate because the patient with this type of injury may have a normal abdominal examination. The trauma patient who exhibits a persistently high amylase level from the time of admission may have pancreatic trauma. This may be confirmed by further diagnostic studies such as CAT scan and hypaque swallow prior to operative intervention.

Diaphragm

Penetrating trauma to the lower chest may also result in trauma to the abdomen. This combination of injuries usually includes trauma to the diaphragm. Blunt diaphragmatic injuries are often missed during the initial evaluation of the patient. The left side of the diaphragm is injured much more frequently than the right. The diagnosis of this injury can be difficult to make on initial physical examination and should be suspected in patients who exhibit decreased breath sounds and audible bowel sounds in the lower chest within a few days or more after admission. Treatment of these injuries consists of surgical repair of the defect. Patients with diaphragmatic tears are at risk for respiratory problems.

GI tract

Injuries to the duodenum are frequently associated with injuries to the pancreas, liver, and biliary systems. They are not easily diagnosed on initial examination and may present later in the patient's hospital course with fever, jaundice, and signs of obstruction. These injuries require surgical repair and drainage. Decompression of the stomach must be maintained postoperatively to allow healing of anastomoses.

Stomach injuries rarely occur as a result of blunt trauma. They do appear frequently in patients with penetrating wounds. Injuries to the mesentery and small intestine may result from either blunt or penetrating trauma. The most common sites of blunt injury to the small bowel are the proximal jejunum and distal ileum. Surgical repair of these injuries is necessary.

Colon injuries carry a relatively high morbidity and mortality. Depending upon the location and extent of the injury, the patient may require varying degrees of operative intervention. Many of these patients will require colostomy.

GU organs

Of these organs, the bladder, urethra (in males), and kidneys are the most frequently injured. Contusion to the kidneys generally does not require operative intervention and is treated with adequate hydration. The urine clears of blood within a few days. A fractured kidney may require resection or nephrectomy.

Bladder injuries require surgical repair of the defect and placement of a suprapubic cystostomy tube. Urethral injuries are usually not repaired emergently, whereas injuries to the ureters are usually repaired immediately. Patients with trauma to the urinary system should be monitored for signs of infection of this system. Those with renal injuries require monitoring of urine output as well as of sp gr and serum indicators of renal function.

Injuries to the uterus occur rarely but are most likely to occur as a result of penetrating abdominal trauma in the pregnant female. As a rule, these injuries necessitate surgical intervention, with the main goal being saving the mother's life.

HEAD INJURIES

Head injuries are responsible for a large number of deaths from trauma. Penetrating injuries to the head place the patient at high risk for infection, if the initial injury is not lethal. Blunt trauma results in injury of varying degrees, but even seemingly minor injuries have been found to have long-term effects on the patient's recovery and life-style.

Skull fractures alone do not account for mortality and morbidity due to head trauma. Rather, it is the damage to the underlying structures that places the patient at risk. Depressed skull fractures may require operative intervention if the fragment is impinging on the underlying tissue. Compound fractures of the skull require debridement and operative intervention.

Basilar skull fractures are common in the multiply injured patient and place the patient at risk for infection if a CSF leak is present. For this reason, prophylactic antibiotics are used in patients with a CSF leak. These fractures may also lead to malplacement of a nasogastric tube into the cranium through the opening created by the fracture. This can be avoided by placing an orogastric tube, if possible, or using extreme caution in the placement of a nasogastric tube.

Concussion is a temporary loss of consciousness without apparent significant injury to the brain. Patients with this injury should be observed for changes in their neurologic examination that would raise the suspicion of more serious, unrecognized injuries. It is common for these patients to have headache, dizziness, nausea, or a period of amnesia; however, the neurologic examination demonstrates no focal neurologic findings.

Cerebral contusion may be minor or quite extensive. Patients with this injury may have focal neurologic findings and alterations in level of consciousness. Neurologic findings are dependent on the area of the brain that is injured. This may be that region directly underlying the point of impact or may be the area directly opposite the site (a contra-coupe injury). Another type of injury is the quadripolar contusion in which several areas of the brain are contused due to "bouncing" of the brain within the skull at the time of impact. Contusions are managed by observation and careful monitoring of the neurologic examination. Delayed bleeding leading to increased intracranial pressure (ICP) may occur and require operative intervention.

There are several types of **intracranial bleeding** that may occur due to trauma. *See* Chapter 5 for a detailed discussion of intracranial bleeding.

Facial fractures pose several problems for the trauma patient. Compound fractures result in high risk for infection. Other fractures can result in nerve damage as well as deformities. Fractures of the zygoma may cause damage to the intraorbital nerve. Orbital fractures may lead to entrapment of the extraocular muscles. Nasal fractures are common and hematoma formation at the septum may lead to impairment of the nasal airway. Mandibular and maxillary fractures may result in malocclusion.

Midface fractures were classified in 1900 by Rene LeFort. These fractures are known as LeFort I, II, and III fractures. The LeFort I fracture is a transverse maxillary fracture; LeFort II is a pyramidal fracture through the nasal bones and maxilla, and LeFort III is a craniofacial separation involving fractures of the maxilla, nasal bones, and zygoma.

Management of facial fractures is dependent upon the extent of the injury. Mandibular and maxillary fractures usually require stabilization with arch bars and wiring. A tracheostomy may be performed if the patient is not alert or requires mechanical ventilation. Other fractures may require open reduction and wiring of the fracture segments. Prophylactic antibiotics are used in patients with open fractures. All patients with these injuries should be observed closely for signs of infection. Those with mandibular and maxillary fractures require careful but frequent oral care.

SPINE AND SPINAL CORD INJURIES

Injuries may occur at any level of the spine or spinal cord. All patients with fractures of the spine do not experience neurologic deficit, but in those who do, the extent of deficit is dependent on location of the injury and the extent of encroachment of the spinal cord.

Cervical spine injuries result not only from vehicular trauma but frequently occur from diving accidents. The mechanism of these injuries may be flexion-extension, hyperextension, or rotational. The most serious injuries result in loss of neurologic function below the level of injury. *See* Chapter 5 for a detailed discussion of spine and spinal cord injury.

EXTREMITY INJURIES

Extremity injuries are common in patients who have experienced blunt trauma. Penetrating trauma may also result in extremity injuries. These injuries may affect bone, vasculature, muscle, or nerve, with fractures being the most common type of injury.

Fractures

Fractures may be simple, compound (open), comminuted, fracture/dislocation, or a combination of these. Simple fractures may only require splinting of the extremity involved. Open fractures require debridement and often, open reduction and internal fixation. Comminuted fractures may also require operative intervention, depending on the position of the fracture segments. Fracture/dislocations require reduction to avoid neurovascular compromise and loss of function. Dislocated joints require prompt reduction and stabilization.

Pelvic fractures result in a high mortality rate if not adequately treated. If the fracture is unstable, external splinting or fixation with an external fixation device may be necessary. Open pelvic fractures place the patient at high risk for infection, especially if associated injuries to the bowel are present. These patients require close monitoring for signs of infection as well as careful positioning and turning.

Methods of stabilization of fractures are many. Open reduction and internal fixation involves the use of metal plates, wires, and pins to realign the fractured bone segments. An external fixation device consists of bars and pins that are placed through the fractured segments and externally connected to other pieces of the device (Fig. 10–2). Traction is frequently used to stabilize fractures of the lower extremities. Pins may be placed through the bones and then attached to the traction device. Splints may also be used as a method of immobilization.

Careful monitoring of the status of the injured extremity is required. This includes serial assessment of distal pulses, sensation, and movement. Alignment of fractured segments must be maintained. Patients with open fractures usually receive prophylactic antibiotics and should be observed for signs of infection. Those with external fixation devices and traction apparatus must also be watched closely for signs of infection at pin sites, and pin site care done a regular basis.

Compartment syndrome

Compartment syndrome (closed space syndrome) can be devastating if not recognized and attended to. The etiology of this syndrome is an increased pressure in the extremity compartment, leading to ischemia and damage to the nerve and muscle. It may not become evident until several hours after injury. Pain may be an early sign of increased pressure. Later symptoms include paresis, paralysis, edema, pallor, and lack of pulse. If any extremity injury is suspected in a multiply injured patient, the patient must be carefully watched for evolution of this syndrome.

Traumatic amputations

Traumatic amputations of any of the extremities are serious injuries. The ability to replant the amputated part is dependent upon several factors, including the condition of the extremity and the patient's overall condition (i.e., presence of other major injuries). Postoperatively, patients who have had replantation require careful, frequent monitoring of vascular and

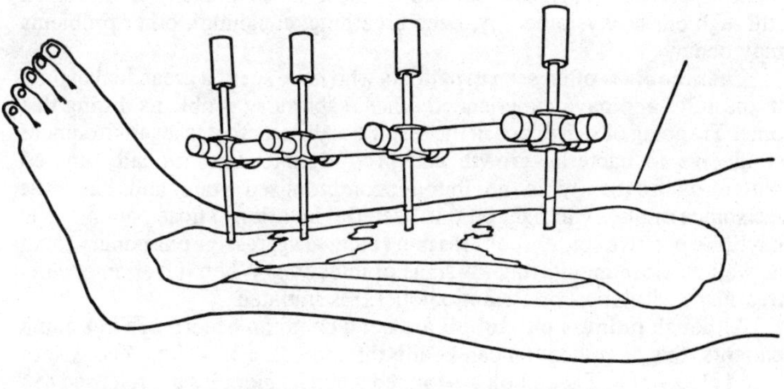

Figure 10–2. External fixation device on a lower extremity.

sensory function distal to the site of replantation. Elevation of the injured extremity will decrease edema. Prophylactic antibiotics are usually required.

Vascular injuries

Vascular injuries require operative repair if the circulation is impaired. After surgery, the patient must be assessed frequently for the presence of adequate circulation and nerve function distal to the injury.

COMPLICATIONS

Survival after serious injury is not only dependent upon the extent of injury itself but also upon predisposition to the development of serious complications, especially failure of single or multiple organs. Patients who are at increased risk of developing these complications are those who have experienced any of the following: (1) hypovolemic shock (systolic BP <90 mmHg); (2) massive blood transfusions; (3) sepsis; (4) thoracic trauma with flail chest, pneumothorax, pulmonary contusion, aspiration, endobronchial bleeding, or myocardial contusion.

PULMONARY COMPLICATIONS

Pulmonary failure is usually related to the occurrence of **adult respiratory distress syndrome (ARDS).** The exact event that triggers the development of this complication is unknown. ARDS can be defined as the inability of the lungs to maintain a PaO_2 of >50 torr despite an increasing fraction of inspired O_2 (FIO_2). The patient with ARDS has a decreased functional reserve capacity and requires continued ventilatory assistance, often with increasing levels of PEEP. *See* Chapter 3 for a detailed discussion of ARDS.

Other, less serious pulmonary complications may precede the development of ARDS. The least serious of these is **atelectasis.** If untreated (through chest physiotherapy, deep breathing, coughing), other problems may occur.

Pneumonia is often seen in patients who have spent a great deal of time in the ICU and have experienced other respiratory problems during this time. Trapping of secretions in the respiratory tract creates an environment conducive to bacterial growth and proliferation. The critically injured patient is frequently in an immunocompromised state and has little resistance or ability to fight off this bacterial invasion. Those patients who have had positive sputum cultures must receive aggressive pulmonary toilet as well as close monitoring for signs of infection. When infection occurs, treatment with appropriate antiobiotic(s) is initiated.

Although **pulmonary emboli** are not a common occurrence in trauma patients, this complication can be life-threatening. Emboli may consist of blood clots or fat. Fat emboli are formed when fat globules are released at a fracture site and travel into the vascular system. The patients who are most at risk for development of fat emboli are those who have suffered fractures of the long bones, especially the femur. Improper alignment and delayed fixation of the bone increases the risk of the development of fat emboli. Thrombotic emboli are more likely to occur in the patient who has undergone a long period of bed rest that has contributed to venous stasis in the lower extremities. To prevent this complication, the patient should be mobilized as early as possible. Immobile patients should have an exercise routine provided for them on a regular basis; this will not only help prevent venous stasis but will also maintain range of motion of the joints.

RENAL COMPLICATIONS

Urinary tract infection (UTI) was once the most frequently occurring complication seen in the ICU. Although the incidence of UTI has decreased, it does occur and in many cases may be preventable. If not treated adequately, it can lead to more serious complications or become chronic in nature. Prevention of UTI consists of avoiding long periods of continuous catheterization of the urinary bladder. An intermittent catheterization regimen has been shown to decrease the risk of UTI when compared with long-term catheterization. In patients in whom continuous catheterization is necessary, meticulous care of the catheter and thorough cleansing of the perineal area is required.

Acute tubular necrosis (ATN) occurs in many patients who have experienced a prolonged period of hypotension after injury, resulting in inadequate renal perfusion and tissue hypoxia. ATN is usually reversible with adequate rehydration, thus increasing renal blood flow. If untreated, acute renal failure is likely to develop. Urine output as well as other indicators of renal function (BUN, creatinine, urine sp gr) in patients who have had episodes of hypotension must be carefully monitored.

Development of **acute renal failure (ARF)** after trauma generally results from one of two etiologies. When ARF develops early in the patient's hospital course, it can usually be attributed to ATN following a period of hypotension (*see* Chapter 7). Late development of ARF is seen as a component of the syndrome of MOF. This usually occurs in conjunction with sepsis and pulmonary failure. The risk for developing ARF at this time is increased for patients who are receiving antibiotics that can cause nephrotoxicity (i.e., gentamicin, tobramycin, amphotericin B). Careful titration of dosages of these drugs is necessary to provide adequate trough levels and avoid excessive peak serum levels. Maintenance of appropriate hydration is also essential.

Dialysis may be necessary to avoid uremia in patients who develop ARF. In patients with hemodynamic instability, however, dialysis may be difficult, if not impossible. Therefore, the prevention of ARF is of utmost importance.

GASTROINTESTINAL COMPLICATIONS

The GI system is also prone to complications after injury. **Gastritis** caused by increased acidity may occur in the patient who is not eating; this is easily avoided by prophylactic administration of antacids at regular intervals. Cimetidine has also been recommended as a prophylactic measure for prevention of gastritis; however, the side effects of this drug are numerous, and it has not been shown to have any clear advantage over antacids. It should therefore, be used only in patients who have a prior history of peptic ulcer disease.

Stress ulcers are relatively uncommon in trauma patients. They occur most frequently in patients with spinal cord injury, especially in those patients who are receiving corticosteroids for treatment of the injury. Again, prophylactic antacid therapy is indicated to prevent this problem.

Upper GI bleeding is occasionally a problem. When it does occur, it is usually a result of stress ulceration. This complication may require replacement of blood loss. It is also a component of the syndrome of MOF.

Ileus commonly occurs in patients who have suffered vertebral or pelvic fractures or have undergone abdominal surgery. Although this problem may be unavoidable, steps can be taken to avoid further difficulties. Placement of a nasogastric or orogastric tube may be of assistance in preventing gastric dilation. This will also allow for drainage of gastric contents and help to prevent aspiration.

SEPSIS

Sepsis is one of the leading causes of late death (after several days) in trauma patients. Trauma patients at greatest risk are those with multiple severe injuries, open pelvic fractures, abdominal injuries with fecal contamination of the peritoneal cavity, major thoracic injuries, and patients who require prolonged stays in the ICU. Inadequate nutrition also contributes to the increased risk of sepsis.

Sources of sepsis include: urinary tract (especially with prolonged catheterization), respiratory tract, GI tract, intra-abdominal organs, wounds, open fractures, and invasive lines (especially central lines). Most cases of sepsis are caused by gram-negative organisms that are present in the hospital environment. Early signs of sepsis include an elevated serum glucose level as well as temperature elevation and tachycardia. When sepsis is suspected, cultures of urine, blood, sputum, wounds, and CSF (if applicable) are done to locate the septic source and identify the invading organism.

Treatment of sepsis is directed toward eliminating the septic focus and preventing the development of septic shock. Patients with intra-abdominal sepsis may require reoperation. Antibiotics that are effective against the causative organism must be used. Prior to identification of the organism, broad-spectrum antibiotic therapy may be initiated. If septic shock develops, circulatory support may be necessary. The patient with sepsis is at increased risk for the development of MOF.

MULTIPLE ORGAN FAILURE

MOF occurs when more than one organ is unable to maintain its own function. The organs fail sequentially, with the lungs usually being the first organs to succumb with ARDS. After this, failure generally occurs in the liver, kidney, GI system, circulatory system, and coagulation system, with sepsis as a contributing factor to this syndrome.

Liver failure may result from hypoperfusion after shock. Other factors contributing to liver failure include hypoxia resulting from ARDS, hepatic vasoconstriction, sepsis, malnutrition, and anesthetic agents. The coagulation system usually fails as a result of sepsis, and the manifestation of this is disseminated intravascular coagulation (DIC). The treatment of coagulopathies such as DIC may require the replacement of clotting factors as well as anticoagulant therapy.

Cardiac failure may be due to arrhythmias, injury to the heart, or inadequate circulation. Treatment is dependent upon the cause of the failure and may include inotropic agents, volume replacement, or antiarrhythmic drugs.

ARDS requires ventilatory support with PEEP. Renal failure is treated through the use of dialysis. GI failure or bleeding necessitates replacement of blood volume lost. Sepsis is treated with appropriate antibiotics. Thus, it is clear that the treatment of MOF requires treatment of individual organs that have failed. When this syndrome occurs, the mortality rate is high, as treatment of one organ system may result in problems with another organ system. Therefore, the prevention of MOF and early treatment of single organ failure is necessary in order to decrease mortality in trauma patients.

STRESS

Stress affects not only the trauma patient, but also the patient's family and the staff who provide care for the patient. It is necessary for the patient to adjust to the ICU environment, which in itself is stressful. The injured patient is faced with the sudden impact of injury on his or her life-style. The patient experiences alterations in body image caused by disfigurement, lack of mobility, and dependence on medical devices for maintenance of body function. Inability to communicate because of intubation or lack of movement adds to this stress.

Many patients do not remember the event that resulted in their injury and may be very concerned about what has happened. In addition, the patient may experience feelings of guilt over what has happened, especially if he perceives himself to be responsible for the accident. This may be even more of a problem if others were injured or killed in the accident. The patient may also verbalize other concerns related to the length of hospitalization that will be necessary, the possibility of returning to work or school, and further treatment that will be necessary.

The family of the trauma victim is under a great deal of stress. The occurrence of an accident is unexpected and unpredictable, and so the family is suddenly faced with a critical event in their lives. They must cope with alterations and adjustments in their daily lives as a result of the patient's hospitalization. These adjustments are not only emotional and social, but may also be financial. The family is frequently concerned with the length of hospitalization as they may need to change future plans or prepare for the patient's homecoming. One of the most important needs of the family in the early part of hospitalization is the need for information. Other needs are similar to those of the family of any critically ill patient.

The ICU staff is also under a great deal of stress when caring for a trauma patient, possibly because many trauma victims are members of the same age group as the staff. The staff may find it difficult to accept a critical illness with a risk of death in someone their own age, as it may force them to face their own mortality. *See* Chapter 19 for a detailed discussion of stress factors in the ICU.

CHAPTER 11

NUTRITIONAL ASPECTS OF CRITICAL CARE

Sally W. Hills

FRAMEWORK

Nutritional support as an adjunctive therapy is a vital component in the care of the critically ill. The patient in the ICU is frequently compromised by many factors that may lead to multisystem body failure. Because of recent medical advances, the patient more often survives the acute phase of illness such as MI, multiple trauma, major surgery, or pneumonia, and long-term survival is dependent on a continued therapeutic response to injury, adequate body defenses, and supportive nutritional therapy.

MALNUTRITION

The human body needs nutrition to maintain homeostasis. When the body is deprived of food, the body tissues are tapped to fuel metabolic processes. Prolonged starvation results in changes in body composition and malnutrition.

Malnutrition, specifically protein-calorie malnutrition, is prevalent among hospitalized patients. Research has shown that as many as 25 to 50% of medical-surgical patients hospitalized for >2 weeks, suffer from protein-calorie malnutrition.

Critically ill patients are particularly prone to develop protein-calorie malnutrition because they are frequently exposed to prolonged periods of limited oral intake, compromised with various types of organ failure, and may require mechanical ventilatory assistance and complicated pharmacologic support.

The three major types of malnutrition are marasmus, kwashiorkor, and marasmic-kwashiorkor. Marasmus (protein-calorie malnutrition) is the result of a chronic decrease in caloric intake over a period of months or years. The clinical features include a starved appearance, extreme wasting of body muscle, and the absence of subcutaneous fat. The marasmic patient is easily identified as malnourished because he is weak, cachetic, and often described as a walking skeleton.

Kwashiorkor (protein malnutrition) is the result of decreased intake of protein and increased stress of illness or injury over several weeks. Clinically the patient appears well nourished. The patient has adequate fat and muscle stores and may even appear obese. The somatic protein compartment may, however, be spared at the expense of the visceral protein compartment, leading to severe depletion of visceral or organ protein. Decreased body proteins are reflected in decreased serum albumin and manifested by clinical signs such as hair that falls out or is easily pluckable, peripheral or abdominal edema, decreased wound healing, and immunoincompetence. Because the signs and symptoms of kwashiorkor are not as conspicuous as marasmus, the potential exists for this patient to suffer from undiagnosed malnutrition.

Marasmic-kwashiorkor is a combined form of protein-calorie malnutrition. It commonly occurs when the critically ill marasmic patient develops kwashiorkor malnutrition from prolonged protein-calorie starvation and the stress of acute illness or injury. This patient is seriously debilitated and will require finely tuned, individualized nutritional support.

NUTRITIONAL REQUIREMENTS

The maintenance of normal body tissues, as well as the repair of injury, requires the availability of various macronutrients and micronutrients. The National Academy of Science establishes a Recommended Daily Allowance (RDA) for each of the nutrients necessary for the maintenance of health (Table 11–1). It is important to remember that these nutrient recommendations are based on studies of healthy persons less than 50 years old. In severely stressed patients, greater requirements of protein and calories are needed to support a major injury response. Conversely, a severely malnourished patient may be subject to complications and death upon sudden administration of nutrients in recommended amounts.

ENERGY METABOLISM

The body produces chemical energy from food by the process of metabolism, which is divided into two phases: (1) catabolism and (2) anabolism. Catabolism is the breakdown phase in which macromolecules, such as protein and glycogen, are converted to smaller molecules at a faster rate than that of resynthesis. This process results in negative nitrogen balance, which is a classic feature of stress and injury. Anabolism, the opposite of catabolism, is the build-up phase during which protein and other

TABLE 11–1

*Daily Nutrient Requirements**

Nutrient	Requirement
Water	1 ml/cal
Energy	2,050–2,700 cal‡
Protein	44–56 g
Linoleic acid	7–9 g
Retinol equivalents	800–1,000
Vitamin D	200–300 IU
Vitamin E, d-α-tocopherol equivalent	8–10
Vitamin K	70–140 μg§
Ascorbic acid	60 mg
Folic acid	400 μg
Niacin	13–19 mg
Riboflavin	1.2–1.7 mg
Thiamine	1.0–1.5 mg
Vitamin B_6	2.0–2.2 mg
Vitamin B_{12}	3.0 μg
Pantothenic acid	4–7 mg§
Biotin	100–200 μg§
Calcium	800 mg
Phosphorous	800 mg
Iodine	150 μg
Iron	10–18 mg
Magnesium	300–350 mg
Zinc	15 mg
Copper	2–3 mg§
Potassium	50–150 mEq§
Fluoride	1.5–4 mg§
Sodium	50–150 mEq§
Chloride	50–150 mEq§
Chromium	50–200 μg§
Manganese	2.5–5 mg§
Molybdenum	150–500 μg§
Selenium	50–200 μg§

*Based on National Academy of Sciences. Recommended Dietary Allowances. NAS, Washington, D.C. 1980. Ninth edition.
‡In young adults doing light work.
§No RDA established. Amounts quoted represent "safe and adequate daily dietary intake."

components of the cell are rebuilt from smaller molecules. The rate of metabolism can be increased by exercise, fever, or hormonal activity. An elevated body temperature can more than double the metabolic rate. Hormonal activity, such as secretion of insulin or epinephrine, can also increase metabolic rate. The hormonal activity of the critically ill patient strongly favors catabolism.

Energy requirements vary. In general, the normal adult need is 25 to 30 kcal/kg of body weight/day. Therefore, the calorie requirement of a normal healthy adult ranges from 1,800 to 2,500 calories/day, depending on height, weight, and physical activity.

Of all the substances that the body requires for optimum functioning, only carbohydrates, fat, and protein are metabolized to provide energy. The body metabolizes **carbohydrates** for immediate needs; ~40 to 45% of total calories are derived from carbohydrates, some of which are stored as glycogen in the liver and are immediately available in periods of stress. The amount of glycogen stored is enough to meet the body's energy needs for one day, and glycogen stores can be depleted within 12 to 24 hr. When body stores of carbohydrate decrease below normal, moderate quantities of glucose can be formed from protein and fat by gluconeogenesis. Some glycogen stores in the muscle cells are available for systemic needs after muscle converts it to lactate via glucose and releases it into the bloodstream. When glycogen storage is filled, excess carbohydrate is converted to lipid for storage as fat or triglycerides in adipose tissue.

Lipid, or **fat**, is the chief stored-energy substrate in the body, and energy is most economically stored in the form of lipid. Fat provides 40 to 45% of total calories and as an energy fuel supplies ~9 kcal/g, more than twice the caloric output per gram of either carbohydrate or protein. One disadvantage of lipid as a fuel is that metabolites such as acids and ketone bodies may accumulate in the blood and lead to ketosis and acidosis. And fat stores cannot totally satisfy the energy requirements of the glucose-dependent organs of the CNS, such as the brain.

In the severely stressed, septic, or traumatized patient, there appears to be diminished fat utilization and an absence of ketone body formation. Although the cause of fat utilization is unclear to date, the net effect is the absence of fat calories for energy.

Protein is not stored in the body. Every molecule of protein is assigned to a specific body function or structure. Proteins have a limited life-span and they are constantly undergoing synthesis, degradation into amino acids, and then resynthesis into new protein. Since amino acids are not stored, the protein compartment must be maintained by daily intake, and the nutritional intervention for the ICU patient is primarily directed toward sparing body protein.

Protein metabolism for energy is available at 4 kcal/g, and the average adult requires ~0.8 g of protein/kg of body weight/day. Depending on the metabolic need, protein may be synthesized or burned for energy. If the body's energy needs exceed the carbohydrate and lipid stores, some body protein may be catabolized for energy; about one-third of the body's total protein is potentially available as an energy source in extreme circumstances. The wasting of protein, or lean body mass, to supply energy is undesirable and may be a serious threat to survival. Protein, in the form of amino acids, is better utilized for critical needs such as replacement, growth, and repair of tissue and maintenance of serum proteins such as albumin, transferrin, fibrinogen, and antibodies or the manufacture of enzymes.

BODY RESPONSE TO STARVATION, INJURY, INFECTION

The human body responds to **starvation** gradually; as carbohydrates are exhausted and subsequently protein breakdown is accelerated, the body adjusts so that life can be supported for many weeks. In contrast, the response to serious **injury** prevents these key adaptions to conserve body tissue from occurring. Therefore, metabolic processes, such as fat mobilization, muscle protein breakdown, urea synthesis, and gluconeogenesis, remain activated as long as the acute catabolic phase is present. This metabolic response to injury results in tissue loss that endangers survival. The body's response to **infection** and, specifically, to acute surgical sepsis is more severe than its response to injury because the metabolic process is accelerated to an even greater extent. For example, the resting energy expenditure will be increased 10 to 30% after a long bone fracture but will be increased from 20 to 60% during major infections such as peritonitis, while a major third-degree burn is associated with an increase of 40 to 100%.

The nutritional needs of the critically ill patient are also increased by major illness or injury. Hypermetabolism and hypercatabolism tend to occur simultaneously in the acutely ill patient. A hypermetabolic response is an increase in energy expenditure and a hypercatabolic response is breakdown that is characterized by loss of tissue and excretion of nitrogen, with negative nitrogen balance that is difficult to reverse. Amino nitrogen is excreted in the urine regardless of the amount of replacement nitrogen. Protein breakdown is greater than protein synthesis. Gluconeogenesis (the production of glucose from the amino acid cycle) and ureagenesis result in weight loss and severe muscle wasting.

RISK CATEGORIES

Patients at risk for inadequate nutritional support fall into certain categories and may be identified early in the acute phase of illness, once the patient is hemodynamically stable and adequately oxygenated. At risk are those patients who are **grossly underweight** or **grossly overweight** (i.e., weight for height <80 to 85% of standard, or weight for height >110 to 120% of standard). The obese person is particularly at risk because he appears well nourished and there is a tendency to overlook protein and calorie needs. Patients who have experienced a recent weight loss are also at risk. Impairment of maximal physical performance occurs in healthy individuals who have lost ~10% of their body weight. It has been observed that a weight loss of 30 to 40% of original normal body weight is usually life-threatening.

Those patients that are **NPO** are at risk nutritionally; those who have been sustained on **IV** solutions such as dextrose/water or normal saline for >7 to 10 days should be reevaluated for nutritional support. In addition, patients experiencing **protracted nutrient losses** are also at risk (those with malabsorption syndromes, short bowel disease, who are on prolonged renal dialysis, or have draining abscesses or open wounds or who have experienced prolonged nutrient losses prior to hospitalization, such as the anorexic, bulimic, and the alcoholic).

Patients with **increased metabolic needs**, such as the extensive burn, infected, septic, or trauma patients, fall into a significant risk category, as do those patients **taking drugs** with antinutrient or catabolic properties, such as chemotherapeutic agents, steroids, or immunosuppressants.

NUTRITIONAL ASSESSMENT

Nutritional assessment is an integral part of the general assessment for the patient in an ICU and should be made as soon as possible after admission. Early assessment allows recognition of the depleted, at-risk patient and provides base-line data for future comparison. Ongoing evaluation, performed at regular intervals, provides comparison data with which to define ongoing prognosis and therapy.

A nutritional profile is developed by assessing the nutrition history, performing a physical examination that includes anthropometric measurements, evaluation of biochemical tests and immunologic data. The final step is to determine nutritional requirements.

History

The nutrition history will provide information about underlying illness, dependencies (such as alcoholism), diet patterns (including food fads), obesity, anorexia, endocrinopathies, and recent weight changes. A medication profile, the existence of allergies, and past weight and height is part of the general information that can be included in the nutrition history.

Historical data may be difficult to gather because the critically ill patient is frequently unable to communicate. The nurse can collect information from various sources other than the patient, such as family members, friends, family physicians, or past medical records from hospital or clinic. Nutrition history is an ongoing process: it will not be complete on admission and will develop from admission through discharge.

Physical examination

Physical examination may show nutritional abnormalities indicative of the various types of malnutrition: marasmus, kwashiorkor, or mixed marasmic kwashiorkor. The condition of the hair may provide information about nutritional status. Easily pluckable, thin, dry, brittle hair and flag sign (light and dark transverse pigmentation of the hair) are positive signs of protein deficiency.

Vitamin and mineral deficiencies may be found in the critically ill patient, particularly those who have been malnourished over a long period of time. Dry, scaly, skin may be indicative of Vitamin A, zinc, or essential fatty acid deficiency. Angular blepharitis, corneal vascularization, and perioral stomatitis or cheilosis may indicate riboflavin deficiency.

The signs of muscle wasting are visually apparent, particularly in the extremities. It may be difficult to differentiate between muscle wastage from protein-calorie malnutrition and muscle atrophy from decreased use or exercise. The wasting of the fine muscles on the dorsum of the hand is usually a positive sign of nutritional depletion.

Deficiencies in ascorbic acid, zinc, and protein are associated with poor wound healing and delayed tissue repair. If these deficiencies are not corrected, the patient may develop complications, such as fistula formation, wound infection leading to dehiscence, decubitus ulcers, and anasarca.

Diagnostic tests

Anthropometric tests may be used to evaluate the patient's nutritional status. The performance of serial objective measurements at regular intervals permits the nurse to identify changes or trends. Caution in the interpretation is essential because factors other than nutrition may influence these measurements.

Anthropometric observations analyze three body tissues: skeletal muscle protein, visceral organ protein, and fat stores. Arm anthropometry is easily performed and is used to determine the status of skeletal muscle protein. The nondominant upper arm is measured for triceps skin-fold (TSF) and for midarm circumference (MAC). TSF is a measure of available calories and sc fat stores. Using Lange calipers, the fold of skin on the posterior arm is grasped midway between the shoulder and the elbow. The average of three successive readings is compared to a standard. Severe sc fat store depletion is indicated by <3 mm. MAC provides information about fat and protein stores. The circumference of the upper arm is measured in cm at the midpoint. To obtain arm muscle circumference (AMC), a measure of muscle protein alone, a formula using MAC and TSF is calculated: $AMC = MAC - (0.314 \times TSF)$. The calculation is compared to normal values. Severe muscle protein depletion is indicated by an AMC of <15 cm.

Visceral protein status is best determined by measuring circulating levels of various proteins synthesized in the liver, such as albumin and transferrin. Depletion in plasma proteins will affect the body's ability to maintain oncotic pressure, carry therapeutic levels of medications, and form antibodies.

Serum albumin has a relatively long half-life (20 days) and decreases slowly during malnutrition. Concentrations of <3.0 g/dl have been associated with hypoalbuminemic tissue edema; concentrations <2.5 g/dl are highly significant and associated with severe protein depletion. All factors must be considered when interpreting a low albumin level; e.g., impaired hepatic function is the primary single cause of pathologically depressed synthesis of albumin.

Serum transferrin has a half-life of 4 to 8 days and thus is a more discriminating index of protein status than albumin. Concentrations of <100 mg/dl are considered indicative of severe protein depletion, whereas concentrations of 100 to 200 mg/dl are marginal. Plasma concentrations of transferrin, like albumin, are dependent on rate of synthesis, utilization, catabolism, excretion, and hydration. Levels are affected by kidney disease, starvation, chronic infection, and severe burn. Also, transferrin levels may be depressed by medications that inhibit protein synthesis, such as cortisone, L-asparaginase, and testosterone.

Total lymphocyte count is a measure of cell-mediated immunity. Measurement of immunocompetence, as determined by total lymphocytes, has been correlated with nutritional status. Total lymphocyte count is calculated by multiplying the total WBC count by the percentage of lymphocytes. A lymphocyte count of <1,000 is of concern, and all clinical factors should be carefully considered.

Body weight is a simple but important measurement of body composition. Although a gross measurement, body weight is a valid indicator of nutritional status. The actual weight is compared to ideal weight by the Metropolitan Life Insurance Company standard chart. The percentage of weight loss may be calculated in terms of a person's age, sex, and height. The percentage of ideal weight, of usual weight, and of weight change over a defined period of time can be calculated to evaluate protein-calorie status. Evaluation of weight gain or loss in the ICU patient is important because the critically ill patient is subject to ascites, pleural effusion, or anasarca from disease states other than malnutrition. The patient who is severely catabolic may not be expected to gain weight. In such instances, the maintenance of body weight is an optimal goal.

Urinary nitrogen balance is used as an indicator of protein catabolism and protein status. On a 24-hr basis, nitrogen intake and urine urea nitrogen are determined. Total nitrogen excretion for 24 hr is calculated by taking the value of urea nitrogen in grams, adding 3.5 g for extraneous losses from stool and skin, and comparing this output to total nitrogen input for 24 hr. Negative nitrogen balance reflects protein catabolism. Normal values should be between positive 4 to 6 g.

Nitrogen balance may be an indicator of severity of catabolism in the ICU patient, and it may also be a marker on which to adjust individualized nutritional support therapy. Urinary nitrogen balance is not a valid marker in patients with renal disease. Nitrogen excretion will be accelerated in patients with severe burns, protracted diarrhea, vomiting, or fistula output.

Nutritional requirements

Energy requirements must be carefully evaluated prior to ordering a nutritional formula for a critically ill patient. One approach is to estimate the basal energy expenditure (BEE) using the Harris-Benedict equations in which W = weight in kg, H = height in cm, and A = age in yr.

BEE (men) = 66.47 + 13.7 W + 5.0 H − 6.67 A
BEE (women) = 655.10 + 9.56 W + 1.8 H − 4.68 A

Once the basal energy requirement is determined, the additional energy requirement associated with stress, injury, physical activity, or disease is calculated. The basal calculation is multiplied by a stress factor to estimate total metabolic needs. The stress factor for a critically ill person ranges from 1.4 to 2. It has been demonstrated that energy expenditure is increased by an average of 32% in patients with skeletal trauma and 61% in patients with head trauma or those taking steroids. Sepsis increases energy requirements by approximately 80%.

Protein requirements for the critically ill patient are determined by the utilization of amino acids and the urinary nitrogen balance excretion. The acutely ill patient has increased requirements for protein synthesis beyond the recommended 0.8 g/day. The goal is to spare endogenous protein stores and to achieve positive nitrogen balance.

Fat requirements for the normal healthy adult are 0.4 g/kg of body weight/day and may be increased for the acutely ill. Although fat consumption under normal circumstances is 30% of energy needs, the acutely ill patient may need 30 to 50% of his energy needs provided by fat replacements. Recent studies demonstrate that using fat calories in place of glucose calories may decrease hyperglycemia and prevent respiratory failure related to excessive glucose calories.

It should be remembered that a person can be harmed by excessive nutrients. A well-planned nutritional program should be individualized and modified to provide adequate protein, carbohydrate, and fat.

ADMINISTRATION OF NUTRITIONAL THERAPIES

The degree of depletion and the rate of metabolism are significant factors to take into consideration when the patient's needs are determined.

Several modes of nutritional therapy are available. Central venous and peripheral venous lines are parenteral methods of providing nutrition. Enteral alimentation provides nutrition via the GI tract. All three routes have distinct advantages and disadvantages, and choosing the appropriate method is often a challenge. The final choice may involve a combination of both.

Enteral nutrition is the preferred method if the GI tract is functional because it is the most natural, efficient, effective, and safe way to administer nutrients. Furthermore, enteral feeding is essential for the maintenance of the normal structure and functional integrity of the small intestine. A GI tract that is not used will require a recuperation time of days to weeks when feeding is restarted; therefore, even though a patient may not receive all his calories from enteral nutrition, a portion of nutrient needs may be given via the enteral route to maintain the small bowel and prevent further complications.

Providing nutrition by the enteral route will also maintain the integrity of the liver. Nutrients supplied via the esophagus, stomach, and bowel are absorbed into the bloodstream through the portal system. This process stimulates a number of GI hormones that signal the metabolic process regulated by the liver. Providing nutrients by a near-physiologic method is preferable so as to maintain near normal bodily function.

Critically ill patients frequently have a dysfunctional GI tract and may be unable to tolerate the enteral method (e.g., abdominal injury, sepsis and prolonged ileus, presence of an oral or nasal endotracheal tube, gastric outlet obstruction, and surgery that requires complete bowel rest). Utilizing the GI tract in these situations may be possible by placing a feeding catheter into the jejunum in early stages of illness. Anticipating nutritional needs and modes of therapy is challenging and often requires an innovative approach.

TOTAL ENTERAL NUTRITION ADMINISTRATION

The traditional method for ICU total enteral nutrition (TEN) has been the intermittent bolus technique of administration through a firm, plastic nasogastric tube. With the increased use of enteral nutrition, alternative routes, techniques, and products have been developed.

Routes

Access routes for TEN are variable. The oral route, the most basic, is selected if oral ingestion of nutrients is feasible; if not, an alternative route is chosen. The nasogastric route is used most frequently for critically ill patients because it is the safest and most efficient. A benefit of gastric feeding is the neutralizing effect on gastric pH, which is specifically important for this group of patients. Nasoduodenal and nasojejunal routes are also used. For the patient with head-and-neck disease, a pharyngostomy or esophagostomy is used.

Passage of a nasogastric tube is a relatively simple technique, and the new nasogastric tubes that are soft, pliable, have various sized lumens, and are compatible with body tissues are well tolerated. The nasogastric tube may be inserted with the use of a guide wire or stylet that is removed once the tube is in place. Caution is recommended to avoid perforation of the GI tract by a misguided wire. Misplacement of a nasogastric tube into the respiratory tract, for those patients who already have an endotracheal tube, is not uncommon because the enteral tube seems to follow the path of the endotracheal tube. Correct placement of the nasogastric tube is verified by auscultation, aspiration, or fluoroscopy.

To facilitate passage of the tube and to maintain placement, many tubes have tips that are weighted with mercury or tungsten encapsulated within the distal end. Various weights, depending on the individual need, may be used. The weight-tipped tube is particularly desirable when duodenal or jejunal placement is required. The weighted tube will move through the pylorus into the duodenum or jejunum by gastric peristalsis, or the tube may be placed into the bowel segment by endoscopy. The major advantages of a small catheter or tube placed in the distal duodenum or proximal jejunum are: less irritation of the gastroesophageal junction, decreased incidence of reflux vomiting and aspiration, and progressive enteral support simultaneous with gastric decompression.

The classic long-term method for delivering enteral nutrition is through a gastrostomy. Various tubes may be used. A rubber Foley catheter is most common because it permits stabilization within the stomach by a balloon built into the end of the catheter. Almost any tube may be inserted through a gastrostomy, and the tip can remain in the stomach or pass into the small bowel, which is accomplished by threading a small-lumen, weighted tube through the larger gastrostomy tube and allowing it to travel to the desired location.

The catheter for the feeding jejunostomy is placed by operative procedure and permits enteral feeding for patients with total gastrectomy or esophagojejunostomy. In the immediate postoperative period, when the small bowel appears to be functional while the rest of the GI tract is not, the jejunostomy tube may be the catheter of choice. More often this method is used for long-term enteral patients.

Modes

Various modes are used to deliver enteral feedings. The **bolus instillation** appears to cause gastric distension or delay in gastric empyting, which increases the risk of vomiting and aspiration. The critically ill patient does not tolerate bolus feedings of hypertonic nutrient formula over a short period of time.

The preferred mode for the acutely ill is the **continuous method** of administration. This technique avoids problems of influx of large amounts of formula into the stomach and reflux of formula, with risk of aspiration. Enteral feedings by continuous method can be accomplished by a gravity drip technique in which a simple flow-control device, such as a roller clamp around the administration tubing, is used to regulate the rate of infusion. Mechanical infusion pumps are recommended for continuous drip over 12- to 24-hr periods because they provide a steadier, more dependable controlled rate.

Formula

Enteral formulas are varied, and there are many commercially available for feeding through enteral tubes. The basis for diet formula selection should be the patient's history of food tolerance, GI function (i.e., digestive and absorptive capacity), indicated route of administration, and nutritional requirements. Additional factors such as osmolality and electrolyte, mineral, and vitamin composition are considered for individual patients. Storage facility and cost are also considerations in formula selection.

Enteral diet formulas can be divided into four general categories: blenderized, general lactose-free, high caloric density, and defined or elemental formulas. Special disease-related formulas are available for enteral nutrition. Care must be taken to individualize any formula that is commercially prepared, because each patient has individualized needs that may not always be met with a standard formula.

Administration techniques for continuous TEN. Nasogastric feedings are better tolerated by an alert patient with an intact gag reflex and competent esophogastric valve. The stomach can tolerate high osmolar formula better than the small bowel. Feedings can be started at half strength at a rate of 25 to 50 ml/hr. The strength of the formula is increased q 24 hr. Once full strength is attained and tolerated, the rate or volume is increased gradually to the desired level.

Duodenal or jejunal feedings decrease the risk of aspiration, but high osmolar feedings are not well tolerated by the small bowel and may cause diarrhea. Therefore, the strength of formula may be diluted by one-fourth or one-third for the initial feedings. Strength is increased gradually as tolerated. Volume and rate are increased once full strength is attained.

Complications

Mechanical complications are related to placement of the tube. Insertion of the feeding tube may produce epistaxis, pharyngoesophageal irritation, mucosal injury, regurgitation, or aspiration. With extended intubation, displacement, ulceration, and aspiration are potential complications. Aspiration is the most frequent and morbid complication. The potential for life-threatening pulmonary aspiration of gastric contents may be avoided by placement of the feeding tube into the small bowel, distal to the lower esophagus and beyond the pyloric sphincter. Erosion of the esophageal, tracheal, nasal, or oropharyngeal mucosa can occur if the enteral tube is left in place for a long period of time without change in position. Tracheoesophageal fistula may occur in the patient who has had both an enteral nasogastric tube and an endotracheal tube in place simultaneously, over an extended time period.

Metabolic complications are hyperosmolarity, hyperglycemia, dehydration, fluid overload, and diarrhea. The latter is the most common. Diarrhea may be seen in patients whose GI tract has not been used for a time when feedings are started abruptly with full-strength hypertonic solutions. Hyperosmolarity, malabsorption, and maldigestion contribute to this condition and may be avoided by reducing the strength and rate or changing the formula until tolerated. Antidiarrheal medications are successfully added to formulas and help to control this common complication.

Dehydration may occur in the absence of adequate free water. All formulas have a predictable amount of free water; however, additional water may be required by some patients. High-density, hypertonic feedings are usually better tolerated with the addition of more water.

Nursing management

Nursing management of a patient with an enteral feeding tube includes maintenance and/or insertion of the nasogastric tube and maintaining patency and correct placement, routine checks for residual volumes, and monitoring the critical parameters such as daily intake and output. Collaboration with other professionals, specifically the physician and dietician, will enhance safe and comprehensive enteral therapy.

Insertion of the nasogastric tube is often the responsibility of the ICU nurse. Explanation may be given to the conscious patient. Measuring the tube prior to insertion is done by placing the distal end of the tube at the patient's earlobe, extending the tube to the bridge of the nose, and from there to the tip of the xiphoid process. A piece of tape may be used to mark this point on the tube. Once the tube is marked, insert the guide wire, coil the tube around the hand for control, and apply a water-soluble lubricant to the distal portion of the tube. With the patient in an upright position—eyes wide open, when possible—insert the distal end of the tube into one nostril and pass it backward toward the patient's ear. Rotate the tube 180 degrees inward, toward the opposite nostril, exerting steady pressure until the tube passes the nasopharyngeal junction into the esophagus. The patient may drop his head forward at this point to facilitate entry into the esophagus. This maneuver will close the trachea and open the esophagus. Advance the tube through the esophagus into the stomach up to the tape mark on the tube. Remove the guide wire or stylet.

Correct tube placement may be verified by aspirating stomach contents with a large syringe and gentle suction. Auscultation is another easy to check for stomach entry. While injecting 15 to 20 ml of air into the tube, auscultate with a stethoscope over the stomach for a rush of air. The position of the enteral tube can also be verified by x-ray. This method may be indicated with patients who are at risk for aspiration or are difficult to intubate.

Comfort measures are suggested for patients with nasogastric tubes. Securing the tube with a clear plastic dressing or tape will anchor the tube securely, yet allow it to move upon swallowing. Tube drag can be minimized by securing it 10 to 15 in from entry by a large safety pin on the patient's clothing. Mouth care may be offered every few hours to freshen the breath, moisturize the mucous membrane, and prevent coated tongue, cracked lips, and parotiditis. Changing the position of the tube against the naris will prevent pressure sores and necrosis.

Patency of the enteral feeding tube is critical. To maintain a functional tube, the nurse can routinely flush with 10 to 30 ml of water. This process may be done before and after crushed or diluted medications are instilled into the tube. (Medications should not be added directly to the formula because of the potential for altering stability or composition.) Flushing with water is particularly important when the tube feeding is interrupted. When the formula is discontinued for any reason, the tube should be cleared and water instilled to prevent coagulation of formula and eventual disruption of tube patency.

Avoidance of aspiration can often be achieved by good nursing management. Feeding tubes alter the normal physiologic response of the antireflex mechanism and subject the patient to regurgitation and aspiration.

Critically ill patients with neurologic impairment are at maximum risk, as well as patients with tracheostomies or those who are heavily sedated. Positioning the patient in semi-Fowler's, on his right side, will enhance emptying of the stomach through the pylorus into the duodenum.

Residual formula may be checked by aspirating stomach contents q 4 to 6 hr. In general, if residuals are greater than 150 to 300 ml, the feeding should be held until residuals are less. Silastic feeding tubes may collapse during aspiration, giving the false impression that no gastric residual is present. Injection of 10 ml of water or air prior to checking residual may prevent this difficulty.

Pulmonary aspiration is a life-threatening complication for the critical patient, and the nurse should check for tracheal aspirate every shift. Glucose oxidase reagent strips are a sensitive measure of pulmonary aspiration because normal sputum contains no glucose, and thus test strips can detect the presence of tube feeding in the tracheobronchial tree. Signs and symptoms of potential aspiration are cyanosis, dyspnea, coughing, wheezing, tachypnea, tachycardia, fever, atelectasis, and hypoxemia. Tracheal aspirate may be easily checked for the presence of glucose and enteral therapy modified to prevent pulmonary complications.

Monitoring the patient on enteral therapy includes observation and accurate documentation. Daily weights, intake and output, evaluating serum electrolytes such as albumin, transferrin, and other blood studies, figuring nitrogen balance, and obtaining fractional urines every shift are part of nursing responsibilities. Collaboration with the physician and the dietician can ensure optimal nutritional support for the critically ill patient.

The cost is a significant factor to consider when planning nutritional therapy. A major portion of the patient's hospital bill may be the result of enteral or parenteral alimentation. IV hyperalimentation solutions cost from five to ten times more than enteral solutions.

PARENTERAL NUTRITION ADMINISTRATION

Parenteral nutrition is the administration of nutrients via the intravascular route. This method remains a mainstay for the critically ill patient. Parenteral nutrition may be partial or total. Patients whose GI tract is functioning may tolerate partial enteral support but often cannot tolerate delivery of their total energy requirement via the enteral route and may benefit from the simultaneous use of parenteral IV alimentation rather than central venous alimentation.

Peripheral IV nutrition provides nutrients via a catheter placed in a forearm vein. This route avoids potentially dangerous complications associated with the insertion of a central venous catheter. Peripheral alimentation does not allow the infusion of high-dextrose solutions because of the irritating effect of hypertonic solution on peripheral vessels and the large volumes required to meet nutritional needs. A more isosmotic solution is desirable for peripheral therapy. Because this technique does not provide sufficient dextrose and protein for anabolism, a lipid solution should be an integral part of the peripheral nutrition program. Provision of a lipid source will supplement calorie needs for a nonstressed patient whose requirements are not excessive.

The critically ill, highly stressed patient is better alimented by the central venous route, via a catheter that has been placed in the subclavian or jugular vein. High percentages of dextrose and protein and fat can be administered via the central vein. The critical patient often requires large amounts of nutrients in a limited volume (e.g., patients with fluid restrictions). Another advantage of the central vein catheter is a long-term access, which eliminates q-24-to-48-hr catheter changes required with peripheral lines. The central line catheter is usually more comfortable for the patient and permits mobility without endangering misplacement of the venous access. The major disadvantage is the risk of infection of the central line catheter, which is potentially dangerous to a patient already compromised. The risks and benefits should be evaluated prior to initiating therapy for the individual patient.

Indications

The indications for parenteral nutrition for the ICU patient are broad. Any patient that presents in a seriously stressed state with extraordinary nutritional needs may be considered for total parenteral nutrition via the central vein catheter. Preoperative states include those patients who are malnourished and are at significant risk for immediate surgery (e.g., esophageal stricture, carcinoma of the esophagus, or severe peptic ulcer disease with gastric outlet obstruction). Parenteral nutrition is more often used on the postoperative surgical patient whose postoperative course is complicated by prolonged ileus, enterocutaneous fistula, abdominal abscess, peritonitis, or GI fistulas. Patients with chronic GI medical diseases, such as Crohn's, radiation enteritis, persistant pancreatitis, severe gastroenteritis, diverticulitis, or short-bowel syndrome, or obstruction by tumor, stricture, adhesion, or fistulas are also candidates for total parenteral nutrition.

The patient with hypermetabolic needs requires a large amount of calories and cannot be supported adequately without central parenteral nutrition (e.g., patients with burns, trauma, and sepsis). Parenteral therapy is also used as an adjunctive support for patients with cancer who are receiving chemotherapy or radiation treatment, for patients in renal failure or hepatic coma, and in some instances for patients with anorexia nervosa.

Solutions

Total parenteral nutrition (TPN), when administered through a central vein catheter, is the administration of high concentrations of glucose, fat, and amino acids plus major electrolytes, trace elements, and vitamins. Other medications such as insulin, heparin, cimetidine, and corticosteroids may be added as indicated. The solutions are hyperosmolar (>1,000 mOsm) and therefore require central vein infusion in an area of high blood flow.

Solutions contain both essential and nonessential amino acids, with the exception of a solution specifically designed for patients in renal failure, which has little or no nonessential amino acid content. Both 8.5%- and 10%-amino-acid solutions are available, and TPN may be individualized to meet patient needs, depending on nitrogen balance and utilization.

The basal amount of glucose necessary to prevent formation of ketone bodies has been estimated to be 100 g (375 kcal), which is 20% of total energy requirement. For the adult patient, glucose is supplied as 5 to 35 g/kg. When large amounts of glucose are given IV, there is a risk of hyperosmolality and hyperglycemia. Adult solutions for central infusion are commonly mixed with a glucose concentration of 12 to 35%/liter.

Fat emulsions provide an excellent source of nonprotein energy and may be given through a peripheral or central vein. The caloric value of fat is twice that of glucose and exerts minimal osmotic pressure. Fat emulsions, available in 10- and 20%-concentrations, are metabolized and utilized as an energy source at 1.1 kcal/ml and 2 kcal/ml respectively. An additional benefit of the fat source is the provision of essential fatty acids. For the ICU patient there may be an altered pattern of metabolism of fats. Serum triglyceride levels should be monitored to determine capacity of utilization and clearance.

Common admixtures found in TPN are sodium, potassium, calcium, magnesium, and phosphate. These additives are mixed into the solutions in varying amounts, according to serum blood levels. Recommended mEq/day may vary according to the institution.

Sodium, an extracellular electrolyte, may be administered in the form of sodium chloride, acetate, or phosphate. The recommended additive to TPN is NaC1 40 to 120 mEq/day. If the patient is experiencing sodium loss by continuous gastric suction or fistula drainage, however, larger amounts may be administered to correct depletion. Patients with cardiac or renal disease, on the other hand, may require cautious addition of sodium.

Potassium, an intracellular electrolyte, plays an important role in glucose uptake and glycogen synthesis. Potassium may be depleted quickly, once TPN is initiated. Low serum levels may be demonstrated clinically by mental confusion, muscle weakness, hypotension, and arrythmias. To assure optimal metabolism, serum potassium should be checked frequently and maintained in the high normal range. The suggested range is KCL 40 to 120 mEq/day.

Calcium is required for transmission of electrical impulses, for proper muscle functioning, and blood clotting. Symptoms of hypocalcemia include tremors, cramps, seizures, laryngospasm, or respiratory distress. A low serum calcium level may appear in a patient who is hypoalbuminic because 60% of serum calcium is bound to protein, primarily albumin. An ionized calcium test can be done to determine calcium level. Calcium may be administered as gluconate, because the chloride salt is less soluble. Recommended calcium additive is gluconate 9.6 mEq/day.

Magnesium levels may drop with TPN initiation, and patients with excessive GI losses, such as multiple draining fistulas, are prone to magnesium loss. Clinical symptoms of hypomagnesemia are nausea, muscle weakness, tremors, confusion, and tachycardia. Magnesium sulfate is added to TPN solutions at 8 mEq/day.

Phosphate functions to enhance energy and O_2 transport. Low phosphate levels cause symptoms such as perioral numbness, muscle weakness, and respiratory distress. Prolonged respiratory intubations may occur in patients who have subnormal phosphate levels. Adequate phosphate levels are important for energy utilization and may be added to TPN as potassium phosphate at 30 to 45 mEq/day.

Multiple vitamin preparation for IV use are critically needed in long-term parenteral therapy. The multivitamin concentrate is available in 5 cc ampules, the suggested addition being twice a week. The multivitamin concentrate includes fat-soluble vitamins A, D, and E, vitamin C, and the water-soluble B vitamins including biotin, folate, and B_{12}. Trace minerals are essential for human nutrition and need to be included in the TPN formulation. Ampules containing chromium, manganese, copper, and zinc are available. Selenium, iron, and vitamin K may be added to solutions as indicated by serum laboratory tests.

Complications

IV alimentation is an effective therapy and nursing management is the key to recognizing problems in the early stages and implementing measures to prevent complications.

Catheter-related complications. Such complications are technical or mechanical problems that are associated with the insertion of the central line catheter or with catheter maintenance. The invasive procedure of placing a central line catheter may cause pneumothorax or hemothorax. Clinical signs of these complications are sudden respiratory distress, chest pain, cyanosis, and shock. Preventive nursing measures are to support the technical skill of the surgeon, prepare and position the patient prior to insertion, and infuse fluids at a keep-vein-open rate until correct placement of the catheter is verified. Incorrect positioning of the catheter can lead to vein laceration, arterial puncture, brachial plexus injury, or thoracic duct injury. Air embolism can occur during insertion and is clinically recognized by dyspnea, chest pain, disorientation, tachypnea, tachycardia, and cyanosis. The nursing management of air embolism is to immediately plug the catheter and/or the exit site and position the patient in Trendelenburg's, on the left side. This is called the Durant maneuver and facilitates the entrapment of air in the right ventricle of the heart, forcing air out of the pulmonary artery.

The two major complications associated with catheter maintenance are catheter-related **sepsis** and venous thrombosis. Aseptic technique is the prime preventive measure; however, critically ill patients receiving parenteral therapy are continuously exposed to the stresses of underlying disease, malnutrition, multiple drug therapy, and immunosuppression. Adherence to protocol should decrease the incidence of sepsis. Nursing measures to prevent infection include laminar flow preparation of all solutions, maintenance of administration procedure using strict sterile technique, and routine dressing change according to established protocol. Treatment of confirmed catheter sepsis involves antibiotic therapy and removal of the catheter if cultures remain positive. Amphotericin-B is the drug of choice for *Candida* septicemia.

For long-term TPN therapy, a Hickman silicone catheter may be used. The placement of this catheter within a subcutaneous tract and stabilization by fibrous tissue around the dacron catheter cuff may help in preventing microorganisms from entering the body. The incidence of sepsis appears to be lower with this type of catheter.

Venous thrombosis occurs in some patients receiving parenteral nutrition over extended periods of time. Despite the high-volume blood flow and the routine use of heparin, thrombosis may develop. The cause is not clearly identified, although localized trauma and vessel irritation are thought to be contributing factors. Clinical signs occur rather late in this complication and include edema of the neck and face on the affected side or pain, tingling, and edema of the involved arm. Treatment with a thrombolytic agent such as streptokinase or urokinase may be effective in clearing an occlusion. Catheter removal, culture of the catheter tip, and anticoagulant therapy is sometimes the unfortunate result of thrombosis.

Metabolic complications. These result primarily from alteration in glucose metabolism and alteration in amino acid metabolism. Electrolyte abnormalities and fluid imbalances are often seen in the critically ill patient who is receiving hyperalimentation.

Glucose intolerance may be a problem during the first 72 hr of infusion. Because the pancreas is adjusting to the high sugar load being infused directly into the systemic circulation, a period of adaptation is seen, and the patient may develop hyperglycemia and glycosuria. Septic or severely stressed patients may not be able to adapt, and insulin may be added to the parenteral nutrition to maintain safe blood glucose levels.

Monitoring for metabolic complications requires testing for urine sugar and acetone q 6 to 8 hr for glycosuria, as well as routine measurements for intake and output. Frequent blood glucose tests should be done for the first few days, then daily, and then two to three times a week, once stability is achieved. Infusion rates of parenteral nutrition can be increased as tolerated to allow pancreatic adaptation. Ongoing infusion rates should be kept at a constant level to permit a balance between insulin release and blood glucose normalcy. The abrupt discontinuation of a high-glucose infusion may cause hypoglycemia; therefore gradual tapering of the infusion rate is recommended. The use of an infusion pump will provide safe, steady control of the rate of delivery.

Hyperosmolar, hyperglycemic, nonketotic dehydration can result from persistant hyperglycemia and serum osmolality of >350 mOsm.

Serum glucose acts as an osmotic diuretic and causes fluid to be pulled from the tissues into the circulation. Circulating glucose exceeds the renal threshold and cannot be reabsorbed by the renal tubules. Increased urinary output and osmotic diuresis leaves the patient dehydrated. Dehydration suppresses the production of insulin leading to a vicious cycle. Clinical symptomatology includes excessive thirst, poor skin turgor, disorientation and lethargy, an increased pulse rate, and decreased BP. Prevention measures are daily weights, strict intake and output measurements, urine sp gr q 8 hr, daily serum glucose, and urine sugar q 6 hr.

Fluid and electrolyte abnormalities are not uncommon in those patients receiving parenteral nutrition. Because critically ill patients are in catabolic or hypercatabolic states, intracellular ions such as potassium, phosphate, and magnesium are exhausted for energy requirements. Early recognition is dependent on routine serum electrolyte studies and observation of clinical symptoms such as neuromuscular parasthesias, weakness, and changes in level of consciousness.

Hyperchloremic metabolic acidosis may occur, caused by crystalline amino acids administered as chloride salts. Early detection of amino acid problems may be picked up by a rise in serum chloride with a drop in serum CO_2 content. Clinical signs are nausea, lethargy, disorientation, and dehydration. Addition of sodium acetate to solution is an accepted treatment.

Azotemia results from the delivery of a high nitrogen load and inability of the body to handle the circulating protein. The increased BUN in the presence of a normal creatinine and urine output is often seen in children and adults with hepatic or renal dysfunction. The amino acid or nitrogen supplement should be adjusted according to tolerance to prevent azotemia.

Essential-fatty-acid deficiency is associated with fat-free IV nutrition. Linoleic acid, one essential fatty acid, can be depleted within a week in the absence of fat supplement. Clinical symptoms include dry, scaly skin, hair loss, thrombocytopenia, and poor wound healing. Although desquamation dermatitis is the primary sign, there is a tendency for hair to fall out prior to skin changes. With the addition of fat to the parenteral regime, fatty acid deficiency improves. Because fat is usually incorporated into nutritional therapy today, the risk of this complication is reduced.

Monitoring trace elements by weekly serum tests is recommended for patients on long-term parenteral nutrition.

Psychosocial manifestations of TPN

Acutely ill patients with high metabolic needs may require parenteral nutritional support for a limited period of time until adequate enteral intake is sufficient. The psychosocial complications in this group manifest as delirium, specifically in the elderly, the substance-abusing, or the septic febrile patient. Other changes noted are apathy, confusion, irritability, and insomnia. These responses appear to be biopsychological, and the patient and family are probably reacting to the ICU regime, rather than to parenteral nutrition as a specific cause. The degree to which nutritional support is disturbing the patient's well-being is difficult to differentiate from the total illness experience.

Seriously ill patients who require parenteral nutrition over a longer period of time to improve anabolic status often manifest psychosocial reactions to the TPN therapy. Because food is a source of security, status, identity, and social acceptability in our society, patients often become anxious and apprehensive about the central line catheter, the infusion pump, the dependence on IV fluids, and the absence of oral intake.

The nursing management for this group of patients is critical. Support and reassurance for the patient and family may focus on educational intervention and comfort measures. Clear explanations of the rationale, mode, and technique of nutrient administration may help to allay fear and anxiety. The patient can be given some control by learning to assist in dressing change, site care, and scheduling. Frequent mouth care, oral substitutions such as hard candy or ice popsicles, and even allowing a patient to chew, taste, and spit out food may help to satisfy oral needs.

A few nutrition-support patients in the ICU develop severe psychotic reactions manifested by total dependency, regression, and paranoia. Professional counseling and intervention may be indicated in these situations.

CHAPTER 12

ARTERIAL BLOOD GAS INTERPRETATION

Kathy Lynn Emanuelsen

Evaluation of the arterial blood gas has become an invaluable aid in the physiologic diagnosis and therapeutic management of critically ill patients. Arterial blood gases (ABGs) provide information about a patient's acid-base balance, alveolar ventilation, and oxygenation status. Therefore, a comprehensive understanding of blood gases and their clinical applications is an essential assessment skill for nurses who work in critical care units. The intent of this chapter is to provide the background information that is necessary to master this complex skill.

FRAMEWORK

ACID-BASE BALANCE

The maintenance of acid-base balance in the ECF and ICF is accomplished by the regulation of the free hydrogen ion concentration.

Acids

Compounds that release hydrogen when placed in aqueous solutions are called acids. Body fluids contain a number of different acids. The most important, in terms of its effect on the acidity of the blood, is carbonic acid (H_2CO_3). Carbonic acid results from the combination of CO_2 and water. As the amount of CO_2 in the blood rises, the concentration of carbonic acid and, consequently of free hydrogen ions, also rises. CO_2, therefore, is an acid-producing substance.

Bases

Body fluids also contain a number of substances called bases, compounds that will accept hydrogen ions when dissolved in aqueous solutions. The most important base found in body fluids, in terms of its effect on the alkalinity of the blood, is bicarbonate (HCO_3^-). Bicarbonate is capable of accepting a free hydrogen ion, resulting in the formulation of carbonic acid. Conversely, carbonic acid is capable of releasing a hydrogen molecule to form bicarbonate and its free hydrogen ion.

Acidosis and alkalosis

If acids release hydrogen ions and bases accept hydrogen ions, then the acidity or alkalinity of a solution is ultimately reflected in the concentration of free hydrogen ion. The pH reflects the concentration of free hydrogen ions in solution. The pH may be thought of as a scale used to measure the degree of acidity or alkalinity of the blood. It demonstrates the relationship of the hydrogen ion concentration to the bicarbonate level in the blood. The pH is inversely related to the hydrogen ion concentration: As the hydrogen ion concentration rises, the pH falls; conversely, as the hydrogen ion concentration falls, the pH rises.

The symbol *p* refers to the negative logarithm which, in the case of the symbol pH, means the negative logarithm of hydrogen. Therefore, a pH of 5 means that there are 10^{-5} (or 0.00001) g of hydrogen in 1 liter of solution.

On the pH scale of 1 to 14, a pH of 7 is electrochemically neutral. Blood is slightly alkaline, with a normal pH range of 7.35 to 7.45. If the pH value goes below 7.35, a state of acidosis exists. If the pH value goes above 7.45, a state of alkalosis exists.

The clinical consequences of an abnormally elevated or decreased pH are extremely serious. Cells depend on a normal concentration of hydrogen ion in surrounding body fluids to function optimally. An abnormally low or high hydrogen ion concentration interferes with cellular metabolism and, at extreme levels, can cause death of the cells, with consequences for the patient that can be fatal.

Ratio of carbonic acid to base bicarbonate

To understand acid-base balance, it is important to know the ratio of carbonic acid to base bicarbonate and their relationship to the free hydrogen ion activity. The normal carbonic acid:base bicarbonate ratio is 1:20, i.e., for every 1 molecule of hydrogen there are 20 molecules of bicarbonate. It is the ratio of the carbonic acid to base bicarbonate that determines the concentration of free hydrogen ions and, consequently, the pH. The chart in Figure 12–1 demonstrates the pH spectrum of plasma in various degrees of acidosis and alkalosis.

COMPENSATION MECHANISMS OF THE BODY

In normal individuals, arterial pH is maintained between 7.35 and 7.45. This homeostatic process is the result of protection of body pH by three

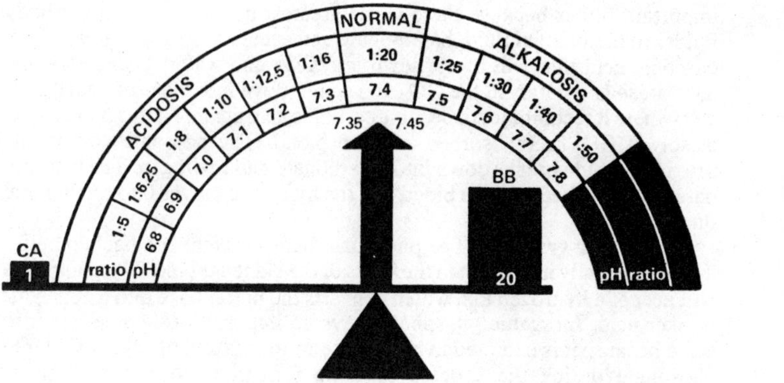

Figure 12–1. The pH spectrum of plasma. CA, carbonic acid; BB, base bicarbonate. *Reprinted with the permission of* Travenol Laboratories, Inc., Deerfield, Ill.

lines of defense: (1) body buffers that provide chemical buffering of an acid or alkali entering the plasma; (2) pulmonary regulation, which allows carbonic acid to be eliminated by the lungs as CO_2; (3) renal reabsorption and excretion of bicarbonate and excretion of acids.

Therefore, chemical buffers, respiratory regulation, and renal reabsorptive, excretory, and metabolic processes cooperate to dispose of the normal daily amounts of carbonic acid and non-volatile acids as well as any addition of alkali to the ECF.

Blood buffer response

The blood buffers are the first mechanism to attempt to correct an acid-base imbalance. The buffers, which are present in all body fluids, act as chemical sponges that begin to work <1 sec after an abnormal pH has been recognized. These buffers are made up of two or more chemical compounds that combine with strong acids or strong bases to form weak acids and weak bases to maintain a stable pH. An example of the buffer effect is demonstrated in the following equations: $HCl + NaHCO_3 \rightarrow H_2CO_3 + NaCl$. In this case, the buffer base (sodium bicarbonate) has changed the strong acid (hydrochloric acid) into a weak acid (carbonic acid), thereby preventing an increase in the hydrogen ion concentration. To take another example: $NaOH + H_2CO_3 \rightarrow NaHCO_3 + H_2O$; in this case, the weak buffer acid (carbonic acid) has changed a strong base (sodium hydroxide) into a weak buffer base (sodium bicarbonate), thereby preventing a decrease in the hydrogen ion concentration.

The four major buffer systems are the bicarbonate system, the phosphate system, the ammonium system, and the protein system.

Bicarbonate system. The bicarbonate buffer system is the most important buffer because there is the greatest quantity of it in the body fluids. In the luminal fluid, bicarbonate can accept a hydrogen ion to form carbonic acid that will break down into CO_2 and water. Using carbonic anhydrase as a catalyst, the CO_2 and water move into the proximal tubule cell, where it recombines to become carbonic acid again. At this point, some dissolved CO_2 is reabsorbed into the blood. The carbonic acid in the proximal tubule breaks down into bicarbonate and hydrogen. The bicarbonate is reabsorbed into the blood and the hydrogen moves into the luminal fluid.

Phosphate system. The phosphate buffer system is a backup buffer and is especially important in the fluids of the kidney tubule. The phosphate will accept a hydrogen ion, which converts the buffer base into a conjugate weaker acid. Inorganic phosphate plays an important role as a buffer in urine because it is excreted in high concentration. Acid titration of filtered phosphate during the process of urine formation permits this buffer substance to play a crucial role in removing hydrogen ions from the body.

Ammonium system. The ammonium buffer system is another backup buffer that will accept a hydrogen ion. Amino acids break down into the very strong base, ammonia, which will accept a hydrogen ion, resulting in the excretion of ammonium. Within the tubular lumen, the great affinity of ammonia for hydrogen ions ensures the rapid conversion of ammonia to nondiffusible ammonium ions, which are trapped in the lumen and eliminated in the urine. This diffusion trapping mechanism for ammonium, coupled with the kidney's ability to alter the rate of ammonia production and secretion, accounts for the kidney's ability to regulate hydrogen ion balance.

Protein system. The protein buffer system is found in blood protein, plasma protein, and cells. Proteins vary considerably in the extent to which they function as buffers. In the living organism, most of the buffer capacity of proteins is attributable to the imidazole group of histidine. Hb is the most important blood protein buffer because it is the principal nonbicarbonate buffer.

Buffering alone cannot maintain homeostasis of the pH. Despite buffering, extra hydrogen ions are continually entering the blood. The respiratory and renal mechanism must function concurrently with the blood buffers if the pH is to remain stable.

Respiratory response

By adjusting the rate and depth of ventilation, the lungs control the hydrogen ion concentration in body fluids. This is accomplished by varying the rate at which CO_2 is removed from the body. Although slower-acting than the blood buffers, the respiratory response to a metabolic abnormality is activated within minutes.

The response by the lungs is controlled by the respiratory center, which is located in the medulla of the brain. The respiratory center is sensitive to changes in the CO_2 content and the pH of blood and CSF. The lungs respond in two ways: If the blood pH has decreased, the respirations will increase in rate and depth to eliminate CO_2. This will reduce the amount of carbonic acid remaining in the blood and, consequently, raise the pH to the normal range. If the blood pH has increased, the respirations will decrease in rate and depth to conserve the CO_2 in the body. This will increase the amount of carbonic acid remaining in the blood and, consequently, lower the pH to the normal range.

Renal response

The kidneys regulate acid-base balance by varying the rate of hydrogen removal from the body via the urine. The renal response to an abnormal pH is a slower one; it requires several hours to several days for the kidneys to attempt to adjust acid-base imbalances to normal. Even so, the kidneys are a powerful mechanism for the removal of large quantities of excess hydrogen and/or bicarbonate from the body. The kidneys play a major role in pH adjustment when hydrogen ion deficit or excess is present in the body.

When ECF is alkalotic, the kidneys conserve hydrogen and eliminate sodium bicarbonate, which results in the elimination of alkalotic urine. When ECF is acidic, the kidneys excrete excess hydrogen, conserve bicarbonate, and excrete ammonium via the kidney tubules, which results in the elimination of acidic urine.

Compensation

Compensation is the term that is given to the body's attempt to return the pH to a normal value when situations occur that alter normal acid-base balance. When there is an abnormality in the respiratory parameter, the body will attempt to correct the acid-base imbalance by altering the metabolic parameter and vice versa. A state of partial compensation exists when there has been an increase or decrease in the compensating parameter and the pH is not yet within the normal range. The body has fully compensated when the assisting parameter is either increased or decreased and the pH is within the normal range. The body rarely, if ever, overcompensates.

Because the respiratory response to metabolic imbalances occurs within minutes, the respiratory compensation will be reflected in the ABGs almost immediately. On the other hand, the renal response to a respiratory imbalance takes from hours to days to occur; therefore, when metabolic compensation to a respiratory imbalance is reflected in the ABGs, the imbalance has invariably existed for a somewhat lengthy period of time.

OXYGENATION

Oxygenation is distinct from acid-base balance. Delivery of O_2 to the cells depends on all of factors that are involved in the transport of O_2 from the atmosphere to the alveolus and across the alveolar capillary membrane. The partial pressure of O_2 in the alveolus, the PAO_2, is determined by the fraction of inspired O_2, atmospheric pressure, and the individual's ventilation. The subsequent partial pressure of O_2 in the arterial blood, the PaO_2, is determined by the surface area available for diffusion, the width of the alveolar capillary membrane, the concentration gradient of O_2 from the alveolus to the capillary, and the solubility coefficient of O_2.

While the PaO_2 does not directly determine the pH, it can both cause and reflect acid-base imbalances. A PaO_2 of <70 mmHg may cause respiratory alkalosis by stimulating hyperventilation. A low PaO_2 may be the result of general or regional hypoventilation or respiratory failure, all of which increase intrapulmonary shunting and venous admixture.

Because ~99% of O_2 is transported in the blood by Hb, effective cellular oxygenation must rely upon factors that govern the association and dissociation of Hb with O_2; therefore, it is possible to bind four molecules of O_2 per Hb molecule. Each gram of Hb has a capacity for 1.34 ml of O_2. As the PaO_2 increases, the saturation of the available Hb receptor sites increases. This relationship is not a linear one. Rather, it is represented by the oxyhemoglobin dissociation curve (*see* Chapter 3). Above 60 mmHg, increases in the PaO_2 can cause only a minimal increase in saturation. Below 60 mmHg, however, even small reductions in the PaO_2 can cause precipitous drops in the percentage of Hb that is saturated with O_2. The body normally operates at the upper flat portion of the curve, which serves to protect against great variations in Hb saturation.

Factors affecting the oxyhemoglobin dissociation curve are discussed in Chapter 3. The reader is referred to this section for additional background information. Table 12–1 displays the clinical implications of the different PaO_2 levels.

CLINICAL INTERPRETATION OF ARTERIAL BLOOD GASES

ABG studies determine the blood pH, $PaCO_2$, the plasma bicarbonate level (HCO_3^-), PaO_2, and oxyhemoglobin saturation (SaO_2). To discuss the acid-base imbalances, it it necessary to have a normal set of ABG values. A suggested range of normal ABG values is shown below. The reader should be aware that there are slight variations in these values in different laboratories.

Suggested range of normal blood gas values

1. The **pH** is a direct measurement that determines the acid-base status of the body. Normal values range from 7.35 to 7.45.
2. The **$PaCO_2$** is a direct measurement that is the best reflector of alveolar ventilation. It measures the partial pressure of CO_2 in blood in mmHg. Normal value is 35 to 45 mmHg. An abnormal $PaCO_2$ reflects a respiratory acid-base imbalance.
3. The **HCO_3^-** is a measurement of acid-base balance that is regulated by the kidneys. Normal value is 22 to 26 mEq/liter. An abnormal HCO_3^-

TABLE 12–1
Clinical Implications of the Arterial Oxygen Level

Arterial oxygen level	Clinical consequence
80–100 mmHg	The O_2 level in the blood is adequate for most body needs.
70–80 mmHg	The O_2 level in the blood is acceptable for the resting patient.
60 mmHg	The O_2 level in the blood is inadequate. At this level the saturation is ~93%, which will cause the hypoxic respiratory drive to become active. The rate and depth of inspiration will increase. The respiratory rate of the resting adult should be 14–19 breaths/min. An increase to 25 should suggest hypoxia.
50–60 mmHg	The organs that require the greatest amount of O_2 will show signs of distress because of hypoxia. Cerebral signs include: anxiety, confusion, agitation, and lack of judgment. Cardiovascular signs include: increased heart rate and BP.
40–50 mmHg	Severe tissue hypoxia exists. Cyanosis will be clearly apparent. Note: this is a late sign of hypoxemia. Hypoxemia is a condition in which the amount of O_2 available is inadequate to meet the needs of most tissues. It affects the brain, heart, adrenals, kidneys, and liver. Severe uncorrected hypoxemia will cause permanent brain damage, severe metabolic acidosis, shock, cardiac arrhythmias, and ultimately death.
30 mmHg	Permanent CNS damage usually occurs. Immediate vigorous intervention is imperative.
20 mmHg	Survival is unlikely. At 20 mmHg the PaO_2 is at or below the physiologic range for many tissues. Immediate vigorous intervention is mandatory.

value reflects a metabolic imbalance.

4. The total CO_2 (**TCO_2**) test is used at some institutions. TCO_2 is composed of dissolved CO_2, H_2CO_3, and HCO_3^-; however, >95% of this value is HCO_3^-, and for this reason, an abnormal TCO_2 reflects a metabolic imbalance. Normal value is 22 to 28 mM/liter.

5. The **PaO_2** measures the partial pressure of O_2 in the blood in mmHg. The normal value is 90 mmHg (75 to 95 mmHg).

6. The **SaO_2** can be measured directly or be plotted on the oxyhemoglobin dissociation curve. Normal value is 94 to 97%. It can be affected by changes in the pH, the $PaCO_2$, and the temperature.

7. The base excess (**BE**) or base deficit is a positive or negative value that indicates the mEq/liter of remaining blood buffer base (plasma HCO_3^- and Hb) after the hydrogen ions are buffered. Normal value is ± 1.

An abnormally positive value will indicate a state of alkalosis, whereas an abnormally negative value will indicate a state of acidosis.

In any clinical assessment of ABG values, a single isolated result is not as significant as the prevailing trend of values. Therefore, one should not make a judgment about which acid-base imbalance is present by analyzing only one value. A guide to interpretation of ABGs is described below.

1. Check pH: determine if it is acidotic, alkalotic, or normal.
2. Check $PaCO_2$ (the respiratory parameter): determine if it is elevated, decreased, or normal.
3. Check HCO_3^- (the metabolic parameter): determine if it is elevated, decreased, or normal.
4. If abnormalities exist, determine which of the major acid-base imbalances is present.
5. Determine whether any compensation mechanisms are involved.
6. Check PaO_2 and SaO_2: determine if they are normal, elevated, or decreased.
7. Observe patient: evaluate vital signs and physical parameters. Are these values normal for this patient?
8. Evaluate why patient presents any abnormal values that are present and implement appropriate actions necessary to correct the acid-base imbalance.

The criteria describing the major acid-base imbalances in Table 12–2 are presented under the assumption that the body is left free to physiologically respond to an imbalanced state. When these mechanisms are interfered with, as with the use of ventilators or electrolyte therapy, these criteria may not necessarily stand. Therefore, the interpretation of ABGs is also dependent upon the awareness of the method of medical treatment.

TABLE 12–2

Major Acid-Base States

State	pH	PCO_2	HCO_3^-
Normal acid-base	Normal	Normal	Normal
Acute respiratory acidosis	Decreased	Increased	Normal
Compensated respiratory acidosis	Normal or decreased	Increased	Increased
Acute respiratory alkalosis	Increased	Decreased	Normal
Compensated respiratory alkalosis	Normal or increased	Decreased	Decreased
Metabolic acidosis	Decreased	Decreased	Decreased
Metabolic alkalosis	Increased	Normal or slightly increased	Increased

ACID-BASE IMBALANCE STATES

RESPIRATORY ACIDOSIS

Respiratory acidosis is initiated by an elevation in the CO_2 tension (hypercapnia). The physiologic mechanism is essentially the same in all forms of respiratory acidosis, i.e., a decrease in effective ventilation at the alveolar level that leads to an increase in CO_2 and, subsequently, to an increase in carbonic acid and free hydrogen ions. The increase in free hydrogen ions leads to a decrease in the pH. If the situation is acute, there is no time for renal compensation; this condition is called acute respiratory acidosis. (The ABG picture is as follows: pH ↓ $PaCO_2$ ↑ HCO_3^-–).

In an attempt to maintain acid-base balance, the body will use its mechanisms (the blood buffers, lungs, and kidneys) to compensate for any abnormal acid-base conditions. The renal response to respiratory acidosis is to increase the excretion of hydrogen and to increase the reabsorption of sodium bicarbonate to restore the pH to normal. When this compensation is evident, the situation is called chronic or compensated respiratory acidosis. (These efforts are reflected in the ABG values as follows: pH – $PaCO_2$ ↑ HCO_3^- ↑).

The cause of respiratory acidosis is alveolar hypoventilation, which can result from a disease or malfunction of any element of the regulatory system controlling respiration. This includes the CNS and peripheral nervous system, the respiratory muscles, the thoracic cage, the pleural space, the lung parenchyma, and the airways. Table 12–3 identifies the many causes of respiratory acidosis.

The clinical signs and symptoms of respiratory acidosis include tachycardia, dyspnea, tachypnea, restlessness, confusion, lethargy leading to coma, diaphoresis, cyanosis, and arrhythmias (particularly ventricular).

Treatment of acute respiratory acidosis must be directed at the prompt removal of the underlying cause of the respiratory problem and providing adequate ventilation to prevent hypoxemia and extreme acidemia. Acute respiratory acidosis poses its major threat to survival not because of hypercapnia or acidemia, but because of the associated hypoxemia. The underlying cause can seldom be removed in the case of patients with chronic respiratory acidosis. Treatment directed toward maximizing alveolar ventilation is often successful. Use of postural drainage, chest physiotherapy, appropriate administration of antibiotics, bronchodilators, and diuretics may be very effective. The patient must be monitored closely and all systems must be maintained throughout the course of therapy.

RESPIRATORY ALKALOSIS

Respiratory alkalosis is initiated by a reduction in the CO_2 tension (hypocapnia). The physiologic mechanism is essentially the same in all forms of respiratory alkalosis, i.e., because of the state of alveolar hyperventilation, CO_2 is "blown off," thereby leaving less end product and

TABLE 12–3
Causes of Respiratory Acidosis

Condition	Acute	Chronic
Airway obstruction	Aspiration of foreign body or vomitus Laryngospasm Generalized bronchospasm Obstructive sleep apnea	Chronic obstructive lung disease (bronchitis, emphysema)
Respiratory center depression	General anesthesia Sedative overdosage Cerebral trauma or infarction Central sleep apnea	Chronic sedative overdosage Primary alveolar hypoventilation (Ondine's curse) Obesity-hypoventilation syndrome (Pickwickian syndrome) Brain tumor
Circulatory catastrophes	Cardiac arrest Severe pulmonary edema	
Neuromuscular defects	High cervical cordotomy Botulism, tetanus Guillain-Barré syndrome Crisis in myasthenia gravis Drugs or toxic agents (e.g. curare, succinylcholine)	Poliomyelitis Multiple sclerosis Muscular dystrophy Amyotrophic lateral sclerosis Diaphragmatic paralysis Myxedema Myopathic disease (e.g. polymyositis)
Restrictive defects	Pneumothorax Hemothorax Flail chest Severe pneumonitis Infant respiratory distress syndrome (hyaline membrane disease) Adult respiratory distress syndrome	Kyphoscoliosis, spinal arthritis Fibrothorax Hydrothorax Interstitial fibrosis Decreased diaphragmatic movement (e.g. ascites) Prolonged pneumonitis Obesity
Mechanical ventilation		

an excess of base, along with an increase in the pH. If the situation were acute, the kidneys would not have time to compensate. This condition is called acute respiratory alkalosis. (The blood gas picture is as follows: pH ↑ $PaCO_2$ ↓ HCO_3^-–.)

In this circumstance, the body will, once again, use its mechanisms to compensate for any abnormal acid-base condition. The renal response to respiratory alkalosis is to decrease the excretion of hydrogen and to decrease the reabsorption of sodium bicarbonate in order to restore the pH to normal. When this compensation is evident, the situation is called chronic or compensated respiratory alkalosis. (These efforts are reflected in the blood gas picture as follows: pH-$PaCO_2$ ↓ HCO_3^- ↓ .)

The major causes of respiratory alkalosis are presented in Table 12–4. Respiratory alkalosis occurs in a wide variety of serious illnesses. It occurs in 45% of all ICU patients.

The clinical signs and symptoms of respiratory alkalosis include lightheadedness, paresthesia, and hyperalkalotic tetany, which leads to contraction of the hands and arms as a result of the pH imbalance.

In general, the only satisfactory treatment of respiratory alkalosis is to remove the underlying cause. If the cause cannot be eliminated, little can be done to alleviate the hypocapnia. Acute hypocapnia can be reversed if the patient breathes into a paper bag, thereby increasing the inspired CO_2. The $PaCO_2$ can be altered readily in patients with ventilator-induced hyperventilation. In such patients, respiratory alkalosis can be avoided if the rate and depth of ventilation are regulated, or if the dead space in the system is adjusted. The patient must be monitored and supported as indicated throughout the course of therapy.

TABLE 12–4

Causes of Respiratory Alkalosis

Condition	Cause
Hypoxia	Decreased inspired O_2 tension
	High altitude
	Ventilation-perfusion inequality
	Hypotension
	Severe anemia
CNS-mediated	Voluntary hyperventilation
	Neurologic disease
	Cerebrovascular accident (infarction, hemorrhage)
	Infection (encephalitis, meningitis)
	Trauma
	Tumor
	Hepatic failure
	Gram-negative septicemia
	Recovery from metabolic acidosis
	Anxiety-hyperventilation syndrome
	Heat exposure
Pulmonary disease	Interstitial lung disease
	Pneumonia
	Pulmonary embolism
	Pulmonary edema
Mechanical overventilation	

METABOLIC ACIDOSIS

Metabolic acidosis is initiated by a reduction in plasma bicarbonate concentration. The resultant acidemia stimulates ventilation that leads to the secondary hypocapnia characteristic of this disorder. (The blood gas picture is as follows: pH ↓ $PaCO_2$ ↓ HCO_3^- ↓). Metabolic acidosis can result from three separate mechanisms: (1) a loss of bicarbonate ions from the body through the GI tract or through the kidney; (2) an increase in the amount of hydrogen ions presented to the body buffers from endogenous or exogenous sources; and (3) a decrease in the kidney's ability to excrete acid.

It is not uncommon for more than one mechanism to be operating at the same time.

The causes of metabolic acidosis can be classified into three categories, each signifying the pathophysiologic mechanism that can produce a reduction in plasma bicarbonate: (1) loss of bicarbonate, (2) addition of acid, and (3) failure of renal excretion.

Loss of bicarbonate. 1. diarrhea;
2. small bowel losses
3. carbonic anhydrase inhibitors.

Addition of hydrochloric acid. 1. Ammonium chloride.

Overproduction of organic acids. 1. Lactic acidosis;
2. diabetic ketoacidosis;
3. starvation ketosis;
4. alcoholic ketoacidosis;
5. methyl alcohol ingestion;
6. ethylene glycol ingestion;
7. paraldehyde ingestion;
8. salicylate intoxication.

Failure of renal tubular function. 1. renal tubular acidosis;
2. mild renal failure;
3. adrenal insufficiency.

Severe renal failure. 1. Acute;
2. chronic.

Clinical signs and symptoms of metabolic acidosis include hyperventilation, a shocklike state, coma, arrhythmia, and if, untreated, death. The lungs will attempt to compensate immediately for the metabolic acidosis by "blowing off" CO_2. Because of this immediate compensation, there is no chronic state of metabolic acidosis.

Many of the clinical circumstances in which metabolic acidosis occurs require specific medical interventions. The following principles are provided as a general guide to the medical treatment of this acid-base disorder:

1. Remove the underlying cause of the disorder whenever possible.
2. Administer alkali therapy only when the severity or the nature of the acidosis warrants it.

3. Use sodium bicarbonate when the administration of an alkali is required in acute metabolic acidosis.
4. Monitor and support the patient throughout the therapy.

METABOLIC ALKALOSIS

Metabolic alkalosis is initiated by an increase in plasma bicarbonate concentration. The resultant alkalemia affects ventilation and leads to the slight secondary hypercapnia that is characteristic of this disorder. (The blood gas picture is as follows: pH ↑ $PaCO_2$ ↑ HCO_3^- ↑). Metabolic alkalosis can result from three separate mechanisms: (1) loss of hydrogen from body fluids, (2) addition of alkali to the body fluids, (3) a disproportionate loss of chloride from the body fluids.

The causes of metabolic alkalosis can be classified into four groups: (1) alkalosis resulting from exogenous alkali; (2) from a disproportionate chloride deficit; (3) from an absence of volume in the presence of abundant dietary chloride; and (4) in which the nature of the alkalosis is not well defined.

Alkalosis secondary to alkali administration. 1. Continuous alkali administration;
2. Milk-alkali syndrome;
3. Ingestion of large quantities of sodium bicarbonate;
4. Ingestion of soybean-formula diet;
5. combined therapy with nonabsorbable alkali and exchange resins;
6. recovery from organic acidosis.

Chloride-responsive alkalosis. 1. Gastric fluid losses;
2. diuretic therapy;
3. posthypercapnic state;
4. stool losses.

Chloride-resistant alkalosis. 1. Primary aldosteronism;
2. Cushing's syndrome;
3. disorders that simulate adrenocortical excess.

Miscellaneous. 1. Secondary aldosteronism: malignant hypertension; renovascular hypertension; renin-secreting tumors;
2. mineralcorticoid excess (other than aldosterone);
3. penicillin therapy;
4. parathyroid disease and hypercalcemia;
5. refeeding following fasting.

Clinical signs and symptoms of metabolic alkalosis include numbness, tingling, muscle twitching, and tetany. As in the state of metabolic acidosis, the lungs immediately attempt to compensate for the metabolic imbalance. There is a minimal retention of CO_2 reflected in the ABGs. Because of this immediate compensation, there is no chronic state of metabolic alkalosis.

The following principles are provided as a general guide to the medical treatment of this acid-base disorder:

1. Remove the underlying cause of the disorder whenever possible.
2. Prevent chloride-responsive alkalosis from developing.
3. Replace chloride deficits when required.
4. Monitor and support the patient throughout the therapy.

MIXED ACID-BASE DISTURBANCES

Mixed acid-base disturbances are defined as the coexistence of two or more simple acid-base abnormalities. These situations pose some of the most challenging problems encountered in the care of patients with acid-base disorders. Mixed acid-base disturbances in which two components can be identified occur quite commonly among hospitalized patients; triple acid-base disturbances are occasionally observed.

The presence of certain underlying disease processes should increase the suspicion that a mixed acid-base disturbance will be found. In septic shock, mixed respiratory alkalosis and metabolic (lactic) acidosis is common; in chronic obstructive pulmonary disease, respiratory acidosis is often complicated by diuretic-induced metabolic alkalosis; in untreated cardiopulmonary arrest, both respiratory and metabolic acidosis are characteristically observed. As with simple acid-base disturbances, the diagnosis of a specific mixed disorder is important not only as a therapeutic guide but also as a clue to the presence of previously unrecognized diseases.

TECHNIQUES FOR OBTAINING ARTERIAL BLOOD GASES

ABGs may be drawn by a percutaneous puncture or from an indwelling arterial line. In either case, the syringe should be heparinized with ~0.5 ml of heparin 1:1,000. The specimen must be placed in an ice-filled container and delivered promptly to the laboratory. The specimen should be accompanied by a requisition slip that gives the following information: the date, the time the specimen was drawn, the patient's temperature, the percentage of O_2 that the patient is receiving, and, if applicable, the type of ventilator that the patient is on. The method for drawing percutaneous ABGs and for drawing arterial blood from an indwelling arterial line are found below.

Percutaneous puncture

1. Select the site to be used for the percutaneous puncture. (Arterial blood can be obtained from the radial, brachial, or femoral artery.)

Precaution. If the radial artery is selected, establish sufficient ulnar collateral circulation. This is done by occluding the radial artery and observing the hand. When there is sufficient ulnar circulation, the hand will **not** become cyanotic.

2. Determine the strongest pulse beat and insert the needle into the artery.

Precaution. Use a 25-gauge ⅝-in needle for radial and brachial punctures and a 22-gauge 1½-in needle for femoral punctures.

3. Withdraw 1 ml of arterial blood for the specimen.

Precaution. When the needle punctures the artery, blood will pulse back into the syringe.

4. Remove the needle from the artery swiftly and place the syringe in the ice-filled container.

Precaution. Be sure to cap the end with a needle cover or rubber stopper to prevent any air from getting into the syringe.

5. Apply pressure over the puncture site for ≥5 min.

Precaution. Observe the site for any signs of bleeding and for sufficient circulation.

Indwelling arterial line

1. Place a syringe in the three-way stopcock that is between the flush device and the short length of tubing.

Precaution. Maintain sterile technique throughout procedure.

2. Turn the three-way stopcock so that it is off toward the flush device.
3. Withdraw ~3 to 5 ml of fluid and discard.

Precaution. Be sure to turn the three-way stopcock so that it is off toward the syringe before it is removed.

4. Insert the heparinized syringe that is to be used for the blood sample into the three-way stopcock.
5. Turn the three-way stopcock so it is off to the flush device.
6. Draw the blood sample (1 ml).
7. Return the three-way stopcock to its original position (off to air).
8. Remove the syringe and place it in the ice-filled container.

Precaution. Be sure to cap the end with a needle cover or rubber stopper to prevent any air from getting into the syringe.

9. Irrigate the system by using the flush device.
10. Flush the three-way stopcock by turning the stopcock so that it is off toward the patient.

Precaution. Place an IV catheter plug in the three-way stopcock opening.

11. Return the stopcock to its original position so that it is off toward the air.

Precaution. Make sure that no air bubbles have been introduced into the system.

CHAPTER 13

OXYGEN THERAPY AND MECHANICAL VENTILATION

Jacqueline McQuay Rosenlicht

Hypoxia is the primary indication for O_2 administration. O_2, a colorless, odorless, tasteless gas, is regarded as a drug. As with any other medication, O_2 administration should be done properly, safely, and with good reason. To ensure optimum results without the underlying harmful effects from excessive use, the dosage and method of O_2 administration must be adapted to the individual needs of each patient.

OXYGEN DELIVERY SYSTEMS

The goal of O_2 therapy is the administration of an adequate concentration of inspired O_2 to allow full use of the O_2-carrying capacity of arterial blood. The adequacy and effectiveness of O_2 therapy is determined by the examination of arterial blood gas (ABG) measurements. Once the decision for O_2 therapy has been made, the method of administration is dependent upon the concentration of O_2 and flow system that is required for an individual patient. There are two methods of O_2 administration: the low-flow system and the high-flow system.

LOW-FLOW SYSTEMS

Low-flow devices allow the patient to inhale room air, which mixes freely with the O_2. The concentration of O_2 varies as the patient's ventilatory pattern changes and is effective only for patients with an intact upper airway. Low-flow systems are comfortable and economical but do not supply an accurate or fixed concentration of O_2.

Nasal cannula

A nasal cannula provides a safe, simple, inexpensive low O_2 concentration to the patient. It is a double-pronged device of soft polyvinylchloride tubing that is placed in both nostrils, extended behind the ears, and secured under the chin (or if it has an elastic strap, around the patient's head). It is the most common method of O_2 administration, and inspired O_2 concentrations can be varied by adjusting the flow rate. Table 13–1 lists flow rates and approximate oxygen concentrations.

The nasal cannula is well-tolerated because it is light and allows the patient to eat and talk without removing it. It is useful for patients who cannot tolerate a face mask and for the chronically hypoxemic. Disadvantages include dryness of the nares—especially with a liter flow >6 liters/min (LPM)— irritation or annoyance with prolonged use, and pain in the front of sinuses with high flow rates. It does not deliver concentrations of O_2 >45%, may dislodge easily, and cannot be used when a patient has a nasal obstruction or when high humidity is needed.

Nursing interventions. (1) Set O_2 flow to desired rate before inserting cannula. (2) Lubricate cannula tips with water-soluble lubricant before inserting into nostrils. (3) Clean cannula q 8 hr. (4) Check openings

TABLE 13–1

Flow Rates and Approximate Oxygen Concentrations

Device	Flow liters/min	FIO_2 %
Nasal cannula	1	23–24
	2	23–28
	3	28–30
	4	32–36
	5	40
	6	44
Simple face mask	2–4	Not recommended
	5	40
	6	45–50
	8	55–60
Partial rebreathing mask	2–5	Not recommended
	6	35
	8	45–50
	10	60
Nonrebreathing mask	2–5	Not recommended
	6	55–60
	8	60–80
	10	90–100

FIO_2, fractional inspired oxygen concentration.

for patency. (5) Give good mouth and nose care. (6) Check for pressure areas under nose and over ears.

Nasal catheter

The nasal catheter is a green, pliable, plastic tube ~12 in long. It has a rounded tip with numerous holes in the end through which O_2 can pass. The nasal catheter delivers low-flow O_2 at concentrations of 23 to 44% at 1 to 6 LPM. The patient will receive O_2 regardless of whether he breathes through his mouth or nose. It is generally used for short-term treatment (e.g., postsurgical patients whose respiratory rate and depth are depressed from anesthesia). The need for frequent changes to alternate nostrils makes the catheter more irritating to patients. It is inexpensive, disposable, and can double as a suction catheter.

The nasal catheter cannot deliver O_2 concentrations >45% and does not permit a high degree of humidification. It may be drying to mucous membranes and may cause headaches or sinus pain if flow rates exceed 6 LPM. The nasal catheter tends to kink easily and may clog with secretions. Because of its invasive insertion route, the nasal catheter is less comfortable than the nasal cannula and gastric distension may occur in patients lacking epiglottal reflexes. Flow rates and approximate O_2 concentrations are the same as those found in Table 13–1 for nasal cannulas.

Nursing interventions. (1) Set O_2 flow to desired rate before inserting catheter. (2) Measure the desired length for insertion (distance from the tip of the nose to the lobe of the ear). (3) Lubricate catheter with water-soluble lubricant before inserting into nostril. (4) Change catheter q 8 hr, alternating nostrils. (5) Avoid trauma to nasal mucosa when inserting. (6) Check frequently to be sure catheter doesn't kink or clog. (7) Use with caution in comatose or debilitated patients.

Simple face mask

To provide O_2 concentration of >40% requires the use of a face mask. These devices fit over the mouth and nose, thereby increasing the volume of the potential O_2 reservoir. Simple, disposable face masks are made of plastic and have no reservoir bag. O_2 is supplied through small-bore tubing and exhaled air is vented through holes on each side of the mask. Consistency of the inspired O_2 concentration is dependent upon the mask fit and O_2 flow rate instead of the patient's inspiratory flow rate. A greater tidal volume and greater inspiratory flow rate will allow more room air to flow through the portholes or around the mask and decrease the actual O_2 concentration inspired.

Simple face masks are lightweight, easy to use, and effectively deliver high concentrations of O_2 of 40 to 60% at 5 to 8 LPM. They don't dry mucous membranes of the nose and mouth and, generally, humidification is adequate for most purposes. (Humidification can also be increased by using large-bore tubing and an aerosol mask.) Face masks are hot and confining, however, and interfere with talking and eating, making long-term therapy impractical. The tight seal necessary for higher O_2 concentration may cause discomfort and produce pressure over bony areas. *See* Table 13–1 for flow rates and approximate O_2 concentration.

Nursing interventions. (1) Mask must fit securely to ensure proper concentration of O_2. (2) Check for redness over bony areas. (3) Remove mask and dry skin when necessary. (4) Don't adjust strap too tightly. (5) Remove and clean mask q 8 hr. (6) Provide patient with an alternate source of O_2 during meals.

Partial rebreathing mask

The partial rebreathing mask is equipped with a bag that acts as an O_2 reservoir and allows the patient to rebreathe his exhaled air. The rebreathed expired air is mainly from anatomic dead space (where no gas exchange occurs) and contains mostly O_2 and no CO_2. The partial rebreathing mask is used when a high concentration of O_2 is needed (35 to 60% at 6 to 10 LPM) and can be set up to deliver 60% O_2. O_2 flow rate to the mask should be at least enough to prevent deflation of the bag so the patient will rebreathe only the O_2 from the reservoir bag, which is high in O_2 content. This increases his fractional inspired oxygen (FIO_2) concentration. The rebreathing mask has a safety valve that allows room air to be inhaled if the O_2 source fails and allows O_2 to be humidified easily.

The rebreathing mask requires a tight seal to ensure accurate O_2 concentrations. It is hot, confining, and may be irritating to the skin and interferes with eating and talking. The bag may twist or kink, and when used with high humidity it will cause water accumulation. It is impractical for long-term therapy. *See* Table 13–1 for flow rates and approximate oxygen concentrations.

Nursing interventions. (1) Always fill bag partly with O_2 before placing mask on patient. (2) Never let bag totally deflate during inhalation. (3) Avoid twisting the bag. (4) To fill bag initially, apply mask as patient exhales. (5) Provide patient with an alternate source of O_2 during meals.

Nonrebreathing mask

The nonrebreathing mask is similar to the partial rebreathing mask but has two one-way valves that prevent the rebreathing of exhaled air. One valve is between the reservoir and the mask. It allows gas flow into the mask from the reservoir but prevents gas flow back into the bag during exhalation. The second valve is at the exhalation port to prevent gas from entering the mask from the room during inhalation. Consequently, the patient breathes in pure O_2 from the reservoir bag and breathes out through the exhalation ports. A safety valve permits inspiration of room air if the O_2 source fails or if the bag collapses during inspiration. The nonrebreathing mask is used used in situations requiring high concentrations of O_2 (55 to 100% at 6 to 10 LPM) while not requiring a high degree of humidity. It delivers the highest possible concentration of O_2 and is indicated for short-term use.

(Patients who require long-term therapy of high concentrations of O_2 usually require intubation and mechanical ventilation.) The nonrebreathing mask can be converted to a partial rebreathing mask if necessary. Its disadvantages are that it requires a tight seal to ensure accurate O_2 concentrations, may irritate the skin, and it interferes with eating and talking. *See* Table 13–1 for flow rates and approximate O_2 concentrations.

Nursing interventions. (1) Always fill bag with O_2 before placing mask on patient. (2) Never let bag totally deflate during inhalation. (3) Avoid twisting the bag. (4) Keep mask snug to prevent inhalation of room air. (5) Make sure all rubber flaps remain in place. (6) Observe patients for signs of O_2 toxicity. (7) Provide patient with an alternate source of O_2 during meals.

Face tent

The face tent is an open, plastic mask that fits under the chin and has a rim that fits around the patient's face. It provides high humidity and is used when only small amounts of O_2 are needed. The face tent also substitutes for a face mask if the patient cannot tolerate having his nose covered. It doesn't dry mucous membranes but is hot and confining and may irritate the skin. It interferes with eating and talking and is impractical for long-term therapy. It is possible for the patient to rebreathe CO_2. The face tent can function as a high-flow system when attached to a Venturi nebulizer. Without the Venturi attachment, the fact tent does not deliver precise O_2 concentrations.

Nursing interventions. (1) Same as for simple face mask. (2) Check temperature of steam periodically to avoid burning the patient. (3) Watch for signs of O_2 toxicity. (4) Provide patient with an alternate source of O_2 during meals.

Trach collar or mask

A tracheostomy collar or mask delivers O_2 and humidity through a tracheostomy. The O_2 concentration depends on the O_2 flow and the type of collar; however, intake of room air through the port lowers O_2 concentration. A swivel adaptor allows tubing to attach on either side, and a frontal port permits suctioning. It is usually well tolerated, and elastic ties allow the mask to be pulled away from the tracheostomy without removing the collar. The collar must be kept clear of condensation because if it is allowed to collect, it can drain into the tracheostomy. The collar must be kept scrupulously clean; if secretions collect, the stoma may become infected. Other disadvantages are that heated aerosol may cause bleeding of a fresh tracheostomy, and intake of room air through the frontal port may decrease O_2 concentration.

Nursing interventions. (1) Check collar frequently to be sure it hasn't slipped away from tracheal opening. (2) Empty condensation buildup q 2 hr. (3) Remove and clean collar q 4 hr. (4) Do not cover exhalation port. (5) Make sure nebulizer delivers constant mist.

T-tube

The T-tube is a plastic, valveless, T-shaped device used to provide constant O_2 and humidity to patients with tracheostomies or endotracheal tubes. One side of the T-tube is connected to large-bore tubing coming from a heated nebulizer and the other side remains open and, with a chimney extension, can function as a partial rebreather. When attached to a Venturi system, the tube can function as a high-flow system. The T-tube must be kept clean and free of secretions to avoid its sticking to tracheostomy or endotracheal tubes. Condensation may collect in the tube and drain into the tracheostomy or endotracheal tube.

Nursing interventions. (1) Avoid contaminating T-tube when disconnecting it to suction the patient. (2) Be sure inspired gas remains at 90 to 100 F. (3) Clean T-tube with hydrogen peroxide and rinse with water to prevent buildup of secretions. (4) Empty condensation buildup q 2 hr. (5) Be sure humidifier or nebulizer has enough water to create a mist.

HIGH-FLOW SYSTEMS

A high-flow O_2 system is one in which the patient breathes only the gas that is being supplied by the appliance. This system allows for the deliverance of exact concentrations of O_2. O_2 enters the tubing at a given flow rate; when it reaches a restricted orifice (Venturi device), room air is entrained through the dilution ports, providing the patients with a constant FIO_2. O_2 concentration is dependent upon O_2 flow rate and the size of the orifice, and changes in depth and/or rate of respirations will not change the FIO_2 value.

Venturi mask

The Venturi mask is a lightweight plastic mask that employs the principles of the high-flow system to deliver predictable, consistent O_2 concentrations. It is helpful for delivering low, constant O_2 concentrations to patients with COPD. Concentration of O_2 is not affected by the patient's respiratory pattern, and diluter jets can be changed to change O_2 concentration. FIO_2 can be directly measured, and temperature and humidity of gases controlled. Venturi masks are well tolerated and do not cause drying of the mucous membranes. They can also be used to deliver humidity or aerosol therapy.

The disadvantages of the Venturi mask are similar to those of other face masks. They are hot and confining and interfere with talking and eating, and condensation may collect and drain on the patient (if humidification is used) and may cause skin irritation. If the mask does not fit snugly, tubing is kinked, if ports are blocked, or less than the recommended flow is used, FIO_2 can be altered.

Nursing interventions. (1) Monitor ABGs frequently. (2) Lubricate skin around mouth to prevent irritation. (3) Remove and clean mask q 8 hr. (4) Provide patient with an alternate source of O_2 during meals.

HUMIDIFIERS AND NEBULIZERS

Air is normally warmed and humidified as it travels through the nasopharynx to the lungs. Pure O_2 has an irritating effect upon mucous membranes, however, because it dries up secretions that normally keep the membranes moist. When the normal humidification system is bypassed because of an airway obstruction and/or endotracheal or tracheostomy tube, there is also not enough humidity in the air being breathed.

Numerous devices that compensate for the lack of humidity reaching the lower respiratory system are available. Water can be administered to the patient by humidification (which delivers water vapor to increase the relative humidity of air) and nebulization (which particulates water in a visible mist). (A suspension of fine solid or liquid particles in a gas is known as aerosol. Because most nebulizers are designed to deliver a maximum number of particles of a specific size, the nebulizer delivers aerosol therapy through nebulization. The term nebulization is commonly used interchangeably with aerosol.)

Cold bubble humidifier

The cold bubble humidifier consists of a plastic jar filled with distilled water and fitted with a cap that is attached to an air/O_2 source by means of a flowmeter. The O_2 passes into the jar and bubbles through the water, where it picks up more moisture, increasing its relative humidity when delivered to the patient. The cold bubble humidifier is relatively inexpensive, easy to use, and can be used with all oxygen masks, nasal cannulas, and nasal catheters. (The exception, however, is the Venturi mask, which doesn't need humidification because enough room air is entrained to maintain adequate humidity.) The cold bubble humidifier delivers 20 to 40% humidity but cannot be used on patients with a bypassed upper airway.

Nursing interventions. (1) Remove and clean equipment q 24 hr. (2) Refill the jar with sterile, distilled water to the indicated level as water evaporates.

Cascade bubble humidifier (heated)

The cascade or heated bubble humidifier utilizes heat to increase humidifier efficiency. This system delivers 100% humidity at body temperature and is the most effective of all evaporative humidifiers. The cascade humidifier is used on most ventilators to humidify inspired gas. It is important to check the water level on the cascade humidifier q 4 hr because the patient's mucosa can become irritated from breathing hot, dry air if the water is not maintained at the indicated level. The temperature control may become defective from constant use, allowing the device to under- or overheat.

Nursing interventions. (1) Check cascade temperature q 2 hr to be sure it doesn't exceed 101.6 degrees F. (2) Check the water level q 4 hr. (3) Refill the cascade with sterile, distilled water to the indicated level as water evaporates. (4) Attach reservoir tightly. (5) If unit overheats, unplug heating element and allow it to cool.

The Puritan Bubble Jet

The Puritan Bubble Jet consists of a wide-mouthed jar fitted with a cap that is attached to an O_2 source through a flowmeter. It is designed in such a way that it can be fitted with either a wide-bore corrugated tubing or with an adaptor for small-bore tubing and has a selector switch that can be set at either "bubble" or "jet." The Puritan Bubble Jet can be used as a bubble humidifier or as a simple nebulizer. The heated nebulizer provides 100% humidity; cool, it provides 40% humidity. When set at "bubble" it acts as a humidifier and when set at "jet" the water is dispersed into a fine mist. This equipment can be used with an aerosol mask, nasal catheter, cannula, or mask. The bubble jet provides adequate humidity for most purposes and is easy to use. It is useful for long-term therapy. Again, care should be taken to ensure that water doesn't fall below the indicated level. Condensation can collect in the wide-bore tubing, and tubing must be checked frequently to remove excess water.

Nursing interventions. (1) If the patient's upper airway is bypassed, use a heated nebulizer. (2) Check water level in reservoir q 4 hr. (3) Drain condensation from wide-bore tubing as soon as it collects. (4) Don't drain water back into the reservoir. (5) Check to be sure nebulizer is always delivering a fine mist. (6) Refill with sterile distilled water to the indicated level as water evaporates.

Mini-nebulizer or Maxi-mist

The mini-nebulizer is used to deliver aerosolized medication. This type of nebulizer conforms to the patient's own physiology and allows him to inhale and exhale on his own. It is a compact, hand-held, disposable device that can be used with compressed air, O_2, or a compressor pump and causes less air trapping than intermittent positive-pressure breathing (IPPB). Disadvantages to this device are that the procedure can take a long time if the patient requires the nurse's assistance, and medication may not distribute evenly if the patient doesn't breathe properly.

Nursing interventions. (1) Instruct the patient to breathe slowly and deeply. (2) Place the patient in sitting or high Fowler's position. (3) Assist by holding the apparatus as needed. (4) Instruct the patient to hold medicine cup upright during treatment. (5) Be sure all tubing connections are tight. (6) Check for a good mist.

Ultrasonic nebulizer

The ultrasonic nebulizer is indicated for use in the patient with thick secretions. It lacks a built-in O_2 delivery system and is used for short therapeutic sessions to mobilize secretions and facilitate a productive cough. The ultrasonic nebulizer produces a very dense mist of 100%

humidity, and 90% of its particles reach lower airways to loosen secretions. Ultrasonic nebulization has proved to be the most clinically effective of all devices in the liquification of thick and tenacious secretions. It may, however, precipitate bronchospasms in patients with asthma, and increased water absorption may cause overhydration leading to pulmonary edema or increased cardiac workload. The patient must be observed during and immediately after therapy and assessed continuously for signs of overhydration (weight gain, pulmonary edema, rales, electrolyte imbalances, etc.).

Nursing interventions. (1) Closely observe patient during and immediately after therapy and assist with secretions. (2) Observe for signs of overhydration. (3) Encourage the patient to take slow, deep breaths. (4) Observe for side effects, such as bronchospasm and dyspnea. (5) Auscultate breath sounds.

Side-stream nebulizer

The side-stream nebulizer attaches to a ventilator or to an IPPB machine to deliver aerosolized medication. The term side stream indicates the way in which the aerosol is injected into the gas stream. The IPPB machine mechanically dilates the bronchi and lungs and delivers bronchodilators to patients who can't generate the adequate tidal volume. It causes expansion of the lungs, which may prevent atelectasis, and counteracts pulmonary congestion of edema by decreasing venous return (as a result of the positive pressure). IPPB therapy helps clear bronchial secretions, and treatment may be given with 40 to 50% O_2 or compressed air, depending on the patient's needs. Some patients with COPD cannot tolerate the treatment. Gastric insufflation may occur, caused by swallowed air. The treatment cannot be used in case of hemoptysis, pneumothorax, active TB, or subcutaneous emphysema. Routine use of IPPB therapy is currently controversial. Some contend that this treatment is costly, complicated, and can be readily replaced by incentive spirometry and deep-breathing exercises. Others believe that these treatments facilitate lung expansion to promote an effective cough, deliver aerosolized medications into deeper air passages, decrease the work of breathing, and assist in the removal of secretions. Hospital policies and physicians' orders govern its use in individual institutions.

Nursing interventions. (1) Encourage the patient to take slow, deep breaths. (2) Don't allow the patient to become tachypneic. (3) Monitor pulse rates before, during, and after treatments; sudden increase could indicate adverse medication reaction. (4) Place the patient in sitting or high Fowler's position. (5) Avoid excess pressures and high flow rates. (6) Monitor COPD patients for CO_2 narcosis (lethargy, decreased respiratory rate). (7) Monitor pulmonary or cardiac deficiency patients for effects of decreased venous return (tachycardia, hypotension, headache). (8) Do not use immediately after pneumonectomy or lobectomy. (9) Avoid administering treatment immediately before or after meals because treatment may induce nausea, and a full stomach reduces lung expansion. (10) Never give treatment without medication in nebulizer because this could dry airways and make secretions more difficult to mobilize. (11) If patient is tolerating treatment, continue until medication in the nebulizer is exhausted (15 to 20 min).

COMPLICATIONS OF OXYGEN THERAPY

As with any other drug, the administration of O_2 is not without some hazards. Contrary to popular belief, O_2 is not an inflammable gas, but it has properties that support combustion. Therefore, policies such as a no-smoking rule must be enforced during its use. Extra precautions must be taken during hyperbaric O_2 therapy where high concentrations of O_2 are used under greater than atmospheric pressures, because any spark may cause a fire.

In addition to these physical hazards, physiologic hazards to the patient exist. In patients with COPD who depend on the hypoxic drive as their stimulus to breathe, high concentrations of O_2 eliminate this stimulus and cause apnea. These patients must be observed carefully, including frequent measurement of ABGs to be sure their FIO_2 are titrated to avoid hypoxemia without causing a respiratory depressive effect.

Absorption atelectasis may also result from the inhalation of high concentrations of O_2. This results from the effects of nitrogen being washed out of the lungs, leaving only O_2, CO_2, and water vapor in the alveoli. If even transient airway obstruction or hypoventilation occurs, O_2 is absorbed from the alveoli by pulmonary blood flow, causing alveolar collapse. When this happens, an increase in the intrapulmonary right-to-left shunt occurs. Absorption atelectasis is best prevented by having the patient properly perform deep-breathing exercises and, if necessary, hyperinflate his lungs.

Pulmonary O_2 toxicity may result in patients who receive high concentrations of O_2 (>50 to 60%) for prolonged periods (3 days to a number of weeks). Pulmonary O_2 toxicity has not, however, been demonstrated in man when 100% oxygen has been breathed for $\leq$24 hr. Therefore, O_2 toxicity should not be a consideration intraoperatively, during resuscitation procedures, or in transport situations. Rather, the relative danger of hypoxia and hypoxemia should predicate the use of essential O_2 therapy as the situation demands. Hypoxia is common, and the damage it can cause is rapid and severe, whereas pulmonary injury from O_2 is less common and relatively slow in developing. The lowest FIO_2 to maintain adequate cardiopulmonary homeostasis should be administered as early as possible in the clinical course. Frequent pulmonary assessment, including measurement of ABGs, is essential for the appropriate administration of O_2 therapy.

The adverse effect of excessive O_2 administration is directly proportional to the concentration of O_2 administered and to the duration of exposure. The brain and myocardium are very susceptible to changes in PO_2, and adequate arterial O_2 levels must be maintained to prevent major organ damage; arterial tensions should be maintained in the near normal range (70 to 100 mmHg) to assure tissue oxygenation. The decision for appropriate O_2 treatment modalities should be based on physical examination, cardiopulmonary assessment, and careful monitoring of essential clinical and serum studies.

AIRWAY MANAGEMENT

A patent airway is the single most important prerequisite in the successful management of respiratory care. Total airway obstruction will cause death from hypoxia within 5 to 10 min, even in a healthy individual who has been breathing room air. Nothing is more important in intensive respiratory care than appropriate assessment and management of the airway. There are many types of artificial airways, and the use of a specific one depends on the general condition of the patient, the reason for which the artificial airway is indicated, and the length of time that it will be needed.

An artificial airway may be needed (1) to bypass an upper airway obstruction; (2) to prevent aspiration of oral and/or gastric secretions; (3) to facilitate the care of chronic respiratory tract infections; or (4) to assist or control respirations over a prolonged period of time.

The types of artificial airways utilized can be divided into four categories: (1) pharyngeal airways, (2) esophageal airways, (3) endotracheal tubes, and (4) tracheostomy tubes.

PHARYNGEAL AIRWAYS

Pharyngeal airways are rigid or semirigid tubes made of rubber, metal, or plastic and are designed to fit into the upper airway. They maintain a patent airway and facilitate the removal of secretions for the unconscious patient who has no other difficulty with ventilation except an obstruction at the pharyngeal level. A pharyngeal airway is indicated for short-term use and must be replaced by endotracheal intubation if the patient is unable to maintain a patent airway. There are two types of pharyngeal airways.

Oropharyngeal airways

These conform to the curvature of the palate and extend from the lips to the pharynx. They lie between the posterior pharynx and the root of the tongue and thereby maintain a patent airway. These airways are designed so that a flange fits outside the lips and a suction catheter can easily be passed to the laryngopharynx. They are used only in the unconscious patient where the gag reflex is absent, because as consciousness returns, the stimulation (by the airway) may produce gagging, vomiting, and even laryngospasm.

Nursing interventions. (1) Select the appropriate-sized airway for the patient, because an oversized airway can obstruct breathing by depressing the epiglottis into the laryngeal opening. (2) To insert, have the patient supine with head tilted back, point the tip toward the roof of the mouth, gently advance the airway by rotating it 180 degrees, slide into place. (3) Tape the airway securely in place to prevent it from slipping out. (4) Position the patient on his side to decrease the possibility of aspiration if he vomits. (5) Suction secretions frequently. (6) Provide mouth care hourly. (7) Remove the airway when the patient can swallow on his own or when he's fully conscious and tries to dislodge it himself.

Nasopharyngeal airways

These are soft rubber or latex catheters that are passed through the nose, extending to the pharynx to just below the base of the tongue. The nasopharyngeal airway is designed as a funnel-shape to prevent slippage into the nasopharynx, and airway diameters range from 26 to 32 French. Its length is usually one inch longer than the distance between the nostril and the tragus of the ear. The nasopharyngeal airway is better tolerated by the semiconscious or alert patient, and it provides a means of suctioning the airway. It may cause pressure necrosis, and it kinks and clogs easily, causing airway obstruction. Other disadvantages include possible injury to the nasal mucosa on insertion, increased airway resistance caused by the catheter lumen, and possible sinus infection resulting from obstruction of sinus drainage. The nasopharyngeal airway should not be used in patients receiving anticoagulant therapy, with hemorrhagic disorders, sepsis, or pathologic nasopharyngeal deformities.

Nursing interventions. (1) Choose an airway with the external diameter slightly greater than the nostril opening. (2) Lubricate the airway with a water-soluble jelly before insertion. (3) Gently insert the airway its entire length through a nostril, and check the tube's position by observing the tip just behind the uvula. (4) Check for adequate breath exchange at the distal orifice. (5) Humidify administered O_2 and instill normal saline when suctioning to prevent mucus obstruction. (6) Suction secretions frequently. (7) Change the airway from one nostril to the other q 8 hr. (8) To remove, suction collected secretions, withdraw the tube in one smooth motion. (9) If tube gets stuck, do not use force but apply lubricant around the tube and nostril and gently rotate until tube is free.

ESOPHAGEAL AIRWAYS

The esophageal obturator airway (EOA) consists of an adjustable, inflatable, transparent face mask with a single port, attached by a snap lock to a blind esophageal tube. It has sixteen perforations at its proximal end through which air or O_2, which is blown into the port of the mask, is transferred to the trachea. The distal end of the tube is closed and circled by an inflatable cuff. When the EOA is inserted into the esophagus, the cuff is inflated with a set volume of air at the level just below the carina. This occludes the esophagus, prevents air from entering the stomach, and acts as a barrier against vomitus and involuntary aspiration.

The EOA is for temporary (2-hr maximum) emergency measures to maintain ventilation in the unconscious patient during cardiac or respiratory arrest. It is easy to place by personnel not experienced in or authorized to do tracheal intubation, but it can only be inserted after successful mouth-to-mouth resuscitation has established patency of the airway. Insertion of the EOA does not require visualization of the trachea or hyperextension of the neck so, therefore, it is useful for patients with suspected spinal cord injuries or facial trauma. The EOA is a desirable alternative to simple face-mask ventilation in circumstances where endotracheal intubation is not immediately feasible, but it should be replaced with intubation as soon as possible. The use of the EOA is frequently seen in the prehospital situation. Its disadvantages are that it is expensive, can be used only in patients $>$age 16 because pediatric sizes are not available, can cause pharyngeal trauma during insertion, can accidentally enter the trachea and occlude the airway, and may cause gastric distension and impaired ventilation if the cuff is not properly inflated or esophageal rupture if cuff pressures are too high. It's use is contraindicated in patients with corrosive poisoning, esophageal disease, or with a foreign body in the trachea.

Nursing interventions. (1) Inflate the esophageal cuff with 35 ml of air to check for leaks; then deflate before insertion. (2) Place the patient in a supine position with the neck in a neutral or semiflexed position before insertion. (Hyperextension may cause tube to enter the trachea instead of the esophagus.) (3) To insert, gently guide the airway over the tongue, into the pharynx, and then into the esophagus without applying any force. If any resistance is encountered, withdraw the tube slightly and readvance. (4) Once the tube is in place, inflate the cuff with 35 ml of air. (5) Perform mouth-to-tube ventilation through the face mask port, or connect the bag to a manual resuscitation bag. (6) To remove, deflate the cuff and withdraw it in one smooth motion following the natural pharyngeal curve to avoid esophageal trauma.

ENDOTRACHEAL INTUBATION

Endotracheal intubation is the oral or nasal insertion of a flexible, cuffed tube through the larynx into the trachea. It provides short-term ventilation when supplemental O_2 is needed, and the cuff provides a seal that permits positive-pressure ventilation and prevents the aspiration of oral secretions and gastric contents. It is indicated for (1) airway maintenance in patients who develop obstruction despite the use of a pharyngeal airway; (2) prevention of aspiration of stomach contents by sealing off the trachea from the digestive tract; (3) removal of tracheobronchial secretions in patients who cannot effectively cough; (4) provision of deep breaths with a manual resuscitation bag or mechanical ventilator; (5) provision of O_2 concentration $>$60% which cannot be adequately done with common face masks; (6) for patients who require controlled mechanical ventilation for 3 to 7 days. It is contraindicated in acute cervical spinal injury, severe local burns, epiglottitis laryngeal obstruction, infection, or vocal cord paralysis.

Nasoendotracheal intubation is the placement of an endotracheal tube into the nose and through the larynx into the trachea and is indicated for patients with jaw fractures, trismus, those requiring long-term intubation, and for the conscious patient. It is not suitable for patients with a deviated septum, fractured nose, or sinusitis. More comfortable for the patient than orotracheal intubation, nasotracheal intubation is more difficult to perform, and the size of the tube that can be used is usually smaller than the oral tube, determined by the nostrils and the turbinates. Disadvantages of the nasotracheal tube include (1) possibility of pressure necrosis in the nose; (2) kinking and clogging of the tube, causing airway obstruction; (3) interference with the cough reflex; (4) preventing the patient from talking when the cuff is inflated; (5) tracheal damage; and (6) respiratory infection, which may result from poor tube care.

Oropharyngeal intubation is the placement of an endotracheal tube into the mouth and through the larynx into the trachea and is indicated for use in situations where thick, copious secretions and/or lung problems exist, or where comfortable nasal intubation would require a tube of <8 mm. Oropharyngeal intubation is preferred in emergencies because insertion is easier and faster than nasotracheal intubation. Disadvantages of the oropharyngeal tube include (1) patient annoyance and discomfort because it stimulates salivation, coughing, and retching; (2) kinking and clogging, causing airway obstruction; (3) preventing the patient from talking when the cuff is inflated; (4) it can be bitten or chewed; (5) pressure sores on the sides of the mouth; (6) tracheal damage; (7) easy dislodgement; (8) respiratory infection, which may result from poor tube care.

Nursing interventions. (1)Adequate stabilization of the endotracheal tube is the highest priority of nursing care. Commercial tube holders and/or various ways of applying adhesive tape to the patient's face can ensure stability; make sure the tube is always securely positioned. Mark clearly the tube's exit port from the mouth with a pen or tape to monitor tube displacement. (2) Frequently assess airway status to maintain patency. (3) To ensure proper tube placement feel the tip for warm exhalations and listen for air movement, observe for chest expansion, auscultate the chest for bilateral breath sounds, obtain chest x-ray. (4) Suction secretions q 1 to 2 hr to prevent obstruction of the tube. (5) Provide frequent nasal or mouth care. (6) Maintain low cuff pressure by measuring pressure with manometer or minimal-leak technique. (7) To remove tube, suction inside and outside the tube, deflate the cuff, elevate the head of the bed 90 degrees, hyperinflate the lungs, auscultate for proper air leak, remove the tube in one smooth, outward and downward motion. (Do not attempt to remove the tube if you do not detect the air leak with the cuff deflated. This may result in total airway obstruction if the tube is removed.) (8) After removal, provide supplemental O_2 to help decrease airway irritation, patient discomfort, and laryngeal edema. (9) Be alert for signs of respiratory distress and/or upper airway obstruction (i.e., stridor, etc.). (10) Keep supplies necessary for re-intubation at the bedside for up to 12 hr after extubation.

Endotracheal tubes are fitted with standard adaptors and allow attachment to all ventilation and O_2 administration equipment. They also have low-pressure cuffs that have significantly lowered the incidence of tracheal erosion and necrosis. By hooking the tail of the pilot balloon to a manometer and measuring the pressure of the balloon (it should register 15 to 20 mmHg) or using the minimal-leak technique, the nurse can monitor cuff pressures to avoid these complications. The object of the minimal-leak technique is to place in the cuff the least volume of air that will allow occlusion of the airway during peak-positive inspiration. The cuff is completely deflated and slowly reinflated during inspiration until no leak is detected when auscultating over the trachea. When no leak is present, 0.2 to 0.3 ml of air is slowly removed from the cuff. A minimal leak should now be detected over the trachea when auscultating during inspiration. If the cuff pressure remains <15 to 20 mmHg and the patient is still getting the prescribed tidal volume, the cuff is adequately sealed. Recording the volume of air needed to inflate the cuff will provide an alert for possible problems. Tracheal dilation or erosion is indicated by a gradual increase in volume; a cuff rupture is indicated by a sudden increase in volume and requires immediate attention. Deflation of the cuff once q 8 hr is sufficient to detect overinflations, tracheal dilation, and erosion. More frequent deflation is not recommended.

Other complications of endotracheal intubation include apnea caused by reflex breath-holding; bronchospasm; aspiration of blood secretions or gastric contents; tooth loss or damage; and trauma to the lips, mouth, pharynx, or larynx. It can also result in vocal cord damage, as evidenced by persistent hoarseness for >7 days; glottic edema, which would require the application of steroids and of a vasoconstrictor directly on the edematous area; subglottic edema, which normally requires reintubation; and tracheal stenosis, erosion, and necrosis.

TRACHEOSTOMY TUBES

A tracheostomy is an opening made into the trachea for any of the following reasons: (1) to provide and maintain a patent airway; (2) to bypass an upper airway obstruction; (3) to facilitate the removal of tracheobronchial secretions in the patient with an ineffective cough; (4) to prevent the unconscious or paralyzed patient from aspirating secretions by closing off the trachea from the esophagus; (5) to permit the use of positive pressure ventilation; (6) to replace an endotracheal tube when such an airway is needed for a prolonged period of time; (7) intolerance of an endotracheal tube; (8) as a prophylactic procedure in anticipation of acute airway management problems (i.e., prior to radical neck surgery, patients with burns of the tracheobronchial tree, Guillain-Barré syndrome, etc.).

The tracheostomy tube is regarded by experts to be the most satisfactory artificial airway because it bypasses the upper airway and glottis and, therefore, avoids any complications in those areas. Tubes are usually fitted with adaptors, which permit proper attachment to respiratory therapy equipment. Tracheostomy tubes also permit administration of high degrees of humidity and ≤100% concentration of O_2; are easy to suction; allow the patient to eat and speak with some adaptation; and are generally well-tolerated. The inflated cuff prevents aspiration. Tracheostomy tubes are less likely to be dislodged than an endotracheal tube. The optimum time for a tracheostomy to be performed is as a controlled procedure in an operating room by a trained professional. The site for the standard tracheostomy is the second cartilaginous ring below the cricoid cartilage. If the airway is maintained with an endotracheal tube in place during the operative procedure, tracheostomy can proceed in an unhurried manner.

Complications of the tracheostomy procedure can be divided into three phases: immediate, late, and postextubation. **Immediate complications** are associated with the surgical procedure itself and generally occur within the first 24 hr. These include hemorrhage at the operative site; aspiration of secretions and/or blood; pneumothorax and pneumomediastinum caused by laceration of the pleural apices; subcutaneous and mediastinal emphysema, and air embolism. When the procedure is performed correctly by a trained professional, however, these immediate complications occur in <2% of all the tracheostomies performed.

Late complications are those that occur after 24 to 48 hr. Their incidence is as high as 40% and are directly proportional to the increasing duration of the tracheostomy. Infection and hemorrhage are always a problem after a surgical procedure. Airway obstruction is a potential danger that always exists in a patient with a tracheostomy and may be secondary to (1) occlusion of the cannula by secretions; (2) overdistension of the tracheal cuff, which allows the balloon to slip over the cannula opening; (3) kinking of the tube; (4) displacement of the cannula; (5) impingement of the cannula tip upon the carina as a result of a cannula that is too long or a low tracheostomy dysfunction; (6) swallowing dysfunction (which generally disappears when the tube is removed).

Postextubation complications include tracheal stenosis, tracheomalacia, and localized tracheal erosions. These problems are all associated with the same pathogenesis—tracheal ischemia caused by the pressure of the tracheostomy tube with or without its inflated cuff. The severity of permanent damage is directly proportional to the incidence of suboptimal airway care, cuff pressures >20 mmHg, tracheal infection, a large tube or cannula diameter relative to the tracheal diameter, damage from prolonged high dosage of steroids, and hypotension. Meticulous medical management and nursing care and the use of high-volume, low-pressure tracheostomy cuffs may decrease the incidence of these occurrences.

There are many types of tracheostomy tubes available, but basically they are all short, curved tubes with a flange that helps anchor the tube on the neck. Both cuffed and uncuffed tubes are available and they can be made of soft plastic or metal. The selection of the tube depends on the individual patient's needs. Several different types of tracheostomy tubes are listed below.

Single-cannula tubes

These tubes (e.g., Portex) have low-pressure cuffs and are used most frequently. They are disposable, and the cuff is bonded to the tube so it won't detach accidentally inside the trachea. Lack of an inner cannula increases the possibility of obstruction with encrusted secretions, but adequate humidification and meticulous pulmonary nursing care eliminate this problem. They are usually supplied with an obturator to facilitate cannulation. These tubes are changed only if there is a problem with the cuff or if accidental decannulation occurs.

Double-cannula tubes

These tubes may be made of plastic or metal. The outer cannula maintains the patency of airway and bears the cuff, whereas the inner cannula is easily removed for cleaning. An obturator is placed in the outer cannula during cannulation and removed immediately after tube placement. The Shiley tube is an example of a plastic, cuffed double-cannula tube. It is disposable and has a swivel adaptor, which facilitates patient mobility. The cuff is a high-residual, low-volume type that is bonded to the outer cannula. The Jackson tracheostomy tube is an example of a cuffless metal double-cannula tube. This tube, however, is becoming less frequently used in ICUs because of its rigid construction; it is usually used for weaning and for the long-term tracheostomy patient.

Fenestrated cannulas

These tubes have a large opening in the outer cannula to permit air to flow through the larynx. The inner cannula can be reinserted into the opening if mechanical ventilation becomes necessary. It also allows the patient to speak when it is plugged because air is passed through the larynx. This tube can be used in preparing patients for extubation because it allows normal breathing when it is plugged.

Regardless of the kind of tracheostomy tube used, the tube should not be changed as long as it is functioning properly, the airway is being humidified, and there are no infections present in the airway or tracheostomy wound. The tracheostomy tube should be changed only as the individual patient's condition indicates. Also, always inflate and deflate the cuff on the tracheostomy tube prior to insertion to ensure its patency.

Nursing interventions. (1) Tracheostomy care is performed using meticulous sterile technique—prn (but at least q 8 hr). (2) Always have emergency equipment close by (i.e., suction, additional tracheostomy tube with obturator). (3) Provide adequate humidity. (4) Observe stomal site for bleeding or signs of infection. (5) Clean inner cannula with cold water and hydrogen peroxide. (Hot water could cause protein in mucus to coagulate making cleaning more difficult.) (6) Suction outer cannula before reinserting cleaned inner cannula.

MECHANICAL VENTILATION

When a patient is unable to maintain alveolar ventilation adequate to prevent abnormalities in gas exchange, mechanical ventilatory therapy is indicated, e.g., when (1) PaO_2 cannot be maintained >50 mmHg by increasing O_2 concentrations; (2) $PaCO_2$ rises >50 mmHg and the pH drops <7.25; or (3) ventilation becomes exhausting and inefficient.

Clinical situations that may indicate the need for mechanical ventilatory support are as follows: (1) acute lung disease (e.g. acute pulmonary edema, adult respiratory distress syndrome, pneumonia, etc.); (2) restrictive lung conditions (e.g., pneumothorax, trauma); (3) neurologic and neuromuscular diseases (e.g., myasthenia gravis, Guillain-Barré syndrome); (4) respiratory center impairment (e.g., drug overdose, administration of respiratory depressants, cerebral injuries, etc.); (5) chronic obstructive pulmonary diseases (e.g., emphysema, asthma, etc.); (6) acute airway obstruction (e.g., foreign body, smoke inhalation, anaphylaxis, etc.); (7) respiratory and/or cardiac arrest; (8) drowning.

The goals of mechanical ventilation are to provide the pulmonary systems with the mechanical power to maintain efficient ventilation, to improve ventilation/perfusion (V/Q) relationships and oxygenation, and to decrease the work of breathing. Mechanical ventilators are divided into two major groups according to the pressure, or type of force, they employ.

NEGATIVE-PRESSURE VENTILATORS

Negative-pressure ventilators mimic the normal mode of ventilation by applying negative pressure to the patient's chest wall, causing the rib cage to expand, increasing intrathoracic subatmospheric pressure, allowing air to be drawn into the lungs. Passive exhalation occurs as soon as the negative pressure ceases.

The patient's body is placed within a chamber that can produce subatmospheric pressure. The head remains outside, permitting the patient to talk and eat in a normal manner. The respiratory rate is preset and the depth of inspirations is determined by the degree of preset negative pressure. The iron lung is a classic example of a negative-pressure ventilator. The cuirass respirator is an adaptation of the negative-pressure principle, but it is more portable than the iron lung because the negative pressure is only applied to the anterior thorax.

Using negative-pressure ventilators, long-term ventilatory support can be provided without the use of an artificial airway, and negative-pressure breathing facilitates normal intrathoracic hemodynamics. These ventilators are uncomfortable for the patient, however, and limit access to him. They are used today primarily for the patient with chronic restrictive lung disease who needs only intermittent periods of assisted ventilation.

POSITIVE-PRESSURE VENTILATORS

Ventilator support in acutely ill patients and in those with primary cardiopulmonary disease is best accomplished with the use of a positive-pressure ventilator. These apply an above-atmospheric pressure by means of an artificial airway (endotracheal tube or tracheostomy tube). The force of the above-atmospheric pressure causes an enlargement of the chest volume, which in turn creates a subatmospheric intrathoracic pressure, resulting in the atmospheric-subatmospheric pressure gradient that allows air to move into the lungs. Expiration occurs by remvoing the positive-pressure from the upper airway, thus providing elastic recoil of the lungs and chest, which creates a driving force from the alveolus to the mouth. There are three basic types of positive-pressure ventilators, each of which terminates inspiration according to a different principle.

Pressure-cycled ventilators

Pressure-cycled ventilators terminate inspiration when a certain preset pressure is reached. They allow the influx of air by the triggering of a valve by the patient or by means of an automatic rate control. The valves close when a preset pressure has been reached. Pressure-cycled ventilators are small, portable, and inexpensive, and they cannot deliver excessive airway pressures to the patient. The major disadvantage is that the volume of gas that the patient receives is variable, depending on changes in airway resistance and pulmonary compliance. Also, O_2 concentrations may vary unless an air-O_2 mixing device (blender) is used. This type of ventilator is best suited for the patient in need of short-term ventilatory support who has no preexisting pulmonary or thoracic conditions and who will not resist mechanical ventilation.

Time-cycled ventilators

Time-cycled ventilators terminate inspiration after a preset time. The volume of air delivered may be determined by the length of inspiratory time, the amount of pressure limit set, the patient's resistance, and compliance parameters. Some devices are capable of providing spontaneous breathing on patient demand between ventilator breaths. Tidal volume in time-cycled ventilators may vary from breath to breath. Many other characteristics of these ventilators are similar to those of volume-cycled devices.

Volume-cycled ventilators

Volume-cycled ventilators deliver a predetermined volume of air for ventilation in spite of intermittent changes in lung compliances or resistance. The preset tidal volume is delivered at whatever delivery pressure is required or that is dialed in, up to the peak pressure capability of the machine. Volume-cycled devices are the most widely used of all mechanical ventilators because they are easier to use and more versatile than pressure- or time-cycled ones. The machines have a number of advantages: (1) the volume of gas delivered is reliably controlled; (2) the tidal volume delivered remains constant despite pathophysiologic changes; (3) when very high pressures are generated and exceed the preset limiting (pop-off) pressure, excess volume will be vented to the outside air; (4) they are adaptable to various monitoring devices; (5) a consistent inspired O_2 concentration can be easily maintained. Disadvantages include: (1) expense; (2) lack of compensation for any leaks in the system; (3) potential for excessive intrathoracic and airway pressures.

Volume-cycled ventilators can be adjusted to meet specific needs of the patient according to his inspiratory effort. A brief description of the ventilatory modes is offered below.

Controlled mechanical ventilation (CMV). This control mode is used when the patient does not participate in the ventilatory cycle. The machine initiates inspiration, provides the power for inspiration, determines the rate of ventilation, and depth of the tidal volume. This mode is useful for an apneic patient, a heavily sedated patient, or one for whom a negative inspiratory effort is contraindicated (as in flail chest). The major disadvantage to CMV is that it does nto allow the respiratory rate to change along with the changing needs of the patient.

Assist-mode. This is a mechanism that allows the patient to control ventilator rate; inspiration will begin when the patient creates a subatmospheric pressure in the circuitry. When the inspiratory effort is strong enough to trigger the ventilator, a preset tidal volume is delivered. This is used for patients who have spontaneous but inadequate ventilation.

Assist/control mode (A/C): This mode allows the patient to trigger the machine to deliver a breath while regulating the machine with a predetermined backup rate. The A/C mode is most commonly used because it allows the patient to initiate an inspiratory breath while providing a fail-safe frequency that takes over if the patient fails to trigger breaths fast enough. This is particularly useful when the patient is subject to fatigue and hypoventilation.

Determination of the mode to be used must be based on the patient's individual clinical situation and not the capabilities of the equipment.

Intermittent mandatory ventilation (IMV): A variation in the augmented mode of ventilator control of breathing, IMV allows the patient to breathe on his own and, at certain intervals, a preset mandatory inspiration is delivered by the machine. All gas inspired (either spontaneous or from the ventilator) has the same temperature, humidity, and O_2 concentration. IMV encourages the patient to use and strengthen his respiratory muscles and is frequently used for weaning. The major difference between IMV and assisted ventilation is that with IMV, each spontaneous breath has a tidal volume that is determined by the patient's own inspiratory effort; with assisted ventilation, the patient initiates the breath and the ventilator delivers the tidal volume.

Synchronized intermittent mandatory ventilation (SIMV): This is similar to IMV except that when a mandatory breath with a predetermined volume is due, the machine waits until the end of the patient's spontaneous expiratory phase before delivering the breath. This eliminates the possibility that a mandatory inspiration could occur at the peak of a spontaneous inspiration and overdistend the lung.

Positive end-expiratory pressure (PEEP). An accessory mode used with positive-pressure ventilation, PEEP maintains positive pressure in the airways and alveoli throughout the expiratory cycle and is effective in patients who have lung units that tend to collapse (e.g., in atelectasis, alveolar instability, etc.). It is generally indicated in clinical situation where the patient is hypoxemic with a PaO_2 of 50 mmHg at a 50% FIO_2. The effects of PEEP are derived from the increase in the functional residual capacity (FRC), which is the volume of gas left in the alveoli at the end of a normal expiration. With an increased FRC, the alveoli remain open and ventilation and perfusion is improved, thus raising the PaO_2. PEEP is measured in cmH_2O.

The primary negative effect of PEEP is decreased CO and resultant decreased blood flows to major organs. Therefore, the recommended end-expiratory pressure is the lowest necessary to achieve a PaO_2 of 60 to 80 mmHg with an FIO_2 of $<50\%$ without interfering with tissue oxygenation. Pulmonary barotrauma is a significant complication of PEEP. It generally refers to lung rupture as a result of overdistension of alveoli by either excessive pressure, volume, or both. Pulmonary barotrauma includes: interstitial emphysema, pneumomediastinum, subcutaneous emphysema, pneumoperitoneum, and pneumothorax. It generally occurs in patients with a preexisting lung abnormality, chest-wall trauma, or those with decreased lung compliance. A significant incidence of barotrauma exists in situations where PEEP therapy of ≥ 10 cmH_2O is required, but therapy should not be withheld for fear of initiating barotrauma.

Continuous positive airway pressure (CPAP) is physiologically similar to PEEP but may be applied with or without a ventilator or use of an artificial airway. Positive airway pressure is maintained in the patient who is breathing spontaneously by means of a tight-fitting mask with an adjustable spring-loaded valve. CPAP is used primarily in the management of neonatal hyaline membrane disease.

POTENTIAL PROBLEMS IN CARE OF THE MECHANICALLY VENTILATED PATIENT

Mechanical ventilation has become an integral part of critical care nursing. This supportive therapy is not without some potentially fatal complications, however. The major goal of nursing management is to restore the patient to his optimal level of functioning while providing physiologic and emotional interventions. Problems commonly associated with the use of mechanical support devices and appropriate therapeutic nursing interventions are listed below.

Nursing interventions

Mechanical malfunction. (1) Make sure all alarms are activated at all times. (2) Each mechanically ventilated patient should have a manual resuscitation bag at the bedside. (3) If a malfunction occurs, immediately disconnect the patient from the ventilator and manually ventilate with the manual resuscitation bag. (4) Notify the respiratory therapy department.

Airway malfunction. (1) Suction patient as needed; instill normal saline to liquify secretions. (2) Empty condensation buildup in tubing frequently. (3) Auscultate breath sounds frequently. (4) Record cuff volumes each time inflated.

Pulmonary barotrauma. (1) Avoid high-pressure settings for high-risk patients (those with COPD, emphysematous blebs, etc.). (2) Observe for: tracheal deviation, triggering of high-pressure alarm, sudden change in breath sounds, tachypnea, tachycardia, hyperresonance to percussion. (3) If this occurs, notify physician and prepare for chest tube insertion.

Hemodynamic alterations (decreased CO and decreased venous return). (1) Observe for: decreased BP, increased or decreased central venous pressure (CVP), decreased pulmonary artery pressure (PAP), restlessness, decreasing level of consciousness, decreased urine output, diminished peripheral pulses, slow capillary refill, pallor, fatigue, chest pain.

Renal malfunctions (positive water balance). (1) Monitor intake and output, daily weights. (2) Examine skin turgor and check for edema. (3) Observe for: changes in ABGs, electrolytes, decreased vital capacity; auscultate breath sounds for rales and/or wheezes. (4) Rotating tourniquets may be necessary.

GI malfunction. (1) Observe for: abdominal distension, decreased Hb and Hct, positive hematest in stool and/or gastric drainage, black tarry stool. (2) Give antacids and other medications as prescribed. (3) Place nasogastric tube. (4) Auscultate bowel sounds.

Pulmonary atelectasis and infection. (1) Provide adequate humidification to inspired air. (2) Auscultate breath sounds. (3) Turn patient q 2 hr. (4) Provide chest physiotherapy; suction and hyperinflate lungs to provide good pulmonary hygiene. (5) Use aseptic technique and sterile equipment when suctioning.

Tracheal tissue trauma. (1) Give mouth care q 2 to 4 hr. (2) Change position of oral tube every day. (3) Provide support for tubing attachments. (4) Give proper cuff care; use high-volume low-pressure cuff. (5) Apply intermittent suction to catheter only during withdrawal, not insertion.

O_2 toxicity. (1) Observe for: burning chest pain on inspiration, dry hacking cough, dyspnea, decreased PaO_2, decreased compliance. (2) Monitor ABGs frequently. (3) Maintain good pulmonary hygiene. (4)

Reduce O_2 concentration as soon as possible. (5) Use PEEP as needed to increase FRC.

Loss of respiratory muscle tone. (1) Use IMV when possible. (2) Encourage patient to cough up secretions if able. (3) Wean as early as possible. (4) Get patient out of bed.

Nutritional deficiency. (1) Give parenteral or enteral nourishment. (2) Check bowel sounds. (3) Monitor weight, intake and output. (4) Initiate bowel regimen as appropriate.

Decreased mobility. (1) Keep skin clear and dry. (2) Change position q 2 hr. (3) Practice passive range of motion qid. (4) Get patient out of bed as tolerated. (5) Ambulate as tolerated. (6) Allow patient to participate in activities of daily living as much as possible.

Psychological trauma. (1) Medicate appropriately for pain and/or sedation. (2) Explain all procedures to patient. (3) Allow patient and family to participate in all therapeutic measures. (4) Provide environmental stimulation. (5) Provide undisturbed rest periods. (6) Provide method for patient to communicate with family and staff. (7) Keep call bell within reach.

Failure to wean. (1) Determine if clinical condition is stable enough for spontaneous respiration. (2) Provide psychological support. (3) Explain all procedures to the patient. (4) Allow for rest periods. (5) Wean during the day, allow patient to rest at night. (6) Use IMV/SIMV.

WEANING

Planning for the weaning process begins when mechanical ventilatory therapy is initiated. The patient should be told at the beginning of treatment that this is a temporary supportive measure only and that he will be able to breathe again spontaneously. Failure to initiate the weaning process as soon as the patient can tolerate it can produce an emotional and/or physical dependence upon the ventilator. Weaning should begin when there is evidence of significant improvement or reversal of the underlying disease process.

When a time is chosen for a trial of spontaneous breathing the procedure is carefully explained to the patient and base-line values for ABGs, pulse rate, respiratory rate, and BP are obtained. The patient should be placed in a sitting or high Fowler's position and the airway well suctioned to prevent aspiration of secretions. Adequate oxygenation and humidification must be provided via a T-tube, making sure connections are tight and adequate flow is provided. Generally, the O_2 concentration needed is ~10% higher than the ventilator FIO_2, unless the PaO_2 is unusually high on the ventilator setting. In patients with a potential for respiratory depression (e.g., COPD patients who depend on the hypoxic stimulus to breathe) the FIO_2 is regulated to maintain PaO_2 50 to 60 mmHg maximum.

When the patient is removed from the ventilator, vital signs and mental status changes are monitored q 5 min for the first 30 min. ABGs are obtained at the end of 30 min; and spontaneous ventilation can be continued if the PaO_2 is $\leq$80% of the preweaning value, the pH is greater than 7.30 and stable, and the patient appears to be tolerating spontaneous ventilation without dyspnea. Weaning should be done during the day, when there is maximum stimulation for the patient, with a return to the ventilator during the night.

An alternate method of weaning may be needed if the patient is not able to tolerate spontaneous ventilation for even short intervals. IMV provides a gradual transition from mechanical ventilation, allowing the patient to breathe on his own and the number of mandatory breaths to be slowly decreased until he can breathe completely independent of the ventilator. The number of mandatory breaths can also be increased during the night, allowing the patient to rest after the work of spontaneous breathing during the days.

Weaning is an important aspect of supportive ventilation, and the main responsibility of the nurse during the first attempts at spontaneous breathing are to decide if the trial should be aborted and the patient returned to the ventilator. Weaning should be terminated if the patient develops tachypnea, respiratory distress, cyanosis, paradoxical movements of the abdomen, extrasystoles, arrhythmias, discomfort, or progressive obtundation agitation. Physiologic parameters that would indicate the need to reinstitute mechanical ventilation are PaO_2 <70 mmHg, $PaCO_2$ increasing at a rate >1 mmHg/min, pH <7.25 or >7.60, pulse rate <60 or >120, respiratory rate <8/min or >30 min, tidal volume <3 ml/kg, BP change of >20 mmHg systolic or >10 mm diastolic, mean arterial pressure change >15 mmHg, or pulmonary capillary wedge pressure >20 mmHg.

Failure to wean may result from increased ventilatory requirement of work of breathing, decreased muscular strength and/or iatrogenic reasons. Successful weaning requires a systematic team approach to help the patient make a successful transition from the mechanical ventilator to spontaneous breathing.

HIGH-FREQUENCY VENTILATION

The general rule of thumb for setting machine parameters on mechanical ventilators to achieve maximum alveolar ventilation is to deliver large tidal volumes combined with slow respiratory rates, which can lead to high inflation pressures, pulmonary barotrauma, and alterations in hemodynamics. A new mode of artificial ventilation is being investigated to reduce or possibly eliminate these complications. High-frequency positive pressure ventilation (HFPPV) utilizes small tidal volumes (3 to 5 ml/kg) at very high respiratory rates (60 to 100/min) under considerable pressure (100 to 3,000 torr or mmHg). This causes little distension of the lung parenchyma and less mean airway pressure change, minimizing the dangers of pulmonary barotrauma and hemodynamic alterations. High-frequency oscillation (HFO) and high-frequency jet ventilation (HFJV) are technical modifications of HFPPV.

High-frequency ventilation has been used during endoscopic and surgical procedures and more recently in patients with acute respiratory failure complicated by bronchopleural or tracheoesophageal fistulas. Nursing care of patients with high-frequency ventilation is complex and demands a new degree of knowledge and expertise. Problems in the clinical use of HFPPV result from the lack of understanding of its mechanism and the difficulties in providing ventilation safely. Problems of inadequate humidification of rapidly flowing gas, inadequate alarm and pressure safeguard systems, mechanical breakdowns, and catheter obstruction need to be addressed during the investigational phase, because HFPPV will be an integral part of respiratory support in the future.

CHAPTER 14

HEMODYNAMIC MONITORING

Thomas Hijeck

FRAMEWORK

A basic understanding of hemodynamic monitoring is necessary for critical care nurses. This should include familiarity with the various pressure wave forms, catheters, their indications for use, complications, and nursing responsibilities. In addition, knowledge of the typical strain gauge transducer, its functioning, and calibration are invaluable to understanding hemodynamic monitoring and to directing intensive nursing care. This chapter discusses many facets of hemodynamic monitoring and will aid the professional nurse in problem solving and caring for the critically ill patient.

THE HEART AS A PUMP

A review of the anatomy and physiology of the heart (*see* Chapter 2) shows that it can be likened to two separate pumps connected consecutively. Each pump consists of two chambers, the atrium and ventricle, separated by a one-way valve—the tricuspid valve on the right and the mitral valve on the left. Blood is prevented from being regurgitated into each ventricle by another set of unidirectional valves, the pulmonary valve on the right and the aortic valve on the left. Proper functioning of the heart is dependent on many variables, including the competence of the valves, the strength of contractions, and the amount of blood available to pump.

Although the heart is a living organ, it is a mechanism conforming to physical laws and properties. The two major laws that affect cardiac function are Starling's principle and the Law of Laplace.

Starling's principle

This principle states that by increasing the length of ventricular fibers at the end of diastole, the stroke volume is increased, up to a finite point. Clinically, this function is demonstrated by measuring left atrial pressures (LAP) or pulmonary capillary wedge pressures (PCWP). These are accurate approximations of left ventricular end-diastolic pressures (LVEDP) (normal: 6 to 12 mmHg). Stroke-volume measurements can be graphically plotted against LVEDP measurements; the resulting curve is known as Starling's curve. The curve will show that at ~18 mmHg pressure, the slope begins to curve downward, and further increases in LVEDP produce a decrease in CO and stroke volume. The Starling curve shifts position, depending on myocardial functioning and metabolism; a normal heart will have a higher CO at 18 mmHg pressure than will a damaged heart. In most situations, however, CO and stroke volume are maximized for everyone at 18 mmHg pressure.

Laplace's law

Laplace's law states that wall tension in a cylindrical container is directly proportional to the radius of the vessel multiplied by the pressure within the vessel. Wall tension has been positively correlated with myocardial O_2 consumption and is essentially equivalent to contractility, the measure that reflects the speed of ventricular muscle-fiber shortening. Pressure and radius can be measured by hemodynamic monitoring and echocardiogram. Clinically, the application of this law tends to modify Starling's principle. As LVEDP increases with administration of fluids (increasing stroke volume), O_2 consumption increases with the enlarging ventricular radius and wall tension. With a compromised heart, administration of unnecessary fluids can lead to decreased contractility and decreased CO.

Cardiac output

CO is the most important parameter with which clinicians are concerned in assessing overall myocardial function. If CO is not sufficient to meet the body's requirements, then a type of failure ensues. The formula for calculating CO is CO = heart rate × stroke volume. Heart rate is measured in bpm. Stroke volume is determined by preload, afterload, and contractility. (Preload is a measure of the filling pressures of the heart and an index of hydration status, usually determined by monitoring PCWP and LVEDP. Afterload is a measure of the pressures that the ventricle must overcome to eject blood, determined by the resistance caused by arteriolar constriction.) Measurement of these parameters provides the clinician with the basis for implementing therapy to improve CO. The application of Starling's principle and Laplace's law affects preload and contractility, whereas systemic vascular resistance (SVR) affects afterload. If preload is increased to the point at which ventricular filling and contractility are maximized, and afterload is decreased to the lower limits of the normal range, then CO is maximized.

Forward flow

Another important point to be considered is the concept of forward flow. For blood to move correctly through the heart, all valves must be fully patent, competent, and unidirectional. Otherwise blood would move in a "to-and-fro" motion as the pressure changed in the chambers and vessels. Furthermore, for forward motion to occur, the pressure in the pumping chamber or vessel must be greater than the pressure in the receiving chamber or vessel. If the pressure in the ventricle were never less than that of the atrium, the atrioventricular valve would never open and the ventricle would never fill.

The heart delivers a pulsatile pressure with each contraction. Pulsatile flow, therefore, oscillates in cycles of amplitude. Variations in the amplitude can be caused by surrounding pressures resulting from the location of the heart and great vessels in the chest cavity. During normal inhalation, the pressure in the cavity is negative, thus aiding venous blood return to the heart, and during normal exhalation, the pressure becomes positive, inhibiting venous blood return. Preload and contractility are altered to some degree, which leads to a rhythmic decrease/increase in pressures. This is most noticeable in pulmonary vasculature.

DISEASE PROCESSES

There are a large number of disease processes that may require hemodynamic monitoring. Monitoring is required whenever it is essential to know the current and precise data of filling pressures, systemic or pulmonary pressures, or output status of the cardiovascular system on a continuous basis. Diseases or situations that require hemodynamic monitoring can be categorized as follows: (1) congenital or developed anatomic anomalies, which include left-to-right shunts (e.g., patent ductus arteriosus, ventricular septal defect), right-to-left shunts (e.g., Fallot's tetralogy), and obstructions to flow (e.g., valvular stenosis); (2) hemodynamic compromise, including pressure overload (e.g., extreme hypertension), volume overload, and volume depletion (e.g., extreme dehydration, gram-negative or gram-positive sepsis); (3) ischemic situations that demonstrate frequent wide vital sign changes, (e.g., infarctions and profound ischemia); (4) metabolic compromise, including profound increase in metabolism, (e.g., gram-negative septic shock, extreme hyperthyroidism) and mechanical or chemical manipulation; (5) surgery, (e.g., major abdominal surgery resulting in third spacing, manipulations of the ANS, or manipulations of the major vessels); (6) trauma resulting in large volume losses; or (7) medication therapies that rapidly and extremely affect preload, afterload, contractility, or BP.

ASSESSMENT

Hemodynamic assessment of the patient can be divided into noninvasive and invasive approaches. Both approaches yield valid, useful information that can dictate therapeutic interventions.

Noninvasive assessment

Urine output. Renal function is to some extent dependent on mean BP. If a patient who is normally hydrated has normal kidneys but low urine output, the BP and CO must be further assessed.

BP. Measurement by sphygmomanometer generally yields accurate results except in patients who have peripheral vasoconstriction.

Pulse amplitude. A bounding pulse can be indicative of rapid blood runoff, typically seen in aortic regurgitation. Weak, thready pulses are seen in low CO states.

Extremity temperature. Temperature can be indicative of vasoconstriction or vasodilation. Markedly cool extremities are associated with shock or the administration of vasoconstrictive medications.

Cardiac auscultation and palpation. These techniques can provide information regarding pump function and explanations for signs and symptoms. Presence of an S_4 is often associated with a noncompliant ventricle during the time of infarction. An S_3 is associated with a ventricle in failure. The presence of murmurs, thrills, or heaves, in specific locations and during specific points in the cardiac cycle, is indicative of pathology and sequelae.

Pulmonary auscultation. The presence of rales often indicates increasing PCWP and decreasing LV function.

Level of consciousness. This parameter may be indicative of cerebral perfusion. A decrease in CO would result in decreased blood flow to the brain, which could cause somnolence.

Peripheral/central vascular examination. Examination of the internal jugular veins can reveal or suggest hyper- or hypovolemia or right-sided heart failure.

Invasive assessment

Invasive hemodynamic assessment is often used in the ICU along with continued noninvasive assessment. Invasive catheters can be used to accurately measure pressures and cardiac function even in the most severely ill patient.

Intra-arterial pressure. Measurement of pressures in the lumen of the vessel is more accurate than measurement with a sphygmomanometer in patients who have marked vasoconstriction.

Central venous pressure (CVP). Measurement of CVP provides similar information to that obtained by measuring the height of the internal jugular vein. The measurement is more accurate because the catheter is placed within the superior vena cava.

PCWP. A catheter is placed in a major terminal branch of the pulmonary artery. The catheter is advanced until the balloon tip (inflated with 1.5 ml of air or CO_2) occludes the branch and measures only pulmonary capillary pressures. When the mitral valve is open (at end diastole), this pressure is reflective of LV function.

LAP. The catheter provides similar information to the PCWP catheter but is placed in the left atrium during open-chest surgery.

CO. Measurements of CO provide information on a goal of hemodynamic assessment: is CO sufficient for the body's needs? With establishment of CO, the basis for calculation of other parameters, such as SVR, is also established.

Table 14–1 lists normal hemodynamic values.

HEMODYNAMIC MONITORING

GENERAL PROCEDURES

Although there is a large variety of equipment available and the required supplies will vary according to the equipment used, the following setup is typical. Equipment needed will include: pressure tubing with Luer Lok

TABLE 14–1

Normal Hemodynamic Values

Parameter	Normal value
Right atrium pressure	
Mean	−1 to +7 mmHg
Right ventricle pressure	
Systolic	15–25 mmHg
End diastolic	0–8 mmHg
Pulmonary artery pressure	
Systolic	15–25 mmHg
Diastolic	8–15 mmHg
Mean	10–20 mmHg
Pulmonary wedge pressure	
Mean	6–12 mmHg
Cardiac output	4–8 liters/min
Cardiac index	2.5–4.0 liters/min/m^2
Systemic vascular resistance	950–1300 dynes/sec/cm^{-5}
Pulmonary vascular resistance	155–255 dynes/sec/cm^5

Adapted with permission from American Edwards Laboratories. Understanding hemodynamic measurements made with the Swan-Ganz catheter. American Edwards Laboratories. American Hospital Supply Corp., Santa Ana, Calif.

connections; catheter (arterial, pulmonary artery, etc.); continuous flush device; disposable transducer dome; transducer; monitor; paper recorder; normal saline, heparinized with 1 U heparin/1 ml of saline; pressure bag; three-way stopcocks.

Under aseptic conditions connect all tubing and stopcocks. Figure 14–1 depicts the typical monitoring system. Starting with the 6 in of tubing extending from the patient, there is a three-way stopcock, 6 ft of pressure tubing, a continuous-flush device with one tail connected to the heparinized saline pressurized to 300 mmHg and the other tail connected to the disposable transducer dome. The dome has a three-way stopcock on each port. All ports that are unused must have a sterile unvented cap in place.

Calibration

For the monitoring system to be accurate, the equipment must be calibrated to known standards. Nurses are usually concerned with three features of equipment accuracy: stability, sensitivity, and linearity. **Stability** refers to the tendency of equipment to drift; that is, once the equipment is set to read zero at atmospheric pressure, it should read zero indefinitely as long that pressure is applied. Any change from that reading is drift.

Sensitivity describes the ratio of the signal in millivolts (mv):the recorded wave form in mm. This ratio is often referred to as gain; it can be adjusted as needed. For example, the nurse has the option of 25 mm displacement equaling 100 mmHg pressure, 160 mmHg pressure, 200 mmHg pressure, etc.

Linearity refers to constancy of the above-described ratio. The system remains linear if the ratio is equal at all ranges of input. Practically, linearity is demonstrated by applying a known pressure to the system and observing the response after a specific gain is selected; e.g., if a gain of 5 mm-equals-20-mmHg-pressure is selected, then in a linear system, when 20 mmHg is applied, a 5-mm deflection is expected; when 40 mmHg is applied, a 10-mm deflection is expected; when 60 mmHg is applied, a 15-mm deflection is expected.

Calibrating procedure. (1) At the dome, turn the stopcock off to the patient and open to the atmosphere. (2) Press the zeroing button on the monitor. The monitor should read zero. If not, adjust the zeroing control until the wave aligns with the zero mark. (3) Adjust the paper recorder to the zero line. (4) Apply a known pressure to the transducer with either a mercury column or electronic calibrator. This known pressure is usually slightly above the highest expected pressure being measured. (5) Observe the monitor pressure reading and adjust the gain to match the pressure. (6) Observe the recorder and adjust its separate gain control if necessary. (7) Continue to apply known pressures at regular intervals through the entire range of expected pressures. Observe the response on the monitor and recorder. If it varies by more than an accepted amount, it must be electronically tested by biomedical engineering.

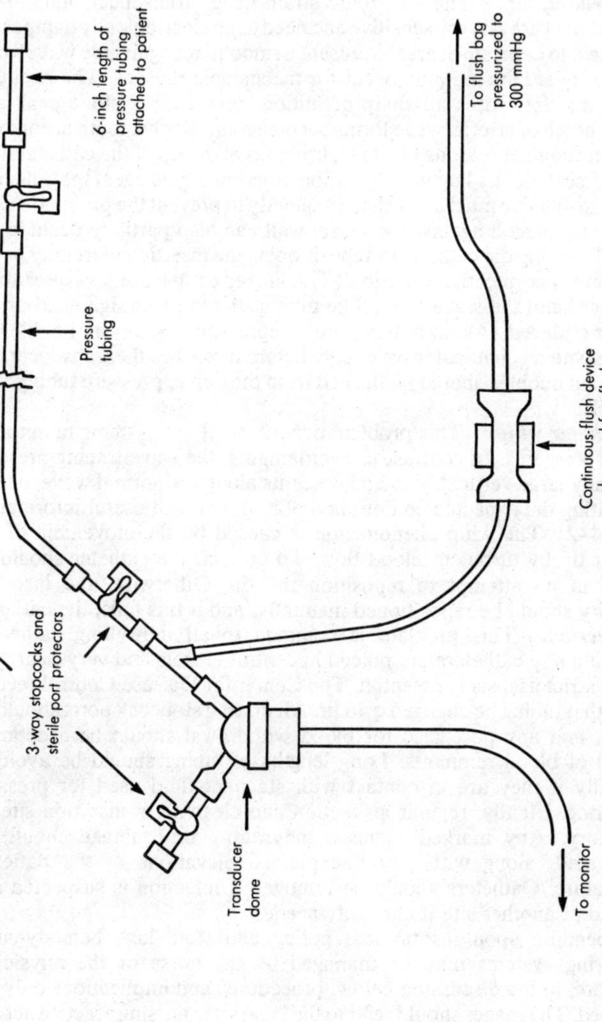

Figure 14–1. A typical hemodynamic monitoring system.

Common problems

There are common problems associated with all hemodynamic monitoring systems. They are overdamping of the wave form, catheter whip, and infection.

Overdamping. The electronic strain gauge transducer, amplifiers, and recorders are all very sensitive and need to be electronically dampened, or blunted, to a certain degree to present a smooth, recognizable wave form; however, overdamping may occur for mechanical reasons. The resulting wave form often loses all sharp definition so that the systolic peak and dicrotic notch of arterial wave forms become rounded or smooth in contour. Some mechanical reasons are: (1) Thrombus at the tip of the catheter may partially occlude the lumen. Aspiration or use of a lytic agent may clear it. Otherwise the line must be flushed frequently to prevent the problem. (2) A catheter tip placed against the vessel wall can also partially occlude the lumen. Flushing the catheter or repositioning the insertion extremity or the catheter may correct the condition. (3) A kinked catheter or pressure tubing may overdamp the wave form. The tubing should be straightened or the catheter replaced. (4) Air bubbles are compressible, so *any* air bubble will absorb some mechanical wave energy before it reaches the transducer. To correct, all bubbles should be flushed from the dome, pressure tubing, and stopcocks.

Catheter whip. This problem occurs mostly in systems monitoring arterial pressures. In contrast to overdamping, the wave tracing presents with many large vertical rises and descents along the normal wave, nearly obliterating the expected contour and obscuring much useful information (Fig. 14–2). The whip phenomenon is caused by the movement of the catheter tip by turbulent blood flow. To correct, the catheter should be flushed in an attempt to reposition the tip. Otherwise, the insertion extremity should be repositioned manually, and if this fails, the catheter.

Infection. This problem is common to all indwelling catheters. Because many catheters are placed in central vessels and very near vital organs, strict asepsis is essential. The Center for Disease Control recommends that tubing be changed q 48 hr. All unused stopcock ports should be capped, and any port used for blood withdrawal should be aseptically cleaned of blood remnants. Long lengths of tubing should be avoided, especially if they are in contact with stagnant fluid used for pressure monitoring. Finally, regular inspection and cleaning of insertion sites is mandatory. Any marked redness, induration, or drainage should be investigated, along with any unexplained elevations of the patient's temperature. Catheters should be removed if infection is suspected and replaced at another site if clinically needed.

Depending upon institutional policy and state law, hemodynamic monitoring systems may be managed by the nurse or the physician. Therefore, in the discussion below, procedures and implications only are described. The reader should refer to the local state nursing practice act and institutional regulations for further information on roles and responsibilities.

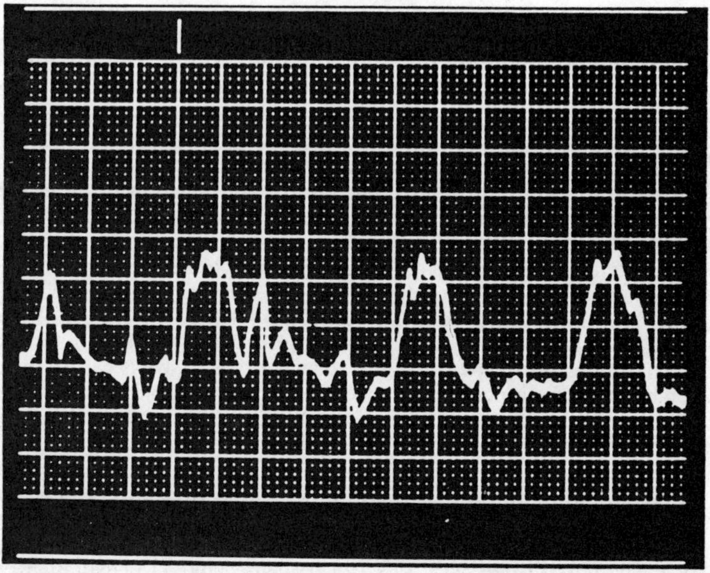

Figure 14–2. Catheter whip. *Reprinted with permission from* American Edwards Laboratories, American Hospital Supply Corp., Santa Ana, Calif.

CENTRAL VENOUS PRESSURE MONITORING

CVP monitoring is instituted when there is concern over right heart function and general fluid status. Very little of the information obtained is useful for assessing left heart function, and therefore it is inadvisable to make any decisions using this data alone. CVP readings are indicated in instances of hyper- or hypovolemia caused by hemorrhage, IV therapy, fluid shifts after surgery, or severe dehydration.

Equipment. Because CVPs are low, there is no need to use pressurized flush bags unless electronic monitoring is being instituted. Otherwise, only a manometer (preferably disposable) marked in centimeters is attached in-line via a three-way stopcock to the IV drip and the patient.

Procedure. The catheter is usually placed by a physician with the terminus just prior to the right atrium (RA). Approaches may be made through the internal jugular, basilic, or femoral veins. The right subclavian vein is preferable to the left because there is less risk of damaging the lymph duct.

Readings. Ideally the patient should be flat in bed and the zero point of the manometer positioned level with the phlebostatic axis, the point that lies level with the RA, located at the left midaxillary line and the fourth intercostal space. Fluid is fed into the manometer from the IV bottle to a level above the expected reading. The stopcock is then opened to the manometer and patient, and the fluid level drops. The level will fluctuate, both with cardiac contractions and with respirations. The point at which the fluid column stabilizes is the correct reading. It should be noted that a single determination is not as important as the *trends* of all determinations, combined with the patient's signs and symptoms.

Wave forms. If the central venous catheter is connected to an analog recorder, one will see three distinct positive waves: *a, c, v* (Fig. 14–3). Each positive wave is followed by a negative wave: *x*, x_1, and *y* respectively. These correspond to the electromechanical action occurring. The positive *a* wave corresponds to atrial contraction, with the *x* descent corresponding to atrial relaxation. If a *c* wave is present, it is reflective of closure of the tricuspid valve, with the x_1 descent occurring when the septum moves downward during ventricular systole. The positive *v* wave is caused by a combination of ventricular contraction bulging the tricuspid valve into the atrium and the concomitant filling of the atrium from the central veins. The *y* descent reflects the opening of the tricuspid valve and blood leaving the atrium.

Abnormal findings. Increased CVPs can be caused by (1) volume overload, (2) right ventricular (RV) failure, (3) tricuspid stenosis, (4) pulmonary hypertension, (5) cardiac tamponade, or (6) inaccurate zeroing or calibration. Decreased CVPs can be caused by (1) dehydration or hypovolemia, (2) misplacement of the catheter, or (3) inaccurate zeroing or calibration.

Complications. Complications include (1) dislocation of the catheter into the RA, (2) hemorrhage produced by disconnected tubing, and (3) air emboli.

Because a central venous catheter is placed with its terminus in the superior vena cava, it is highly possible that air emboli can be drawn into the catheter during inhalation. To prevent this condition, the patient should exhale or cough whenever the catheter is being disconnected or opened. If the patient is unconscious, he should be placed in Trendelenburg's position so that venous pressure will increase. If, despite these precautions, air does enter the line, the nurse may immediately apply a sterile syringe and withdraw the air. Unless the patient has a right-to-left shunt, it is unlikely

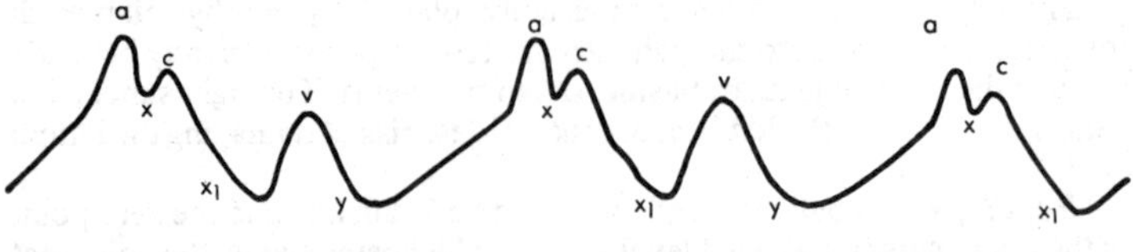

Figure 14–3. Central venous pressure wave forms.

that a small bubble will cause any harm. Nonetheless, caution should be taken to avoid air introduction.

ARTERIAL LINES

Direct arterial pressure readings are indicated when continuous recordings of pressures are warranted because of inaccuracy of sphygmomanometry, severe hypo- or hypertension, or potent vasoactive medications are utilized.

Equipment. Commonly a catheter-over-the-needle system identical to systems for IV puncture is used. In addition, because pressures are high, a continuously pressurized and heparinized flush system must be connected to the catheter with pressure tubing (*see* Fig. 14–1).

Procedure. Once the catheter is inserted, either percutaneously or by cutdown, it is sutured in place. Common sites include radial, brachial, axillary, and femoral arteries.

Readings. Ensure that the system is zeroed and calibrated accurately. The transducer should be level with the phlebostatic axis. Both systolic and diastolic values should be measured, both digitally from the monitor and by analog from a recorder. An average of 3 to 5 waves should be taken to arrive at a systolic and diastolic value.

Wave forms. The placement of arterial catheters contributes greatly to the contour of the wave form. The more distal the catheter from the aorta, the more distorted the wave form becomes. The upstroke is delayed, but when it occurs, it is more vertical, rises to a higher peak, and then has a steeper descent than those seen at the aorta. All arterial wave forms have some similarities (Fig 14–4). Shortly after the systolic peak there is a dip on the downslope, the dicrotic notch. This is a reflection of the closure of the aortic (or pulmonary) valve. Arrhythmias and drugs can have dramatic effects on the amplitude and contour of waves. Ventricular tachycardia can

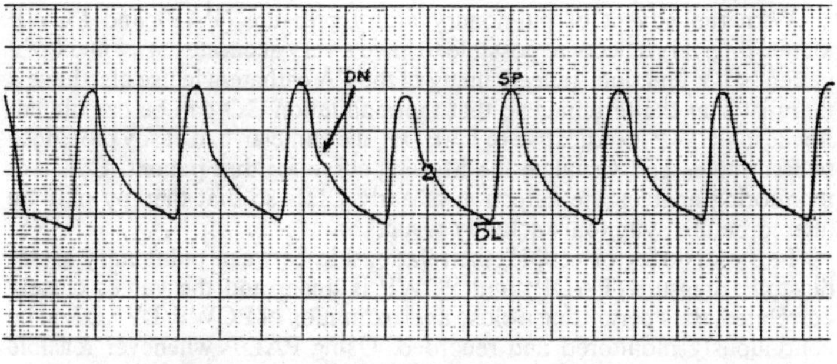

Figure 14–4. Arterial (aortic) pressure wave form. DN, dicrotic notch; DL, diastolic low; SP, systolic peak.

greatly decrease the amplitude because of decreased filling and output; atrial fibrillation can make values extremely variable because of the filling times and loss of atrial kick; and vasodilators decrease resistance, which changes the upstroke and descent contours.

Abnormal findings. High arterial pressure may be caused by hypertension, atherosclerosis, or inaccurate zeroing or calibration. Low arterial pressure may indicate hypovolemia, low CO, shock, arrhythmias, partial occlusion of catheter by thrombus or vessel wall, or inaccurate zeroing or calibration.

Complications. Complications include circulatory problems, hemorrhage, or dislocation of the catheter.

Diminished or inadequate circulation distal to the catheter can occur immediately after insertion or develop hours later. This condition is often caused by arteritis or thrombus formation. Circulatory status should always be assessed prior to catheter insertion and every effort should be made to avoid placing a catheter at the terminus of an extremity. The radial artery is usually preferred because the vessel is easily accessible and the hand is also perfused by the ulnar artery. Circulation may be diminished because of the size of the catheter and artery, because of vasospastic reaction to the catheter, inflammation, or emboli. Catheter removal is the only acceptable treatment if circulation is severely diminished.

External hemorrhage is a complication of any catheter system. It is usually caused by separation of catheters and/or open stopcocks. Interlocking catheters, dead-end caps on unused ports, and actuated alarms should be in use at all times, so as to prevent accidental exsanguination.

Dislocation of the catheter occurs because of improper immobilization of the catheter system. The catheter should be sutured in place, with a loop of tubing taped securely to the skin for strain relief. Dislocation can result in external hemorrhage or hematoma.

PULMONARY ARTERY PRESSURE MONITORING

With the advent of pulmonary artery pressure (PAP) and PCWP monitoring, it has become possible to have a very accurate assessment of a patient's LV function. Indeed, many of the PA catheters in use also have a thermistor at the terminus so that thermodilution CO can be calculated. Because PCWP is indicative of LVEDP, the clinician can easily plot those two variables and visualize the Starling curve for that patient. Constant monitoring enables the detection of early CHF so that therapy may be altered before symptoms actually result.

In the majority of people, the relationship between pulmonary artery diastolic pressure (PADP) and PCWP is linear and the valves closely correlated, thus permitting a close approximation of PCWP/LVEDP to be continuously monitored and recorded. Using PADP whenever feasible decreases the potential for morbidity secondary to repeated wedging of the pulmonary catheter into a small branch of the artery.

PAP monitoring may be used when it is necessary to measure hemodynamic parameters on a frequent basis. The proper catheter allows measurement or calculation of CVP, RV pressure (RVP), pulmonary systolic (PAS) and PADP, preload reflected by PCWP, afterload reflected by SVR, CO, and cardiac index (CI). Figure 14–5 depicts the major hemodynamic formulas used.

Some conditions that require frequent collection of these measurements are MI, shock, hypovolemia, and vasodilator therapy for hypertension or afterload reduction.

Equipment. The equipment needed includes (1) a flow-directed, balloon-tipped catheter (thermodilution catheter is advantageous); (2) a continuous flush device connected to the distal port; (3) a continuous flush device or IV drip connected to the proximal port; (4) transducer(s) and monitoring equipment; (5) a cutdown tray with introducer, sutures, etc.

Procedure. The typical flow-directed, balloon-tipped, thermodilution catheter has four lumens: a proximal exit in the RA, a distal exit in the PA, a lumen for inflating the balloon, and a lumen that carries the thermistor wires. Both proximal and distal lumens should be flushed and connected to the desired monitoring/flush systems. The physician will insert the catheter

$$\text{Cardiac output} = \text{heart rate} \times \text{stroke volume}$$

$$\text{Cardiac index} = \frac{\text{cardiac output}}{\text{body surface area in m}^2}$$

$$\text{Systemic vascular resistance} = \frac{80 \times (\text{mean arterial pressure - mean right atrial pressure})}{\text{cardiac output}}$$

$$\text{Pulmonary vascular resistance} = \frac{80 \times \left(\text{mean pulmonary artery pressure} - \text{pulmonary capillary wedge pressure}\right)}{\text{cardiac output}}$$

$$\text{Mean arterial pressure} = \frac{\text{systolic pressure} + (\text{diastolic pressure} \times 2)}{3}$$

Figure 14–5. Hemodynamic formulas.

through an introducer, placed usually in the brachial, subclavian, or internal jugular veins. The catheter is advanced while wave forms and pressures are being monitored. Changes are noted and recorded as the catheter tip is advanced from the central vein to the RA and RV (Fig. 14–6). At this time the need for mixed venous blood gases is determined. Once the catheter is in the RA, the balloon is partially inflated and allowed to be floated or "flow-directed" through the right side chambers. When the wave forms show that the terminus is in the PA, the catheter is slowly advanced, with balloon inflated, until a wedged tracing occurs. Then the balloon is deflated; the PA wave forms should return. If they do not, the catheter must be withdrawn slightly. A chest x-ray should be obtained to verify position, even though fluoroscopy may have been used during insertion.

Wave forms. The nurse should be familiar with the various contours and amplitudes of wave forms typically observed during insertion of a PA catheter. With the catheter tip in the RA, the *a, x, v,* and *y* waves are seen with an amplitude of 1 to 7 mmHg pressure (*see* Fig. 14–6). As the catheter is advanced through the tricuspid valve into the RV, a very sharp upstroke and descent is observed, with a systolic peak in the range of 15 to 30 mmHg and a diastolic low of 0 to 5 mmHg pressure normally. Further catheter advancement thorugh the pulmonary valve into the PA will show a wave somewhat similar to the RV wave except for two distinct differences: the dicrotic notch is present, and the PAD low is 8 to 10 mmHg higher than the RV diastolic low. Finally, as the catheter is wedged, the PA wave disappears and a wave form similar to RA appears. *A, x, v,* and *y* waves can often be distinguished but are now reflective of LAP and LVP fluctuations. It is very important that the catheter not remain in a wedged position for any length of time because this may result in a pulmonary infarction.

Abnormal findings. High values of PCWP or PAD may indicate LV failure, fluid overload, COPD, pulmonary hypertension, or positive-pressure ventilation. Low values of PCWP or PAD may be caused by hypovolemia, RV failure, or an inaccurately zeroed or calibrated transducer.

Complications. Potential complications of PAP monitoring include PA perforations, balloon rupture, air emboli, pulmonary infarction, catheter knotting, volume overload, and ventricular arrhythmias.

Pulmonary artery perforations are caused either by the catheter's directly puncturing the artery wall or by the continuous pressure exerted on the pulmonary artery wall by the inflated balloon. Immediate signs and symptoms of the tear will be hemoptysis, dyspnea, tachypnea, BP decline, hemothorax, and progressive shock states. To avoid perforation, the catheter should not be pushed to advance it but allowed to float into position. The balloon should not be overinflated, but inflated only until a wedge wave form is seen or until 1.5 ml of air is inflated.

The **balloon** may **rupture** because of manufacturing defects (rare), overinflation, frequent inflation, or torsion placed on the balloon membrane by active evacuation of air. The longer the catheter is in place, the more opportunity blood-borne enzymes have to weaken the balloon material.

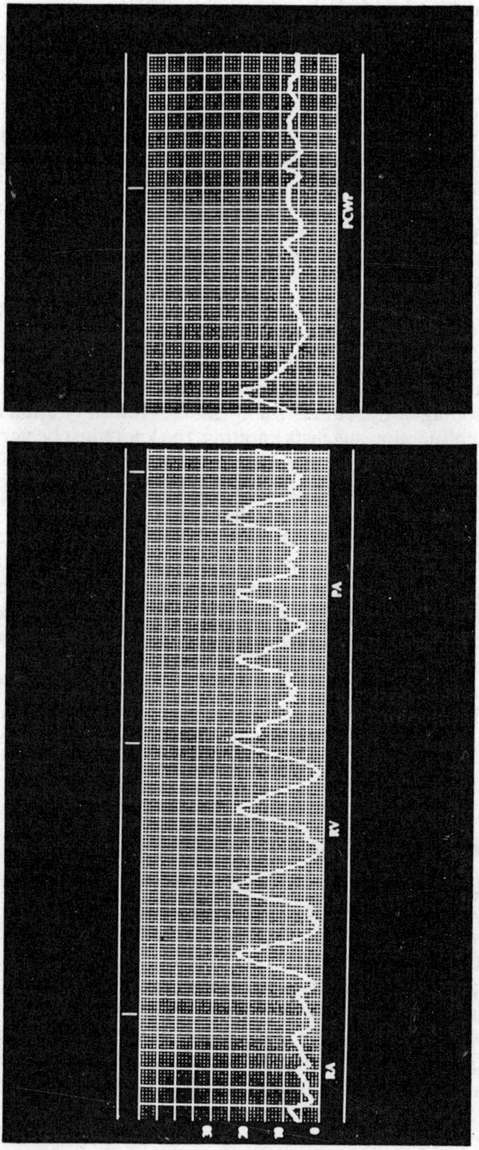

Figure 14–6. Hemodynamic wave forms seen during pulmonary artery catheter insertion. PA, pulmonary artery; PCSP, pulmonary capillary wedge pressure; RA, right atrium, RV, right ventricle. *Reprinted with permission from* American Edwards Laboratories, American Hospital Supply Corp., Santa Ana, Calif.

This activity, combined with frequent inflation/deflation may eventually weaken the balloon enough so that it tears. The consequence of a ruptured balloon is air embolus. While 1.5 ml of air would probably not cause harm in most patients, it should be avoided. For any patient with a right-to-left shunt, CO_2 should be the inflating gas. If a ruptured balloon is suspected (because 1.5 ml of air does not wedge the catheter) *gentle* aspiration with the syringe should be attempted; presence of any blood will indicate that there is a balloon rupture and blood has entered the lumen. Avoid vigorous aspiration because this could damage the balloon membrane if it is not already ruptured.

Air embolus can be caused by an open proximal port, which entrains air during inspiration.

Pulmonary infarction is usually caused by the catheter's being left in the wedge position for extended periods. The wave form should be checked frequently to see whether it is in the PA or wedge position.

Catheter knotting occasionally occurs; usually it is produced by frequent repositioning of the catheter and catheter retromigration into the RV. If catheter malfunction suggests knotting, the knot must be verified by fluoroscopy visualization or x-ray. Surgery is usually not necessary because the catheter can be manipulated under the fluoroscope sufficiently to untie the knot.

Volume overload tends to occur through incorrect interpretation of hemodynamic parameters or inadequate monitoring of infusing fluids. In instances in which multiple determinations of CO are being made, requiring 50 to 60 ml of fluid, caution must be taken not to overhydrate the patient. If numerous determinations need to be made, changes in injectate volume and temperature should be considered.

Ventricular arrhythmias often occur when the catheter tip is advanced into the RV and irritates the tissue. In most situations ectopy ceases as soon as the catheter travels into the PA. Emergency equipment, including IV medications and defibrillators, should be available in case ectopy continues or worsens.

MEASUREMENT OF CARDIAC OUTPUT

In the ICU, CO measurements are performed using a PA thermodilution catheter. The catheter has a proximal port in the RA, a distal port in the PA, and a thermistor located near the distal port. Usually 10 ml of D5W at a known temperature is injected into the proximal port. Simultaneously, the thermistor, which is connected to a computer, measures the temperature change of the circulating blood as the D5W is mixed and pumped by. The computer stores the values of blood temperature, fluid specific gravities and specific heats, and certain correction factors and finally calculates the CO.

There continues to be a controversy over the use of iced D5W injectate versus use of D5W injectate at room temperature. Early literature recommended iced injectate because it increased the temperature change in PA blood and hence increased the signal:noise ratio the computer received.

Recent data suggests that—probably because of more sophisticated equipment—this matter is of concern only in very low output states.

Equipment. The equipment needed includes a thermodilution PA catheter in place, a CO computer, 3 to 5 10-cc syringes of D5W, either at 0-to-5 degrees C or at room temperature.

Available equipment allows for attaching a 10-cc syringe via tubing to a bottle of D5W and the proximal port of the catheter. There are closed systems available for both room-temperature and iced injectate methods.

Procedure. The correct constant must be entered into the computer. (This depends on catheter brand, temperature of the injectate, and the amount of the injectate). With minimal handling of the syringe and/or tubing and as quickly and smoothly as possible, a prefilled syringe is connected to the proximal port of the catheter, the computer is started, and the fluid is quickly injected. The computer will display the output in liters/min after 30 to 45 sec. Three to five determinations are performed. It is recommended that any result varying by ≥10% from the other determinations be discarded.

Abnormal findings. Results may be higher or lower than expected or may vary by >10% for some of the following reasons: (1) Arrhythmias present during determinations (including those caused by rate changes, prematurity, or conduction abnormalities) may change actual outputs radically. (2) Change in patient position may alter venous return to the heart. (3) Change of interventions such as administration of vasoactive medications or the increase of positive end-expiratory pressure may change preload. (4) The presence of intracardiac shunts, either interatrial or interventricular, can produce a dramatic change in hemodynamics.

Complications. Once the catheter is in place, virtually the only complication is fluid overload caused by frequent CO determinations.

INTRA-AORTIC BALLOON PUMP

Intra-aortic balloon pumping (IABP) is a therapeutic intervention that greatly reduces the afterload on the LV. This decreases the LV work, O_2 demand, and increases LV emptying. The IABP works on the principle of counterpulsation: inflating a helium-filled balloon in the descending aorta during diastole and subsequently deflating the balloon immediately prior to systole. Mechanically, the inflating balloon increases coronary perfusion pressure by increasing diastolic pressure at the aortic root. This additional pressure is referred to as diastolic augmentation. It also increases forward BP toward the brain and mesentery. Mechanically, the deflating balloon lowers the EDP in the aorta. The lowest diastolic pressure is referred to as end-diastolic dip. The LV, responding to the lowered EDP, then generates a lower pressure to eject blood and thereby works less hard to maintain a sufficient CO. The lowest diastolic pressure that occurs without balloon assistance is termed the diastolic low.

Assisted systolic peak refers to the systolic pressure immediately following the balloon inflation. The systolic pressure should be lower than both the unassisted systolic pressure and the diastolic augmentation. The change in contour of the arterial wave form that signifies closure of the aortic valve is called the dicrotic notch.

The IABP is typically considered as a treatment when it is believed that the patient is in a reversible but severe low CO state that is not being treated effectively by usual means, or if the patient has preinfarction angina and there is hope of either preventing the infarction from occurring or of limiting its size (e.g., temporary CHF related to cardiac trauma and/or coronary artery bypass graft surgery); acute MI associated with mitral regurgitation, papillary muscle injury, or ventricular septal rupture; temporary but intractable CHF related to MI; intractable ventricular arrhythmia related to ischemia. IABP therapy is contraindicated in situations in which anatomic or physiologic defects, when combined with balloon insertion or pumping, would cause probable patient deterioration. Such conditions include dissecting aortic aneurysm, aortic aneurysm, aortic insufficiency, severe aortoiliac occlusive disease, and severe coagulopathies.

Equipment. The equipment needed includes (1) The IABP console; (2) an IABP catheter of appropriate size; if the catheter can also measure aortic pressure, a pressurized flush system is also needed; (3) sterile drapes, gowns, gloves, masks; (4) cutdown set with sutures; (5) medications such as heparin (prior to arterial puncture or arteriotomy), lidocaine, diazepam, antiemetics, vasopressors; (6) emergency equipment nearby; (7) 2 sets of ECG leads for triggering the balloon cycles and for monitoring the patient.

Procedure. There are several methods the physician can use for inserting the catheter. One of the methods involves performing an arteriotomy in either the iliac artery or the descending aorta and attaching a dacron side-arm graft through which the balloon catheter passes. With the advent of smaller or thinner-walled catheters and balloon membranes, this technique has been largely replaced by the percutaneous approach.

With the percutaneous insertion, the balloon catheter is threaded into the femoral artery and into the descending aorta through an introducer sheath. If these methods are not feasible, other approaches are usually performed in an operating room. These include antegrade insertion through the ascending aorta or a retroperitoneal approach to the aortic bifurcation.

Timing: Because counterpulsation is dependent on identifying systole and diastole, correlating the timing of the machine with the patient's heart is of critical importance. Indeed, if the machine is mistimed and not synchronized properly, the patient will deteriorate faster than if the IABP had never been implemented. The reader is referred to the extensive available literature devoted to IABP therapy; several principles essential for proper timing procedures should, however, be stressed here.

With inflation and deflation markers set for approximately the middle third of diastole and the console on a 1:1 ratio of cycles per cardiac contraction, the **inflation** marker should be slowly moved to the left. At the same time, the arterial wave form should be observed for (1) inflation of the balloon beginning at or slightly before the dicrotic notch (the wave should form a *V* shape); and (2) simultaneously, the height of the diastolic augmentation wave should be maximized (Fig. 14–7).

For **deflation**, the console should be switched into the 1:2 pumping ratio. The deflation marker is moved to the right (toward later deflation) and the wave form observed for (1) the end-diastolic dip to become lower than the diastolic low; and (2) the height of the assisted systolic peak to be lower than the unassisted systolic peak. (There are several manufacturers of IABP equipment. Their respective operating manuals should be consulted for any alteration of this procedure.) Continue to adjust the machine until the end-diastolic dip is at its lowest point without either the mean blood pressure or the diastolic augmentation decreasing.

Weaning. Initiation of IABP therapy is predicated on the belief that the patient's condition is reversible, at least for the short term. Once the patient's condition improves and CO returns to the normal range along with signs of improved renal, cerebral, and coronary perfusion, the process of weaning should begin. The console is placed in a 1:2 pumping mode (one balloon inflation for every two patient systoles) and the patient's response is monitored. If chest pain recurs, BP drops to an intolerable level, or lethal arrhythmias occur, the console should be returned to the 1:1 mode. If these symptoms do not recur, then the patient should remain in the 1:2 mode for 4 to 8 hr. The ratio should then be reduced and the patient's condition reassessed. If a ratio of 1:3 or 1:4 is tolerated for 8 hr, the catheter can be removed. There are some consoles that can reduce the ratio to less than 1:4; because this low ratio greatly increased the chance of thrombus formation around the balloon, a lower ratio should be used only if there is great difficulty weaning the patient. If a low ratio needs to be maintained, the console should be returned to a 1:1 ratio for 5 min q hr to dispel any blood trapped in the folds of the balloon.

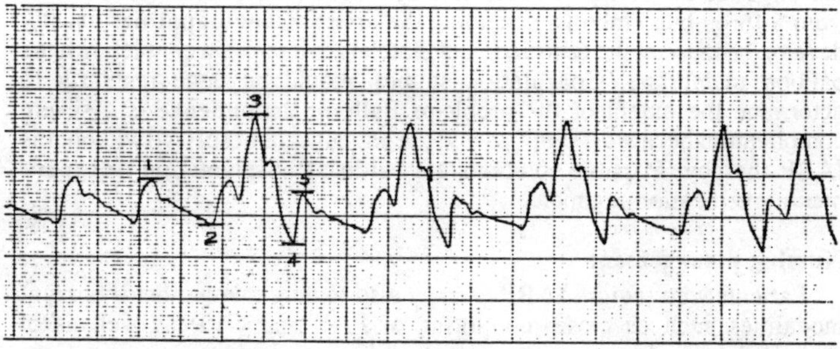

Figure 14–7. Intra-aortic pressures with intra-aortic balloon pump therapy. 1, unassisted systolic peak; 2, diastolic low; 3, augmented diastolic pressure; 4, end-diastolic dip; 5, assisted systolic peak.

Psychological preparation of the patient for weaning from the IABP is extremely important, especially when it is determined that no other pharmaceutical or surgical therapy will improve or stabilize his condition. The patient and family need to accept the eventual separation from therapy, whether or not weaning from the balloon pump is successful. This can only fully be accomplished if teaching about the patient's condition and IABP therapy is begun early and reinforced regularly.

Catheter removal. Removal depends largely on the insertion method. If the balloon catheter was inserted using a dacron side-arm graft, a minor surgical procedure under local anesthesia is required to remove the introducer and catheter and close the graft and cutdown site. If insertion was percutaneous, the balloon is simply deflated, rewrapped, and pulled back. Some physicians leave the balloon partially inflated to act as an embolectomy catheter. The exit site will require pressure to control bleeding and perhaps a suture. Any cutdown site is sutured closed.

Complications. Complications include aortic dissection, balloon rupture, emboli, catheter displacement, ischemia, coagulopathies, and balloon dependence.

Aortic dissection can occur through complete rupture of the aorta by the catheter during insertion or through partial tearing of the vessel, thereby threading the catheter into a false lumen. **Balloon rupture** can occur because of contact of the catheter with foreign matter that damages the membrane or by the constant rubbing of calcified plaque against the membrane. **Embolus** can occur through a thrombus breaking away from the catheter or through helium leaking from a ruptured balloon. Antegrade balloon **catheter displacement** can occur if the catheter is not sutured to the skin or if the patient's hips are flexed more than 30 degrees. Displacement can result in occlusion of the subclavian, innominate, and carotid arteries. **Ischemia** distal to the insertion can result from the insertion of a catheter too large for the diameter of an atherosclerotic iliac or femoral artery or from a thrombus/embolus occluding the artery. **Coagulopathies** usually develop because of the destruction of platelets that come in contact with the balloon membrane. Coagulation studies should be done regularly to determine the extent of the problem. **Balloon dependence** is a severe complication because it signifies that the patient cannot survive without the IABP therapy. Possible solutions are cardiac transplantation or experimental medication regimens.

Nursing management

Patients who require IABP therapy also require many other treatment modalities such as close monitoring of PAP and CVP as well as of neurologic, peripheral vascular, renal, and hematologic functioning. Concerns that are specific to balloon pump therapy include the problems listed below.

Timing. (1) If the heart rate varies by 10% from the previous timing, the IABP should be retimed, using the same timing procedure. (2) Monitor hemodynamic parameters closely and evaluate the accuracy of the balloon timing. (3) Maintain stable ECG rhythm recording to ensure proper IABP triggering.

Catheter displacement. (1) Do not raise the head of the bed higher than 30 degrees to avoid shifting the position of the catheter.

Coagulopathies. (1) Monitor coagulation studies carefully because the presence of the catheter destroys platelets.

Ischemia. (1) Monitor pulses, temperature, and color distal to the catheter to assess adequacy of blood flow.

Immobility. (1) Turn (log roll) patient regularly being careful to turn no more than 30 degrees on the catheter side because the IABP generally restricts movement.

CHAPTER 15

ADVANCED LIFE SUPPORT

Deborah Chyun

Basic life support (BLS) through CPR includes artificial ventilation, accomplished by opening the victim's airway and providing rescue breathing, as well as external chest compression. Advanced life support (ALS) as defined by the American Heart Association (AHA) consists of BLS plus four additional elements: (1) equipment to provide effective ventilation and circulation; (2) cardiac monitoring and arrhythmia recognition; (3) an IV infusion route; and (4) treatment of the patient with suspected or actual MI, both during and after the cardiac arrest.

ASSESSMENT OF LIFE-THREATENING EVENTS

Cardiac or respiratory arrest may be induced by any condition that causes hypoxia or metabolic or chemical abnormalities: i.e., MI, airway obstruction, drug overdose, electrocution, suffocation, and/or trauma. Either cardiac or respiratory arrest may initially occur as an isolated event, but without reversal of one, the other must soon follow. Although sudden cardiac death is likely to be the result of atherosclerotic coronary artery disease, acute MI cannot alone claim responsibility for all instances of sudden death. Selective myocardial cell necrosis, often associated with a variety of intracranial events, has been implicated in causing a high percentage of deaths as a result of ventricular fibrillation (VF). Both lethal and nonlethal cardiac arrhythmias, as well as ECG changes, have been documented to occur with various primary neurologic conditions.

The cardiac and respiratory status of patients with neurologic problems should be carefully assessed. These patients should be placed on a cardiac monitor, at least until their neurologic status has stabilized. Hourly rhythm strips should be taken with measurement of P-R, QRS, and Q-T intervals, along with the heart rate. Daily ECGs and serum enzyme levels, particularly a fractionated creatine phosphokinase (CPK) level should be followed. Antiarrhythmics should be at hand and standing orders available for their administration. When intracranial pressure is being monitored, it should not be allowed to rise precipitously, because a rise in BP and bradycardia will result.

Patients at risk of developing respiratory failure should be observed closely for changes in their respiratory status. Attention should be focused on the patients' subjective complaints, results of arterial blood gas (ABG) analyses, and chest x-ray reports. Respiratory and metabolic acidosis, unless partially compensated, should be promptly corrected. If the patient is unable to mobilize his own secretions, suction should be applied to prevent airway obstruction. Caution should be exercised when administering drugs that have been associated with causing respiratory arrest, such as aminophylline, epinephrine, digitalis preparations, potassium penicillin G, and chlorpromazine (Thorazine). Caution should be used in moving intubated patients or handling their tubings to prevent accidental dislodgement. Alarms should be functioning on the ventilator-dependent patient.

Finally, patients with known or suspected coronary artery disease should be carefully assessed for the occurrence of chest pain or silent MI. The stress generated by a concurrent illness or surgery that has placed the patient in the ICU setting may precipitate myocardial ischemia. Because of the interrelatedness of the body systems, all patients within the ICU setting should be regarded as potential candidates for either a cardiac or respiratory arrest.

BASIC LIFE SUPPORT

The concept of BLS has been expanded to include not only the physical acts involved in performing CPR but also prevention through recognition and intervention in situations that might potentially lead to an arrest. It is assumed that readers are already familiar with the techniques involved in performing CPR.

ADVANCED LIFE SUPPORT

Effective ventilation

The use of special equipment and techniques such as O_2 therapy, artificial airways, and manual resuscitation bags is the first element of ALS. Endotracheal intubation and mechanical ventilation, which are discussed in Chapter 13, are also used to provide ventilatory assistance to the patient when it appears that prolonged ventilatory support will be required.

Endotracheal intubation by a skilled professional should take <30 sec, the maximum time allowed for a break in providing ventilation to the victim.

The nurse not only assists in readying the equipment necessary for intubation but monitors the time required for insertion. Following intubation the nurse should ascertain correct placement by watching for bilateral chest expansion and auscultating for bilateral breath sounds or verifying that the person who has placed the tube does so. Following a successful resuscitation, the location of the endotracheal tube should also be confirmed by x-rays. The tube should be secured in place with adhesive tape or by other measures.

Suction, either wall-mounted or portable, should be readied, along with various sized suction catheters, nonkinking tubing, collection bottles, and sterile water. A nasogastric tube should also be on hand.

O_2 therapy. Supplementary O_2 should be delivered to the patient as early in the arrest as possible to reverse the hypoxic process. Hypoxemia causes anaerobic metabolism and metabolic acidosis, which in turn limit the effectiveness of both drugs and defibrillation used to terminate the arrest. Supplemental O_2 may be delivered through a manual resuscitation bag with or without endotracheal intubation or through mechanical ventilation. Although a time-cycled ventilator can be used with external cardiac compressions, the intubated patient is usually ventilated by means of the manual resuscitation bag until chest compression is no longer required. Supplemental O_2 is usually given at the highest delivery rate possible, i.e., 100%, and adjusted according to the patient's response to resuscitative efforts and the results of ABG analysis.

Artificial airways. An oropharyngeal airway may be placed prior to endotracheal intubation. Care must be observed to place the airway properly so as to prevent airway obstruction. As depicted in Figure 15–1, the tongue should be held forward by the airway. If the patient is still conscious, a nasopharyngeal airway should be placed, because an oropharyngeal airway may precipitate vomiting or laryngospasm. Rescue breathing should not be delayed while obtaining an artificial airway or in struggling to place it correctly. If the critical care nurse is skilled in proper placement of the airway and it is *immediately* at hand, this—along with a manual resuscitation bag—can be used in the initial resuscitation attempt.

Manual resuscitation bag. The manual resuscitation bag can be used with an oral airway or a nasotracheal or endotracheal tube. While this unit is capable of delivering high O_2 concentrations, there is often difficulty in obtaining a tight seal around the victim's mouth, thereby limiting its usefulness. Current recommendations are that manual resuscitation bags be used with an endotracheal tube or esophageal obturator airway, because these tubes can be fitted directly to the unit via an adaptor. The method for properly holding this device prior to endotracheal intubation is depicted in Figure 15–2.

In the event of airway obstruction, ventilation can be performed by means of a catheter that has been placed through the cricothyroid membrane into the trachea (cricothyrotomy). Tracheostomy is usually reserved for the operating room.

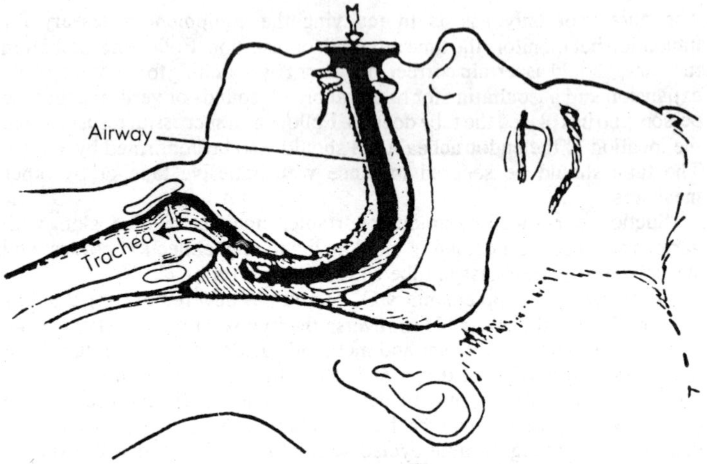

Figure 15–1. Placement of oropharyngeal airway: Tilt head backwards. Enter mouth in "upside down" position. Rotate airway into proper position as base of tongue near posterior pharyngeal wall is reached. Improper placement pushes the tongue against posterior pharynx, resulting in airway obstruction.

Effective circulation

Maintenance of circulation is accomplished by use of bed boards, manual and automatic chest compressors, antishock garments, intra-aortic counterpulsation, and internal cardiac compression. Bed boards provide firm support under the victim who is lying on a surface such as a mattress. They should be large enough to extend from the patient's shoulders to waist, wide enough to lie across the full width of the bed and be readily accessible. BLS should not be delayed while waiting for the board or assistance to place it. It is often difficult for one or even two nurses to lift the patient in order to position the board.

Manual or automatic chest compressors driven by a source of compressed gas may be useful in prolonged resuscitation attempts. Automatic compressors may be used and synchronized with tracheal ventilation. These units, however, are time-consuming and cumbersome to set up. A rigid backboard is placed under the patient and an overhead arm with a plunger attachment must be adjusted over the patient's chest. The correct height of the plunger must be maintained so that chest compressions are effective while minimizing the risk of rib fracture.

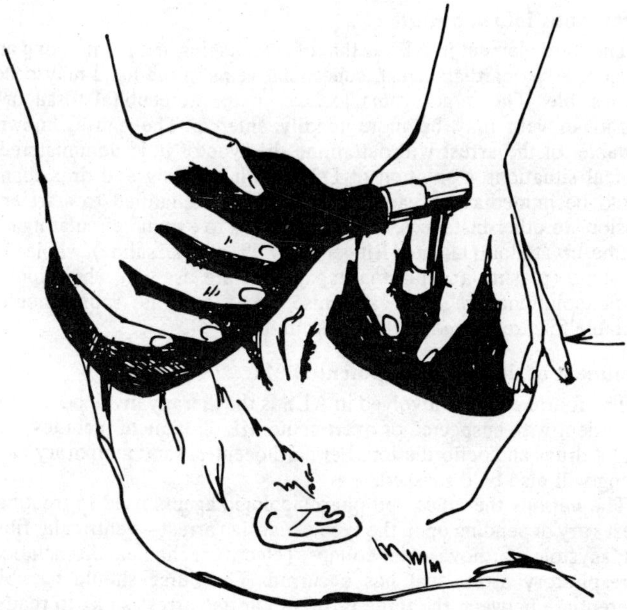

Figure 15–2. Proper positioning of the manual resuscitation bag: Hold head in extension and elevate lower jaw by pulling up on mandible with last three fingers. Place thumb and index finger on either side of valve while exerting pressure downward to assure a tight seal.

Cardiac monitoring and arrhythmia recognition

Cardiac monitoring and arrhythmia recognition is the second element involved in ALS. The patient in the ICU is usually monitored, so that an immediate record of the cardiac rhythm can be established. In addition, most of the newer-model defibrillators are combined with a cardiac monitor that allows for visualization of cardiac rhythm directly through the paddles placed on the patient's chest or through standard lead placement. The limb leads for a standard ECG are applied when assistance becomes available.

Cardiac monitoring can only be successful when staff are able to correctly interpret and treat the arrhythmia and when the equipment is used properly. Alarms should always be turned on. Limits should be set realistically and not far above or below rates that could prove to be life threatening. Patients with cardiac pacemakers should have the alarm low limits set at the pacemaker rate so as to detect pacemaker malfunction promptly.

Intravenous infusion route

The third element in ALS is that of establishing and maintaining an IV infusion. After cardiac arrest, superficial veins in the hand may become inaccessible. The larger veins located in the antecubital fossa or the subclavian vein may be more readily entered. The cause, known or probable, of the arrest will determine the type of fluid administered. In medical situations a solution of D5W with a tubing and drip chamber should be immediately readied for the person qualified to start an IV infusion. In other instances, where the aim is to expand circulating blood volume, crystalloid (lactated Ringer's or 0.9% normal saline), whole blood, or colloid (plasma and plasma expanders) are used. If whole blood or colloid solutions are to be administered, a separate route should be available for drugs used in the resuscitation.

Treatment of diagnosed or potential MI

The fourth element involved in ALS is the therapy involved in treating the patient with suspected or overt acute MI. Treatment includes the use both of drugs and defibrillation. Pericardiocentesis and temporary cardiac pacing will also be discussed.

The various therapies and pharmacologic agents used in treating the arrest vary depending upon the type of cardiac arrest—ventricular fibrillation, asystole, cardiovascular collapse (electromechanical dissociation)—or respiratory arrest that has occurred. The nurse should be able to differentiate between the three types of cardiac arrest so as to ready the appropriate interventions for terminating the arrhythmia.

Ventricular tachycardia (VT) or VF is treated with electrical defibrillation and antiarrhythmic drugs such as lidocaine, bretylium, procainamide, and quinidine. In addition, inotropic agents such as isoproterenol or epinephrine may be utilized in attempting to convert a "fine" VF into a "coarser" variety, which may then be more amenable to defibrillation. In cases of actual or suspected digoxin toxicity, phenytoin may be administered. Potassium may also be administered when serum levels are low, because potassium depletion may significantly alter the efficacy of many of the antiarrhythmics used and predispose the patient to digitalis-induced arrhythmias.

In **asystolic arrest**, epinephrine, calcium, isoproterenol, and atropine may be injected IV, and if restoring a rhythm is unsuccessful, transvenous or transthoracic pacing may be attempted. Although there is some question regarding the usefulness of defibrillation in this setting, it is thought that what may appear to be asystole may in fact be a "fine" VF, making defibrillation an appropriate response.

Electromechanical dissociation tends to have the worst prognosis of the three types of cardiac arrest. Drug therapy is identical to that involved in treating asystolic arrest, often using calcium as a first measure. Cardiac tamponade may be a cause of electromechanical dissociation, and in this case pericardiocentesis is attempted.

Sodium bicarbonate is used throughout the course of the arrest, although its use has become more conservative over the past few years. In the past, it was common to administer it q 5 to 10 min. With rapid ABG determination available, it is advisable to use sodium bicarbonate only in response to pH, $PaCO_2$, and base-deficit determinations, because overzealous administration may cause metabolic alkalosis.

If, during the course of an arrest, the intracardiac route of drug administration is attempted, the following potential complications should be assessed for postarrest: coronary artery laceration, pneumothorax, or cardiac tamponade. Intracardiac administration of drugs also demands that CPR be interrupted.

In addition to these drugs, agents may be required to support arterial BP. Although it is safest to instill these vasoconstrictor agents through a central line, in most instances, this may not be accomplished immediately. If administered peripherally, close attention should be given to the IV site, because infiltration into the subcutaneous tissues can cause severe necrosis and sloughing. Frequent BP determinations should be made to determine the effectiveness of the vasoconstrictors and prevent overshoot.

The drugs commonly used in an arrest are outlined in Table 15–1. The drug interactions that are listed are only for those medications that are apt to be administered during an arrest and are not inclusive of all medication that the patient may have been receiving. As soon as sufficient assistance is available or the patient is stabilized, careful assessment of all previous and current medications should be made in order to detect potential incompatibilities or drug interactions.

Defibrillation. Defibrillation is the application of direct current to the heart in an attempt to depolarize the myocardium and allow the sinus node to regain control of the heart rate. Defibrillation is the treatment of choice for terminating VF, VT associated with absence of pulse, BP, and consciousness (decompensated VT), and may be occasionally used in asystole in hopes of starting up a lower pacemaker.

Ideally, defibrillation should be accomplished within 30 sec after the onset of VF. In practice, the countershock should be applied in $\leq$2 min of identifying this lethal arrhythmia to maximize its effectiveness. In most ICUs, the nurse is responsible for defibrillating the patient immediately upon recognition of VF or decompensated VT. If the patient has been in VF >2 min, the AHA recommends that BLS be initiated and performed for $\geq$2 min prior to a defibrillation attempt.

In some institutions, "blind defibrillation" in the unmonitored patient is also the responsibility of the nurse responding to the arrest with a defibrillator. This usually occurs outside the ICU, where the patient is unmonitored. Prior to delivering the shock, the nurse should question those in attendance as to whether the patient has been on a digitalis preparation. The possibility of digoxin toxicity would necessitate that lower energy levels be used.

The amount of energy used in the initial attempt at external defibrillation

TABLE 15–1

Pharmacologic Agents Used in Advanced Life Support

Drug name	Action	Dose	Side effects	Drug interactions	Nursing implications
Atropine sulfate	Parasympatholytic; increases heart rate by blocking vagus; increases SA node discharge rate and increases conduction through AV node	IV bolus: 0.5–1.0 mg q 3–5 min until desired result or maximum dose (2.0 mg)	Tachycardia; mydriasis; flushed, dry skin; dry mucous membranes; urinary retention	Incompatible with Levarterenol (Levophed), metaraminol (Aramine), sodium bicarbonate.	Use cautiously with myocardial ischemia or MI; potential for VT or VF after IV injection; use cautiously with prostatic hypertrophy or COPD; contraindicated in acute glaucoma, asthma; may cause adverse reactions with cholinergics, digitalis preparations, antihistamines.
Bretylium tosylate (Bretylol)	Antiarrhythmic; inhibits release of norepinephrine and raises VF threshold	IV bolus: 5 mg/kg (500 mg) undiluted over 15–30 sec for VF; increase to 10 mg/kg (1 g) at 5–10 min intervals to max of 30 mg/kg Intermittent infusion: 5–10 mg/kg over 20 min (500 mg-1 g in 50 ml D5W or normal saline) Continuous infusion: 1–2 mg/min (1 g in 500 ml D5W or normal saline)	Postural hypotension; nausea, vomiting; vertigo; syncope	May cause initial release of norepinephrine and aggravate digoxin-induced ventricular arrhythmias in the digoxin-toxic patient.	Monitor BP closely for hypotension and keep supine.

Calcium chloride	Increases myocardial contractility and automaticity	IV bolus: 5–10 ml (500 mg-1 g) of a 10% solution (6.8–13.6 mEq Ca) q 10 min at 1 ml/min Intracardiac: 2–4 ml (200–400 mg)	Hypotension; tissue extravasation and necrosis	Incompatible with sodium bicarbonate. (It is essential to flush IV line between these two medications.)	Monitor injection site carefully (extravasation will cause tissue necrosis); keep patient recumbent to avoid hypotension; monitor for ECG evidence of hypercalcemia-prolonged QRS complex and Q-T interval.
Calcium gluconate	Same as calcium chloride	IV bolus: 10–15 ml (4.8–7.2 mEq Ca) at 1.0 ml/min			
Dopamine hydrochloride (Intropin)	Synthetic sympathomimetic amine; stimulates alpha- and beta-adrenergic receptors to increase myocardial contractility and produce mild vasoconstriction; in low doses its dopaminergic effect dilates renal and mesenteric blood vessels	Continuous infusion: 2–30 μg/kg/min (400–1,600 mg in 500 ml–1,000 ml D5W or 0.9% normal saline)	Tachyarrhythmias; at doses greater than 15 μg/kg/min peripheral vasoconstriction occurs and overrides dopaminergic effect on renal and mesenteric dilation; nausea, vomiting; angina; headache	Incompatible with sodium bicarbonate or other alkaline solutions. May cause bradycardia and hypotension with IV phenytoin (Dilantin). Beta effects can be blocked by beta blockers.	Solution should be tapered gradually rather than discontinued abruptly; avoid extravasation—tissue necrosis and sloughing may occur; maintain adequate fluid volume replacement and treat hypovolemia; carefully monitor heart rate and BP response; observe for myocardial ischemia with increased ventricular rates.
Epinephrine hydrochloride, adrenalin chloride	Synthetic sympathomimetic amine; alpha- and beta-adrenergic stimulator; increases cardiac con-	IV bolus: 0.5–1.0 mg (5–10 ml of 1:10,000 solution) over 1 min; may repeat q 5 min	Hypertension; tachycrdia; ventricular arrhythmias; angina; headache	Incompatible with any other drug in syringe; do not mix with alkalis, alkaline solutions, or oxidizing agents.	Do not use if brown in color or contains sediment; protect from light; may increase blood glucose levels; check BP fre-

Drug name	Action	Dose	Side effects	Drug interactions	Nursing implications
	tractility and CO; increases AV conduction; raises BP in large doses due to alpha-effect				quently; administration via central line preferable; may be administered via endotracheal tube.
Isoproterenol hydrochloride (Isuprel)	Synthetic sympathomimetic amine; beta-receptor stimulator causing increased inotropism and chronotropism; increases CO	IV bolus: 0.02–0.06 mg (Dilute to 10 ml with normal saline and administer very slowly over 1 min) Intracardiac: 0.02 mg (.1 ml of 1:5,000 solution) Continuous infusion: 2–20 μg/min (2 mg in 500 ml D5W)	Tachycardia; ventricular ectopy; hypotension; headache, flushing; angina	Incompatible with sodium bicarbonate, barbiturates. Antagonized by beta blockers.	Do not run solution "wide open" (may cause VF); maintain heart rate <130 bpm; do not use concomitantly with epinephrine (may cause arrhythmias); maintain adequate blood volume; monitor BP.
Lidocaine hydrochloride (Xylocaine)	Antiarrhythmic; used for treatment of ventricular ectopy	IV bolus: 1 mg/kg (50–100 mg) over 1 min and repeat in 5 min for total dose of 100–200 mg Continuous infusion: 1–4 mg/min (2 g in 250–500 ml D5W)	Drowsiness; dizziness; visual disturbances; tremor; paresthesias; convulsions	Incompatible with dopamine, norepinephrine, beta blockers, isoproterenol (Isuprel) and cimetidine.	Wean slowly while watching for arrhythmias; use cautiously with severe liver or cardiac failure, hypovolemia, shock, heart block, and untreated bradycardia.
Naloxone hydrochloride (Narcan)	Narcotic antagonist	IV bolus: 0.4–0.8 mg over 15 sec	Nausea, vomiting	Incompatible with alkaline solutions.	Precipitates acute withdrawal symptoms in narcotic addicts; continued observation of patient

					who responds to naloxone is necessary because duration of action of overdosed drug may exceed duration of action of naloxone.
Norepinephrine, levarterenol bitartrate (Levophed)	Sympathomimetic amine; alpha-stimulating agent causing peripheral vasoconstriction; beta-stimulating inotropic agent and coronary artery dilator	Continuous infusion: Begin at 2–4 μg/min and titrate according to BP response (2–4 amps [8 mg-16 mg] to 500 or 1,000 ml in D5W or saline)	Hypertension; headache	Incompatible with heparin, metaraminol (Aramine), phenobarbital (Luminal), phenytoin (Dilantin), sodium bicarbonate, aminophylline, lidocaine.	Central infusion preferred route; causes severe tissue necrosis, sloughing, and gangrene with extravasation; phentolamine (Regitine) 5–10 mg in 10–15 ml saline should be available and infiltrated into area should solution leakage occur; use with caution in patients with peripheral vascular disease; check infusion site frequently and for evidence of blanching along course of vein; to avoid this problem, phentolamine may be added to the norepinephrine solution.
Phenytoin sodium (Dilantin)	Anticonvulsant with antiarrhythmic properties; used in the management of ventricular ectopy	IV bolus: 100–250 mg at rate of 25–50 mg/min Administer 100 mg q5 min until arrhyth-	Hypotension; asystole; tissue extravasation and necrosis; dizziness; ataxia; nystagmus	Incompatible with all other parenteral medications.	Do not administer solution if hazy or precipitate evident; may be light yellow in color; check IV patency before adminis-

Drug name	Action	Dose	Side effects	Drug interactions	Nursing implications
		mia or seizure is controlled or to maximum 1–1½ g			tering (irritates vein); precede and follow with normal saline flush to decrease the chance of phlebitis and/or extravasation; hypotension may occur with rapid IV administration; use closest possible injection port to the insertion site.
Procainamide hydrochloride (Pronestyl)	Antiarrhythmic; used for ventricular ectopy	IV bolus: 100 mg q 5 min until the arrhythmia has been controlled or until maximum 1 g Continuous infusion: 2–6 mg/min (1–2 g in 250 ml D_5W)	Hypotension; asystole; nausea, vomiting; fever; chills; urticaria	Incompatible with phenytoin (Dilantin).	Monitor BP carefully with IV loading; measure base-line P-R, QRS, and Q-T intervals and compare throughout therapy (QRS prolonged >50% of base-line [or >25% in patient with BBB] and Q-T increase may necessitate discontinuance or dosage decrease); decrease dosage with renal or liver disease; photosensitive—protect from light and discard if darker than light amber; use caution with first- or second-degree heart block.

Sodium bicarbonate	Inorganic buffer; used in treating metabolic acidosis associated with cardiac arrest	IV bolus: 1 mEq/kg (50–100 mEq) over 1–3 min	Metabolic alkalosis; hypernatremia; hyperosmolality, tetany	Incompatible with atropine, calcium chloride, calcium gluconate, dobutamine (Dobutrex), dopamine, 5% dextrose in lactated Ringer's injection, levarterenol (Levophed), phenytoin (Dilantin).	Follow results of arterial blood pH, $PaCO_2$, and base deficit; use cautiously with cardiac, renal, or liver disease resulting from sodium retention; because of incompatibilities, flush IV line before and after administration.

AV, atrioventricular; BBB, bundle branch block; SA, sinoatrial; VF, ventricular fibrillation; VT, ventricular tachycardia. *Adapted with permission* Gahart, B.L. Intravenous Medications. C.V. Mosby Co., St. Louis. 1981. Third edition.

remains controversial. The AHA recommends that 200 to 300 joules be delivered for the first two countershocks. If a third attempt is required, after administration of epinephrine and sodium bicarbonate for metabolic acidosis, the countershock should be increased to no more than 360 joules. For recurrent VF after successful conversion, the energy level need not be increased. During open-chest resuscitation, energy levels of 5 joules should be used initially and should not exceed 20 joules.

Prior to paddle placement, gel should be applied to the paddles, or conductive pads or saline-soaked 4 x 4-in. gauze pads applied to the patient's chest. One paddle is then placed to the right of the sternum below the clavicle and the other to the left of the left nipple in the anterior-axillary line.

It has been suggested that for patients with pacemakers, the anterior-posterior paddle placement be adopted. One paddle is placed over the left precordium and the other, flatter, "posterior" paddle under the left scapula. Each paddle should be positioned 10 cm from the pulse generator and leads to lessen the possibility of damage to the pacemaker during defibrillation. When a patient who has a temporary pacer is defibrillated, the unit should be shut off prior to defibrillation. The anterior-posterior approach may also prove more successful for patients with a large chest.

Precautions to observe when defibrillating are as follows: Once the unit is charged, the nurse should not leave it unattended. Avoid getting conductive gel on hands or handles of the paddle, or allowing a bridge to form on the skin where it might cause a short circuit. When ready to discharge the current, make sure that everyone is off the bed, away from the patient or any piece of equipment that is connected to the patient—IV pole, ECG machine, etc. State as loudly as possible that you are about to defibrillate. Make sure that neither you nor the patient are in contact with any grounded metal object or with any fluid while operating defibrillator. While most equipment used in the ICU should be electrically safe to operate with the defibrillator, it may need to be disconnected prior to delivering the shock. Know the policy in your unit. If the patient is restrained, release the restraints before applying the countershock. Apply paddles firmly to the patient's chest. If chest is wet, wipe dry first. If unit cannot be discharged from the paddles, the person releasing the discharge has responsibility for making sure others are not in contact with the patient. Paddles should be wiped clean of gel *immediately* after resuscitation. Follow manufacturer's recommendations for testing equipment. Check patient for burns. Do not use alcohol in the presence of the defibrillator. If the patient is being resuscitated on the floor, do not kneel while defibrillating—knees are not well insulated.

Temporary pacing. A temporary pacemaker may be inserted in the setting of an acute MI, for overdrive pacing with tachyarrhythmias, or to treat bradysystolic arrest that is unresponsive to pharmacologic intervention. In the arrest situation it is often difficult to utilize a transvenous approach, so that a transthoracic approach is often necessary. A large-bore needle is passed either from the cardiac apex toward the right shoulder for a left ventricular puncture, or from the subxiphoid area toward the left shoulder for a right ventricular puncture. The angulated tip of a transthoracic pacing wire is then passed through and the needle withdrawn over the wire. The wire is then connected to a pacing unit by means of an adaptor.

Placement is determined either by pacing at full output until capture occurs or through ECG guidance. Complications of transthoracic placement include laceration of the lung or coronary artery, pericardial tamponade, or intramyocardial hemorrhage. These should be assessed for in the immediate postresuscitative phase.

Transvenous pacemaker insertion may be accomplished under fluoroscopy or through ECG guidance via an antecubital, subclavian, internal jugular, or femoral vein approach. During the procedure, the patient should be attached to an ECG machine and have an IV running. The defibrillator and a bolus of lidocaine should be at hand, and the nurse should constantly monitor the patient for ventricular ectopy.

After preparing the skin with the appropriate solution and anesthetizing the area, a needle with an introducer and syringe is inserted into the vein. When adequate blood flow is returned, the needle is pulled back over the introducer and the pacing catheter is inserted. With a bipolar electrode, the distal electrode (cathode, negative pole) is connected to the V lead via well-insulated alligator clamps and an intracardiac ECG recorded to determine placement. When the catheter comes in contact with the endocardium of the right ventricle, ST segment elevation occurs.

Once the electrode is secured in position, it is connected to a pacing box, which should have been tested prior to attaching it to the patient. The stimulation threshold is ascertained by turning the milliampere (MA) setting down until capture is lost and up until 1:1 capture occurs (usually at levels <1.0 MA). The MA setting is then set at two to three times threshold. Heart rate and mode of pacing—demand or fixed-rate (asynchronous)—are set. The connectors should be firmly placed in the box, which is then placed in a secure, conspicuous place.

Pericardiocentesis. Pericardial tamponade, resulting from a variety of causes, may lead to cardiac arrest. Measures used in attempting to terminate an arrest, such as intracardiac drug administration or pacemaker insertion, may themselves lead to tamponade. Pericardiocentesis, the insertion of a needle or catheter into the pericardial sac, relieves fluid accumulation.

Acute fluid buildup within the pericardial sac causes compression of the myocardium. Ventricular filling is restricted and CO falls, giving rise to the classic signs and symptoms of pericardial tamponade—increased central venous pressure, equalization of all intracardiac pressures, neck vein distension, hypotension, narrowed pulse pressure, pulsus paradoxus, tachycardia, enlarged cardiac contour on chest x-ray, muffled heart sounds, and diminished ECG voltage.

A subxiphoid-subcostal approach is the preferred route. A large-gauge needle, with or without a catheter, is inserted in either the left or right xiphocostal angle or beneath the xiphoid tip and advanced until fluid is aspirated. The needle can be attached to the V lead of the ECG machine to detect the ST segment or P-R interval elevation and ectopic beats that occur when the myocardium is contacted. This necessitates needle withdrawal.

Surgery may be required if fluid cannot be removed by needle aspiration or if tamponade is not relieved. As with pacemaker insertion, an IV route, the defibrillator, ECG machine, equipment for tracheal intubation, and O_2 should be at hand. In addition, rapid administration of fluid and beta-adrenergic stimulants, such as isoproterenol and dopamine, may be required to maintian CO. After pericardiocentesis, the patient should be assessed for the following complications: laceration of lung, coronary artery, or myocardium, hydrothorax or pneumothorax.

CHAPTER 16

INFECTION CONTROL IN THE ICU

Barbara Goldrick

The nature of ICUs makes them important areas for infection control. Patients in the ICU are usually at higher risk for nosocomial infections for a number of reasons: (1) They often have underlying conditions that compromise their host defenses; (2) they are exposed to invasive procedures, some of which may be performed in emergencies and thus not under ideal aseptic conditions; (3) they are clustered in a confined area, often near other highly susceptible or colonized/infected patients; and (4) contacts between patients and personnel are frequent, providing a situation that allows ample opportunity for cross-infection. Because of the widespread use of antibiotics, ICUs often become reservoirs of multidrug-resistant microorganisms, presenting an intrahospital and an interhospital problem, as well.

Critical-care nurses are particularly instrumental in identifying real and/or potential problems of infection in their own unit because they have knowledge of the unit in aggregate and can look for patterns and trends of infection in patients, spot the emergence of an organism not previously seen in a particular unit, and identify organisms with the same sensitivity pattern that are isolated from culture specimens of different patients. Although the hospital infection control team is responsible for the hospital as a whole, it may not be able to provide detailed surveillance of individual units. Therefore, observation of these occurrences and trends are the first line of defense against infection in the ICU. Any suggestion of such trends should be reported to the infection control team, who can then evaluate and investigate them further if necessary.

EPIDEMIOLOGY

Epidemiology is defined as the study of the determinants, occurrence, and distribution of health and disease in a population. It defines the relationship of disease to the population at risk—i.e., in this case, the ICU population, including patients and personnel—and is concerned with the factors involved in morbidity and mortality associated with infections in the ICU. Once these factors have been identified, effective prevention and control measures become apparent.

Morbidity measures the amount of illness in a population by relating cases to a given population base. **Mortality,** on the other hand, refers to the number of deaths in a time period for a population in a given area.

Incidence defines the number of people who develop an illness (infection) within a specified period of time, i.e., all *new* cases that occur. **Prevalence** measures the number of people in the population who have the illness (infection) at a given point in time, i.e., *all* cases, new and old.

The infectious process

One of the most important principles in epidemiology is that of the infectious process—a chain of relationships among the causative organism, its transmission, and the host. This interaction may be likened to links in a chain in which each element must be present in an orderly sequence to produce an infection. For purposes of review, these elements are (1) causative agent, (2) reservoir, (3) portal of exit, (4) transmission, (5) portal of entry, and (6) susceptible host.

The causative agent. While most nosocomial infections are caused by bacteria and viruses, fungi occasionally are the cause of nosocomial problems, and rarely, are parasites.

The reservoir. Reservoirs for the causative agent may be persons, animals, or inanimate objects (fomites) in the environment. Viruses generally survive and multiply better in animate reservoirs, whereas certain bacteria can survive and multiply in both animate and inanimate reservoirs. When we speak of contamination, we refer to organisms that transiently are present on body surfaces (such as hands) or on inanimate objects (such as respiratory therapy equipment).

An important concept to keep in mind is the distinction between infection and disease. While the two terms may be used interchangeably, epidemiologically speaking, they refer to different phenomena. *Infection* is the process whereby an organism invades the host and replicates in the tissue of that host. *Disease* results when the invasion of the organism produces overt clinical manifestations; however, if the infection causes an immunologic response without clinical disease, we refer to this as an inapparent, or subclinical, infection. When organisms are present in or on the host but without any overt clinical expression of an immune response detected, the person is considered to be *colonized*. To detect subclinical infection, special serologic tests may be necessary. Colonization (also called the carrier state) may be transient (short-term), intermittent (occasional), or chronic (long-term, persistent, or permanent). A carrier can be the reservoir of infection for another individual, or may develop an autoinfection.

Portal of exit. Portals of exit associated with human reservoirs are: (1) the respiratory tract, (2) the GU tract, (3) the GI tract, (4) open wounds, and (5) the bloodstream.

Transmission. Knowledge of how organisms are transmitted can be very helpful in the prevention and control of their spread within the ICU. There are four primary routes of transmission: (1) contact, (2) airborne, (3) vehicle-borne, and (4) vector-borne.

The contact route: In the ICU, contact occurs among patients, personnel, and equipment during hands-on care. Transmission of infection can be controlled by having an appropriate number of sinks in the unit to allow persistent and careful hand-washing between patients. Fomites, such as pressure-monitoring devices and respiratory therapy equipment, act as intermediary mechanisms for the transmission of infectious agents from patient to patient. Therefore, invasive equipment (e.g., pressure-monitoring devices) that is to be used by other patients must be appropriately sterilized or disinfected before being used again.

Spacing patients ≥4 ft apart, preferably by cubicles, will minimize the spread of infection from patient by droplet spread.

The airborne route: Organisms contained within evaporated droplets (droplet nuclei) or dust particles may remain suspended in the air for long periods of time. TB is an example of an infection that can be transmitted by airborne route to other patients several feet away.

The vehicle-borne route: Food, water, drugs, IV fluids, and blood that become contaminated are vehicles for infection. Hepatitis B is a viral infection that is transmitted via blood from an infected person.

The vector-borne route: By this route, organisms are transmitted through an intermediary such as an insect, a tick, or a mite. With the exception of scabies, infections transmitted by vector-borne spread are rarely, if ever, found in ICUs in the USA.

Portal of entry. The portals of entry into the new host are the same as those listed above for the portals of exit: (1) the respiratory tract, (2) the GU tract, (3) the GI tract, (4) open wounds, and (5) the bloodstream.

Host susceptibility. A variety of host factors influence whether or not an infection occurs and disease develops. A major factor is the host's defense mechanisms. These may be nonspecific or specific. **Nonspecific defense mechanisms** include the skin, mucous membranes, body secretions, and the local inflammatory response.

Specific defense mechanisms result from specific immunity. To protect it from microorganisms, the body has two systems: the humoral immune system and the cell-mediated immune system. These interdependent systems derive from B-lymphocytes and T-lymphocytes, respectively.

B-lymphocytes: The B-lymphocytes, which originate from stem cells in the bone marrow, differentiate into plasma cells producing five types of immunoglobulins (Ig), or antibodies: IgM, IgG, IgA, IgD, and IgE. When the body first encounters an antigen, the primary response by the plasma cells is the production of IgM within 24 to 72 hr, followed by production of IgG and IgA. B-lympocytes live for ~16 days. Therefore, it is important that the bone marrow remain intact and in good condition throughout life to protect against infection.

IgG is the predominant antibody produced by subsequent exposure to a particular antigen; it elicits a response (secondary immune response) within 24 to 48 hr. Antibodies can be transferred from one individual to another through blood serum.

IgA, a secretory antibody, is found in colostrum, tears, saliva, and the mucous membrane linings of the respiratory, GU, and GI tracts.

IgE is capable of attaching itself to basophils, neutrophils, and most tissue cells, causing those cells to become sensitized to allergens. Upon contact with these allergens, histamines and histamine-like substances may be released by the cells. The results could be anaphylaxis, hay fever, allergic asthma, hives, or atopic dermatitis.

The function of IgD is unknown at this time.

When antibodies are triggered by antigens, opsonization and neutralization occur. Phagocytosis by microphages is facilitated by antibodies that coat pathogenic organisms (opsonization). When the antigen is a toxin rather than an organism, it will be neutralized by antibodies.

The interaction between antibody and antigen is also triggered by the complement system. The complement system consists of nine components found in the bloodstream that are activated sequentially. After the original antibody-antigen response, the action of the complement system further enhances phagocytosis.

T-lymphocytes: T-cells, derived from the thymus gland, cannot produce and secrete antibodies. They do, however, contain chemicals called lymphokines. Like B-lymphocytes, T-cells are programmed to recognize specific antigens. When triggered by a specific antigen, T-cells release these lymphokines, producing the inflammatory response of erythema and induration by pulling macrophages into the area.

T-cells provide the body with cell-mediated immunity by producing delayed hypersensitivity. They are responsible for the immunosurveillance of the host. Malignant cells carry tumor-specific antigen on their membranes, which T-cells are genetically programmed to recognize and kill. When the integrity of the T-cell is interrupted by drugs or disease, the risk of cancer increases. Therefore, when transplant patients receive large doses of drugs to prevent T-cells from rejecting the new organ, the T-cell's ability to reject tumors is also affected. The recipient is also placed at risk for viral and fungal infection, because T-cells supply the major protection against viral and fungal infections.

RISK FACTORS FOR NOSOCOMIAL INFECTIONS

The advent of biomedical technology is a two-edged sword. Although this sophisticated technology has decreased morbidity and mortality for certain diseases, the use of drugs and invasive instrumentation in ICUs has increased morbidity and mortality caused by infection. The risk factors associated with nosocomial infection in critical care units are: (1) invasive devices; (2) resistant microorganisms; (3) altered host immunity; (4) antimicrobial therapy; and (5) underlying chronic or debilitating disease.

Of the outbreaks investigated by the Center for Disease Control (CDC) between 1970 and 1975, 42% were associated with invasive devices. Five categories—urinary catheters, intravascular catheters, pressure monitoring devices, respiratory therapy equipment, and hemodialysis equipment—accounted for 83% of the outbreaks reported.

CATHETER-ASSOCIATED URINARY TRACT INFECTION

Urinary tract infection (UTI) is a general term referring to any type of urinary infection (e.g., cystitis, pyelonephritis, or asymptomatic bacteriuria). It is defined as the presence of significant numbers of bacteria in the urine (≥100,000 bacteria/ml in noncatheterized patients; ≥10,000 bacteria/ml in catheterized patients). Of all nosocomial infections, 40% are UTIs; 75% of these are associated with instrumentation, whether it be for urethral dilation, bladder catheterization, or cystocopy.

Epidemiology

The incidence of catheter-associated UTI (UTIC) is directly related to the length of time the catheter is in place. After ~2 wk of catheterization, 50% of patients are infected. After a month, nearly all catheterized patients become infected. Additional risk factors for patients with catheters include: sex (females have a higher incidence of UTI because of the shorter female urethra, which facilitates the introduction of bacteria into the bladder), periurethral colonization with gram-negative rods, severe underlying illness, and improper catheter-care techniques.

Asymptomatic bacteriuria may persist for long periods of time in both catheterized and previously catheterized patients. Subsequently, these patients can serve as reservoirs for the spread of infection to other patients in ICUs, as well as provide a source for the intrahospital and interhospital spread of multiresistant bacteria. The causative organisms associated with UTIC can be bacteria, fungi, or viruses. Bacteria are the most common cause, however. They include *Serratia, Pseudomonas, Proteus,* and *enterococci.* Because of the widespread use of antimicrobials in hospitals, these microorganisms are often multiresistant.

The sources of entry for bacteria into the bladder can be periurethral or intraluminal. **Periurethral** colonization can originate either from the patient's own bowel flora or from the hands of hospital personnel manipulating the catheter or touching the perineal area. By ascending the thin mucous layer between the outer catheter surface and the urethra, bacteria can enter the bladder and multiply.

Intraluminal ascent of bacteria into the bladder most probably occurs when the distal catheter and collecting system are disconnected for irrigation, sample collection, or by accident. Contamination of the collection system may also occur during emptying of the drainage bag. In either case, organisms are able to ascend into the bladder via the column of urine in the collection tube and catheter or by reflux from an improperly placed collection bag.

Clinical manifestations and complications

At least one half of patients with UTIC lack symptoms. Those patients who do develop symptoms may complain of suprapubic pain and urethral burning. Typical findings of cystitis in noncatheterized patients (urgency, frequency, dysuria) are obscured because of the catheter. In most cases uncomplicated UTIC does not cause fever. If secondary bacteremia develops, however, fever, chills, sweats, and in severe cases, septic shock may ensue.

Gram-negative sepsis is the major complication of UTIC. The mortality rate is 25% to 30% of cases. If shock also occurs, this rate increases to 80%. One study reported that 50% of patients who developed gram-negative sepsis had had an indwelling urinary catheter within 10 days of developing bacteremia.

Another complication of bacteriuria is the development of acute or chronic pyelonephritis with its resultant problems of renal dysfunction and hypertension.

Prevention

The best way to prevent UTIC is to use a catheter only when it is essential, never solely to accommodate nursing care. Alternative techniques of urinary drainage (e.g., a condom catheter collecting system for cooperative male patients) should be considered first. Once it has been determined that catheterization is essential, the most significant measures for the prevention of urinary tract infection are as follows:

1. Educate, and periodically reeducate, personnel in correct techniques of catheter insertion and catheter care.
2. Insert catheter using aseptic technique, sterile equipment, and atraumatic insertion.
3. Use smallest-bore catheter suitable.
4. Secure catheter properly.
5. Maintain closed sterile drainage system.
6. Maintain unobstructed urine flow.
7. Avoid intermittent irrigation.
8. Obtain urine samples aseptically.
9. Avoid daily application of antimicrobial agents to the urethral meatus.

10. Change catheter only if it is leaking, malfunctioning, or if concretion can be felt in the lumen.
11. Provide each patient with a separate measuring receptacle when emptying the drainage system.
12. Segregate infected and uninfected patients with indwelling catheters.
13. Avoid continuous bladder irrigation with antiseptics as a routine infection control practice.

INTRAVASCULAR INFECTIONS

The second major source of nosocomial infection in ICUs is intravascular devices, such as IV infusion and pressure-monitoring devices. These devices are also one of the major sources of primary bacteremias. Other infections related to intravascular devices include suppurative thrombophlebitis, and possibly phlebitis. Nonetheless, despite the significant risks of infection associated with them, these devices have become an integral and necessary component of critical care.

Epidemiology

Most IV-associated infections are cannula related. Regardless of cause, phlebitis occurs in an estimated 1.3 million patients annually; those patients with plastic catheters have a tenfold greater risk than those with "scalp-vein" steel needles. Other factors that influence a patient's risk for an IV-catheter-associated infection include (1) patient susceptibility (e.g., burn patients and immunocompromised patients are more susceptible to these infections); (2) the method of insertion (e.g., cutdowns and central catheters, used for monitoring central venous pressure [CVP], are associated with comparatively higher rates of infection than cannulas that are inserted percutaneously); (3) duration of cannulation (e.g., peripheral cannulas that have been in continuous use for >48 to 72 hr are associated with a markedly increased rate of infection).

Infections related to microbial contamination of infusate occur much less frequently than cannula-related infections, but when they do occur, they generally are associated with an epidemic. Contamination can occur during manufacture of the infusate (intrinsic contamination) or during hospital preparation or use (extrinsic contamination), which occurs when organisms are introduced during manipulation of the IV bottle, tubing, or devices connected to the tubing (e.g., "piggyback" infusions, stopcocks, pressure-monitoring equipment).

Infections associated with contaminated infusate are almost exclusively caused by gram-negative bacilli, primarily *Klebsiella, Enterobacter,* and *Serratia;* however, *Citrobacter* and *Pseudomonas* also have been implicated in epidemics. Isolation of one of these organisms from the bloodstream of a patient believed to have an IV-related infection would suggest that the infusate had been contaminated rather than the cannula, although either may be responsible.

Hyperalimentation fluids, especially those containing crystalline amino acids, on the other hand, inhibit the growth of most microorganisms. *Candida* can, however, proliferate in these fluids. Lipid emulsions support rapid growth of a variety of microorganisms.

Intravascular pressure-monitoring systems, widely used in ICUs, have been implicated in infectious complications resulting in significant morbidity and mortality in the patients being monitored, as reported by the CDC. Bacteremia is the most common complication associated with intravascular-pressure monitoring. This can result from either contamination of the fluid and monitoring components external to the skin or from infection of the cannula insertion site. Most epidemics of bacteremia were related to reusable transducer domes. Once contaminated, these transducers acted as a reservoir for microorganisms because they received inadequate disinfection between patients. These epidemics abruptly ceased when measures were taken to assure proper reprocessing of equipment between patients and the use of disposable domes.

Since 1975, however, several infectious outbreaks involving patients monitored with transducers fitted with disposable domes have been reported. Contamination of the interspace between the protective dome membrane and the transducer head has been reported consistently in these outbreaks. Similar contamination of stopcocks and sampling ports in the system also have been documented. It is hypothesized that contamination of the exterior of the system, perhaps at assembly, leads to contamination of the flush fluid and subsequently, to bacteremia, although the precise mechanism remains undocumented.

Cannula-associated bacteremia also occurs in pressure-monitoring systems. With arterial lines, infection is more common with insertion by surgical cutdown than by percutaneous puncture. The frequency of infection related to arterial pressure monitoring, both local and systemic, increases significantly when the cannula is left in place for >4 days.

Clinical manifestations

Cannula-related infections are frequently preceded by, or associated with, phlebitis (usually characterized by warm, erythematous skin over an indurated or tender vein). Suppurative thrombophlebitis is characterized by gross or microscopic evidence of suppuration within the lumen of the vessel as well as by the signs and symptoms of phlebitis; pus may drain spontaneously from the cannula wound or may be expressed with pressure.

When other causes for a sudden elevation in temperature cannot be explained, the IV site should become suspect. The IV should be discontinued or restarted with an entire new setup at a different site.

Prevention of IV-associated infections

Because cannula-related infections account for most IV-associated infections, the CDC recommends that when initiating IV therapy, steel needles be used in preference to plastic cannulas because they are associated with a lower risk of infection. Percutaneous punctures are preferred over cutdowns for the same reason, and upper extremities, subclavian, and jugular sites are preferred to lower extremity sites for cannula insertion in adults. Hands must be washed carefully before inserting an IV cannula. Preparation of the insertion site with an antiseptic, preferably tincture of iodine, is recommended prior to cannula insertion. Application of topical polyantibiotic ointments appears to reduce infections when used for insertions requiring a cutdown. Antiseptic ointments (e.g., povidone-iodine) provide little, if any, benefit for most insertions. Covering the IV site with a sterile dressing reduces the risk of contamination. Securing of the cannula after insertion reduces the possibility of motion that can injure the vein and prevents the migration of microorganisms deeper into the cannula wound. Antiseptic compounding of parenterals, preferably in a controlled environment (i.e., under a laminar flow hood in the pharmacy), will control contamination of the infusate. Inspection of IV containers for cracks, leaks, or precipitants is recommended prior to use. Admixed IV fluids should be refrigerated at 4 degrees C until use. In-use fluids should be discarded after 24 hr. IV tubing should be changed at 48-hr intervals. Hyperalimentation tubing should be changed q 24 hr. Inspection of the IV insertion site q 24 hr and central cannula sites at 24-to-48-hr intervals will detect early complications associated with intravascular cannulas.

Prevention of pressure-monitoring-device-related infections

Invasive pressure-monitoring systems should be reserved for clinical situations in which information gathered by their use is necessary for patient management. When it is necessary to monitor intravascular pressure, recommendations for insertion and maintenance are similar to those for IV cannulas described above. In addition, it is recommended that strict sterile technique be observed during cannula insertion, including gowns, gloves, masks, etc. It is also recommended that pressure-monitoring systems that are used for a period of days should be replaced at regular intervals, such as q 48 hr. Patency of cannulas should be maintained through use of a closed-flush system rather than an open system that requires use of a syringe and stopcock. Taking of routine blood samples through the system should be discouraged, because this increases the risk of contamination. The use of non-glucose-containing solutions is recommended to flush lines whenever possible, because glucose solutions are known to support the growth of many microorganisms. Cannula sites should be inspected and redressed with a new sterile dressing at 48-to-72-hr intervals. Between dressing changes, patients should be evaluated at least daily for evidence of cannula-related complications. This includes gentle palpation of the insertion site through the intact dressing. Should the system be implicated as a source of infection, clinical sepsis, or bacteremia, it should be promptly discontinued or placed at another site. Cannulas for pressure monitoring should not be replaced over a guide wire if this is done solely for infection control.

Intravascular pressure-monitoring systems should be removed when they are no longer medically indicated. Disposable components of the pressure-monitoring system should not be resterilized and reused. Transducers should be cleaned and, preferably, sterilized with ethylene oxide. If ethylene oxide is not available or not recommended by the manufacturer, high-level disinfection with a chemical agent is the second method of choice for decontamination. The chamber dome, administration tubing, and continuous-flow device (if used) should be replaced at 48-hr intervals. As with IV solutions, flush solutions should be changed q 24 hr.

LOWER RESPIRATORY TRACT INFECTIONS

Lower respiratory tract infections are the third most frequent nosocomial infection in the USA.

Epidemiology

According to the CDC, 51% of nosocomial pneumonias are caused by aerobic gram-negative bacilli such as *Klebsiella, Enterobacter, Proteus, Pseudomonas,* and *Serratia.* Gram-positive bacilli, such as *Staphylococcus aureus* and *Streptococcus,* can also cause nosocomial bacterial pneumonia.

The incidence of gram-negative colonization in patients admitted to ICUs has been found to be 22% within 24 hr of admission. Susceptibility to colonization increases when the pulmonary defense mechanisms are compromised by instrumentation of the respiratory tract, e.g., intubation, tracheostomy, and suctioning. Other factors contributing to the development of nosocomial pneumonias include: (1) antibiotic therapy, which predisposes patients to colonization of the oropharynx with resistant gram-negative microorganisms; (2) aspiration of upper airway organisms and GI tract contents; (3) hematogenic spread of infectious organisms to the lungs from distant foci (e.g., UTI); and (4) debilitating conditions, such as acidosis, hypotension, coma, leukocytosis, or leukopenia.

The case fatality rate for nosocomial pneumonia is ≥30%, even with appropriate antibiotic therapy.

Clinical manifestations

Clinically, the onset of nosocomial pneumonia generally begins with a temperature spike. On physical assessment, signs of pulmonary consolidation (rales, bronchial breathing, or egophony) may be present, along with tachypnea. Laboratory data reveal an increase in the WBC. In some cases, however, particularly in immunosuppressed patients, signs and symptoms may consist only of fever and tachypnea; the differential blood count may not reflect an increase in WBCs in immunosuppressed patients. Findings on chest x-ray will show the presence of an infiltrate in the lungs. It must be noted, however, that there are many other causes of fever, cough, dyspnea, and pulmonary infiltrate in ICU patients. These include CHF, pulmonary embolus, adult respiratory distress syndrome (ARDS), atelectasis, and aspiration.

The presence of purulent sputum, along with the signs and symptoms described above, is highly suggestive of the presence of nosocomial pneumonia. Sputum Gram stains that show ≤10 epithelial cells and ≥25 WBCs in association with bacteria suggest the presence of pneumonia; cultures of the sputum will identify the etiology of the pneumonia. In most cases, however, without a properly collected sputum specimen, a mixture of organisms will be present on culture. Because most hospitalized patients develop upper airway colonization with gram-negative bacilli, these microorganisms contaminate the expectorated sputum specimen. In ICUs it should be possible to collect tracheal secretions (e.g., with sputum traps) to assist in the identification of the causative organism. Transtracheal aspiration or use of a triple lumen bronchoscope may be necessary to ascertain the presence or absence of bacteria in the lower respiratory tract, particularly in the immunosuppressed patient.

Prevention

One of the common sources for the colonization of the upper airways of critical care patients is via the hands of ICU personnel. Therefore, rigorous hand-washing procedures must be emphasized to reduce this risk. Strict adherence to aseptic technique in procedures such as tracheostomy or endotracheal suctioning will also prevent the transmission of microorganisms by the hands of health-care personnel.

Frequent coughing, deep breathing, and incentive spirometry, along with postural drainage and percussion, facilitates the removal of respiratory secretions and also reduces the risk of nosocomial pneumonia in high-risk patients.

Nasogastric tube feedings are often employed for critically ill patients. Careful management of patients with tube feedings can reduce the risk of aspiration, i.e., proper positioning of the patient after feedings and small, frequent feedings.

Respiratory therapy equipment has been implicated in outbreaks investigated over the past 20 years. Therefore, prevention is also directed toward control measures for the handling of ventilatory equipment. Equipment posing the greatest hazard is apparatus that nebulizes heated or warmed liquids and is used for a long period of time. The risk increases when aerosols produced are very small (1 to 2 μm). These small particles bypass the respiratory defense mechanisms, reaching the bronchioles and alveolar surfaces. Ultrasonic nebulizers on positive-pressure ventilators, as well as on intermittent positive-pressure breathing circuits, produce an effluent of small particles. Should the reservoir become contaminated, millions of microorganisms may be directly introduced into the lungs. Therefore, only sterile fluids should be nebulized or used in a humidifier. These fluids should be dispensed without allowing contaminated equipment to enter the fluid, and any unused fluid should be discarded within 24 hr of being opened. Room-air humidifiers that create droplets to humidify should not be used in an ICU because of their environmental risk.

Liquid medications delivered via a nebulizer also must be sterile and, preferably, in single-dose vials. If multiple-dose vials are used, they should be refrigerated between uses and discarded 24 hr after they are opened.

Several other areas of respiratory circuitry from patient to ventilator are possible sites of system contamination. These include the circuit tubing, the nebulizer manifold, the t-tube adapter, and the cascade humidifier. Indeed, any part of a respiratory apparatus in which fluid collects and is subject to manipulation is a potential source of infectious organisms.

Corregated circuit tubing can become contaminated with the patient's own microflora, making it a reservoir for the microorganisms to multiply and be transmitted back to the patient. Therefore, it is recommended that the patient's ventilatory circuit be changed at regular intervals. While the issue of frequency of ventilator tubing changes remains controversial and further study is needed, the CDC recommends changing the tubing q 24 hr.

Another possible source of microorganisms is in the effluent from the exhalation valve, which can contaminate the environment around the patient. This increases the risk of colonization for patients in close proximity to the effluent. The use of hydrophobic-type filters on inspiratory and expiratory lines to filter out bacteria is recommended to control this possible source of contamination.

Placement of an artificial airway, such as endotracheal tube or tracheostomy, also increases the risk of lower respiratory tract infection because of interference with the normal defense mechanisms of the upper respiratory tract. Endotracheal intubation provides a short-term airway, usually no longer than three to ten days. Tracheostomy involves long-term airway management. Tracheostomy should be performed in an operating room, except when strong clinical indications for emergency or bedside operation intervene.

Endotracheal and tracheostomy tubes have an inflatable cuff at their distal end to prevent air leakage around the tube. Constant pressure from an inflated cuff can cause damage to the tracheal tissue. Therefore, normal procedures sometimes require deflation of the cuff at regular intervals to allow for intermittent circulation. There is, however, the hazard of aspiration of pooled oral secretions that have accumulated above the cuff; oropharyngeal suctioning prior to deflation of the cuff removes this risk. Aseptic technique should be employed when suctioning both endotracheal and tracheostomy tubes. This requires the use of sterile gloves on *both* hands and a sterile catheter each time the procedure is done. Suctioning should be as atraumatic as possible to reduce the risk of infection.

Suction collection tubing (up to the canister) should always be changed between patients. High-efficiency bacterial filters between the collection bottle and the vacuum source are recommended for portable suction devices; however, such filters have not been shown to be useful for infection control when used with wall suction units.

Mouth care decreases the risk of infection in patients with an artificial airway by preventing breakdown in the integrity of the oral mucosa caused by dehydration. Frequent mouth care is an important nursing intervention because it also prevents the risk of infection caused by aspiration of oral secretions.

Tracheostomy care requires aseptic technique. Sterile gloves should be worn on both hands for all manipulations at the tracheostomy site. Patient education prior to the tracheostomy procedure should include what is to be expected, the importance of keeping the area as clean as possible, and advising the patient not to touch the site. The tracheostomy outer tube should not be changed until 4 to 5 days after initial insertion to allow for stabilization of the tissue. It is then recommended that it be changed q 2 to 4 days, using strict aseptic technique.

Patients with potentially transmissible respiratory infections should be isolated according to the latest recommendations from CDC (e.g., contact isolation for patients with multidrug-resistant bacteria, infected or colonized).

ANTIMICROBIAL THERAPY

While it is not within the realm of nursing practice to prescribe antibiotics, an understanding of their actions and the significance of antimicrobial resistance in infection control will provide the critical care nurse with a knowledge base important in patient management.

Epidemiology

Despite the lifesaving benefits of antimicrobial agents over the past several decades, their widespread use has brought about the selection of resistant strains of microorganisms. This selection occurs when antibiotic pressures suppress sensitive microflora and facilitate colonization and/or superinfection with resistant bacteria. This is particularly significant in the immunosuppressed patient. Resistance occurs most commonly through the mechanisms of (1) enzymatic inactivation of antibiotics; (2) changes in cell-wall permeability or cell-binding sites; (3) changes in metabolic pathways; or (4) alterations in drug-receptor sites.

Resistance to antimicrobials also may be genetic, occurring either by the bacterial chromosome or by extrachromosomal DNA. The former occurs by spontaneous mutation and the natural selection of organisms resistant to single (or closely related) agents. Extrachromosomal DNA (plasmids), called R factors or resistance plasmids, allow the transfer of coding for antibiotic resistance between bacteria. Plasmids may spread rapidly across species lines as well as between genera, often encoding multiple resistance.

Multiple-resistance is defined as resistance to two or more unrelated antibiotics to which the bacteria are usually susceptible. The identification of multidrug-resistant bacteria is an epidemiologic marker for real or potential problems in ICUs, and should not be overlooked. When multidrug-resistance in patients (infected or colonized) is identified, appropriate control measures should be instituted and it should be reported to the hospital infection control team. These nursing interventions can prevent the epidemic spread of multiple resistant bacteria both within the ICU and throughout the hospital.

Adverse manifestations

Two infectious processes directly related to the administration of antimicrobial agents are (1) mucocutaneous candidiasis, and (2) pseudomembranous colitis. *Candida* (a fungus) is part of the normal flora of the mucous membranes and the skin; however, its presence does not become clinically apparent until antimicrobial therapy has eliminated the normal flora.

Pseudomembranous colitis occurs when normal anaerobic flora in the intestinal tract are suppressed, permitting the growth of the bacterium *Clostridium difficile. C. difficile* produces a toxin that has a cytopathic effect and may lead to fatal hemorrhagic colitis. If diarrhea develops in a patient who is being treated with antibiotics, the physician should be notified immediately.

Other reactions to antimicrobial therapy include: (1) allergic reactions, and (2) intrinsic toxicity of the agent to body tissues, e.g., *ototoxicity* (aminoglycosides, vancomycin, streptomycin); *nephrotoxicity* (aminoglycosides, polymyxin B, amphotericin B, colistin, methicillin, tetracycline); *hemotoxicity* (chloramphenicol, penicillin, nafcillin, carbenicillin, sulfonamides).

Prevention of adverse effects

The nurse plays a critical role in avoiding potential toxic reactions or drug interactions. If drugs that are administered by IV infusion are given too fast or too early, excessively high blood levels may occur, leading to toxicity or transient peak levels beyond effective therapeutic levels. Serum levels should be drawn on time and documented to avoid dosage changes based on incorrect data, which could lead to toxicity.

With certain drugs (e.g., vancomycin) rapid IV infusion may cause a histamine release, resulting in flushing of the patient and cardiovascular collapse. The nurse must be aware of drug interactions that could result in inactivation of one antibiotic when being administered in association with another. For example, penicillins can inactivate the aminoglycosides; administration of the two in the same IV line may result in subtherapeutic levels. It is advisable to administer antimicrobial agents through different IV lines, at separate times, or by a different route (e.g., one IV and the other IM).

INFECTION CONTROL IN CRITICAL CARE PERSONNEL

An important aspect of infection control in the ICU is the prevention and control of infection in and by personnel. Nurses working in adult ICUs are at risk of exposure to certain infectious diseases. Exposure to any infectious disease is always possible; the more common ones, viral hepatitis type B and herpes simplex, are discussed below.

VIRAL HEPATITIS TYPE B

Patients admitted to the ICU who are hepatitis-B-surface-antigen (HB_sAg) positive constitute a reservoir of hepatitis B virus (HBV) that can be transmitted to staff members and other patients. Although HB_sAg has been detected in many body fluids (e.g., saliva, semen, breast milk, synovial fluid), blood is the most consistently effective vehicle of HBV transmission. The prevention and control of hepatitis B in ICUs thus deals with mechanisms of transmission via the blood. Because non-A, non-B (NANB) hepatitis is similar epidemiologically to hepatitis B, it represents the same hazards.

There is an extraordinary amount of circulating infectious HBV in the blood of individuals who are either in the acute phase of infection or are chronic HB_sAg carriers who also have positive hepatitis B e antigen (HB_eAg). The amount of inoculum of HBV necessary for the transmission of the disease is relatively small. The following mechanisms for transmission are listed in order of their efficacy of disease transmission:

1. Direct percutaneous inoculation by stick from a needle contaminated with serum or plasma of an infected individual.
2. Percutaneous transfer of infective serum or plasma by contamination of minute cutaneous scratches, abrasions, or other lesions.
3. Contamination of mucosal surfaces by infective serum or plasma (e.g., mouth pipetting, splashes to the eyes or mouth).
4. Transfer of infective material via fomites contaminated with HBV.
5. Contamination of mucosal surfaces by infective secretions other than serum or plasma (e.g., by sexual activities and other forms of physical contact involving secretions, such as saliva and semen).

The last category has little significance in the transmission of HBV between patients and staff; however, it does have significance for the counseling of patients and staff who have positive HB_sAg and thus bears mentioning. ICU personnel exposed to HBV through any of the mechanisms described above should report it to Personnel Health and/or the infection control nurse (team) in their hospital. Personnel health policies and protocols should be established for follow-up assessment after exposure to hepatitis and other communicable diseases.

Patients admitted to the ICU with a diganosis or possible diagnosis of hepatitis B or of NANB hepatitis should be placed on Blood/Body Fluid

Precautions recommended by the CDC. These precautions include: (1) use of gowns if soiling with blood or body fluids is likely; (2) avoidance of needle-stick injuries by handling used needles cautiously; (3) immediate hand-washing if hands become contaminated with blood or body fluids; (5) bagging and labeling of articles contaminated with blood or body fluids; (6) prompt cleaning up of spills with a 1:10 sodium hypochlorite solution. Isolation precautions appropriate for any infectious disease should be employed as soon as the diagnosis, or potential diagnosis, is made.

HERPES SIMPLEX

Several reports suggest that health-care personnel, especially those who have direct contact with respiratory tract secretions, acquire herpes simplex virus from patients with occult infection. In one survey, one-third of the nurses caring for critically ill patients developed herpetic whitlow during the study period. Personnel with herpetic whitlow should not have direct contact with patients until the lesions are healed. Personnel with primary or recurrent orofacial herpes simplex should not care for high-risk patients (e.g., severely immunocompromised patients). The risk of spread and/or acquisition of herpes simplex is minimized by careful hand-washing and the use of gloves on *both* hands when handling respiratory tract secretions.

Health-care personnel with any infectious disease in an acute phase (e.g., chickenpox; infectious diarrhea; upper respiratory infections, including influenza) should not be in contact with high-risk patients.

ISOLATION PRECAUTIONS

The reader is referred to the revised isolation precautions published by the CDC in 1983. These guidelines represent the first major revision in isolation techniques for use in hospitals since 1975.

Isolation practices are directed toward the prevention of the spread of infectious diseases and are designed to (1) control or eliminate the infectious agent; (2) control or eliminate the reservoir; (3) interrupt transmission; (4) protect the largest number of susceptible persons in the area.

Variations in precautions used are based on the epidemiology of the disease or infection involved. To ensure compliance with isolation practices, inservice education must be provided to all health care staff, including physicians.

CHAPTER 17

SHOCK

Susan DeGroot Emanuelsen

INTRODUCTION

Circulatory shock is a devastating syndrome and one of the leading killers of hospitalized patients. Although common to ICUs, shock is a potential threat to any patient in any area of the hospital. Its acute and lethal nature requires highly skilled and knowledgable nursing care to prevent and/or keep up with its rapidly progressive changing course. The key to management is early recognition; the ability to detect the subtle signs of shock may mean the difference between the survival or death of the shock victim. Any patient who is a potential victim must be observed continuously for the elusive and insidious signs of shock.

Some patients are more likely to develop shock than others. The list of likely candidates is wide and varied indeed. They include: the very young, the very old, the chronically ill, the trauma patient, the postsurgical patient, the diabetic, the patient with cardiac disease, those patients with burns and/or infections, those patients receiving immunosuppressive therapy, those patients with vessel lines or urinary catheters, and those patients who have had instrumentation.

Shock varies in its onset but, more often than not, it is acute, precipitous, and insidious. The course shock takes varies with the underlying etiology; hypovolemic shock usually takes time to develop and has a more predictable course, whereas the victim of anaphylactic shock may succumb in a matter of minutes. Septic shock may overwhelm the victim before it is even recognized.

Definition

Shock is a group of syndromes representing mixed etiologies. The core problem is at the cellular level, a reason that the early signs often go unnoticed. Basic to the concept of shock is that circulatory insufficiency causes an unevenness of flow at the level of the microcirculation, resulting in low tissue perfusion and derangements in the metabolic and hemodynamic balance of the body. Low tissue perfusion leads to cellular hypoxia and inadequate removal of metabolic wastes, the end result being cellular deterioration and death.

Shock occurs as a result of an alteration or failure of one or more major components of the circulatory system: (1) the heart and its ability to pump, (2) the peripheral vascular resistance of the vessels, and (3) the circulating blood volume. A temporary shift in one or more of these components can occur and be compensated for by the regulatory mechanisms of the body, but when the shifts are profound, the regulatory mechanisms are inadequate.

There are essentially two main conditions that allow for shock to occur: (1) the inability of the heart to pump adequately and (2) a decrease in venous return caused by diminished circulating volume, decrease in vasomotor tone, or an increase in resistance to flow.

Physiology of circulation

A basic understanding of the physiology of circulation is necessary before one can begin to comprehend the nature of shock and the complexities of its treatment. As the focus of the effects of shock is at the level of the tissues, knowledge of the physiology of the microcirculation is essential (*see* Chapter 2). It is equally important that the nurse be familiar with the cellular anatomy and physiology.

PATHOPHYSIOLOGY

Shock impinges on every aspect of normal body functioning. When one system malfunctions, others follow. In response to the shock state, the body launches all of its defenses to compensate for the malfunction. The course of shock can be divided into three stages. How fast or slow the condition progresses depends upon its etiology. It cannot be overemphasized, however, that regardless of the etiology, early recognition and management contributes greatly to the victim's ability to survive.

Compensatory stage

In the initial stage of shock, the compensatory stage, the CO is sufficiently diminished to cause decreased tissue perfusion but not enough to cause cellular deterioration. Compensatory mechanisms are initiated to cause vasoconstriction in an effort to raise and maintain arterial BP. The catecholamines, norepinephrine and epinephrine, are released to increase blood flow to the heart, brain, and skeletal muscle and decrease blood flow to less vital areas. Humoral factors are released to constrict vessels and to increase blood volume through the conservation of water. Ventilation is increased to compensate for the decreased O_2 levels in the arterial blood. Initially, the two most striking physiologic responses to shock are evidenced by increased activity in cardiorespiratory function. Heart rate and myocardial contractility are increased to increase CO. Increased respiratory rate strives to improve alveolar ventilation.

Although overall blood supply to the kidneys is diminished, the kidneys have their own local regulation and can maintain glomerular filtration in the early stage of shock. With the decrease in arterial BP, however, the amount of glomerular filtrate is reduced.

If this stage is recognized, the shock treated, and its cause eliminated, no damage at the cellular level will result and the prognosis is very good.

Progressive stage

The body's ability to compensate for decreases in arterial BP has a limit. Once the limit is reached, the compensatory mechanisms fail and the victim goes into the second stage, the noncompensated, or progressive, stage of shock. It is believed that the single most important factor in the progression of shock is the deterioration of the heart. As the compensatory mechanism fails, circulatory and cellular deterioration begins. The heart becomes increasingly weak and is unable to maintain adequate CO. This in itself reduces the blood supply to the myocardium, further compromising cardiac functioning. It is in this noncompensated stage that the vicious and deadly cycle of shock begins. It is important to note that the initial cause of the shock may not, at this point, be getting worse, but the numerous responses of the body are causing an increase in the degree of the shock.

As arterial BP falls and blood flow is diminished, severe tissue hypoxia makes the syndrome self-perpetuating. The cells deteriorate, metabolism is impaired, waste products accumulate, and finally the cell dies. The effects of hypoxia are seen systemically.

Vascular integrity is severely damaged when ischemia is present. The vessel walls become weak, unable to constrict, allowing for venous pooling and diminished venous return. Relaxation of the precapillary sphincter allows blood in, but not out. The result is pooling and sludging of blood and eventually thrombosis in the small vessels. The clotting mechanism (*see* Chapter 4) becomes deranged with the terminal result being disseminated intravascular coagulation (DIC).

Diminished blood flow to the brain results in damage to the vasomotor and respiratory centers. Vasomotor tone is lost, further contributing to tissue hypoxia.

Impaired cell membrane function results in an increase in capillary permeability. Transudation of fluid into the interstitial spaces further reduces blood volume, diminishes venous return and CO.

Hypoxia and anoxia lead to the release of toxins and substances that potentiate the severity of the shock state. The breakdown of cells frees substances that activate histamine and bradykinin, resulting in severe vasodilation and depression of cardiac function. Bacterial invasion as well as vasoconstriction in the liver and subsequent hypoxia result in impaired ability to detoxify. Prolonged ischemia and anoxia result in the loss of integrity of the intestinal mucosa, allowing for the release of toxins and bacteria into the systemic circulation. Release of toxins from liver, intestines, and muscle contributes to the development of DIC, alters the functioning of the reticuloendothelial system, and destroys the integrity of the microcirculation.

Cellular hypoxia results in a shift from aerobic metabolism to anaerobic. Metabolic acidosis results when there is a decrease in the oxidative metabolism of foodstuffs, an increase in extracellular lactic acid caused by anaerobic metabolism, and an increase in CO_2 in the tissues resulting in the formation of carbonic acid.

Irreversible stage

The third and final stage of shock is the irreversible stage. It is at this point that cellular and circulatory destruction is so widespread and complete that no amount of therapy can correct the damage. The patient in this stage may seem to improve for a time but eventually succumbs to the effects of shock.

It is believed that lack of O_2 is the stimulus for the development of irreversible shock because the less available the O_2, the more rapid the onset of irreversible shock. Failure of the cardiorespiratory system is characteristic of this stage. The heart is unable to meet the demands made upon it; the lungs become "stiff," interstitial edema develops, respiratory drive decreases, and finally, terminal hypoxia and hypercarbia occur.

CLINICAL PICTURE

Generally, the signs and symptoms of shock are classic, and the nurse can rely on their appearance. (There are some exceptions that will be noted throughout this discussion.) It is of utmost importance, however, to note *patterns* of development. Reliance on the textbook picture can lead a practitioner down the wrong path when, instead, significant *changes* should be noted. Continuous assessment of the patient at risk may be all that stands between the life or death of thc patient. If one waits to see a sign or note a symptom, the shock syndrome may be so far advanced that treatment is either very difficult or impossible in order to save the life of the victim.

Skin

Decreased skin temperature is usually present in all types of shock except in septic shock. The usual cool skin of shock is caused by vasoconstriction, a compensatory mechanism used to divert the skin's blood supply to more vital areas. The warm skin of septic shock occurs early in shock and is temporary, for as the shock progresses, the signs of hypovolemia occur.

Skin color is usually pale; however, in the case of septic shock, the skin may be flushed. In cases of shock caused by pulmonary embolus or heart failure, the skin may be cyanotic. In late hemorrhagic shock, the victim may also appear cyanotic because of pooling of unoxygenated blood in the capillaries of the skin and the sludging of blood.

Clammy skin is noted more often than not and suggests a deficit of vascular fluid. Diaphoresis is an occurrence of the late shock state. Those patients in shock caused by infection may have dry skin.

Collapsed veins are another sign, although a patient in heart failure or with pulmonary emboli may have distended veins.

Blood pressure

Hypotension is usually present in most forms of shock. A systolic BP <80 mmHg usually suggests shock and that adequate coronary circulation cannot be maintained. This number is relative, however, and means little when assessing a normally hypertensive patient for shock. Again, change is the key, and knowing a base-line assessment figure is essential. The person in septic shock may have a normal or elevated arterial BP in the early stages. Generally, the pulse pressure narrows during shock as the systolic BP falls faster than the diastolic. In septic shock, the pulse pressure widens initially but then falls as shock deepens. Peripheral resistance is indicated by the level of the diastolic BP. When resistance is increased, the diastolic BP increases. When vasoconstriction stimulus is lost, marked vasodilation occurs, causing a decrease in resistance and a fall in the diastolic BP.

Cardiac status

Tachycardia is a common sign of shock. The heart rate increases as a compensatory mechanism to increase venous return and CO. In most forms of shock, the pulse is also weak and thready; in septic shock the pulse may be full and bounding. In the irreversible stage of shock, the pulse rate may become very slow and irregular.

Respiratory status

Because of decreased tissue perfusion, the respiratory rate in all forms of shock is increased and becomes shallow. This occurs as a compensatory mechanism to increase the O_2 level in the blood and also, as the amounts of CO_2 increase, the respiratory center is stimulated. Once the compensatory mechanism fails, the respirations become slow. This is a late sign. In septic shock, respiratory rate increases as the condition worsens.

Mentation

Early in the shock state, because of overstimulation of the sympathetic nervous system, the patient appears nervous, anxious, agitated, and his facial expression reflects this anxiety. Whether or not the victim becomes unconscious early in shock depends on the rate of onset and the severity of the shock condition. Most often the patient becomes lethargic, drowsy, and confused because of decreased blood flow to the brain. Some patients, however, are quite agitated, restless, and unusually alert. As the shock state deepens, the patient becomes less alert, more lethargic, apathetic, and finally comatose. Drowsiness and stupor are more characteristic of shock states caused by sepsis. The blood vessels in the brain do not respond to the vasoconstricting stimulation of the sympathetic nervous system. Therefore, blood from peripheral organs is diverted to the brain. The systolic blood BP must be >40 mmHg to maintain circulation to the brain.

Renal function

Urinary output is very sensitive to changes in BP and is usually a reliable indicator in shock. Because vasoconstriction takes place in the kidneys when BP falls, the volume of urine produced is diminished. Decreased urinary output is an early sign of shock and indeed, may occur before a decrease in arterial BP is noted. If the output falls too low, renal shutdown will occur. Urine output <30 ml/hr is critical.

Metabolic function

Metabolic acidosis is a late sign of shock. As aerobic metabolism gives over to anaerobic because of stasis of blood and inadequate circulation, the by-products—mainly lactic acid—accumulate and produce a severe state of acidosis. Initially, the body attempts to compensate. In early septic shock, the patient may be in metabolic alkalosis. The reason for this is unclear at this time. Respiratory alkalosis is most often caused by tachypnea.

Circulation

Observation of hemodynamic changes is essential. In hypovolemic shock, the central venous pressure (CVP) is almost always reduced. In cardiogenic shock, the CVP will usually be elevated. Pulmonary arterial wedge pressure (PAWP), which reflects left ventricular end-diastolic pressure (LVEDP), will be elevated in cardiogenic shock and reduced in hypovolemic shock.

Acid-base balance

In early shock the PO_2 and the PCO_2 fall and the alveolar-arterial oxygen difference ($AaDO_2$) rises. The fall in PCO_2 reflects the patient's tachypnea; the fall in PO_2 and the rise in $AaDO_2$ represents increased physiologic shunting in the lungs.

Patients in shock also manifest extreme thirst caused by hypovolemia from blood loss or fluid shifts.

Generally, the accepted clinical criterion for determining whether or not a patient is in shock and treatment should be initiated is when any two of the following conditions exist: (1) systolic BP of ≤80 mmHg; (2) pulse pressure of ≤20 mmHg; (3) pulse rate of ≥100. Again, it must be stressed that *changes in patterns* must be observed, for a normally hypertensive individual may not tolerate pressures of 80 mmHg and may already be in irreversible shock by the time the systolic BP reaches such a low level. On the other hand, patients on vasodilators may have a normal systolic BP of ≤80 mmHg, and the initiation of shock treatment would be inappropriate for these individuals.

GENERAL MANAGEMENT

The general management of shock requires the expertise of many members of the health team. Essentially, there are three goals in the management of shock: (1) to restore or increase CO to meet the demands of the tissues; (2) to distribute blood flow to vital organs if the CO cannot be increased effectively; (3) to maintain the arterial BP so as to assure perfusion of the brain and heart and maintain glomerular filtration.

The initial step is to identify the underlying etiology. A rapid review of the patient's history and a quick assessment will assist the practitioner in determining the basic mechanism. Some parameters are common to management of all forms of shock.

Ventilation

Because O_2 deprivation in the cells is considered to be the most important stimulus for the development of irreversible shock, adequate ventilation of the patient in shock is of utmost importance. Delivery of O_2 depends on the condition of the patient. The goal is to assure airway patency and provide adequate ventilation. This may require endotracheal intubation, tracheostomy, and/or assisted ventilation. As soon as shock is considered a possibility, O_2 via mask should be initiated.

Circulation

Restoration of blood volume is essential so that adequate nutrients can be delivered unhampered to the tissues to deter the deterioration of the cells. In the case of hemorrhagic shock, the bleeding must be stopped. CVP or PAWP monitoring is essential to deliver proper fluid replacement therapy. Measurement of arterial BP, either direct or indirect, must be frequent. Urinary output measurement is vital; output of ≥30 ml/hr is essential. Fluid challenge is commonly ordered by the physician. CVP and arterial BP are measured and lungs auscultated just prior to the fluid challenge. These assessments are continued frequently throughout the time of the fluid challenge.

Cardiac function

Cardiac function is observed throughout via monitoring and 12-lead ECG determinations and laboratory values. CO can be measured by various methods, most commonly in a thermodilution pulmonary artery catheter. Arrhythmias (mostly ventricular) are common when the systolic BP falls below 80 mmHg and myocardial action becomes weak. O_2 must be provided and fluid replacement vigorously accomplished.

Laboratory values

Laboratory values commonly obtained include: Hb, Hct, type and cross matching, serum electrolytes, CBC, arterial blood gases (ABGs), urinalysis, and blood cultures when sepsis is suspected.

Pharmacologic agents

Drugs play an essential role in increasing the CO by changing the degree of peripheral resistance. The drugs used are vasopressors and vasodilators and are classified as to their effect on the sympathetic nervous system receptor sites (alpha or beta receptors). The use of these drugs, however, depends on the basic mechanism involved in the shock syndrome. Vasopressors are alpha-adrenergic and act to constrict the peripheral blood vessels. On the other hand, beta-adrenergic drugs dilate the peripheral vessels but increase the heart rate and myocardial contractility. Then there are drugs that are both alpha and beta stimulators, such as dopamine, that constrict skeletal muscle vessels but dilate the vessels of the vital organs (heart, brain, and kidneys). A fine line exists between the predomination of one effect or the other. In all cases, these drugs are administered cautiously because of their extreme potency, and a continuous infusion device is required. Continuous monitoring of vital signs, CVP, and urinary output is essential when these agents are used.

CLASSIFICATION OF SHOCK

The most accurate and concise classification of shock is based on the three major physiologic mechanisms that support circulation: the pump, the volume, and the vascular tone. Therefore, there are three major pathophysiologic events that precipitate the shock syndrome: (1) decreased blood volume (hypovolemic shock); (2) pump failure (cardiogenic shock); and (3) decreased vascular tone (vasogenic [septic] shock and neurogenic shock).

Hypovolemic shock

Hypovolemic shock is caused by a decrease in circulating blood volume because of actual blood loss, plasma loss, or protein-free fluid and electrolyte loss, all of which cause a decrease in venous return and thus a decrease in CO.

Actual blood loss from hemorrhage is by far the most common cause of hypovolemia. Plasma loss occurs as a result of burns or any condition that causes rapid shifts of plasma from the vascular compartment to the interstitial spaces. Loss of protein-free fluids and electrolytes occurs in diabetic ketoacidosis or dehydration caused by diarrhea and vomiting or any condition where losses occur from every compartment: intravascular, intracellular, and interstitial.

As volume decreases, arterial BP falls and the body's compensatory mechanisms take over. Peripheral vascular resistance increases to raise arterial BP, veins and venous beds constrict in order to increase volume, and heart rate increases to improve CO. The compensatory mechanisms are effective as long as the loss does not exceed 10 to 15% in the previously healthy individual. Symptoms of shock occur when losses become >15 to 25%.

Clinical picture. Clinical features depend upon the precipitating etiology (bleeding, trauma, burns, polyuria, copious vomiting, diarrhea, abdominal distension, etc.). Some of the clinical signs include a decrease in arterial BP, flat neck veins, cool and clammy skin caused by peripheral vasoconstriction. Loss of skin turgor is evident, especially in the case of protein-free fluid loss. Heart rate and respiratory rate are increased. Severe alterations in mentation usually do not occur, although the patient may become drowsy and confused and express feelings of impending doom. Orthostatic hypotension is common and may be evident before systemic hypotension manifests itself. Urine output is decreased. As the shock condition worsens, all the clinical signs become worse: arrhythmias, shallow respirations, systolic BP <60 mmHg, cyanosis, anuria, coma; CVP, PAWP, and LVEDP are all reduced in hypovolemic shock. Patients in hypovolemic shock often have extreme thirst. In hemorrhage, the Hb falls rapidly; the Hct is also low, but it takes a few hours for Hct to accurately reflect the amount of blood loss. Hct is elevated in other types of fluid loss.

Medical management. It is essential to observe for shock in any patients at risk (i.e., those who are postoperative or have burns, diabetes, trauma). The degree of fluid loss is critical and the sooner it is treated, the easier it is to treat. Medical management consists of replacing lost circulating blood volume. The type of solution used depends on the nature of the fluid loss. The most commonly used solutions are lactated Ringer's, saline, serum albumin, dextran, whole blood, or packed cells. Fluid replacement must be monitored by following PAWP and CVP measurements and urinary output. Measurements of serum Hb, Hct, and electrolytes are also essential. Appropriate chemistries are done to ascertain alterations in blood volume, potassium, and bicarbonate. ABGs are taken at appropriate intervals to ascertain the ventilatory status of the patient. O_2 (per mask) is usually given. Diuretics, such as furosemide, are administered if urinary output does not increase with administration of fluids. Usually the use of vasopressor drugs is contraindicated in hypovolemic shock because of the intense vasoconstriction produced in the microcirculation. Pharmacologic agents used are those that increase cardiotonicity, CO, and provide dilation of renal vascular bed to increase urinary output. These include digitalis, isoproteronal, and dopamine hydrochloride.

Nursing management. Initial nursing care of a suspected or actual shock victim is to assess ventilation and circulation, ensure an airway, and provide O_2 via mask; if the patient is bleeding, attempt to control and estimate blood loss; establish an IV line and administer fluids as ordered to provide volume expansion; insert an indwelling urinary catheter; place the patient in the horizontal position with legs elevated ~20 degrees; move him gently and keep him warm, but not overly so; obtain appropriate serum studies and ABGs. Assist the physician in the insertion of monitoring lines and administer drugs as ordered. Parameters to be measured frequently (q 15 min to 1 hr) include: BP, heart rate and quality, respiratory rate and quality, CVP, pulmonary artery pressure (PAP), PAWP, and urinary output. Be alert to alterations in mentation. It is essential that the patient be kept calm, as excitement and fear increase the demands on the heart. Give support and alleviate apprehension.

The nurse should constantly be alert to the possibility of complications. Pulmonary edema and adult respiratory distress syndrome (ARDS) are not uncommon. Renal failure should be suspected if urinary output does not respond to fluid therapy.

Cardiogenic shock

Cardiogenic shock is a pump-failure syndrome associated with inadequate cardiac filling or inadequate cardiac ejection. Cardiogenic shock occurs with any situation that interferes with the pump action of the heart, including pericardial tamponade, MI, pulmonary embolism, metabolic derangements, valvular disease, and arrhythmias. Characteristics of cardiogenic shock include an increase in pressure of venous beds and increased peripheral resistance.

Owing to the wide variety of underlying conditions, this syndrome is most difficult to treat and carries an 80 to 85% mortality. Symptoms mimic those of heart failure and, very often, the shock goes unnoticed until it is well advanced. Unless detected early, treatment is rarely successful. Once the shock has progressed, the already damaged heart becomes further damaged by the added effects of shock. Death can occur rapidly, in <1 hr or over a period of days.

When the heart becomes damaged by whatever underlying mechanism, its ability to contract adequately is impaired and CO reduced. Hypotension develops along with compensatory peripheral vasoconstriction. Coronary and collateral circulation is reduced, adding to myocardial ischemia. Indeed, in the patient who has infarcted, the decrease in perfusion may increase the size of the infarcted areas. CO and arterial BP are further reduced when cardiac afterload is increased.

Clinical picture. The cardinal signs of cardiogenic shock are hypotension, depressed mentation, and oliguria, along with engorgement of neck veins and peripheral or pulmonary edema. The CVP and LVEDP are elevated. Very often the initial signs of cardiogenic shock may be changes in mentation, agitation, anxiety, disorientation, lethargy, and apathy. The skin is cool, clammy, often cyanotic; body temperature is decreased; respirations are rapid, and rales are heard as the pump failure affects the lungs. Tachycardia usually occurs in the early stages of shock unless heart block is present. The pulse will be feeble and thready. Other arrhythmias develop as shock progresses because of a decrease in coronary perfusion and increase in metabolic derangements. Urine output falls <30 ml/hr. The systolic BP drops to 80 to 90 mmHg or 30 mmHg below the patient's usual BP.

Medical management. The key to management and successful therapy is to prevent even short periods of hypotension. Therapy focuses on reducing the work of the heart, increasing myocardial contractility and CO. The underlying etiology must be removed as well. Monitoring of fluid volume is most accurately accomplished with the use of a Swan-Ganz line to measure PAP and PAWP. Any administration of fluids must be done judiciously, based on these measurements. Measurement of arterial BP with an arterial line is preferred. Adequate ventilation is essential to promote oxygenation and is accomplished with the use of an O_2 face mask or mechanical ventilation, depending upon the results of ABGs and the patient's own ability to provide effective ventilation (*see* Chapter 13).

Metabolic derangements contribute to the progression of shock and circulatory collapse; hypoxemia, hypercapnia, and acidosis may interfere with the ability of myocardium to respond to treatment. Treatment with sodium bicarbonate and O_2 is essential.

Heart rate, whether it is rapid or slow, must be controlled. Isoproteronal is used to increase the cardiac rate and force of contraction. In pronounced bradycardia, atropine is used to increase the rate. Rapid rhythms may be controlled with digitalis. This drug may improve CO, but its effect is compromised in those patients receiving catecholamines. Conditions such as acidosis and any myocardial ischemia increase the risk of digitalis-induced arrhythmias. Cardiac pacing may be indicated. Dopamine, a mixed alpha-beta stimulator, is the drug of choice for increasing arterial BP by its ability to increase CO. It improves the strength of cardiac contraction as well as dilates the renal, splanchnic, and coronary vessels. Vasodilators, such as sodium nitroprusside, are helpful in reducing cardiac afterload. Large doses of prednisone may be useful for their effects on the microcirculation and capillary permeability.

Norepinephrine increases arterial BP and slows the heart rate to increase myocardial perfusion. Norepinephrine, epinephrine, isoproteronal, and dopamine are all sympathomimetics but have different cardiovascular effects.

Mechanical life-support devices, such as the intra-aortic balloon counterpulsation device, have been more successful than any other therapy. The use of this device increases coronary blood flow, decreases left ventricular filling pressure, and decreases myocardial O_2 demands.

Vasodilators are usually used when the CVP and PAWP are elevated. Treatment should not increase peripheral vascular resistance. Arrhythmias are treated appropriately, so continuous cardiac monitoring is essential.

Nursing management. Alteration in mentation may be the very first clue that the patient is in cardiogenic shock. Any patient with underlying heart disease who experiences a sudden, sharp drop in BP and urine output should be considered in cardiogenic shock.

Immediate establishment of adequate ventilation is essential. O_2 via mask is initiated. ABG analysis assists in determining the need for mechanical ventilatory assistance. The horizontal position utilized in other forms of shock is contraindicated in cardiogenic shock because it interferes with the patient's ability to breathe properly; the patient's trunk should be elevated. Continual assessment of lung sounds to detect rales is indicated. Alterations in heart sounds signal a worsening condition. An indwelling urinary catheter is necessary for frequent measurement of urinary output and sp gr. Establishment of a dependable IV line is essential. Measures must be taken, however, to prevent accidental fluid overload. Vital signs are measured frequently (q 15 min). More frequent measurement of BP is indicated when the patient is receiving vasopressors or vasodilators. Assist the physician with the insertion of Swan-Ganz line and measure PAP and PAWP frequently. Administer pharmacologic agents as ordered while continually assessing their effects.

It is equally important that the nurse provide a quiet and comfortable environment so as to reduce the work of the heart.

Septic shock

Septic, or vasogenic, shock occurs as a result of profound vasodilation secondary to the loss of vasomotor tone caused by the release of toxic substances that produce vasodilation of the blood vessels. The septic shock syndrome is probably the most complex because it alters all mechanisms that support circulation. It is subtle, often going unrecognized until the shock state has progressed to a dangerous level. The mortality rate is high (80%), and treatment is only successful when it is recognized early. The clinical signs of septic shock are the opposite of those for hypovolemic shock and cardiogenic shock. The effects on the microcirculation occur early in the condition and therefore are more rapidly devastating.

Septic shock results from a widely disseminated infection (most frequently a gram-negative organism), carried through the blood from one area of the body to another. Underlying etiology includes peritonitis, generalized gangrene, and generalized infection from a simple skin wound. Again, the patients at risk include the very young or very old, those debilitated with infections, the postsurgical, burn, or trauma patient, the malnourished, the chronically ill, and those with vessel lines or urinary catheters; those patients with defects in host resistance or on immunosuppressive therapy are also at risk.

The consequences of septic shock occur as endotoxins are released from bacteria. The endotoxins cause an increase in capillary permeability, with a subsequent increase in filtration pressure. Circulating blood volume is lost with a fluid shift from the capillaries into the interstitial spaces. Along with the alteration in capillary permeability, peripheral vasodilation occurs. To compensate for the vasodilation and resulting hypovolemia, CO is initially increased, BP rises, heart rate is increased as well as the force of the contraction. A widened pulse pressure is evident. Alteration in cellular perfusion occurs early in septic shock, and widespread cellular damage is often severe by the time the condition is recognized. The capillaries of the lungs are especially vulnerable to damage by the bacterial endotoxin, and hypoxia occurs early, leading to hyperventilation. Respiratory alkalosis occurs, and as the shock progresses and anaerobic metabolism takes place, a combination of respiratory and metabolic acidosis exists. This situation increases capillary permeability further, with decreased venous return, resulting in pulmonary edema and ARDS. Respiratory failure is a main cause of death.

The bacterial endotoxin also causes intense vasospasm in the lungs, liver, and kidneys. Presence of bacterial endotoxins interferes with adequate cell metabolism, and there is inadequate nutrient exchange.

Sludging of blood is another characteristic problem. As the bacterial endotoxins are released, RBCs agglutinate in response to the degeneration of tissues. In the late stage of septic shock, the symptoms become more consistent with the other forms of shock. Massive cardiovascular deterioration is evident, with hypotension, decreased CO, and narrowing pulse pressure.

Clinical picture. Characteristically, the patient in early septic shock has a significant increase in CO, and a normal to rising BP. The skin is warm. (Septic shock is also referred to as "warm shock" because the skin is warm secondary to vasodilation and temperature elevation.) The pulse is full and bounding. Urine output may be normal to increased. Tachypnea is present. The ABGs may be normal. Trends that occur early and give clues to the problem include widening pulse pressure and early and significant deterioration of mental status (lethargy, apprehension, restlessness, confusion, cloudy sensorium, and coma). Urine sodium is decreased. Hypoxemia is almost always a constant feature in septic shock because of pulmonary venoarterial admixture. The patient may have nausea, vomiting, abdominal distension and cramping. WBCs and BUN are elevated. Proteinuria is present.

In the late stage of septic shock, the symptoms come more into line with those of other forms of shock. Hypovolemia is evident; skin is cool, clammy; the patient may be hypothermic; the pulse becomes rapid and thready; oliguria and cyanosis are present. Hypotension with a narrowing pulse pressure and all the other late signs signify massive circulatory deterioration. Whereas initially the ABGs may have been normal although the patient was tachypneic, later the ABGs show respiratory alkalosis, metabolic alkalosis, and finally a combination of respiratory and metabolic acidosis. The patient who is not tachypneic may need early ventilatory assistance, because tachycardia and tachypnea are compensatory mechanisms, and the prognosis may be especially poor for the patient who does not exhibit these compensatory mechanisms. It is increasingly thought that the survival of the septic shock patient is determined in great part by the pulmonary response to the shock.

Medical management. The management of septic shock involves (1) treating the shock and (2) treating the sepsis. The key to success depends on *very* early recognition and treatment. If septic shock is even a remote possibility, treatment should begin while definitive diagnosis is being made.

Assessment modalities include ABGs, blood cultures, PAP, PAWP, arterial pressures, CBC, appropriate serum electrolytes, and chemistry studies.

First, the most important treatment is to provide adequate ventilation because the lungs are a primary target of the endotoxin, and respiratory complications are the main cause of death. Restoration of circulation is accomplished by establishing a dependable IV route and appropriate infusion of fluids according to PAP and PAWP measurements. Monitoring of urine output, sp gr, and urine sodium is indicated.

Treatment of metabolic acidosis is initiated. Volume challenge is necessary to obtain the most rapid influence on tissue perfusion. Steroids in large doses are given because it is thought that these increase circulation at the capillary level. Antibiotics are begun as soon as all cultures are obtained, inotropic agents are given as indicated, and vasodilators are administered to increase renal perfusion and improve mental status.

Nursing management. The key to nursing management is knowing which patients are at risk for septic shock and recognizing the subtle and insidious signs of early septic shock. Early recognition challenges all the nurse's skills of observation and assessment. Base-line assessment of these patients is essential, for it may be the subtle trends that provide the clues to the presence of septic shock.

Once septic shock has been recognized or suspected, immediate blood cultures must be obtained. All tubes must be removed from the patient and must be cultured. All wounds, dressings, drainage, mucus, and urine must be cultured as well. A dependable IV route must be established; the physician must be assisted in the insertion of a Swan-Ganz line to measure PAP. Serum electrolytes and BUN are also obtained. Accurate intake and output records are maintained; urine sp gr and pH are measured. Frequent vital signs and continuous ECG monitoring is indicated as well as CVP, PAP, PAWP.

Antibiotics are administered IV and must be initiated as ordered as soon as all cultures are obtained. Drugs to improve myocardial contractility and CO and steroids are administered as ordered, and nursing care specific for the administration of these pharmacologic agents is carried out.

The patient must be kept quiet, and continuous reassurance for the patient and his family is a must. Skin care and relief of pain, along with other comfort measures, is provided.

Neurogenic shock

Neurogenic shock is a syndrome resulting from a change in blood vessel capacity secondary to decreased peripheral vascular resistance. The marked decreased in peripheral vascular resistance results in venous pooling and stagnant circulation.

Anytime there is a sudden cessation of sympathetic impulses from the CNS to the peripheral vascular system, the result is a sudden loss of vasomotor tone, a decrease in pressure in all areas of the vascular system, decreased venous return, and finally, a decreased CO. If left untreated, the same results associated with other forms of shock will ensue, such as tissue anoxia, cellular destruction, and death.

Conditions contributing to the development of neurogenic shock are many and varied, ranging from general anesthesia to strong emotional excitement. Probably the most frequent causes of neurogenic shock are deep general anesthesia and spinal anesthesia. The most serious cause is brain damage, particularly damage to the brainstem or vasomotor areas. Other contributing factors include instrumental manipulation, severe pain, and strong emotional excitement. Neurogenic shock may also be the result of excessive catecholamine effect caused by excessive use of vasoconstrictors. Fainting is a mild example of neurogenic shock.

Clinical picture. The major clinical finding is sudden hypotension. The patient may or may not remain alert, depending upon the underlying etiology. If the cause is excessive catecholamine effect, the patient remains alert even though his BP may not be detectable. Other signs and symptoms include: cool and clammy skin, nausea, initially a slow heart rate that soon increases as a compensatory response to increase the CO.

As the condition progresses, the late signs of neurogenic shock are consistent with those seen in all types of shock.

Medical management. The goal of treatment is to restore effective blood volume, i.e., to fill the dilated vessels. Adequate ventilation is of primary importance. Early fluid administration is indicated. Vasoconstrictors may be administered, particularly when fluid administration does not restore adequate tissue perfusion. The patient is positioned flat. Identification and treatment and/or removal of the underlying etiology is essential as the prognosis largely depends on the underlying process. Neurogenic shock in the brain-damaged patient is a cause for grave concern, and treatment becomes more complex and is aimed at maintaining circulatory and ventilatory integrity in the hope that once the cerebral edema subsides, the vasomotor tone will return. If the cause is severe pain, the prompt relief of the pain will reverse the shock condition.

Nursing management. Ensure adequate ventilation by establishing an open airway and administering O_2 by mask. Position the patient flat. Monitor vital signs q 15 min initially. Assess vital signs, skin temperature and color, and mentation frequently. Establish an IV route and administer fluids as ordered. Administer pharmacologic agents as ordered. Assess hydration through accurate recording of intake and output and sp gr. Observe for signs of progressive shock. Keep the patient calm and quiet and provide emotional support for the patient and his family.

CHAPTER 18

LEGAL ISSUES IN CRITICAL CARE

Antoinette E. Grenier

This chapter will contain an overview of the law on issues raised in critical care. Because each state has, and will continue to develop, its own case law (decisions rendered by the court) and its own statutory law (law created by the legislature of that state), this chapter cannot be authoritative for any state. Contrary to popular belief, the law is extraordinarily dynamic and can and will change from year to year. The reader, therefore, must be cautioned to refer to her own state law for any specific answers to any specific questions raised by this chapter.

PRINCIPLES OR NURSING LIABILITY

It has become a hackneyed expression that we live in a litigious society. Fear of suit, however, cannot interfere with the professional nurse's responsibility. For the professional nurse, the best offense to litigation is a good defense. Defense involves—or requires—the nurse to know the basic concepts of the law as they relate to negligence and malpractice. Negligence is a term that is frequently used but is rarely explained. Legally, an attorney must prove four elements to justify a judgment for his client in a malpractice or negligence action. Negligence presupposes that a person (1) had a duty recognized by law that requires that person to conform to a certain standard of conduct, and that (2) the person with the duty failed to conform to that standard and (3) her failure to conform was the proximate cause of an injury to another party, and (4) that injury to the other party caused actual damages. Negligence by a professional person in the practice of her profession is called malpractice. The nurse, under the terms of the licensor in the particular state in which she practices, has a professional duty; her election to become a nurse and to meet the state qualifications to practice her profession has created in her a duty to the people under her care. Her standard of conduct, as in all negligence actions, is the reasonable person standard. In other words, her actions will be judged by the opinion of what another reasonable nurse would do in the same set of circumstances. Her care may also be judged by the actual written standards found in the facility within which she works. It is very important that the professional nurse be aware of the written standards created by the hospital that employs her and that she strenuously insist that those standards conform with the actual traditional or customary care given within her facility.

Since the 1950s it has been possible for hospitals to be sued. Suits brought by patients against the employer hospital and the employee nurses are relatively new, given the history of the negligence action. One of the first theories of law used in the medical malpractice field was the concept of respondeat superior, which holds the employer liable for the acts of its employees. A literal translation of the legal concept of respondeat superior is "let the master answer." Respondeat superior was not developed to meet the medical malpractice need but was quickly used by the attorney to justify suit of a hospital for the negligence of its nurses and other employees. The concept of respondeat superior is founded on an employee-employer relationship. Using this concept, a nurse's negligence would be used as a conduit to reach her employer hospital for damages. Other courts have relied on the agency theory to support a conclusion that the hospital is ultimately responsible: a corporation, being an artificial entity, can only act by its agents and is thus responsible for the acts of its agents when they are performed in the course of duty. The nurse or physician employee can be considered the agent of the hospital corporation.

The nurse must be aware, however, that the gains she has made in the last 20 years in the medical setting can become a two-edged sword in the legal setting. Once it is established that the nurse indeed may make a nursing diagnosis, that the nurse indeed uses independent judgment, her exposure to suit increases. It is possible for a nurse to be liable for her failure to follow a doctor's order, but given her present status as a professional with independent judgment, she could be liable for following a doctor's order if a reasonably prudent nurse would not have done so.

Thus, it becomes clear that a nurse must always remember that *she works for the hospital and not for the physician.* She must at all times conform to the standards of care set by her employer and not by the independent contractor physician who uses the facility. Traditionally the nurse must respond to the written orders of the physician. When, however, the physician's order—or the physician's failure to write the appropriate order—contradicts the hospital policy or standards, the nurse must pursue the appropriate chain of command set up for the supervision of the staff. When necessary, the nurse must report conduct contrary to established standards to the chief of the medical service in which the physician functions. The nurse must also seek relief within her chain of command.

Although it is true that hospitals do not generally scrutinize the treatment given by a duly certified physician who has been granted permission to practice at the facility, the "hands off" approach may not be acceptable in the future. Certain courts have determined that a hospital may be liable for improper treatment rendered by a physician who has privileges at its facility. The legal doctrine that underlies this increase in responsibility and liability by a hospital or its board of governors is termed "corporate responsibility." It should be noted that under the law a corporation is a person. It may sue or be sued.

In order to find liability, however, it must be shown that the hospital had knowledge that an attending physician using its facility rendered care that deviated from the standards of care established in the medical community. Once it has this knowledge, or should have had this knowledge under the circumstances, it is obligated to protect the patient from any subsequent harm that might occur as a direct result of the unqualified physician's treatment of the patient.

The legal theory is not yet universally accepted but will most certainly be used by attorneys whenever the factual background supports a conclusion that the hospital had notice that an attending physician at its facility was not qualified to treat a patient admitted to the hospital.

Despite the fact that it is the hospital or the physician who is generally the defendent in a legal action, it should not be forgotten that the professional nurse will always be responsible for her own actions. Certainly the attorney representing a client will seek out a defendant with "deep pockets," i.e., a defendant who has the financial ability to satisfy any judgment rendered by a court or a jury. This quest for a solvent defendant, however, does not create immunity for the nurse, nor does it lessen the likelihood that she will be sued if she deviates from the standards expected of the reasonably prudent nurse.

CONFIDENTIALITY OF RECORDS

Each patient in a hospital setting has a right to expect that his records and any information obtained by the health-care provider during the course of his stay in the hospital will be held in confidence, for each patient in a facility has a constitutional right to privacy, which he does not relinquish because of his illness or need for care. Information obtained during his hospitalization should not be transmitted to any person without authorization by the patient. Courts have ruled that the patient's medical information is protected by the rights of privacy afforded by a confidential relationship.

CONSENT FOR MEDICAL AND SURGICAL PROCEDURE

Any attempt to render treatment or care of a patient in a nonemergency situation without the prior consent of that patient constitutes assault. The patient must not only consent to the treatment rendered, the patient must have a clear understanding of the reasons why the treatment has been ordered and any alternative form of treatment that might be appropriate. He must have knowledge of the total situation in order to make an informed decision as to what he wishes done to his own body. It must be kept in mind that informed consent is a responsibility of the physician, not of the nurse. In an emergency situation, the unconscious patient may have treatment rendered after review by more than one of the physicians on the staff or by court order, depending on the jurisdiction in which the hospital is located. In a nonemergency situation, the facility may seek legal relief by way of an appointment by a guardian or conservator to make decisions for the incompetent person. In a nonemergency situation, the ultimate determination should be made through the legal process.

Refusal of consent

Courts have consistently ruled that the competent person may refuse treatment based on his religious beliefs. This is not to say that a parent may refuse treatment for a child based on his personal belief, or that a family member may refuse treatment for an incompetent relative based on religious beliefs. Only the competent adult will have that right. One can also conceive of instances where the competent would be limited in his right to follow his religious belief by the state's right and responsibility to intercede to protect children within its jurisdiction. A Jehovah's Witness who is six months pregnant may not refuse treatment if the final result of that refusal would be the proximate cause of the death of the fetus.

In recent years, owing to the advances within the medical field, a new problem has developed in this area. The competent person's right to refuse treatment under any circumstance has become a heavily debated issue in both the medical and legal communities. The media quickly focuses on any individual who deviates from the norm. The person who seeks the right to determine when treatment should be stopped generally bases that decision on the terminal nature of the diagnosis or the extraordinary treatment that would be required to prolong life. Intrinsic to a decision to refuse treatment is the patient's acceptance of the end result and a determination as to the quality of life that would be acceptable to the individual.

From a legal perspective, there is no question that a competent adult has the right to refuse treatment. As early as 1914, Justice Cardozo, sitting on the Court of Appeals in the State of New York stated, "Every human being of adult years and sound mind has a right to determine what shall be done with his own body." Although black-letter law is not easily applied to the gray area of reality, the courts have consistantly reaffirmed the basic premise. A patient can refuse to allow intrusions on his person, even though they are intended to save his life, and the physician is not to be held liable.

For the nurse working in the critical care area, the probability that she will be presented with the nonconsenting patient at some point in her career increases yearly. Certainly a critical care nurse should reflect upon the dilemma and attempt to reconcile any problems she may have arising from her own personal bias. She must also be acutely aware that the person who elects to refuse treatment may present a far greater challenge to the professional than the patient who works with the staff to fight the inevitable.

There is some evidence that the competent adult's refusal of treatment, standing alone, has been used to support a decision that the patient is incompetent. Without benefit of a judicial or psychiatric opinion, these patients can be stripped of their constitutional rights. A family member is then selected to make a "correct" decision for the recalcitrant patient. The nurse should not be persuaded that this procedure is legal or ethical. There are *competent* adults who will elect to forego further treatment. Such a decision unquestionably interrupts the status quo; the nurse may quite likely find herself in the middle of a *cause célèbre.* The nurse, however, must be alert to the patient's legal rights and not be an accessory to a deprivation of those constitutional rights, however it may be justified as "good intentions" or "in the best interest of the patient."

Certainly the decision to forego treatment by the patient's request cannot be made without careful thought and a thorough investigation of the situation. It is essential that all members of the health team, the patient, and his family work together to support the patient's decision once it is determined that the patient is competent to make that decision. From a legal perspective, it is essential that the family fully understand the situation and that the patient's refusal could ultimately lead to the patient's death. Once the consenting adult has died, it is the family who may seek legal redress for an alleged negligent act. The best witness the medical team would have to support their decision to forego treatment has died. Every effort must be made to document the patient's decision, but the most effective method to prevent litigation is to educate and support the family during the decision-making process. If the family feels it participated in the decision, it is less likely to dispute the end result in a court of law. Although the ultimate decision to discontinue treatment within the hospital setting lies with the physician, the nurse must actively participate in the process. She is responsible to the patient and her employer. As a member of the profession of nursing, she also has a responsibility to maintain the integrity of her profession.

If, at any time, it becomes clear that there is a conflict between the family and the patient, the physician and the patient, or the family and the physician, the decision should be left to a court of law. The exposure to the nurse, hospital, and the physician to litigation in this area cannot be emphasized enough. A good example can be seen in the case of *Barber v. Superior Court,* decided by the California Court of Appeals, Second District in 1983. A patient was admitted to a Los Angeles hospital for routine abdominal surgery in 1981. In the recovery room he suffered a cardiac arrest, suffered brain damage, and was subsequently maintained on a respirator. At his family's request, he was removed from the respirator. The patient, however, was not brain dead and continued to maintain respiratory function after removal from the machine. The physician then discontinued IV therapy. A few days later the patient expired from dehydration. The state brought a criminal charge of murder against the physician. The charges were finally dismissed in 1983. The court concluded that "a physician has no duty to continue treatment once it has proved to be ineffective." This decision has not been published and cannot be relied upon to protect the health-care provider. It does, however, point out the dangers present whenever a facility is presented with a person or family who vigorously pursues the constitutional right to privacy and refuses treatment.

One other important aspect of this developing area is the "living will." This document notifies the world that the person who has signed it does not want the medical profession to use "extraordinary" means to keep him alive. Certain states have enacted laws that validate this document. In most states, however, the legislature is hesitant to allow a person to enter into an agreement with unknown persons based on unknown contingencies in the future. Even without the legal stamp of approval, however, the "living will" can be invaluable. It can be used in a court of law as evidence of the person's belief that life support systems should be terminated in certain circumstances. It also serves another purpose, in that it lessens the guilt felt by many families of unresponsive patients when the ultimate decision is left in their hands.

The term "extraordinary means" requires clarification. One court in New York has adopted the definition of extraordinary care used by Gerald Kelly, a well-known Catholic ethician. Extraordinary care includes "all medicines, treatment, and operations which cannot be obtained or used without excessive pain, expense, or other inconvenience, or if used, would not offer a reasonable hope or benefit." This definition, however, is very broad and subject to many different interpretations. Each case must be handled individually; it is not an area in which the courts or the legislature can set down clear-cut standards to be followed by the medical profession.

Legislatures in some states have begun to respond to the problems created by advanced medical science. The legal definition of death recently enacted by the Connecticut legislature in Public Act No. 84–261 provides a good example of the type of statutes that are being promulgated:

> AN ACT CONCERNING THE DEFINITION OF DEATH AND LIFE SUPPORT SYSTEM.
>
> Be it enacted by the Senate and House of Representatives in General Assembly convened:
>
> Section 1. (NEW) For purposes of making a determination concerning the continuation or removal of any life support system in a general hospital licensed under section 19a-491 of the general statutes, an individual who has sustained either (1) irreversible cessation of circulatory and respiratory functions, or (2) irreversible cessation of all functions of the entire brain, including the brainstem, is dead. Determination of death shall be made in accordance with accepted medical standards.
>
> Section 2. (NEW) For the purpose of this act, "life support system" means any mechanical or electronic device utilized by any medical facility in order to replace, assist or supplement the function of any human vital organ or combination of organs.

It should be noted that the legislature ultimately relies on the accepted medical standard.

AUTOPSY AND DONATION

The legislature of each state has also promulgated laws that govern state residents as to the procedures to be followed to determine if an autopsy is required. All residents are charged with the responsibility of notifying the chief medical examiner of any death that would require postmortem investigation. Although notification of the medical examiner's office will be handled by the pathology department or an administrative assistant in the hospital setting, the nurse should have a general knowledge of which deaths mandate autopsy. Most states require an autopsy when the death is violent in nature; when the death is sudden or unexpected and not caused by a readily recognized disease; when the death occurs under suspicious circumstances; when the body is to be cremated, buried at sea, or otherwise disposed of so as to be unavailable for examination; when the death is related to disease resulting from employment; or when the death relates to a disease that might constitute a threat to public health.

The legislatures have also promulgated laws governing the procedures to be followed by a person who wants to donate all or part of his body. The law in this area has been standardized in that all states have adopted the Uniform Anatomical Gift Act. It should be noted that each state has the right to make minor changes in the act to adapt it to the particular state; although variations will be found, the main theme is consistent throughout the country.

All competent persons over 18, and all competent persons from 14 yr to 18 yr with the consent of the parent, may make a gift of his body, which gift takes effect upon death.

If the person during his life has not indicated opposition to a donation, the act sets out who may give consent for the deceased. Authorization to consent, in the order of priority, may be given by the spouse, an adult son or daughter, either parent, an adult brother or sister, the guardian of the person of the decedent at the time of his death, or any other person authorized or under an obligation to dispose of the body after death.

It is recommended that a nurse in a critical care area have a thorough knowledge of the law governing anatomic gifts. Certain aspects of the law will be highlighted here but cannot be considered the final word on this subject.

The statute requires that the gift be made by a competent person. Competency is a difficult concept to define. If the nurse has any question as to a person's competency, a psychological evaluation is definitely in order.

If the person is clearly incompetent to make the decision, the order of priority of authorization noted above must be followed. Problems occur when there is more than one person in a class and the people in the class cannot agree that a donation should be made. For example, say the unresponsive person is a widow with a daughter, a son, and a brother. Under the order of priority, the brother's decision is not controlling. The daughter and son have the right to veto any decision made by the brother. If the daughter and son cannot reach agreement, the gift cannot be accepted.

At the present time, anatomic donations have not been subjected to close judicial scrutiny. News coverage of organ transplants focus on the donee, not the donor.

By way of contrast, suits filed by families on behalf of a family member requesting permission to discontinue a life support system, despite a finding that the patient is not brain dead, continue to be front page material.

Careful monitoring of this new area of health care by the professionals working in it will decrease the possibility of intervention by the legal profession. The courts may be hesitant to interfere, but cases of clear abuse with factual situations heavily laden with emotion require the judicial system and, frequently, the legislature to react in a strenuous manner. When made aware of the court decisions that have been rendered on actual cases that have occurred, the professional nurse might well think "I would never be in that situation" or "I would never stand by and let that happen to my patient." With awareness of the rights of patients, her responsibilities to those patients, and the laws of the state governing her practice, that might very well be so.

CONCLUSION

Nurses today have a professional responsibility to be aware of the areas of the law that directly affect the health-care provider and the patient. If each nurse would carefully read the applicable statutes in her state and the standards set forth in her facility, she would decrease the odds of further court intervention into her profession. If each nurse would carefully read the First Amendment to the Constitution and remember that this right applies to each of her patients, she would decrease the odds of being sued by that patient, and, in so doing, bring further respect to her chosen profession.

CHAPTER 19

PSYCHOSOCIAL IMPLICATIONS IN CRITICAL CARE

Melissa Mesick Meth and Constance S. Weiskopf

The psychosocial aspects of critical illness pose a unique challenge for the critical care nurse. Nurses must balance their own and their patient's demanding physical and emotional needs in an environment that can be both stressful and dehumanizing. To achieve this balance, the nurse must have a working knowledge of how the critical care experience affects the psychosocial health of patients, their families, and the caregiver.

THE STRESS PHENOMENON

ICUs are frequently described as stressful, not only for the patient and family but for the nurse as well. A solid understanding of stress and its sequelae is helpful when working in critical care. This understanding can enable nurses to mitigate the destructive effects of stress and augment the positive potential of stress both in their patients and themselves.

Stress

Stress is defined as the physical and emotional response to *any* demand made upon the individual that is interpreted as a threat to homeostasis. Stress is a complex phenomenon, a collection of interacting components that work in unison. When there is a requirement for change in one component subsystem, the whole system is affected. If the demand for change causes disequilibrium in the system, stress occurs. The individual then mobilizes coping resources to deal with the stress and reestablish equilibrium. Ideally, stress combined with the proper coping behaviors will promote a *positive* change in the individual. When stress overcomes a person's ability to cope, then the potential for crisis occurs.

Stressors are internal and/or external factors that demand change in the individual and result in the phenomenon of stress. Stressors originate in the biophysical, psychosocial or societal subsystems. Biophysical stressors are such things as infectious organisms, disease processes, or poor nutrition. Examples of psychosocial stressors are low self-esteem, problematic interpersonal relationships, and developmental crises. Those stressors originating from society at large are such things as economic fluctuations, pollution, and high technology.

How people experience a stressor depends on their perception of the stressor and on their coping resources. Stress is also additive. If a person is bombarded with multiple stressors, the stress response will be more intense.

The stress response

The stress response can be induced by any biophysical, psychological, or social stressor. Hans Selye is considered the founding father of stress research. Selye incorporated his findings into a model of stress called the General Adaptation Syndrome (GAS). The GAS consists of three stages. The **alarm response** is the first stage and is characterized by an instantaneous, short-term, life-preserving response in which there is total sympathetic nervous system activity. A common term for this stage is the fight-or-flight response. The second stage is the **stage of resistance.** It is the body's way of adapting to the disequilibrium caused by a stressor. The body stays in this stage until the noxious stressor disappears and the body is able to return to homeostasis. If the body has consumed all of its coping energy, the **stage of exhaustion** occurs. This third stage results in physical illness, major psychological disturbances, or death.

THE PATIENT

Patients who are sick enough to warrant admission to the ICU are not only suffering from the stress of physical illness but from concomitant psychosocial stress as well. Consequently, critical care nurses perform nursing care designed to maintain or restore all vital physical and psychosocial functions that have been disrupted by the illness.

Psychosocial response

The patient's psychosocial response to the critical care experience may be mediated by internal phenomena such as emotional state and coping mechanisms or by external phenomena such as the quantity and quality of environmental stimulation.

Emotional reactions. The intensity of emotional reactions can be best understood if it is recognized that ICUs are places where patients attempt to literally fight off death. Critical care patients exhibit predictable emotional reactions that share common features, regardless of the illness. **Fear and anxiety** are generally the first reactions to appear. The patient may be fearful of pain, uncomfortable procedures, body mutilation, loss of control, abandonment, and/or dying.

Depression is another commonly seen emotion and usually comes after the initial fear and anxiety. The depression is frequently in response to grief and loss. Experiencing loss may evoke memories of past losses, which in turn can intensify the feelings of sadness.

Anger may surface after or during depression. Frequently anger masks a depression and serves to prevent the patient from falling into a deeper depression. Patients may feel angry and resentful about being sick and often lament that life is not fair to have dealt them such a blow.

Coping mechanisms. Coping mechanisms are a collection of conscious and unconscious mental strategies that are used to stabilize a potentially threatening situation and recreate equilibrium. Patient coping strategies are those attempts to produce emotional stability, environmental mastery, redefinition of life goals/tasks, and resolution of problems created by the illness.

Some examples of coping behaviors are humor, distraction, asking for information, talking with others about concerns/feelings, redefining problems in more favorable terms, confronting a problem by taking some action, negotiating possible alternatives, reducing tension by drinking, eating, or taking medications, withdrawing, blaming someone or something, blaming oneself, seeking direction from authority, acting-out, and seeking religious counsel.

Patients who cope well are able to establish positive relationships with staff. They are optimistic, resourceful, flexible, and directly confront problems or revise them in more tolerable terms.

Patients who have difficulty coping are more likely to display heightened emotional distress, do not clearly recognize relevant psychosocial concerns, avoid issues, deny or disguise problems, are less communicative, blame others or themselves, and have trouble building alliances with the staff.

Defense mechanisms are part of a person's coping repertoire. They operate at an unconscious level and are used by people to protect themselves from being overwhelmed by internal impulses and feelings. Common defense mechanisms seen in critical care are denial, distortion, regression, acting-out behavior, and projection.

Denial occurs when a patient blocks out a real situation that is too frightening or overwhelming to tolerate. **Distortion** occurs when a patient twists a threatening real situation to conform to internal needs or wishes. **Regression** occurs when a patient returns to a developmentally earlier level of functioning that was more satisfying. **Acting-out** behavior is defined as the external manifestation of an internal need that the patient cannot tolerate or does not want to admit. **Projection** occurs when patients attribute to others those unacceptable thoughts or feelings they can't acknowledge in themselves.

Environmental stimulation. The phenomenon of sensory and perceptual stimulation has received much attention since the early days of ICUs. Health professionals noted alterations in the mental status of their previously lucid patients. Those alterations eventually were labeled ICU Syndrome. There are multiple factors that contribute to this syndrome, such as the disease process itself, the effects of medication, the cardiopulmonary bypass pump, sensory overstimulation or understimulation, and sleep deprivation.

Sensory deprivation is a reduction in the variety and strength of sensory stimuli with or without a change in pattern, e.g., immobility. **Sensory overload** is defined as two or more sensory stimuli that act concurrently at high levels of intensity and usually begin suddenly, such as machine alarms and flashing lights. **Perceptual deprivation** occurs when the amount of the stimulus remains the same but its characteristics and meaning change, e.g., listening to monotonous beeping. The phenomena of sensory and perceptual disturbances can lead to distortions in body image, depersonalization, disorientation, problems with concentrating and paying attention, hallucinations, and such emotional reactions as fear, panic, labile moods, and depression.

Sleep deprivation can also cause mental status changes. Subjects in experimental sleep deprivation studies have shown symptoms such as slurred speech, irritability, and disorientation after 2 to 5 days of sleep deprivation. When sleep deprivation continued, the symptoms progressed to psychotic behaviors, such as delusions and paranoia. When subjects in sleep deprivation studies were allowed one night of recovery sleep, all signs of psychosis disappeared.

Implications for nursing care

The role of the nurse in meeting the patient's psychosocial needs is threefold: (1) the nurse assesses how her patients are coping with illness; (2) the nurse evaluates their emotional reactions to the illness; (3) the nurse evaluates those environmental factors that are impinging on her patients. Once this data is collected, the nurse can then plan interventions to meet the psychosocial needs of her patients.

Coping behaviors. The nurse needs to help the patient free up coping energy that is being inefficiently consumed by undue stress. To assess coping behaviors, nurses can ask themselves: Which coping strategies and defense mechanisms is this patient using? What coping behaviors did this patient use in the past? How effective are this patient's coping behaviors?

Next, the nurse decides whether to support the patient's coping style or whether to modify it by teaching new coping behaviors. If the patient's coping behaviors are not containing the problem, the nurse may want to explore other coping strategies. It is often valuable to include the patient in this process, using his perceived strengths.

When evaluating coping behaviors, it is imperative that the nurse preserve the patient's self-esteem, not stripping patients of coping behaviors before they are ready. The nurse must also try to remain nonjudgmental when assessing coping behaviors, realizing that patients may choose different ways of handling a situation from those the nurse would choose.

Some questions to ask the patient to elicit coping information are: What is most stressful for you being in the ICU? Have you ever had to handle a problem like this in the past? What are you doing now to cope with your problem? Is it working for you?

Another aspect of the coping process is the patient's need for control. Stresses in ICUs can result in learned helplessness. Patients learn that they have no control over what is happening to them and they feel helpless. As they perceive greater and greater degrees of helplessness, they will lose their initiative to assert any control, thus creating a downward spiral. Studies illustrated that although people are not able to control a stressful situation completely, providing some opportunity for personal control—even a perception that personal control is possible—has beneficial results.

Nurses can intervene to help patients take as much control as possible in their care, even in the most helpless of situations. It is important to convey the message that there are certain things, no matter how small, that patients can do if they so choose. The nature of personal control activities should be very specific and made explicit, e.g., when to have a bed bath or certain medications. Also, activities for personal control should be personally relevant and not require complex judgments or the expenditure of excessive energy if the patient is not ready.

Emotional reactions. **Fear and anxiety** may continue in varying degrees throughout the patient's stay. Even though fear of dying may not be in the patient's awareness, it is frequently the basic concern.

Fear is displayed in many ways, ranging from overtalkativeness to withdrawal. Explanations and calm dialogue can be helpful. The nurse should try to elicit from patients what they know about their disease so any misconceptions can be clarified. Patients should be encouraged to specify what their fears are. Specific, valid reassurances should be offered; false reassurances should be avoided because they harm credibility and trust. Positive aspects of the treatment plan can be mentioned. An air of competence in the nursing role helps patients feel confident that they are receiving quality care. It is important to remember that patients may hide their fears so as to be seen as "good patients." Nurses may even unconsciously foster this behavior, but it is counterproductive in the long run.

Depression is a response to feelings of real or threatened loss; it may stem from disappointment with what has not been and may never be accomplished by the patient. Failures and vulnerabilities may haunt the patient.

The nurse can reassure the patient that depression is a normal reaction to serious illness and that it is time-limited. As patients feel better physically, so will they feel better emotionally. Patients can be encouraged to articulate what may be precipitating their sense of loss. The nurse can focus on bolstering the patient's self-esteem by helping them feel like people rather than objects. Capitalizing on any signs of improvement, no matter how small, also helps the patient to feel better.

Though **anger** is a normal response to loss and illness, it is especially difficult for patients to find an appropriate way to express anger without endangering relationships with health personnel. Angry patients can be difficult to manage because they may threaten the staff. Nurses need to hear out the gripes patiently and take them seriously, taking the time to show that they are trying to understand patient's concerns.

Another aspect of patients' anger may result from feeling ambivalent about needing and wanting to be taken care of yet resenting that they must be taken care of. The nurse should be sensitive to this independent/dependent struggle.

Environmental factors. The nurse can use a two-level approach when assessing and intervening with environmental stress factors: (1) planning to control or prevent environmental stressors; (2) planning to help the patient tolerate the environment better.

The nurse is the patient's link to **reality.** She should introduce herself to the patient and orient the patient to time, date, place, and person. This measure is particularly important for the elderly, who may be more likely to manifest stress by confusion. Clocks, calendars, radios, and televisions are additional ways to help the patient maintain orientation. The nurse should be aware whether patients normally wear eyeglasses or hearing aids. If the ICU has no windows, it is helpful to dim the lights at night so patients can tell day from night. Patients should be familiarized with their surroundings and family should be encouraged to bring familiar objects from home to be placed in the room.

If nurses relate to patients on a personal as well as a clinical basis, the resultant trust can prevent alienation and augment **communication.** Communication skills include verbal, nonverbal, listening, and touch. Frequent supportive, consistent, face-to-face contact can alleviate some of the adverse effects of sensory and perceptual deprivation. Encouraging patients to express feelings they harbor about their ICU experience may prevent some problematic behavior, such as acting-out and withdrawal.

Because of patients' high level of fear and anxiety, they may not process or retain information well, so the nurse should repeat information when necessary and assess what patients know about their illness, clarify misconceptions, and relieve unsubstantiated fears, without overloading them with information they can't assimilate. Patients should be kept informed of the future plans for treatment.

Immobility is a primary factor in sensory deprivation, so early mobilization is very important. **Exercise** can provide stimulation to help counteract other forms of deprivation.

Nurses as well as other hospital personnel can be a major source of **sensory overload.** Sensory overload can be controlled by such interventions as preventing overcrowding, attending to patient's spatial and privacy needs, proper lighting, controlling noise level, and if possible, placing monitoring equipment outside the room. Rounds should be conducted out of earshot. Many patients suffer misconceptions based on snatches of conversations that don't even apply to them.

Nurses need to organize their activities to allow for the maximum number of **uninterrupted sleep** periods, remembering that 60 to 90 min are needed to complete one sleep cycle, and completion of an entire cycle is needed to benefit from sleep.

THE FAMILY

The family plays a significant positive or negative role in the patient's response to illness. If nurses are adequately prepared to identify and meet family needs, the nurse can foster the families' positive contribution to the total nursing care of the patient. Conversely, if the nurse ignores the families' needs, the families could become a source of stress for the patient and the nurse.

Studies have shown that the most common family needs fall into three general categories: information, emotional, and physical/personal needs.

Informational needs

The patient's family uses information to help them rally their coping strategies as well as to give them some sense of stability and control. Information needs include such things as the need to know concrete facts about the patient's illness, progress, and expected outcome in understandable terms; to know exactly what is being done for the patient and why; to have questions answered honestly; to know what emotional and behavioral reactions to illness they can expect from the patient and themselves; to talk about the possibility of the patient's death but to balance this with the need for hope; and for an orientation before entering the ICU for the first time.

Emotional needs

The primary emotional needs of the family include: relief from anxiety; confidence that the patient is getting quality care and that the hospital staff are truly concerned about the patient; to be called at home if there are changes in the patient's condition; to be given information at least once a day; for support and ventilation of their concerns; to initially relive the critical incident that led to the patient's admission; and to be told about transfer plans from the ICU to another unit.

Physical/personal needs

Physical/personal needs of the family do not consistently rank as highly as information or emotional needs, even though they may be very important for certain families. The major physical needs of the family are such things as the need to visit anytime, the need to feel useful, the need to have a telephone nearby, the need to have a place to rest, the need to be alone, and the need to have help with financial concerns.

Implications for nursing care

Even though the direct care of the patient is the nurse's priority, the patient is an extension of a family who can have a major impact on the patient's recovery from illness. Therefore, it behooves the nurse to incorporate the needs of the family as part of the total patient care plan.

Because illness disrupts family roles, it is useful to determine what roles were held by the patient and who will assume those roles while the patient is ill. The patient's primary support person, as well as the primary spokesperson for the family, should be identified because these roles may be filled by two different people, e.g., the primary support person may be the spouse, but the spokesperson may be a son-in-law.

Base line information about the family's previous experience with the patient's illness, especially if it involved any previous ICU admissions, should be gathered. The nurse needs to assess the family's level of fear and anxiety, as well as what coping resources they are using.

Two other considerations to include as part of the total assessment process are cultural and ethnic issues and information about social and economic resources.

Information needs. Nursing interventions for meeting the information needs of the family include (1) explaining facts about the patient's condition and progress in concrete understandable terms; (2) encouraging questions and feedback about what has been said to help determine if the family is understanding the information; (3) repeating information at different intervals; (4) avoiding medical jargon; (5) presenting information to the family as a doctor-nurse team; (6) allowing adequate time to spend with the family so feelings and questions can surface, especially if the patient's prognosis is poor; (7) setting up periodic family/doctor/nurse meetings to update information; (8) remaining nonjudgmental so the family will not be too intimidated to ask questions; (9) and educating families about how to go about getting needed information.

Emotional needs. Nursing interventions designed to meet the emotional needs of the family are initially directed at reducing family anxiety. These interventions include: (1) helping the family clarify what they see as the immediate problem to give them some sense of intellectual mastery of the situation; (2) reassuring the family that the staff working with the patient are competent and empathic; (3) identifying the roles of the different health personnel working with the patient; (4) making every effort to keep the patient comfortable and as pain-free as possible; and (5) keeping the family informed of any changes in the patient's condition.

In notifying the family about changes in patient condition, it is helpful to work out a mutually agreed upon communication system, such as designating one family member to call the ICU at a specific time each day or to have the nurse call the family at a specific time each day. Another method of sharing information is planning to meet with the family each shift. These meetings also provide the family with a forum for ventilation and the opportunity for support.

One important way for the nurse to provide support is to recognize the families' feelings, reassure them that they are entitled to have such feelings, and help them work through the shock and denial of the initial grief reaction. By helping the family to focus on feelings of anger, depression, and guilt, the nurse may help the family avoid a delayed grief reaction.

When discussing a prognosis such as impending death or a permanent loss of function, the nurse should determine the family's perception of the situation and look for signs of anticipatory grief. It is extremely useful to meet jointly with the physician and family to discuss the use or nonuse of extraordinary measures or advanced life support systems (*see* Chapter 18). Nurses should be aware of their own feelings about loss and death because this will surely influence how comfortable they will be discussing these sensitive issues with families.

When the patient is ready for transfer out of ICU, the nurse should discuss these plans with the family and educate them about the new unit and what the transfer means in terms of patient care. Also the family should tour the new unit and meet the staff who will be working with them.

Physical/personal needs. To meet this category of needs the following interventions should be considered. Even though every ICU has basic visiting guidelines, they will need to be flexible based on individual needs. Families can feel useful if they are involved in the planning and providing of patient care even if it is something small such as feeding, bathing, or providing reality orientation to the patient. This inclusion will decrease the family's feelings of helplessness and also strengthen the relationship between the family member and the nurse.

The nurse should educate the family about other resources available to them such as chaplains, psychiatric liaison nurses, and social workers. If the nurse feels the family has special needs, a referral should be made to the appropriate resource after discussing it with the family.

Managing families during an emergency. During an emergency it is best to escort the family out of the critical care area so they do not interfere with the provisions of care. If possible have someone stay with the family for at least several minutes to explain the nature of the emergency and allow for questions.

THE DYING PATIENT

ICUs are usually thought of as places where efforts are made to preserve life and facilitate healing. Yet the paradox is that they are also places where patients may die and, in fact, the dying process may be prolonged. As a result, nurses may experience a sense of loss and failure when the patient does not recover.

The nurse can face the challenge of caring for dying patients and their families by cultivating the positive and constructive aspects of a painful experience. She can learn to deal with the patient and family honestly, yet be sensitive enough to allow them to maintain their hope and integrity. She will want to examine her own feelings about death.

A model of emotional adaptation to the dying process has been developed by Kübler-Ross. The model consists of five stages: (1) shock and denial—"No, it can't be true"; (2) anger—"why me?"; (3) bargaining—"Yes, it is me but give me more time to . . . ."; (4) depression—"Yes, it is me and the sadness is so painful"; (5) acceptance—"Yes, it is me and I'm ready."

The nurse's main concern is to be aware of the patient's emotional level of adaptation to the dying process and its fluctuations from shift to shift.

Nursing implications

There are five major treatment considerations in the nursing care of the dying patient. They are presence and perseverence, caring, comfort, communication, and dignity.

Presence and perseverence. Because fear of abandonment is usually a major concern of the dying patient, the nurse needs to maintain her presence when the patient is dying. Sometimes nurses and families feel helpless. But just the presence of a caring person relaxes and comforts the dying patient. To prevent feelings of isolation in both the family and patient, flexible visiting times should be allowed.

Caring. Caring is conveyed when the nurse is actively involved with the patient and family. The nurse learns to cultivate the concern and empathy that are already an integral part of the nurse's emotional makeup.

Comfort. Pain relief is an important part of providing comfort for the dying patient. When a patient is in continuous pain, it is appropriate to give pain medication on a fixed schedule, rather than prn. Concerns for comfort override concerns for problems with addiction. The nurse needs to know the patient's wishes about his pain experience so the medication can be properly regulated.

Other important comfort measures are mouth care, positioning, skin care, and massage. The family may choose to participate in this care, which can be a highly meaningful experience for the grieving family.

Communication. Patients will deal with death in many different individualized ways. Some patients will not want to talk about dying whereas others may wish to. The nurse's role is to create an atmosphere that allows patients and families the freedom and flexibility to deal with dying in their own personal way.

The most comfortable atmosphere is created when the nurse talks to the patient in her usual style, remembering that one of the most effective communication tools is being a good listener. Touch can also be an effective way of communicating concern. Dying patients may enjoy cheerfulness; well-timed humor can sometimes help people relax.

Dignity. The dying patient's dignity should be respected and his requests about his care should be honored. It is in the best interest of the patient for the health team to know how aggressive the patient and family want treatment to be. A collaborative approach to care is certainly the most effective way to deal with the dying patient's treatment issues.

When the patient dies

When death seems imminent, the nurse needs to ensure that the family is notified and told honestly the details surrounding the patient's death. It is helpful to provide a private place for the family to grieve. If the family chooses to view the body, the nurse can accompany the family to the bedside, but if the family wants to be left alone with the body, this wish should also be respected. The nurse should be prepared to refer the family to the appropriate resources either for emotional or spiritual support or to answer any practical questions they may have about funeral arrangements.

THE STAFF

ICUs are among the most stressful of workplaces. While working in such a setting, the nurse should learn to recognize and reduce her own stress, thus significantly affecting her performance as a professional caregiver.

Stressors

Critical care nurses feel the responses connected with stress repeatedly during the working day. Stressors within the critical care setting can originate from the environment, the workload, the medical staff and administrators, and the psychological and social experiences.

Environment. The ICU setting offers a number of sensory stimuli, from the intricate machinery with the accompanying beeping, buzzing, whooshing, and flashing lights, the rushing around of a variety of staff, amid a mixture of patient voices and/or screams, to the smells of disease, excreta, and antiseptics. The patients the critical care nurse cares for are in various stages of dying or recovery. In the midst of providing ongoing physical care to the patient, the nurse must deal with the other needs of the patient and his family. In addition to all of this is constant contact with death.

Workload. Another formidable stressor is the repetitive routine of critical care nursing, of collecting, recording, and evaluating data. Most nurses comment that no sooner have they completed the tasks for one patient then it is time to start them again. In the midst of these routines, judgments must be made and appropriate action taken. Staff shortages and/or illness compound the demands because shortages are difficult to fill. Three major environmental stressors identified by nurses related to their workload are: (1) heavy lifting, amount of physical work; (2) hectic pace of the unit, and (3) the varied responsibilities of the nurses.

Doctors and administrators. Those who may be in a position to provide support to critical care nurses in actuality may often cause them stress. Physicians may respond to stress by avoiding the nurses or their reports or suggestions about patients; misunderstandings and misinterpretations may result from ineffective communication. Sudden changes in treatment without explanation or inappropriate monitoring measures for a dying patient are examples of high stressors for nurses.

Hospital and/or nursing administrators are sometimes viewed as nonsupportive because services do not always meet nursing needs. Nurses in administrative roles are often enmeshed in an assignment of two incompatible roles: that of the caring mother and of the law enforcer. They are in a position where they may easily become a target for the staff nurses' frustrations arising from their unmet needs.

Psychological experience. In addition to external stressors, the nurses must deal with their own emotions, fears, anxieties, and pain. Mistakes are inevitable and quick decision-making is routine. Anxiety is a latent companion, often exceeding minimal levels, reducing efficiency and the decision-making capacity. The nurse's self-esteem takes a beating as she deals frequently with patients that die and the patient's grieving family members in need of understanding and comfort. This repetitive object-loss is a major stressor.

Social experience. The critical care experience provides an opportunity for the staff to work together on a common job, albeit one of the most difficult in the hospital. The very stressfulness of the job is a source of pride. Cooperation is essential for unit function and can lead to group pressures that create uncomfortable feelings. Guilt because of an illness or error, conflicts between wanting help from others and fear of those giving it add to stress. With so many strong-willed, independent nurses, personality conflicts can lower team spirit and decrease trust.

Often, critical care nurses isolate themselves from other nursing staff, and this situation can be made worse by the physical isolation of some of the units.

Within this social experience the issue of change cannot be avoided. Patient status and technology change quickly. Critical care nurses take pride in identifying themselves as change agents and pace-setters, while the workload and the stress associated with these changes may actually hamper them from being so.

Coping with stress

When a stressor is identified, either individually or as a group, preparation takes place for the action termed fight-or-flight response. That energy can produce creative approaches to change if constructively channeled. On the other hand, the energy in the stress response can be detrimental if misdirected.

Some of the physiologic indicators of stress the nurse experiences are insomnia or lethargy, muscular tension and aches, headaches, nausea, hyperactivity, constant fatigue, and elevated BP. Psychologically the nurse may feel frustrated, helpless, depressed, anxious, withdrawn, irritable, critical of self and others. Intellectual responses may include forgetfulness, indecisiveness, errors in judgment, and lack of attention to details. If not addressed, these responses may lead to physical or emotional disturbances, such as ulcers, MI, depression, or addiction.

Group indicators of stress are interpersonal and can include behaviors such as arguing with others, scapegoating staff members, responding to others with silence, busy behavior, intolerance of other's ideas or behavior. Patterns of lateness, absenteeism, and rapid staff turnover may also indicate the presence of stress.

Identifying signs of stress is the first step in managing it successfully. Individually, the nurse must learn what triggers stress for her and to appraise which stimulus is threatening. Within the nursing group, the staff must look at their behaviors as an interlocking system where one behavior acts as a stimulus for another behavior. In addition to identifying the stressors, the nurse must take into account the number to be coped with simultaneously and the time she is exposed to the stressor.

Management of the stress response will vary, depending on basic personality style and the defensive style unique to each individual. The nurse can reduce stress by either decreasing the stressors or increasing her ability to cope.

Coping describes a successful adjustment to challenge or the ways the ego attempts to maintain internal stability during times of increased stress. Coping mechanisms include: (1) conscious stress management devices to reduce feelings of tension, and (2) the unconscious use of defense mechanisms. When defense mechanisms are maladaptive, they can lead to coping failure. If adaptation is successful, and there is relief in a stressful situation, the nurse will most likely try the same approach in other stressful occurrences.

Coping strategies. Nurses in the ICU use a variety of defense mechanisms and coping strategies to deal with the many feelings they encounter within their setting.

Denial can interfere with the nurse's ability to recognize the stressors in the environment. She may perceive a stressful event through her senses but using the mechanism of denial shuts out the external reality that is too threatening to tolerate. **Laughter** and **joking,** many times associated with friendly behavior, may also be a product of denial as a defense against the stressful situation. These responses are especially evident at times of crisis. **Rationalization** may interfere with the nurse's ability to identify stressors by detaching the normal feeling connected with either the feeling or idea. It is usually the uncomfortable feeling associated with the stressor that is repressed. Another common defense mechanism used is **displacement.** Feelings about one object are redirected to another. The pressure of the job often places great constraint upon the expression of anger; nurses may direct displaced anger toward family or coworkers. **Isolation** or **withdrawal** is sometimes exhibited toward patients. On an intellectual level the nurse is aware of what the patient and/or family are experiencing but may treat them impersonally.

Other coping strategies cited by nurses are: seeking out their coworkers; partying more; exercising; thinking about changing jobs; taking more time off from work; drinking; talking with spouses or roommates.

The burnout phenomenon. One of the possible results of working in a stressful environment is burnout, a state in which the nurse feels that no matter what she does or how hard her effort, she cannot change a situation; feelings of hopelessness prevail. For critical care nurses, this may mean that the nurse either leaves the job or functions ineffectively in it.

One of the most positive methods of reducing stress and avoiding burnout is by increasing the person's ability to cope. One study (Albrecht) discovered that common strategies used in coping with burnout were behaviors that tended to draw nurses away from their present role as nurses (over-eating, thinking about changing jobs). In a sense there was a "flight," both physically and emotionally, from the unit. This contrasted with strategies that involved the nurse in creatively and actively managing stressors at work. Successful coping—decreasing or avoiding burnout—was achieved by nurses who followed strategies that involved them in the hospital environment. Their patterns seemed to suggest that once they thought about the nature of the difficulties, they talked about them with other staff nurses involved in the same situation. This suggested a healthy level of relational bonds among the staff nurses and supervisors, who were perceived as approachable, helpful, and able to be trusted.

Recommendations

It is unrealistic to work in the ICU without expecting to experience stress. Many stressors cannot be eliminated or reappraised as harmless; the stress response is essential in preparing the nurse to deal with the environment. Any change that improves the physical and emotional states of ICU nurses must be initiated by the nurses themselves. For the most part, many stressors can be addressed if the nursing staff is unified and the individual nurse has a knowledge of what triggers stress for herself.

Taking care of self. Nursing is a predominantly female profession. The feminist movement, with its strong emphasis on selfhood, has made men and women increasingly aware of their right to experience their lives fully. Nurses, by nature of their profession, are in the role of giver, nurturer, and caretaker—often at an expense to themselves. With increased awareness of the possible ill effects this all-encompassing giving role can have nurses must realize that permission to stop giving has to come first from the giver. It is desirable to give, but nurses must allow themselves to take as well. They can then be more effective in balancing their own time and energy. For example, restricting professional time will allow the nurse to have more time for self, family, or friends.

Taking time for self on a daily basis provides space to feel free and spontaneous. It is a time that is needed to "play," as a break from the work-oriented cycle.

Critical care nurses have a variety of roles. Understanding the roles one plays (e.g., nurse, daughter, father, wife, husband) can be crucial in setting reasonable expectations for these roles. It is up to the individual nurse to impose role expectations on self that determine what others can expect of her or him.

Another way to care for self is to eat wisely. Providing the body with resources it needs allows the system to work more efficiently, especially in times of stress.

Effective communication. The way nurses express their feelings can influence how they manage their work-related stress. Being able to speak up for what one needs, saying what one thinks and taking a stand for what one believes can be difficult for nurses who have traditionally taken a passive or nonassertive role.

Assertiveness can help nurses effectively communicate their feelings. Assertiveness is often confused with aggressiveness, however, and viewed as unfeminine and intimidating. But the assertive nurse need not be offensive or infringe on the rights of other people or institutions. Assertive nurses are aware of their own needs and the treatment they are entitled to as human beings. They express these needs when appropriate in an open, honest manner. Through assertiveness nurses can learn to train intellect to rule, instead of unchecked emotions, which can assist in controlling the guilt nurses often feel about things that are out of their control. When the intellect takes charge, the nurse can set priorities more objectively.

Nurses may not always be able to release the many emotions associated with critical care work on the job. Burying them can increase stress, therefore, it can be helpful to release them when alone (e.g., crying about a dying patient) or through other activities. Learning to express real feelings in an assertive way can help nurses earn respect from themselves and others.

Group meetings. A solution presented by many authors who have addressed the problem of stress in the ICU is to have the nursing staff meet regularly with an objective outsider who is trained in individual and group dynamics, preferably a nurse, who can best understand the specific issues that are of concern to nurses.

Group dynamics play an important role in the appraisal of stressors. Within the group setting, a warm, safe environment can be provided where staff members can ventilate their concerns and receive helpful feedback that is especially meaningful because it is derived mainly from peers. It is important that the request for such a group come from nursing staff.

Exercise. Exercise provides a direct outlet for the physiologic stress response. Relaxation techniques are also valuable personnel tools and can be effective especially in situations where control of stressors is not possible.

Other functional coping behaviors suggested are music, reading, or daydreaming—distracting the person emotionally from the stress situation. In response the body relaxes.

Physician director. It is frequently recommended that a full-time physician be employed as permanent critical care director. This position can play a key role in alleviating stress imposed on nurses by monitoring conflicts among medical colleagues and keeping avenues of communication open between medicine and nursing. Promoting a policy of team patient care with collegial association between medical and nursing personnel can enhance the recognition of present and potential levels of stress in the critical care area.

Organizational changes. When examining possible alternatives to current stressors, the critical care staff must translate their concerns about work into objective evaluation of continuing policies. Control/participation rewards include control over work pace and input into decisions affecting the ICU. Intrinsic rewards include learning opportunities, a chance to use one's own skills and abilities, an opportunity to do what one does best, and observing the results of one's work (Harris).

Managing work-related stress can be a difficult task for the critical care nurse and is best begun slowly, so the very management does not become stressful. Integrating one's own style is paramount to initiating any of these recommendations. The critical care nurse can best do this by giving herself permission to make mistakes and begin again.

APPENDIX A

INTERPRETATION OF ECG RHYTHMS AND ARRHYTHMIAS

Sylvia G. Talkington

THE ELECTROCARDIOGRAM

The ECG is the graphic recording of the heart's electrical activity, particularly atrial and ventricular events. This electrical activity is generated by chemical changes within the myocardial cells of the conduction system. It is measured by the placement of electrodes in variable positions on the chest wall. As the heartbeat occurs, representative deflections are marked on recording paper.

TABLE A–1
Location of Leads

Lead	Positive	Negative
Limb leads (bipolar)		
I (Fig. A–1)	Left arm	Right arm
II	Left leg	Right arm
III	Left leg	Left arm
Augmented leads (unipolar)		
a_VR	Right arm	
a_VL	Left arm	
a_VF	Left leg	

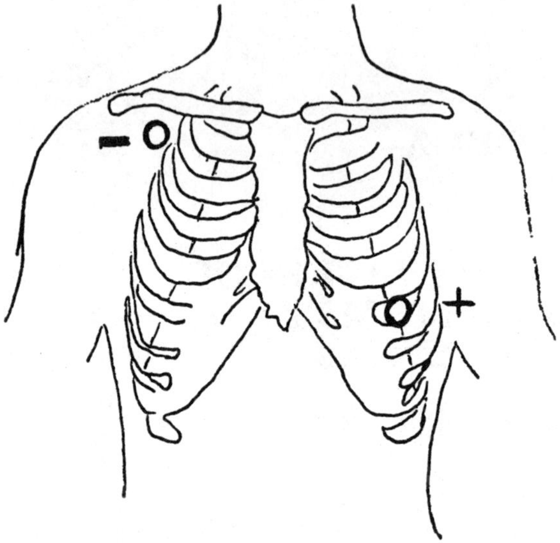

Figure A–1. Limb lead II.

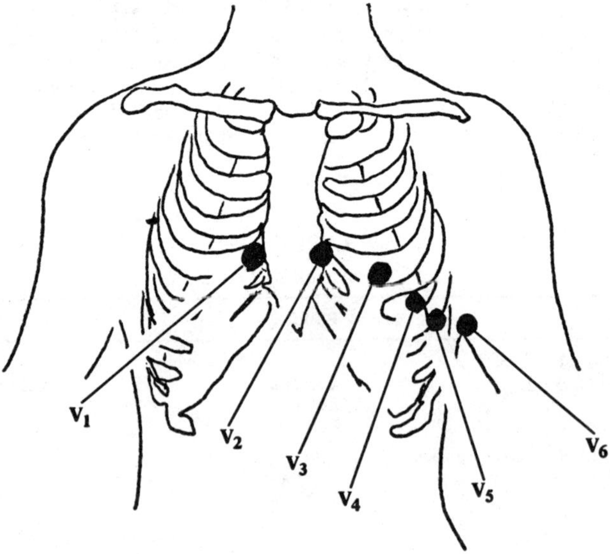

Figure A–2. Precordial chest leads.

TABLE A–1
Location of Leads

Lead	Positive	Negative
Precordial leads (unipolar) (Fig. A–2)		
V_1	Right sternal border, 4th Ic	
V_2	Left sternal border, 4th Ic	
V_3	Halfway between leads V_2 and V_4	
V_4	Left midclavicular line, 5th Ic	
V_5	Anterior axillary line (left), 5th Ic	
V_6	Midaxillary line (left), 5th Ic	
Other		
MCL_1 (bipolar) (Fig. A–3)	Right sternal border, 4th Ic	Left arm

Ic, intercostal; MCL, modified chest lead.

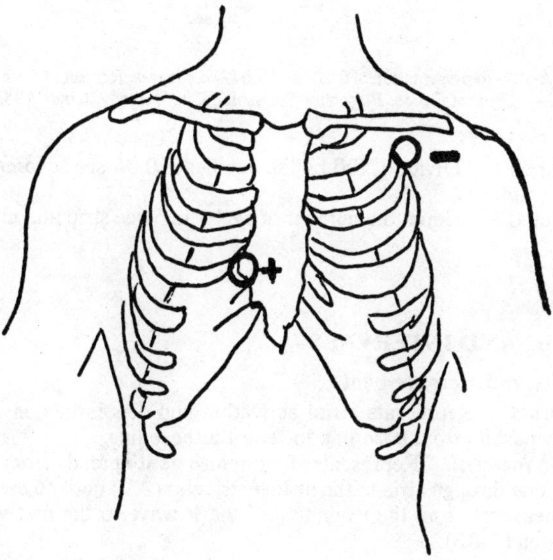

Figure A–3. Modified chest lead (MCL_1).

DETERMINATION OF HEART RATE

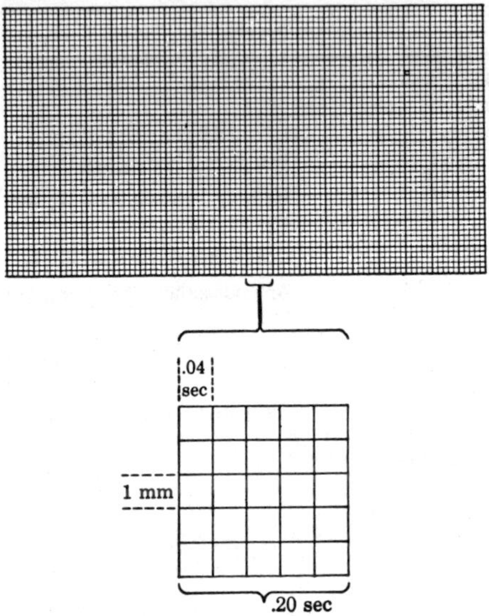

Figure A–4. Representation of 0.20- and 0.04-sec squares. *Reprinted from* Talkington, S. ECG—A Pocket Guide. Fleschner Publishing Co., Bethany, Conn. 1982, p. 4.

Method 1. Divide 1,500 by the number of 0.04-sec squares between QRS complexes.

Method 2. Count the number of cycles in 6-sec strip and multiply by 10.

WAVES AND INTERVALS

Activity and measurement

P wave. Represents atrial activation and depolarization; measured from departure from base line to return to base line.

P-R interval. Represents the impulse as it spreads from sinoatrial (SA) node through atria to the atrioventricular (AV) node to the bundle of His; measured from the beginning of the P wave to the first ventricular deflection (QRS).

TABLE A–2

Determination of Heart Rates

A No. of 0.04-sec squares between QRS complexes	B Corresponding heart rate (1,500 ÷ no. in Column A)
	bpm
5	300
10	150
11	136
12	125
13	115
14	107
15	100
16	93
17	88
18	83
19	78
20	75
21	71
22	68
23	65
24	62
25	60
26	57
27	55
28	53
29	51
30	50
31	48
32	46
33	45
34	44
35	42
36	41
37	40
38	39

Reprinted from Talkington, S. ECG-A Pocket Guide. Fleschner Publishing Co., Bethany, Conn. 1982. p. 5.

QRS complex. Represents activation and depolarization of the ventricles; measured from the end of the P-R interval to the end of the S wave.

ST segment. Represents complete ventricular depolarization; measured from the end of the QRS complex (J point) to the beginning of the T wave.

T wave. Represents ventricular repolarization; measured from the end of the ST from departure from base line to return to base line.

Duration and shape

P wave. Normal duration: 0.11 sec. Shape upright in leads I, II, a_VF; variable all other leads; rounded contour; amplitude 2 to 3 mm.

P-R interval. Normal duration: 0.12–0.20 sec, normally shortened with rapid rates or increased age or weight. Shape determined by the shape of the P wave that comprises it.

QRS complex. Normal duration: 0.05–0.10 sec. Shape of variable amplitude, variable component waves: Q wave = initial negative deflection, R wave = first positive deflection, S wave = negative deflection following R wave.

ST segment. Duration variable. Shape usually isoelectric; normal variation: upward 2 to 3 mm (if concave and succeeded by tall T wave).

T wave. Duration variable. Shape upright in leads I, II, V_3 to V_6; inverted in lead a_VR; slightly rounded and asymmetric.

Characteristics

P wave. Abnormal characteristics in patients with atrial arrhythmias, atrial abnormalities, and electrolyte imbalance. Prolonged duration and notched contour: left atrial enlargement. Normal duration but tall and peaked in leads II, III, and a_VF: perhaps right atrial enlargement. Prolonged duration and decreased amplitude: hyperkalemia.

P-R interval. Abnormal characteristics in patients with atrial arrhythmias, electrolyte imbalance, digitalis toxicity, and conduction disturbances in the Av node, atria, bundle of His, or bundle branches. Prolonged duration: digitalis toxicity and serum potassium alterations. Shortened duration: rapid atrial pacing and Lown-Ganong-Levine syndrome or Wolff-Parkinson-White syndrome.

QRS complex. Abnormal characteristics in patients with heart disease, heart block, electrolyte imbalance, and conduction disturbances of the bundle branches and/or ventricles. Prolonged duration: aberrant conduction, hyper- or hypokalemia, hypercalcemia, and bundle branch block. Deep, pronounced Q wave: perhaps MI.

ST segment. Abnormal characteristics in patients with MI, pericarditis, pulmonary embolism, electrolyte imbalance, and/or left ventricular enlargement. Elevation >0.5 mm: perhaps myocardial ischemia. Depression: perhaps hypokalemia. Prolonged duration: hypocalcemia. Shortened duration: hypercalcemia.

T wave. Abnormal characteristics in myocardial ischemia, electrolyte imbalance, and ventricular enlargement. Inverted: right or left ventricular enlargement, myocardial ischemia, and hypocalcemia. Peaked: hypercalcemia or hyperkalemia. Decreased amplitude: hypokalemia.

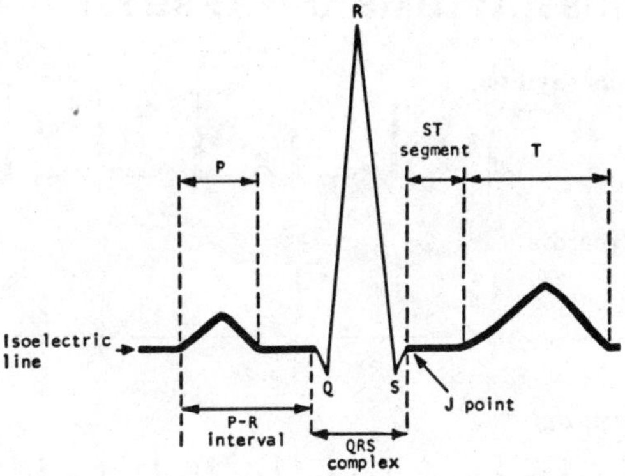

Figure A–5. Schematic representation of ECG wave forms. *Reprinted from* Talkington, S. ECG—A Pocket Guide. Fleschner Publishing Co., Bethany Conn. 1982, p. 11.

Wave-form interpretation

1. Determine lead placement and skin integrity.
2. Determine rhythm: regular or irregular.
3. Determine rate:
   Atrial: Regular if duration from P wave to P wave remains constant.
   Ventricular: Regular if duration from R wave to R wave remains constant.
4. Evaluate atrial function: note P wave in all leads for height, contour, and duration.
5. Evaluate AV function: note P-R interval.
6. Evaluate ventricular function: note QRS complex component waves, amplitude, and duration.
7. Determine if atrial activity is related to ventricular activity. (Is there a P wave for each QRS complex, and does the P wave precede or follow the QRS complex?)
8. Determine if there are ectopic complexes and/or beats (different configurations from the commonly observed complexes).
9. Consider the clinical setting: What is the significance of the rate, rhythm, or arrhythmia?
10. Decide how the rate, rhythm, or arrhythmia should be treated.

SINUS RHYTHMS AND ARRHYTHMIAS

Normal sinus rhythm

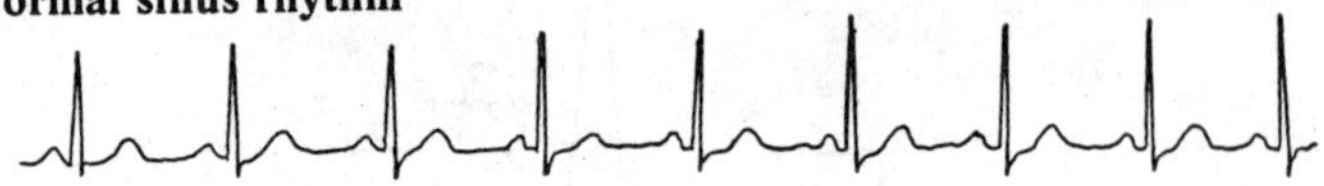

Sinus bradycardia

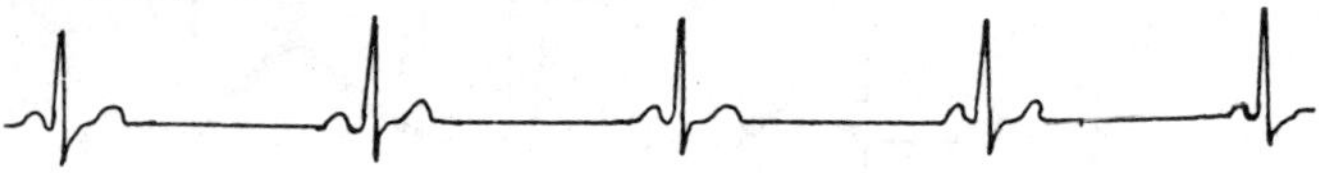

Sinus tachycardia

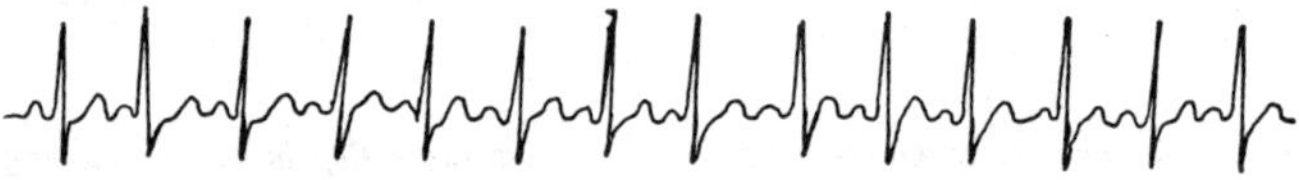

Sinus arrhythmia

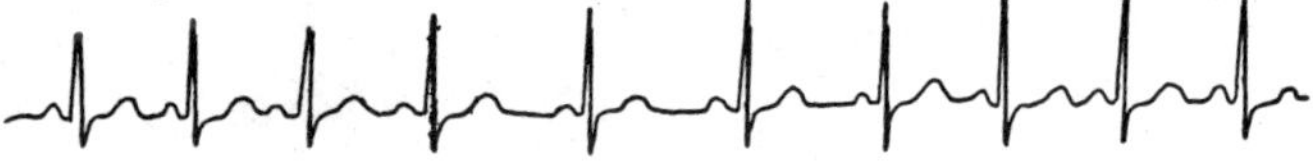

Wandering pacemaker

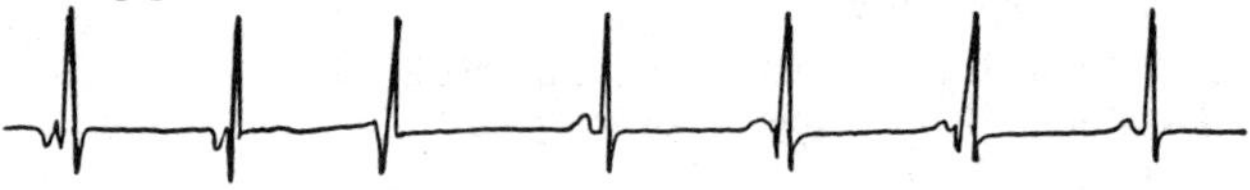

Sinus block

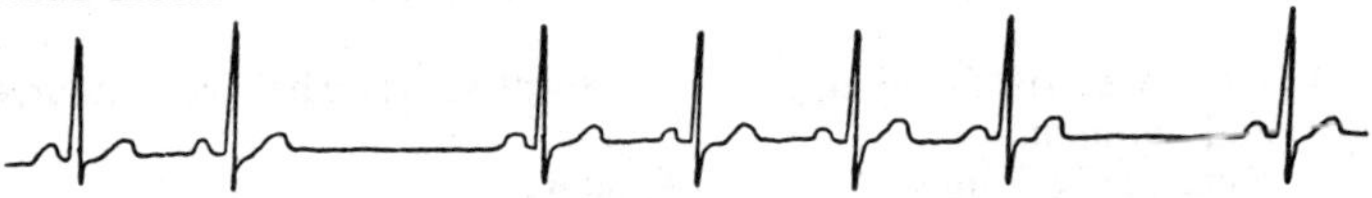

Sinus arrest

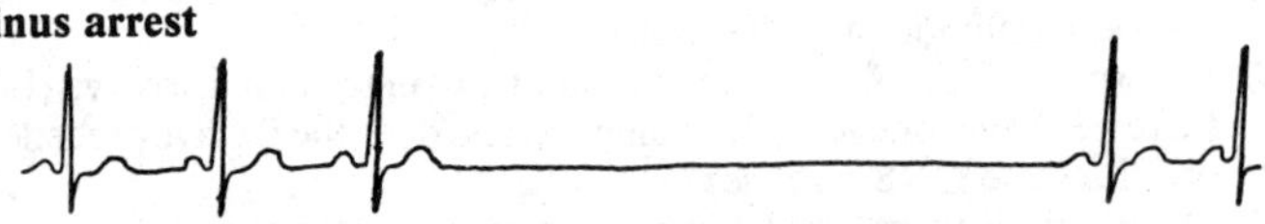

Sick sinus syndrome

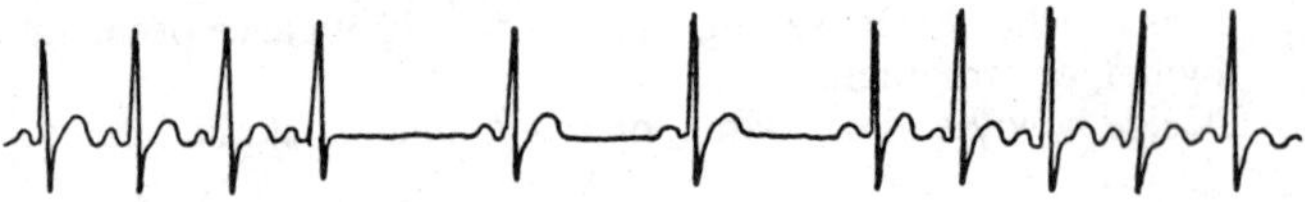

INTERPRETATION

Normal sinus rhythm

Atrial and ventricular rates regular: 60 to 100 bpm; each P wave is related to and followed by a QRS complex; P-R interval is of normal duration; QRS is normal or prolonged.

Sinus bradycardia

Rate is <60 bpm; P-P interval is regular; R-R interval is regular; each P wave is related to and followed by a QRS; P-R interval is of normal duration; QRS is normal or prolonged; sinus arrhythmia may be present.

Sinus tachycardia

Rate is 100–160 bpm; each P wave is related to and followed by a QRS; P-R interval is normal; QRS is normal or prolonged; gradual onset and termination.

Sinus arrhythmia

Normal: irregularity of the heartbeat under control of the SA node. Phasic: irregularity related to phases of respiration (rate increase on inspiration, rate decrease on expiration). Nonphasic: irregularity not related to respiration.

Wandering pacemaker

Passive arrhythmia (type of multifocal atrial pacemaker); rate is 60 to 100 bpm; P wave changes in shape, contour, and deflection; possible variable P-R interval; QRS normal or prolonged.

Sinus block

A failure or delay in conduction from the SA node that results in P-QRS-T sequences that are occasionally absent or in abnormally long cycles. Types of SA block: (1) failure of impulse to emerge from the SA node (exit block); (2) failure of the emerging impulse to activate the atria. Length of block or pause in cycle is recorded in seconds.

Sinus arrest

Complete sinus block. Absent P-QRS-T intervals. Atrial standstill. Failure of sinus node to form the impulse.

Sick sinus syndrome

SA node dysfunction, including marked sinus bradycardia, prolonged sinus pauses, sinus block, sinus arrest, and tachycardia-bradycardia ("tachy-brady") syndrome.

CAUSES

Normal sinus rhythm

Normal function of the conduction system.

Sinus bradycardia

Normal variation, especially in athletes. Physiologic reaction to sleep, fright, carotid sinus sensitivity, increased intracranial pressure, or disease (e.g., obstructive jaundice or glaucoma). Associated with acute MI. Drugs: e.g., digitalis and/or beta blockers.

Sinus tachycardia

Normal reaction to stress, hemorrhage, shock, fever, infections, or thyrotoxicosis. Common reaction to heart disease (MI and CHF). Drugs: stimulants, atropine, or quinidine.

Sinus arrhythmia

Normal variation.

Wandering pacemaker

Shift in pacemaker focus among SA node, other atrial foci, and AV node.

Sinus block

Drugs: e.g., digitalis, quinidine, salicylates, or procainamide hydrochloride. Diseases, such as coronary artery disease, acute infection. MI involving the sinus node. Increased carotid sinus and/or vagal tone.

Sinus arrest

As with sinus block.

Sick sinus syndrome

Temporary (reversible): digitalis, quiniddine, beta blockers, or aerosol propellants.

Chronic (progressive): ischemic disease, collagen disease, metastatic disease, or cardiomyopathy.

EFFECTS

Normal sinus rhythms

Sinus rhythm indicates integrity of the cardiac conduction system and provides for effective CO.

Sinus bradycardia

Symptomatic sinus bradycardia may decrease CO or increase number and frequency of various arrhythmias. Chronic sinus bradycardia may induce CHF.

Sinus tachycardia

Rapid rates (>160) may decrease coronary artery perfusion, decrease CO, or have deleterious effects on persons with CHF, hypoxia, or ischemia.

Sinus arrhythmia

None usually encountered.

Wandering pacemaker

None usually encountered if ventricular rate remains ≤60 to 100 bpm.

Sinus block

None, unless abnormally long cycles produce symptomatic bradycardia.

Sinus arrest

Lower pacemaker site takes over. Syncope if the lower pacemaker fails. Prolonged episodes may decrease CO with resulting hypotension, weakness, pallor, coolness of extremities, and diaphoresis.

Sick sinus syndrome

May cause weakness, intermittent hypotension, and variable pulses. Symptoms of tachycardia and bradycardia.

TREATMENT

Normal sinus rhythm

Observe and document the assessment of an acceptable cardiac rhythm.

Sinus bradycardia

Increased activity or exercise. Atropine: 0.5 mg by IV push initially (if symptomatic). Isoproterenol (Isuprel): 1 mg in 250 ml of D5W at 2-20 μg (mcgs)/min, then adjusted to increase heart rate (if markedly symptomatic). Temporary pacemaker.

Sinus tachycardia

Evaluate underlying cause and eliminate or treat if symptoms persist. Primary sinus tachycardia: administer sedatives, reserpine, or propranolol hydrochloride (Inderal).

Sinus arrythmias

No treatment necessary.

Wandering pacemaker

Withdraw digitalis or reduce dosage if digitalis toxicity exists. Close observation of rhythm and continued clinical assessment.

Sinus block

Evaluate underlying cause and eliminate, or treat if symptoms persist.

Sinus arrest

Atropine (IV) followed by isoproterenol (continuous IV). Atrial and/or ventricular pacing.

Sick sinus syndrome

Temporary: Evaluate underlying cause and eliminate, or treat if symptoms persist.

Chronic: Insert permanent pacemaker.

SUPRAVENTRICULAR RHYTHMS AND ARRHYTHMIAS

Premature atrial contraction (PAC)

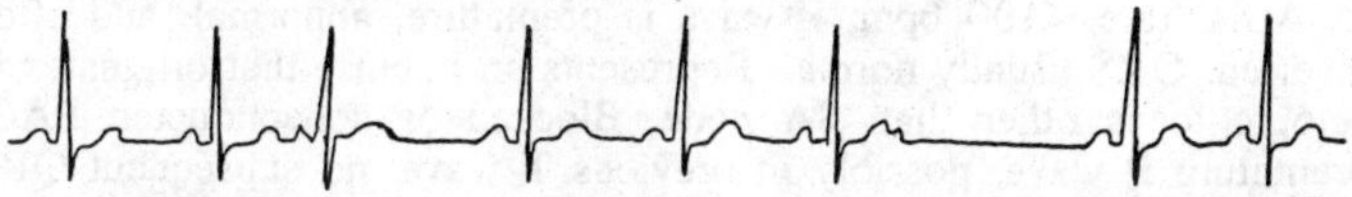

Paroxysmal atrial tachycardia (PAT) (supraventricular tachycardia [SVT])

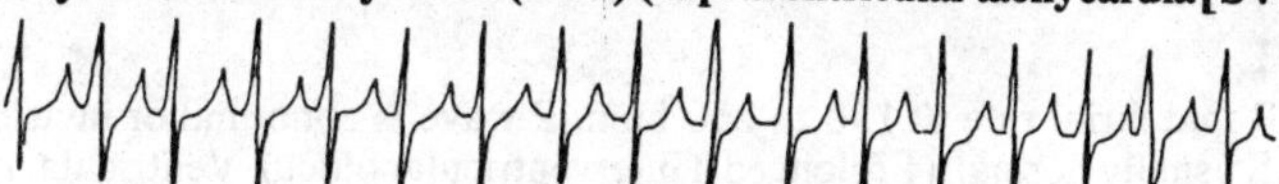

Atrial flutter

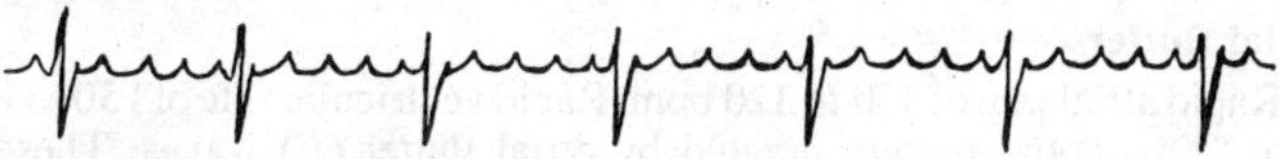

Atrial fibrillation

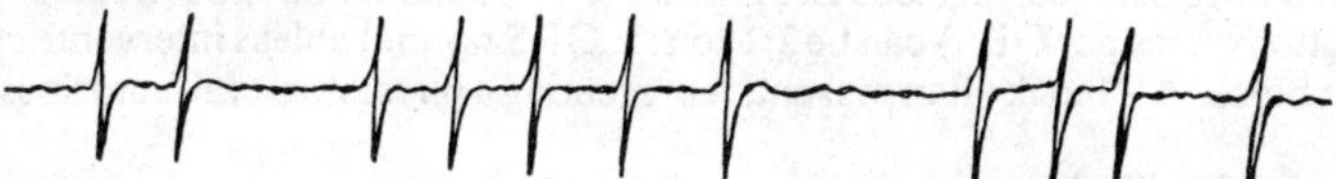

AV-JUNCTIONAL RHYTHMS AND ARRHYTHMIAS

Premature junctional contraction (PJC)

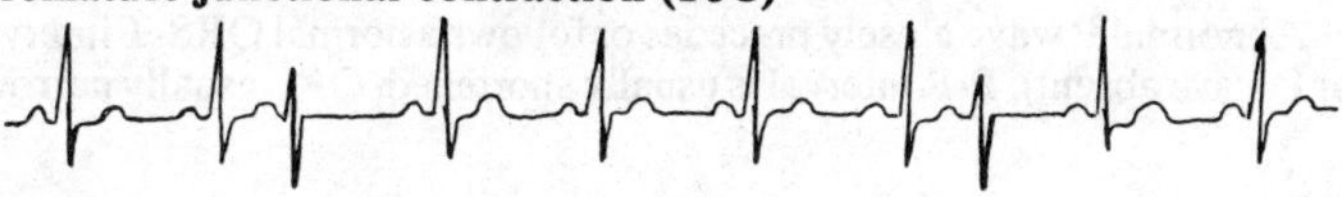

AV-junctional tachycardia

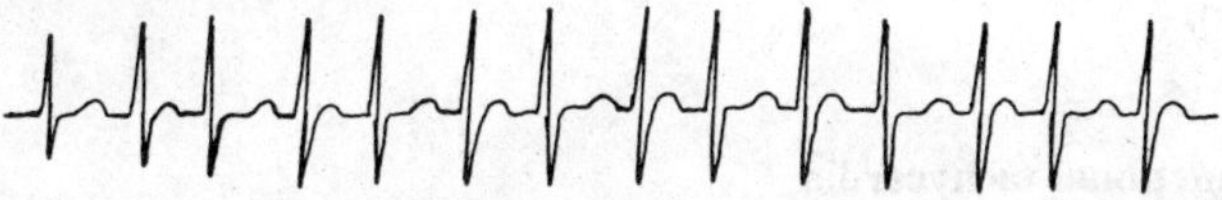

Nonparoxysmal junctional tachycardia (accelerated junctional rhythm)

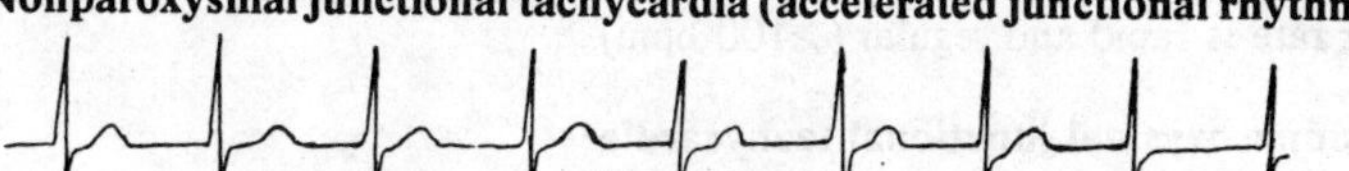

AV-junctional rhythm (AV-junctional escape rhythm)

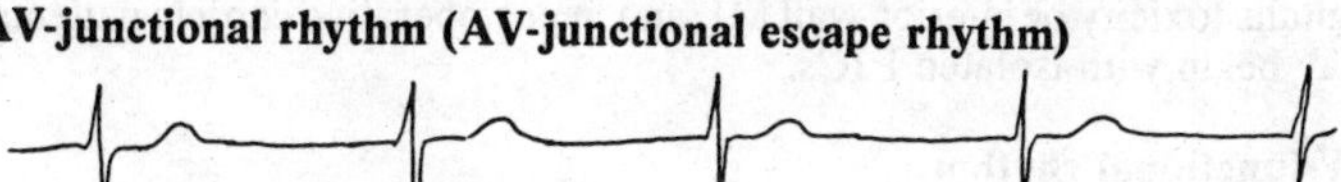

INTERPRETATION

PAC

Atrial rate <100 bpm; P wave is premature, abnormal, and often inverted; QRS usually normal. Represents an impulse that originates in ectopic focus other than SA node. Blocked or nonconducted PAC: premature P wave, possibly in previous T wave; no subsequent QRS complex. *Most common cause of pause.*

PAT

Rapid atrial rate of 150 to 250 bpm. P wave is abnormal or invisible; QRS usually normal. (Prolonged if interventricular block). Ventricular rate is usually regular. ST segment and T wave depression possible.

Atrial flutter

Rapid atrial rate of 300 to 320 bpm. Rapid ventricular rate of 150 to 160 bpm. "Sawtooth" pattern created by atrial flutter (F) waves. These F waves are best seen in leads II, III and V_1. The conduction ratio (number of flutter waves per QRS) can be 2:1 to 8:1. QRS normal unless interventricular block. AV block often present, representing a physiologic refractoriness.

Atrial fibrillation

Atrial rate of ≥350 bpm, indicating a rapid, irregular, ectopic atrial rate. P wave is unobservable or invisible. Fibrillation (f) waves indicate the atrial activity. QRS normal. *Ventricular response is irregular.*

Abnormal P wave closely precedes or follows a normal QRS-T interval (or P wave absent). P-R interval is usually shortened. QRS usually narrow.

PJC

P wave closely precedes or follows normal QRS-T interval (or P wave absent).

AV-junctional tachycardia

P wave absent, inverted or retrograde. P-R interval shortened. Ventricular rate is rapid and regular (>100 bpm).

Nonparoxysmal junctional tachycardia

Ventricular rate 62 to 100 bpm. This arrhythmia is seen in patients with digitalis toxicity or inferior-wall MI, and in postoperative cardiac patients. May begin with isolated PJCs.

AV-junctional rhythm

45 to 60 bpm (rate will increase with atropine administration). His bundle rhythm: 30 to 40 bpm (not affected by atropine).

CAUSES

PAC

Acute infection, myocardial ischemia, organic heart disease, or stimulation from medication, tobacco, caffeine, or tension.

PAT

Single repetitive atrial focus. Circus movement impulses (reentry). Short P-R interval syndromes: Wolff-Parkinson-White or digitalis toxicity (especially with AV block). Overexertion or coronary artery disease (CAD).

Atrial flutter

Ectopic atrial focus with enhanced rate of discharge. Organic heart disease. Or rhythm may occur normally.

Atrial fibrillation

Rheumatic heart disease with mitral disease. Hypertension. Thyrotoxicosis. Atrial septal defect. Constrictive pericarditis.

SA node depression caused by medications (e.g., digitalis or quinidine), disease, or congenital absence.

PJC

Occurs in response to stimuli (emotion, tobacco, coffee). Associated with atrial dilation or hypertrophy, hypoxia, MI, CHF, electrolyte imbalance.

AV-junctional tachycardia

As with other AV-junctional rhythms and arrhythmias.

Nonparoxysmal junctional tachycardia

Digitalis toxicity the primary cause when junctional rate is >60 bpm.

AV-junctional rhythm

Occurs in response to depressed or low sinus rhythm or when complete AV block is present.

EFFECTS

PAC

May precipitate SVT or PAT. Physical symptoms of palpitations if recurrent SVT or PAT.

PAT

Decreased diastole with decreased CO. Decreased coronary artery perfusion. Increased O_2 consumption. May increase angina, CHF, or shock. May cause syncope, anxiety, or palpitation, all of which may vary according to duration, rate, and/or presence of heart disease.

Atrial flutter

May cause atrial fibrillation. Often recurrent. May produce visible "waves" on the neck ("cannon a waves").

Atrial fibrillation

May be associated with systemic emboli or pulmonary embolism, especially in rheumatic heart disease and mitral disease. When accompanied by a rapid ventricular rate, may cause symptoms of PAT or cardiac decompensation.

Symptoms vary according to type of rhythm, rate, and clinical situation.

PJC

May initiate accelerated AV junctional rhythm.

AV-junctional tachycardia

May precipitate symptoms of atrial tachycardia, especially if heart disease present.

Nonparoxysmal junctional tachycardia

With accelerated rate (70 bpm), loss of atrial contribution to CO.

AV-junctional rhythm

Symptoms of decreased CO.

TREATMENT

PAC

In patients with MI (if symptomatic): digitalis, quinidine, or procainamide hydrochloride.

PAT

Treatment is administered according to duration of the rhythm, presence of heart disease, and symptoms. Vagal maneuvers: carotid sinus massage, Valsalva maneuver, or gagging. Cholinergics: edrophonium chloride (Tensilon). Calcium antagonists: verapamil hydrochloride. Vasopressors: metaraminol bitartrate (Aramine), phenylephrine hydrochloride (Neo-Synephrine), or methoxamine hydrochloride (Vasoxyl). Digitalis, propranolol hydrochloride, or procainamide hydrochloride. DC cardioversion.

Atrial flutter

Synchronous DC cardioversion (≤50 watt sec). Digitalis or quinidine to terminate. Verapamil for temporary reduction of ventricular rate. Propranolol hydrochloride or variable combinations of digitalis, quinidine, and procainamide hydrochloride for long-term reduction of ventricular rate. Rapid atrial pacing may be initiated in a few uncommon situations (e.g., when the flutter is resistant to digitalis routines or cardioversion).

Atrial fibrillation

Treatment is administered according to rate of ventricular response, assessment of patient's symptoms, and evaluation of the underlying disease. DC cardioversion if ventricular rate increases with symptoms (50 to 100 watt sec). Verapamil for temporary reduction of ventricular rate. Digitalis to maintain resting ventricular rate (60 to 80 bpm) except in patients with Wolff-Parkinson-White syndrome. Combined digitalis and quinidine for long-term reduction of ventricular rate or return to normal rhythm.

PJC

Close observation of rhythm and continued clinical assessment.

AV-junctional tachycardia

Close observation of rhythm and continued clinical assessment.

Nonparoxysmal junctional tachycardia

Close observation of rhythm and continued clinical assessment. Remove digitalis if indicated.

AV-junctional rhythm

Close observation of rhythm and continued clinical assessment.

VENTRICULAR RHYTHMS AND ARRHYTHMIAS

Premature ventricular contraction (PVC)

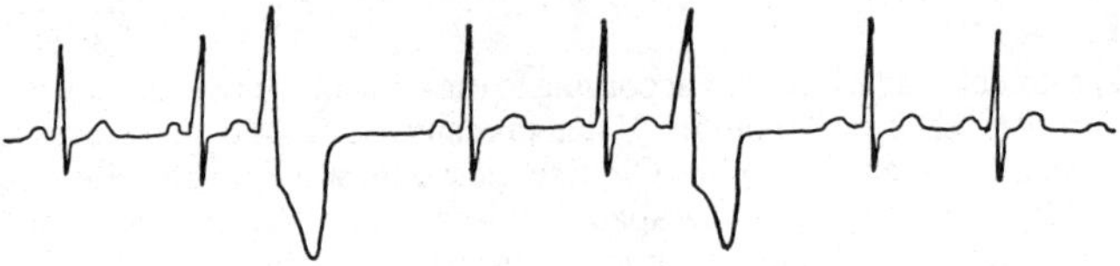

Ventricular tachycardia (VT)

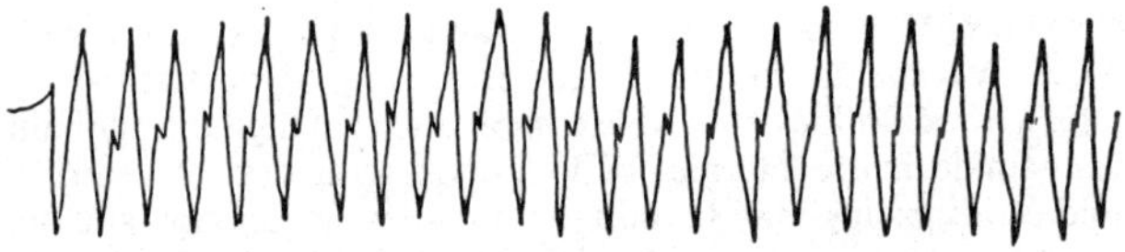

Ventricular fibrillation (VF)

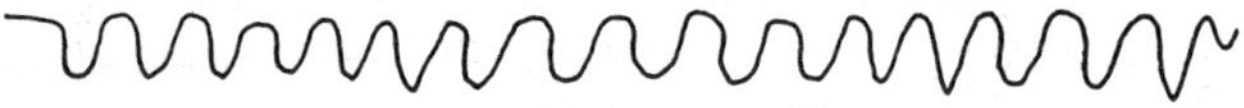

Accelerated idioventricular rhythm

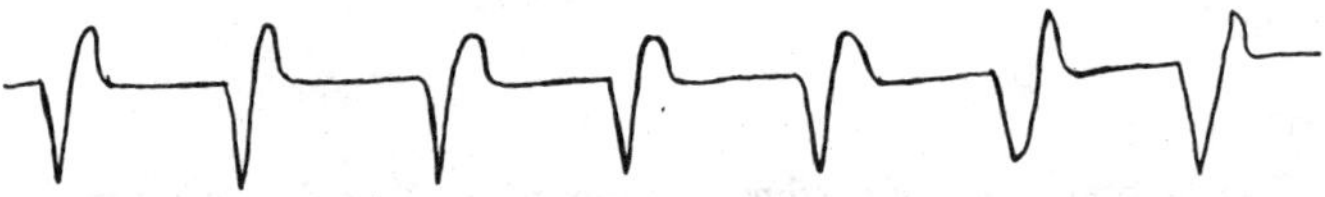

Ventricular asystole/standstill

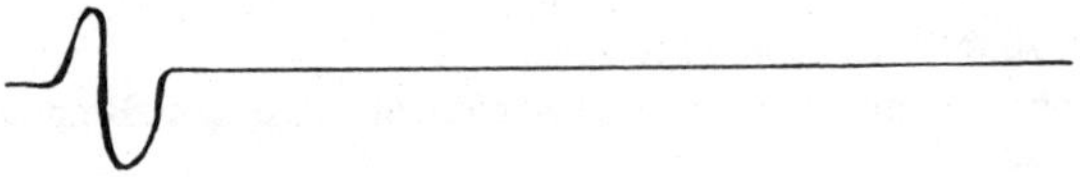

INTERPRETATION

PVC

Impulse originates in the ventricle below AV node in the His-Perkinje network. Also called extrasystole, ventricular premature beat, premature ectopic beat, or ventricular ectopic beat. P wave may be invisible before PVC or may be in previous QRS or in the terminal portion of the PVC (retrograde). QRS is broad, bizarre, and prolonged. ST segment slopes in opposite direction from the QRS. Compensatory pause (the distance from R wave before PVC to R wave after PVC equals the distance between two normal cycles). Fixed coupling exists (a fixed relationship exists between PVC and preceding beat). Types include interpolated, bigeminy, trigeminy, unifocal, multifocal, coupled, Ron T phenomenon, right ventricular, left ventricular.

VT

Repeating PVCs (three or more). Often occurs in short bursts (repetitive VT) and is interrupted or initiated by fusion beat (beat that exhibits characteristics of sinus-initiated beat and a PVC). Rapid rate: 110 to 240 bpm. QRS is wide, bizarre, and usually regular. P waves present but not easily visible.

VF

Numerous impulses in ventricle initiating depolarization. May be preceded by bradycardia, PVC, or VT. Coarse fibrillation: zigzag tracing of increased amplitude with sharp peaks. Fine fibrillation: zigzag tracing of decreased amplitude and less sharp peaks. No observable P wave, QRS, or T wave.

Accelerated idioventricular rhythm

Absent P wave and P-R interval. Wide QRS complexes. Ventricular rate: 50 to 100 bpm and regular; often similar to preceding sinus rate. Occasionally initiated by PVC or often preceded by fusion beat.

Ventricular asystole

Isoelectric tracing evidencing no intervals or complexes.

CAUSES

PVC

May occur in normal hearts or with isometric exercise. May occur in acute MI. May occur with hypoxia and/or altered electrolyte states.

VT

Results from enhanced automaticity or reentry occurring in the His-Perkinje network. Occurs with significant heart disease (acute MI or CAD). May result from electrolyte imbalance. Can be initiated by a premature beat, a pacemaker stimulus, or DC shock.

VF

Seen in ischemia with MI, advanced heart disease, severe digitalis or quinidine toxicity, or severe hypo- or hyperkalemia. May occur during cardiac pacing or catheterization, or during cardioversion.

Accelerated idioventricular rhythm

May be benign. Seen frequently in digitalis toxicity or MI.

Ventricular asystole

Complete heart block.

EFFECTS

PVC

May be asymptomatic. May increase angina or decrease BP in patients with heart disease. May cause palpitations, dyspnea, or neck or chest discomfort. Increased risk of sudden death in patients with MI.

VT

May be asymptomatic. May cause hyypotension, variable heart sound, CHF, shock, or VF. Symptoms of angina, palpitations, weakness, confusion, restlessness, or dyspnea. At high rates or long duration, may decrease CO, or coronary artery perfusion.

VF

Loss of consciousness, heart tones, and respiration. Complete cardiovascular collapse leading to pronounced shock and immediate death if not treated.

Accelerated idioventricular rhythm

May be asymptomatic. Symptoms of bradycardia may develop if a low rate of discharge persists.

Ventricular asystole

Intermittent: weakness, hypotension, and dyspnea. Prolonged: loss of peripheral pulses, consciousness, and respiration.

TREATMENT

PVC

Asymptomatic: no treatment necessary (or evaluate possible underlying causes). Symptomatic or in patients with heart disease or MI: Lidocaine hydrochloride: 1 to 2 mg/kg/min IV bolus, followed by 1 to 4 mg/min via continuous IV infusion pump. Procainamide hydrochloride: 375 to 500 mg PO q 3 to 4 hr; 50 to 100 mg (25 mg/min) IV bolus; 750 to 1,000 mg (25 mg/min) IV loading dose; 2 to 6 mg/min via continuous IV infusion pump. Bretylium tosylate (Bretylol) if no response to other medications.

VT

Evaluate the underlying cause and eliminate or treat. Asymptomatic: Lidocaine as with PVCs. Procainamide hydrochloride as with PVCs. Bretylium tosylate 5 to 10 mg/kg over 10 min. Quinidine, propranolol hydrochloride, or phenytoin sodium (Dilantin). Potassium may be administered when digitalis toxicity induces VT. Symptomatic: prompt cardioversion.

VF

Immediate cardiopulmonary resuscitation (CPR) with defibrillation at 200 watt sec. Continued advanced cardiac life support. Lidocaine or bretylium tosylate (IV bolus). Treatment of resulting severe metabolic acidosis.

Accelerated idioventricular rhythm

Evaluate underlying cause and eliminate, or treat if symptoms persist. Close observation of rhythm and continued clinical assessment.

Ventricular asystole

Immediate CPR and advanced cardiac life support. Probable pacemaker.

HEART BLOCK (CONDUCTION DISTURBANCES)

First-degree AV block

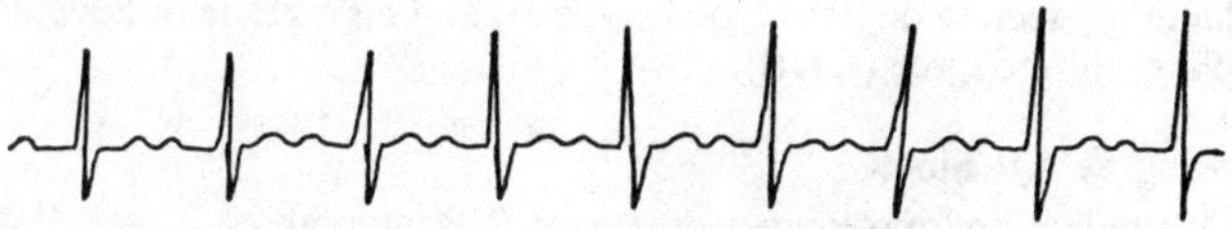

Second-degree AV block Type I (Wenckebach)

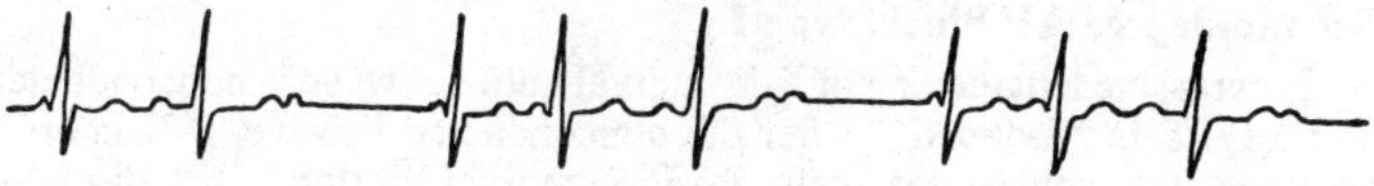

Type II

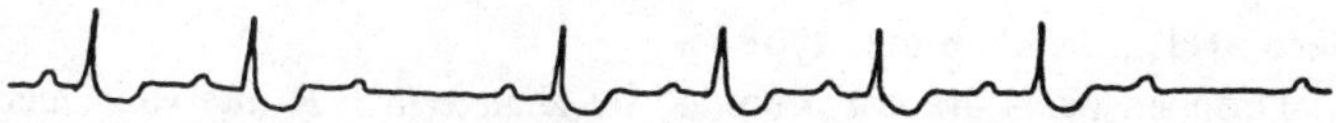

High-grade or advanced AV block

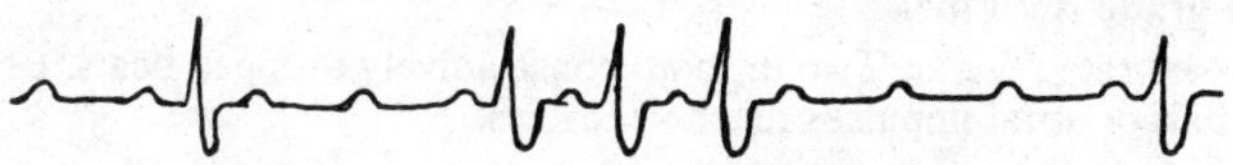

Third-degree AV block (complete heart block [CHB])

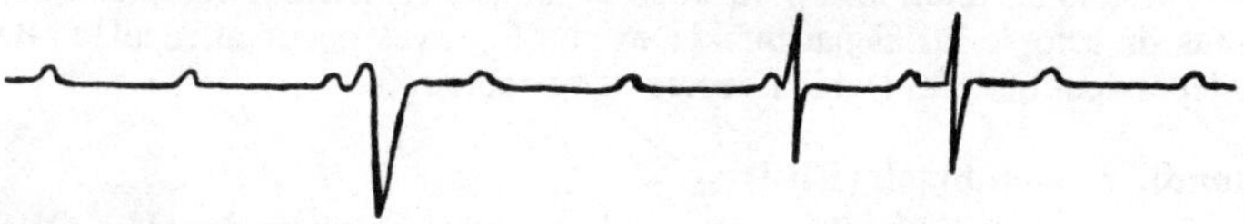

Right bundle branch block

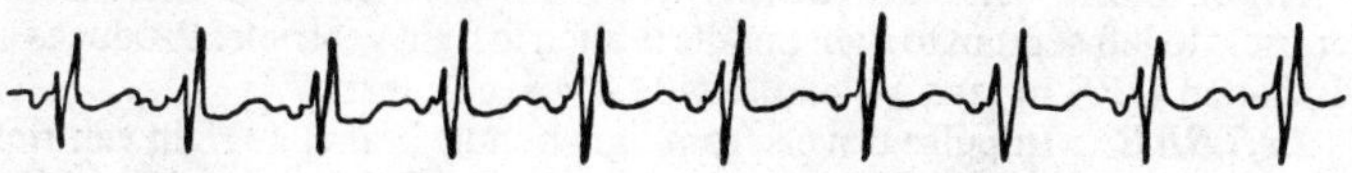

Left bundle branch block

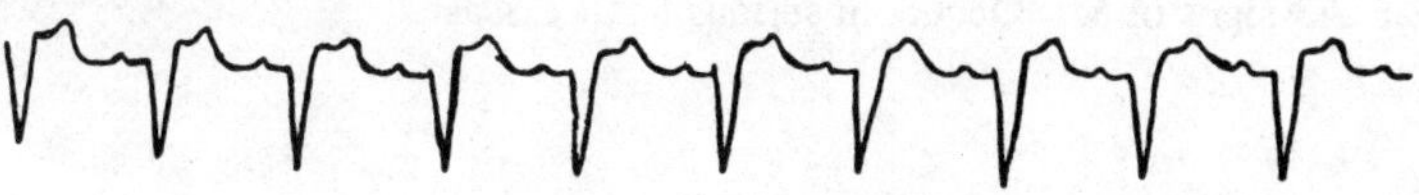

INTERPRETATION

AV block may be a permanent or transient condition. The severity is related to heart rate. Types include incomplete: first degree (prolonged conduction); second degree (type I, type II, and high-grade or advanced); complete: third degree (CHB).

First-degree AV block

AV conduction is prolonged, creating a P-R interval >0.20 sec. P wave exists for every QRS. Ventricular rate is regular.

Second-degree AV block, type I

Progressive lengthening of P-R interval until a P wave is nonconducted and a QRS is "dropped." After the nonconducted P wave, P-R interval shortens and cycle begins again. As P-R interval shortens, R-R shortens. QRS usually normal. Characterized by groups of beats.

Second-degree AV block, type II

Dropped beats are not preceded by change in P-R interval. Occurs frequently with bundle branch rhythms (QRS >0.12 sec).

High-grade AV block

Atrial rate regular. Two or more consecutively dropped beats. Fewer than half of atrial impulses reach ventricles.

Third-degree AV block (CHB)

There is no relationship between atrial and ventricular complexes. A sinus or ectopic atrial pacemaker exists. P waves occur at regular rate independent of QRS (which occurs at variable rate).

Bundle branch block (BBB)

Occurs when disease blocks one or both branches of bundle of His. QRS prolonged. ST slopes in opposite direction from QRS.

Right BBB. Impulse travels from the left bundle branch to left ventricle to left septum to right bundle branch to right ventricle. Produces an M-shaped QRS in lead V_1 and a wide S wave in lead V_6.

Left BBB. Impulse travels from right bundle branch to right ventricle to septum to left bundle branch to left ventricle. Produces a Q-S or R-S wave in lead V_1 and may cause the Q wave to be absent in V_6. Can obscure ECG signs of MI. Occurs in serious heart disease.

CAUSES

In children: mal- or nonformed AV valve or rheumatic fever. In adults: digitalis, propanolol, or quinidine toxicity; infections; myocarditis, arteriosclerotic heart disease; MI, left CAD, or Lev's and Lenegre's diseases.

First-degree AV block

Seen in patients with inferior-wall MI, rheumatic heart disease, and digitalis toxicity.

Second-degree AV block type I

As above.

Second-degree AV block, type II

As above.

High-grade AV block

As above.

CHB

As above.

BBB

CAD, rheumatic heart disease, syphilis, aortic stenosis, trauma, cardiomyopathy, tumors, congenital lesions, right ventricular hypertrophy, or hypertension.

EFFECTS

First-degree AV block

Rarely symptomatic; frequently transient.

Second-degree AV block, type I

If ventricular rate is slow, symptoms of bradycardia and decreased CO may occur. May be transient in patients with inferior-wall MI.

Second-degree AV block, type II

Less common than type I but may be more serious. May precipitate Stokes-Adams attacks. May cause right BBB, CHB, asystole, or shock in patients with acute anterior MI.

High-grade AV block

As with Type II above.

CHB

Symptoms of angina, CHF, or syncope may develop. Nodal or ventricular escape beats may occur. Ventricular standstill can occur if rhythm is not treated.

BBB

May be asymptomatic or may cause symptoms of the underlying disease.

TREATMENT

First-degree AV block

Close observation of rhythm and continued clinical assessment. Remove digitalis if toxic.

Second-degree AV block type I

Asymptomatic: no treatment necessary. Symptomatic: remove digitalis if indicated, or administer atropine per IV bolus. Pacemaker is indicated if no response to medication or prolonged symptomatic episodes occur.

Second-degree AV block, type II

Atropine not usually administered. Isoproterenol: 1 to 2 μg/kg/min. Usually a temporary pacemaker in patients with acute anterior MI.

High-grade AV block

Temporary pacemaker.

CHB

Isoproterenol (titrated by continuous infusion via control pump to achieve ventricular rate of 60 to 80 bpm). Temporary or permanent pacemaker.

BBB

Close observation of rhythm and continued clinical assessment.

MYOCARDIAL INFARCTION

RHYTHM

Death or necrosis of cardiac muscle caused by interrupted or blocked blood supply will exhibit particular tracings according to how the cardiac muscle is being affected (Figure A–11).

INTERPRETATION

Area of ischemia

T-wave inversion.

Area of injury

ST segment elevation.

Area of necrosis

Appearance of Q wave (previously absent) ≥0.04 sec and >4 mm depth.

In addition, the particular leads of the cardiogram will exhibit characteristics.

Indicative changes

Noted in leads facing area of damage; Q wave present; ST segment elevation; T wave inversion.

Reciprocal changes

Noted in leads opposite area of damage: Q wave absent; R wave and T wave taller; ST segment depression.

TYPES

Transmural

Involves entire thickness of myocardium; ST segment large and elevated; Q wave abnormal.

Subendocardial

Involves inner portion of myocardium; Q wave absent; ST segment depression; T wave inversion. Clinical symptoms of MI; high mortality.

Inferior-wall MI (IWMI).

Indicative changes occur in leads I, II, and a_VF; reciprocal changes occur in leads I and a_VL.

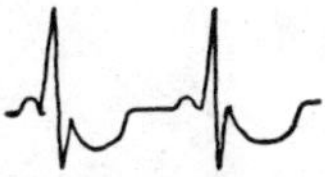
Area of ischemia

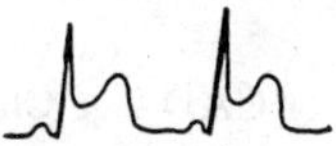
Area of injury

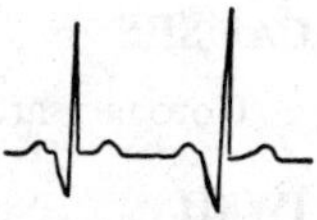
Area of necrosis

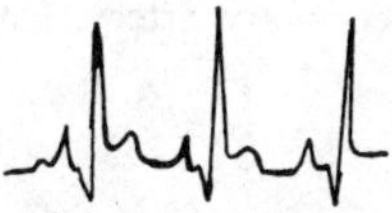
Indicative changes

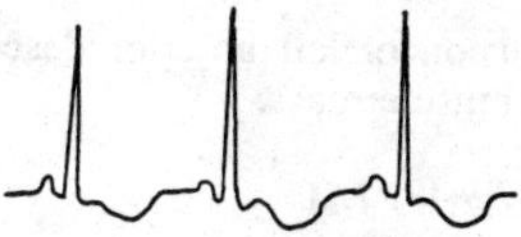
Reciprocal changes

Inferior-wall MI

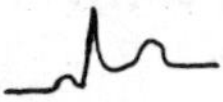
Lead II

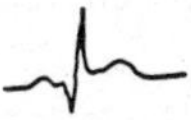
Lead III

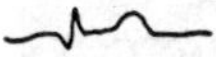
Lead a_VF

Anterior-wall MI

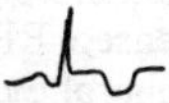
Lead I

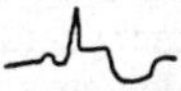
Lead a_VL

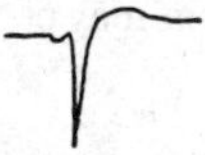
V_1

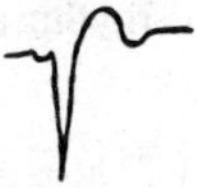
V_2

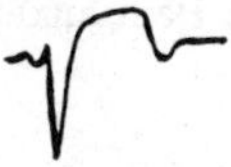
V_3

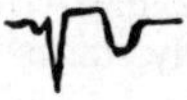
V_4

Anterior-wall MI (AWMI)

Indicative changes occur in leads I, a_VL, and V_1 to V_4; reciprocal changes occur in leads II, III, and a_VF.

True posterior MI

ST segment depression with developing R wave; reciprocal changes in anterior leads (especially V_1 and V_2).

Lateral-wall MI

Indicative changes in leads I and a_VL.

CAUSES

Coronary artery injury or CAD (*see* Chapter 2).

IWMI

Occlusion of right coronary artery.

AWMI

Occlusion of left anterior descending coronary artery. Involves the greatest muscle mass.

True posterior MI

Occlusion of circumflex coronary artery or right coronary artery.

Lateral-wall MI

Occlusion of left circumflex coronary artery.

EFFECTS

Chest pain (substernal): heavy, crushing, tight, or burning; may radiate to shoulders, arms, neck, or jaw; and usually persists >30 min. (Silent MI: no chest pain.) Possible dyspnea, nausea, diaphoresis, weakness, fatigue, or vomiting. Either tachycardia and increased BP or bradycardia and decreased BP. With decrease in CO: peripheral cyanosis and increasing shock. Advancing symptoms: third heart sound, murmurs, or rales. Increased blood levels of cardiac enzymes: SGOT, lactic dehydrogenase (LDH), and total creatine phosphokinase (CPK) with positive CPK-MB isoenzyme. Arrhythmias. Pain, anxiety, and rhythm alterations may persist in early stages.

Complications

Persistant pain, serious arrhythmia, pulmonary embolism, persistant hypotension, CHF, pericarditis.

TREATMENT

Continuous ECG monitoring with serial 12-lead electrocardiograms. *See* Chapter 2 for further discussion.

APPENDIX B

PHARMACOLOGIC ASPECTS OF CRITICAL CARE

Joyce B. Comer

INTRODUCTION

This appendix is designed to be a quick reference for the nurse. It is not intended to be all-inclusive, but instead it should serve as a reference or supplement to other educational materials. For a more detailed discussion concerning pharmacology, dosage, or adverse effects, the reader should refer to a pharmacology text. The medication sections provide information concerning pharmacology, dosage, adverse effects, and nursing parameters to monitor.

CONVERSION TABLES

Many medications require a calculation before they can be prepared or administered. The following conversion tables have been provided to assist in these calculations.

TABLE B–1

Metric System Conversions

Weight		
1.0 kilogram (kg)	=	1,000 grams (g)
1.0 gram	=	1,000 milligrams (mg)
1.0 milligram*	=	1,000 micrograms (μg)
Volume		
1.0 liter	=	1,000 milliliters (ml)
1.0 milliliter†	=	1,000 microliters (μl)
Comparative terms (using weight)		
1.0 microgram	=	0.000001 gram
1.0 milligram	=	0.001 gram
1.0 centigram	=	0.01 gram
1.0 decigram	=	0.1 gram
1.0 gram	=	1.0 gram
1.0 dekagram	=	10.0 gram
1.0 hectogram	=	100.0 gram
1.0 kilogram	=	1,000.0 gram
	=	
	=	

*0.001 g = 1.0 mg = 1,000 μg.
†1 ml = 1 cc (cubic centimeter).
Reprinted from Comer, J.B. Pharmacology in Critical Care. John Wiley & Sons, Inc., New York. 1981. p. 3.

TABLE B–2

Apothecary System Conversions

	Metric	Approximate apothecary equivalent
Weight		
	30 grams	1 ounce
	1 gram	15.4 grains
	65 milligrams	1 grain
Volume		
	1.0 liter	1 quart
	0.5 liter	1 pint
	30 milliliters	1 ounce

Data from Remington's Pharmaceutical Sciences (Mack Printing Co.).
Reprinted from Comer, J.B. Pharmacology in Critical Care. John Wiley & Sons, Inc. New York. 1981. p. 4.

TABLE B–3
Commonly Used Measuring Equivalents

Weight		
1 pound (avoir)*	=	454 grams
1 pound (avoir)	=	16 ounces
2.2 pounds	=	1 kilogram
1 ounce (avoir)	=	28 grams
1 ounce (apoth)†		31 grams
Volume		
1 pint	=	16 ounces
1 pint	=	473 milliliters
1 ounce	=	30 milliliters
1 teaspoonful §	=	5 milliliters
1 tablespoonful	=	15 milliliters

*avoir, avoirdupois system.
† apoth, apothecary system.
§ The actual size of a teaspoon may vary from 4 to 6 ml.
Reprinted from Comer, J.B. Pharmacology in Critical Care. John Wiley & Sons, Inc., New York. 1981. p 4.

INFUSION RATE CHARTS

Many medications that are administered by continuous IV infusion require calculation. The calculations usually involve several steps. To minimize these calculations, conversion charts are given below.

Aminophylline Infusion Rates

		Concentration (per milliliter)		
Volume	Infusion rate	500 mg (0.5 mg/ml)	1,000 mg (1.0 mg/ml)	2,000 mg (2.0 mg/ml)
ml	*ml/hr*	*mg/hr*	*mg/hr*	*mg/hr*
1,000				
	5	2.5*	5.0	10.0
	10	5.0	10.0	20.0
	15	7.5	15.0	30.0
	20	10.0	20.0	40.0
	25	12.5	25.0	50.0
	30	15.0	30.0	60.0
	40	20.0	40.0	80.0
	50	25.0	50.0	100.0
		500 mg (1.0 mg/ml)	1,000 mg (2.0 mg/ml)	2,000 mg (4.0 mg/ml)
500				
	5	5.0	10.0	20.0

Volume	Infusion rate	500 mg (1.5 mg/ml)	1,000 mg (2.0 mg/ml)	2,000 mg (4.0 mg/ml)
	10	10.0	20.0	40.0
	15	15.0	30.0	60.0
	20	20.0	40.0	80.0
	25	25.0	50.0	100.0
	30	30.0	60.0	120.0
	40	40.0	80.0	160.0
	50	50.0	100.0	200.0

*To obtain the dose in milligrams per kilogram per hour, divide this number by the patient's ideal body weight.
Reprinted from Comer, J.B. Pharmacology in Critical Care. John Wiley & Sons, Inc., New York. 1981. p. 126.

Dobutamine Infusion Rates

Volume	Infusion rate	Number of ampules* (concentration)		
		1 (250 mg/1,000 ml)	2 (500 mg/1,000 ml)	4 (1,000 mg/1,000 ml)
ml	*ml/hr*	*µg/min*	*µg/min*	*µg/min*
1,000				
	10	41.6†	83.3	166.6
	20	83.3	166.6	333.3
	30	125.0	250.0	500.0
	40	166.6	333.3	666.6
	50	208.3	416.6	833.3
	60	250.0	500.0	1,000.0
		1 (250 mg/500 ml)	2 (500 mg/500 ml)	4 (1,000 mg/500 ml)
		µg/min	*µg/min*	*µg/min*
500				
	10	83.3	166.6	333.3
	20	166.6	333.3	666.6
	30	250.0	500.0	1,000.0
	40	333.3	666.6	1,333.3
	50	416.6	833.3	1,666.6
	60	500.0	1,000.0	2,000.0

*One ampule of dobutamine is equal to 250 mg of dobutamine.
†All doses are given in micrograms per minute. To obtain the dose in micrograms per kilogram per minute, divide the dose given in micrograms per minute by the patient's ideal body weight:

ideal body weight = 50 kg

$$\frac{83.3\ \mu g/min}{50\ kg} = 1.6\ \mu g/kg/min.$$

Reprinted from Comer, J.B. Pharmacology in Critical Care. John Wiley & Sons, Inc., New York. 1981. p. 23.

Dopamine Infusion Rates

Volume	Infusion rate	Number of ampules* (concentration) 1 (200 mg/1,000 ml)	2 (400 mg/1,000 ml)	4 (800 mg/1,000 ml)
ml	*ml/hr*	*μg/min*	*μg/min*	*μg/min*
1,000				
	10	33.3†	66.6	133.3
	20	66.6	133.3	266.6
	30	100.0	200.0	400.0
	40	133.3	266.6	533.3
	50	166.6	333.3	666.6
	60	200.0	400.0	800.0
		1 (200 mg/500 ml)	2 (400 mg/500 ml)	4 (800 mg/500 ml)
		μg/min	*μg/min*	*μg/min*
500				
	10	66.6	133.3	266.6
	20	133.3	266.6	533.3
	30	200.0	400.0	800.0
	40	266.6	533.3	1,066.0
	50	333.3	666.6	1,333.3
	60	400.0	800.0	1,600.0

*One ampule of dopamine is equal to 200 mg of dopamine.
†All doses are given in micrograms per minute. To obtain the dose in micrograms per kilogram per minute, divide the dose given in micrograms per minute by the patient's ideal body weight:

ideal body weight = 50 kg

$$\frac{33.3\ \mu g/min}{50\ kg} = 0.66\ \mu g/kg/min.$$

Reprinted from Comer, J.B. Pharmacology in Critical Care. John Wiley & Sons, Inc., New York. 1981. p. 26.

Heparin Infusion Rates

Volume	Infusion rate	Concentration (per milliliter): 10,000 U (10 U/ml)	20,000 U (20 U/ml)	40,000 U (40 U/ml)
ml	*ml/hr*	*U/hr*	*U/hr*	*U/hr*
1,000				
	5	50	100	200
	10	100	200	400
	15	150	300	600
	20	200	400	800
	25	250	500	1,000
	30	300	600	1,200
	35	350	700	1,400
	40	400	800	1,600
	45	450	900	1,800
	50	500	1,000	2,000
		10,000 U (20 U/ml)	20,000 U (40 U/ml)	40,000 U (80 U/ml)
		U/hr	*U/hr*	*U/hr*
500				
	5	100	200	400
	10	200	400	800
	15	300	600	1,200
	20	400	800	1,600
	25	500	1,000	2,000
	30	600	1,200	2,400
	35	700	1,400	2,800
	40	800	1,600	3,200
	45	900	1,800	3,600
	50	1,000	2,000	4,000

Reprinted from Comer, J.B. Pharmacology in Critical Care. John Wiley & Sons, Inc., New York. 1981. p. 130.

*Lidocaine Infusion Rates**

Infusion rate	Concentration (per milliliter): 1 g/425 ml (2.5 mg/ml)	2 g/450 ml (4.4 mg/ml)	4 g/500 ml (8.0 mg/ml)
ml/hr	*mg/min*	*mg/min*	*mg/min*
10	0.39	0.73	1.33
20	0.78	1.46	2.66
30	1.17	2.19	4.00
40	1.56	2.92	5.33
50	1.95	3.65	6.66
60	2.35	4.40	8.00

*Average dose is 25–30 μg/kg/min. To obtain the dose in micrograms per kilogram per minute, multiply the dose (in milligrams per minute) by 1,000 and divide by the patient's ideal body weight.

Reprinted from Comer, J.B. Pharmacology in Critical Care. John Wiley & Sons, Inc., New York. p. 49.

Nitroglycerin Infusion Rates

Infusion rate	Concentration 50 μg/ml	100 μg/ml	200 μg/ml
ml/hr	*μg/min**	*μg/min**	*μg/min**
5	4.1	8.3	16.6
10	8.3	16.6	33.3
15	12.5	25.0	50.0
20	16.6	33.3	66.6
30	25.0	50.0	100.0
40	33.3	66.6	133.3
50	41.6	83.3	166.6
60	50.0	100.0	200.0

*The dose is given in μg/min.

50 μg/ml	100 μg/ml	200 μg/ml
—	25 mg/250 ml	50 mg/250 ml
25 mg/500 ml	50 mg/500 ml	100 mg/500 ml
50 mg/1,000 ml	100 mg/1,000 ml	200 mg/1,000 ml

*Nitroprusside Infusion Rates**

Infusion rate	Concentration 100 μg/ml	200 μg/ml
ml/hr	*μg/min*	*μg/min*
5	8.3	16.6
10	16.6	33.3
15	25.0	50.0
20	33.3	66.6
25	41.6	83.3
30	50.0	100.0
40	66.6	133.3
50	83.3	166.6
60	100.0	200.0
70	116.6	233.3
80	133.3	266.6
90	150.0	300.0
100	166.6	333.3

*One vial is equal to 50 mg of nitroprusside:
1 vial 250 ml = 200 μg/ml.
1 vial 500 ml = 100 μg/ml.
2 vial 500 ml = 200 μg/ml.
2 vial 1,000 ml = 100 μg/ml.

To obtain the dose in micrograms per kilogram per minute, divide the dose given in micrograms per minute by the patient's ideal body weight.

Reprinted from Comer, J.B. Pharmacology in Critical Care. John Wiley & Sons, Inc., New York. 1981. p. 82.

*Norepinephrine Infusion Rates**

Infusion rate	Micrograms of base/ml. . . .	1 amp/500 ml 8.0	2 amps/500 ml 16.0	2 amps/1,000 ml 8.0
ml/hr		*μg/min*	*μg/min*	*μg/min*
5		0.66	1.33	0.66
10		1.33	2.66	1.33
15		2.00	4.00	2.00
20		2.66	5.33	2.66
30		4.00	8.00	4.00
40		5.33	10.66	5.33
50		6.66	13.33	6.66
60		8.00	16.00	8.00

*Levophed bitartrate, brand of norepinephrine bitartrate (formerly called levarterenol bitartrate) 1 amp = 4 ml = 4 mg norepinephrine base.
Reprinted from Comer, J.B. Pharmacology in Critical Care. John Wiley & Sons, Inc., New York. 1981. p. 29.

*Procainamide Infusion Rates**

Infusion rate	Concentration (per milliliter)		
	1 g/500 ml (2 mg/ml)	2 g/500 ml (4 mg/ml)	4 g/500 ml (8 mg/ml)
ml/hr	*mg/min*	*mg/min*	*mg/min*
10	0.33	0.66	1.33
20	0.66	1.33	2.66
30	1.00	2.00	4.00
40	1.33	2.66	5.33
50	1.66	3.33	6.66
60	2.00	4.00	8.00

*Average dose is 25–30 μg/kg/min. To obtain the dose in micrograms per kilogram per minute, multiply the dose (in milligrams per minute) by 1,000 and divide by the patient's ideal body weight.
Reprinted from Comer, J.B. Pharmacology in Critical Care. John Wiley & Sons, Inc., New York. 1981. p. 53.

AUTONOMIC NERVOUS SYSTEM

Many of the medications that are collectively known as "pressors" act pharmacologically on the ANS.

An overview of the ANS is presented in Table B–4.

TABLE B–4
Organ Effects of the Sympathetic and Parasympathetic Systems

Structure	Sympathetic	Parasympathetic
Neurotransmitter	Norepinephrine	Acetylcholine
Anatomy		
Outflow of CNS	Thoracolumbar	Craniosacral
Location of ganglia	Close to CNS	Close to effector organ
Heart		
SA node	Increase rate	Decrease rate
AV node	Increase automaticity Increase conduction	Decrease automaticity Decrease conduction
Atria	Increase contractility	Decrease contractility
Ventricles	Increase automaticity Increase contractility	Decrease contractility
Blood vessels		
Arterioles		
Skeletal muscle	Constrict and dilate	Dilate
Skin and mucosa	Constrict	Dilate
Renal	Constrict	—*
Coronary	Constrict and dilate	Dilate
Abdominal	Constrict and dilate	—
Cerebral	Constrict	Dilate
Veins		
Systemic	Constrict	—
Intestine		
Motility	Decrease	Increase
Secretion	Inhibit	Stimulate
Sphincter	Contract	Relax
Urinary bladder		
Detrusor	Relax	Contract
Trigone	Contract	Relax
Sphincter	Contract	Relax
Lung		
Bronchial muscle	Relax	Contract
Bronchial gland	—	Stimulate
Salivary gland	—	Secrete
Sweat gland	—	Secrete
Eye		
Radial muscle of iris	Contract	—
Ciliary muscle	Relax	Contract
Stomach		
Motility	Decrease	Increase
Sphincter	Contract	Relax
Secretion	Inhibit	Stimulate
Uterus	Relax	Contract

AV, atrioventricular; *—, no data; SA, sinoatrial.

Reprinted from Comer, J B. Pharmacology in Critical Care. John Wiley & Sons, Inc., New York. 1981. p. 19.

Many of the medications to be addressed are sympathomimetics and sympatholytics; an examination of Table B–5 will demonstrate the specificity of the sympathetic system.

TABLE B–5

Sympathetic Receptor Sites, Location, and Responses

Tissue	Receptor	Response
Heart		
SA node	β-1	Increase automaticity
Atria	β-1	Increase contractility Increase conductivity
AV node	β-1	Increase conductivity Increase automaticity Decrease effective refractory
His-Purkinje	β-1	Increase automaticity
Ventricles	β-1	Increase contractility
Blood vessels		
Pulmonary arterioles	α and β-2	Constrict and dilate
Cerebral arterioles	α	Constrict
Skin and mucosa arterioles	α	Constrict
Skeletal muscle arterioles	α and β-2	Constrict and dilate
Abdominal viscera arterioles	α and β-2	Constrict and dilate
Renal arterioles	α	Constrict
Coronary arterioles	α and β-2	Constrict and dilate
Vein/peripheral	α	Constrict
Lung		
Bronchial smooth muscle	β-2	Relax
GI		
Stomach		
Motility and tone	β-2	Decrease
Sphincter	α	Contract
Intestine		
Motility and tone	α and β-2	Decrease
Sphincter	α	Contract
Uterus	α and β-2	Contract and relax

AV, atrioventricular; SA, sinoatrial.

Reprinted from Comer, J.B. Pharmacology in Critical Care. John Wiley & Sons, Inc., New York. 1981. p. 20.

Sympathomimetics are medications that mimic epinephrine or stimulate the sympathetic nervous system. A general overview of the sites of actions of sympathomimetics is presented in Table B–6. For a detailed examination of sympathomimetics, consult Table B–7.

TABLE B–6

Sympathomimetics and Receptor Site Activity

Sympathomimetic	α	β-1	β-2
Dobutamine	+	++++	++
Dopamine*	+++	+++	+
Epinephrine	++++	++++	++
Isoproterenol	0	++++	++++
Norepinephrine	++++	++	0

0, no effect; +, least effect; ++++, greatest effect.
*Dopamine is the only sympathomimetic that also stimulates dopaminergic receptors, which are located in mesenteric, intracerebral, coronary, and renal vascular beds.
Reprinted from Sonnenblicke, E., W.H. Frishman, and T.H. LeJemtel. Dobutamine: a new synthetic cardioactive sympathetic amine. New England Journal of Medicine (January 1979). p. 18.

The sympatholytics are medications that block or inhibit the actions of epinephrine or the sympathetic nervous system. A detailed review of sympatholytics is given in Table B–8.

TABLE B–7
Sympathomimetics

Generic name	Trade name	Mechanism* of action	Dosage range	Adverse effects	Nursing parameters
Dobutamine hydrochloride	Dobutrex	β_1, β_2	2.5–10.0 μg/kg/min continuous IV infusion	Cardiac: arrhythmias, anginal pain. Headache.	ECG, HR, BP, CVP, PAWP
Dopamine hydrochloride	Intropin	α, β_1, β_2 dopaminergic	2.5–30.0 μg/kg/min continuous IV infusion	Cardiac: arrhythmias, anginal pain. If extravasation occurs, dermal necrosis may result.	Renal function tests, ECG, urine output, CVP, PAWP, HR, BP
Epinephrine hydrochloride	Adrenaline chloride	α, β_1, β_2	0.1–0.5 mg IM/SC for anaphylaxis, bronchospasm; 0.5–1.0 mg IV for cardiac standstill	Cardiac: arrhythmia. Hyperglycemia, tremor, headache.	ECG, HR, BP, blood sugar
Isoproterenol hydrochloride	Isuprel	β_1, β_2	0.02–1.0 mg IM or 0.15–0.2 mg SC for bronchospasm; 0.02–0.2 mg IV for cardiac standstill	Cardiac: anginal pain, tachycardia, arrhythmia. Tremor, agitation, diaphoresis.	ECG, HR, BP, CVP
Norepinephrine bitartrate	Levophed	α, β_1	2–4 μg base/min	Cardiac: arrhythmia, anginal pain. Decrease perfusion of liver, brain, kidney. If extravasation occurs, dermal necrosis may result.	ECG, renal function tests, urine output, CVP, HR, BP, liver function tests, change in mental status
Phenylephrine hydrochloride	Neo-synephrine	α	40–180 μg/min continuous IV infusion	Reflex bradycardia. Decrease perfusion of liver, brain, kidney.	ECG, HR, BP, liver and renal function tests
Terbutaline hydrochloride	Brethine Bricanyl	β_1, β_2	0.25–0.5 mg SC q 4–8 hr 2.5–5.0 mg PO q 6–8 hr	Cardiac: arrhythmia, anginal pain. Tremor, agitation.	ECG, HR, BP

CVP, central venous pressure; HR, heart rate; PAWP, pulmonary artery wedge pressure.
**See* Table B–6.

TABLE B–8
Sympatholytics

Generic name	Trade name	Mechanism* of action	Dosage range	Adverse effects	Nursing parameters
Atenolol	Tenormin	$\beta_1 > \beta_2$	50–100 mg PO q 24 hr	Bradycardia, CHF, bronchospasm, mental confusion	ECG, HR, BP, change in mental status; do not discontinue abruptly
Labetolol	Trandate Normodyne	α, β	100–400 mg PO q 12 hr	Hypotension, bradycardia, bronchospasm, nasal congestion, impotence, fatigue, mental confusion	ECG, HR, BP, change in mental status
Metoprolol	Lopressor	$\beta_1 > \beta_2$	50 mg PO q 12 hr	Bradycardia, CHF, bronchospasm, mental confusion	ECG, HR, BP, change in mental status; do not discontinue abruptly
Nadolol	Corgard	β_1, β_2	40–120 mg PO q 24 hr	Bradycardia, CHF, bronchospasm, mental confusion	ECG, HR, BP, change in mental status; do not discontinue abruptly
Phentolamine	Regitine	α	50 mg PO q 6 hr; 0.1–2.0 mg/min continuous IV infusion	Hypotension, nasal stuffiness, flushing of skin, reflex tachycardia	ECG, HR, BP; to prevent dermal necrosis and extravasation from a norepinephrine infusion, add phentolamine 5–10 mg/500–1,000 ml of IV solution
Pindolol	Visken	β_1, β_2	5–10 mg PO q 12 hr	Bradycardia, CHF, bronchospasm, mental confusion	ECG, HR, BP, change in mental status; do not discontinue abruptly

Generic name	Trade name	Mechanism* of action	Dosage range	Adverse effects	Nursing parameters
Propranolol	Inderal	β_1, β_2	10–600 mg PO q 6–8 hr; 1 mg IV	Bradycardia, CHF, bronchospasm, mental confusion	ECG, HR, BP, change in mental status; do not discontinue abruptly
Timolol	Blocadren Timoptic	β_1, β_2	10 mg PO q 12 hr; 1 gtt of 0.25% in eye(s) q 12 hr	Bradycardia, CHF, bronchospasm, mental confusion	ECG, HR, BP, change in mental status; do not discontinue abruptly

Gtt, drop; HR, heart rate.
*Receptor site that is blocked or antagonized. Where there is a greater effect on a particular site, it is noted by >.

ANTIARRHYTHMICS

Table B–9 is a general overview of antiarrhythmic medications. It classifies the antiarrhythmics and examines their effects on the action potential and the ECG.

The individual antiarrhythmics are reviewed in Table B–10.

TABLE B–9

Antiarrhythmics: Classification

	Type I	Type II	Type III	Type IV	Digoxin
Automaticity	↓	↓	o ↑		↓ (SA node)
Conductivity	↓ ↑	↓	o	↓	↓(AV node)
Refractory period	↑[a], ↓[b]	↓	↑	↑	↑(AV node)
P-R interval	o ↑ ↓	o ↑	o ↑	↑	↑
QRS complex	o ↑	↑ ↓	o	o	o
Q-T interval	o ↑[a] ↓[b]	o ↓	o ↑	o	o ↓

AV, atrioventricular; SA, sinoatrial; ↓, depression, decrease, reduce; ↑, prolong; o, no effect, no change.

Type I: a: disopyramide, procainamide; quinidine; b: lidocaine, phenytoin, tocainide

Type II: sympatholytics, beta blockers (see Table B–8)

Type III: bretylium

Type IV: calcium channel blockers: diltiazem, nifedipine, verapamil

TABLE B–10
Antiarrhythmic Medications

Generic name	Trade name	Mechanism of action	Dosage range	Adverse effects	Nursing parameters
Bretylium tosylate	Bretylol	Alters norepinephrine release	5–10 mg/kg IV/IM q 6–8 hr; 1–2 mg/min continuous IV infusion	Orthostatic hypotension, vomiting, bradycardia	ECG, BP
Digoxin	Lanoxin	Direct decrease in AV node conduction	0.125–0.25 mg IV/PO q 24 hr	GI: vomiting, diarrhea; cardiac: bradycardia, PVCs, AV block; CNS: confusion, hallucinations	ECG, HR, serum potassium; toxicity with serum level >2.0 ng/ml
Disopyramide phosphate	Norpace	Decreases cellular membrane conductance of sodium	100–150 mg PO q 6 hr	GI: vomiting, anorexia; cardiac: QRS widening, AV block, CHF; anticholinergic: constipation, urinary retention	ECG, urine output, number of stools
Lidocaine hydrochloride	Xylocaine	Increases cellular membrane conductance of potassium	25–100 mg IV at 25–50 mg/min; 20–55 μg/kg/min continuous IV infusion	CNS: drowsy, paresthesia, slurred speech, euphoria, seizures	ECG, change in neurologic status; toxicity with serum level >6 μg/ml
Phenytoin sodium	Dilantin	Increases cellular membrane conductance of potassium	300 mg IV/PO q 8–24 hr; IV, administer at 25–50 mg/min	Cardiac: hypotension, bradycardia; CNS: ataxia, nystagmus, lethargy	ECG, BP, change in neurologic status; toxicity with serum level >20 μg/ml

Procainamide hydrochloride	Pronestyl	Decreases cellular membrane conductance of sodium	100 mg IV at 25–50 mg/min; 25–50 μg/kg/min continuous IV infusion; 250–500 mg PO q 3–6 hr	Dose-related: AV block, QRS widening, psychosis; non-dose-related: lupus syndrome, agranulocytosis	ECG, BP: toxicity with serum level >8 μg/ml
Quinidine	—	Decreases cellular membrane conductance of sodium	200–400 mg PO q 6 hr; 0.3–0.4 mg/kg/min continuous IV infusion	Allergy: drug fever, thrombocytopenia; idiosyncratic: diarrhea, tinnitus, syncope; toxicity: AV block, prolongs; Q-T, widens QRS	ECG, platelet count, Hct, toxicity with serum level >12 μg/ml
Tocainide hydrochloride	Tonocard	Decreases sodium and potassium conductance	400 mg PO q 8 hr	CNS: vertigo, tremor, confusion; cardiac: prolongs Q-T; GI: vomiting, anorexia	ECG, change in neurologic status
Verapamil hydrochloride	Calan Isoptin	Inhibits slow channel (calcium channel)	5–10 mg IV over 2 min; 80–120 mg PO q 6–8 hr	Cardiac: hypotension, heart-block, bradycardia; CNS: dizziness, headache	ECG, BP, HR

AV, atrioventricular; HR, heart rate; PVC, premature ventricular contraction; SA, sinoatrial.

ANTIHYPERTENSIVES

Drugs that are prescribed for the treatment of essential hypertension and hypertensive crisis are listed in Tables B–11 and B–12.

Because diuretics are frequently prescribed, they are presented separately in Table B–11. The antihypertensive dosages given are for the treatment of essential hypertension; however, those drugs that are primarily used in treating hypertensive crisis (diazoxide and nitroprusside) provide dosages for that indication.

TABLE B–11

Antihypertensives: Diuretics

Generic name	Trade name	Mechanism of action	Dosage range	Adverse effects	Nursing parameters
Amiloride hydrochloride	Midamor	Interferes with exchange of sodium for potassium in distal tubule and collecting duct; "potassium-sparing"	5–10 mg PO q 24 hr	Dehydration, hyperkalemia	Serum potassium, fluid balance, BP
Bumetanide	Bumex	"Loop"; inhibits sodium and chloride reabsorption in ascending limb of loop of Henle	0.5–2.0 mg PO/IV/IM q 24 hr	Hypokalemia, hyperglycemia, hyperuricemia, dehydration	Serum potassium, blood sugar, serum uric acid, fluid balance, BP
Chlorothiazide	Diuril	Thiazide; inhibits sodium and chloride reabsorption in distal portion of ascending limb of loop of Henle	500–1,000 mg PO/IV q 12–24 hr	Hypokalemia, hyperglycemia, hyperuricemia, dehydration, hyperlipidemia	Serum potassium, blood sugar, serum uric acid, serum cholesterol and triglyceride, fluid balance, BP
Ethacrynic acid	Edecrin	"Loop"; inhibits sodium and chloride reabsorption in ascending limb of loop of Henle	50–100 mg PO/IV q 12–24 hr	Hypokalemia, hyperglycemia, hyperuricemia, dehydration, ototoxicity	Serum potassium, blood sugar, serum uric acid, fluid balance, BP

Furosemide	Lasix	"Loop"; inhibits sodium and chloride reabsorption in ascending limb of loop of Henle	20–320 mg PO/IV q 6–12 hr	Hypokalemia, hyperglycemia, hyperuricemia, dehydration, ototoxicity	Serum potassium, blood sugar, serum uric acid, fluid balance, BP
Hydrochlorothiazide	HydroDIURIL Esidrix	Thiazide; inhibits sodium and chloride reabsorption in distal portion of ascending limb of loop of Henle	50–100 mg PO q 12–24 hr	Hypokalemia, hyperglycemia, hyperuricemia, dehydration, hyperlipidemia	Serum potassium, blood sugar, serum uric acid, serum cholesterol and triglyceride, fluid balance, BP
Metolazone	Zaroxolyn	Thiazide; inhibits sodium and chloride reabsorption in distal portion of ascending limb of loop of Henle	2.5–10 mg PO q 24 hr	Hypokalemia, hyperglycemia, hyperuricemia, dehydration, hyperlipidemia	Serum potassium, blood sugar, serum uric acid, serum cholesterol and triglyceride, fluid balance, BP
Spironolactone	Aldactone	Aldosterone antagonist; "potassium sparing"	25–100 mg PO q 6–12 hr	Dehydration, hyperkalemia, gynecomastia, impotence, menstrual irregularity	Serum potassium, fluid balance, BP
Triamterene	Dyrenium	Interferes with exchange of sodium for potassium in distal tubule and collecting duct; "potassium-sparing"	100 mg PO q 12 hr	Dehydration, hyperkalemia	Serum potassium, fluid balance, BP

TABLE B–12

Antihypertensives

Generic name	Trade name	Mechanism of action	Dosage range	Adverse effects	Nursing parameters
Beta-blockers*		Negative chronotropic and inotropic			
Captopril	Capoten	Inhibits angiotensin-converting enzyme	25–75 mg PO q 6–12 hr	Hyperkalemia, proteinuria, blood dyscrasia	Urinalysis, serum potassium, BP
Clonidine	Catapres	Central-acting inhibitor of sympathetic nervous system	0.1–0.2 mg PO q 12 hr; Catapres—TTS-1 transdermal q 7 day	Dry mouth, sedation, constipation, headache, dizziness; rebound hypertension if abruptly discontinued	BP, change in neurologic status; do not discontinue abruptly
Diazoxide	Hyperstat	Vasodilator	5 mg/kg IV (300 mg); repeat after 30 min if no response	Sodium/water retention, tachycardia, hyperglycemia, hypotension	BP, ECG, HR, blood sugar
Guanethidine	Ismelin	Peripheral-acting inhibitor, which inhibits norepinephrine release and depletes norepinephrine stores	10–50 mg PO q 24 hr	Diarrhea, impotence, sodium/water retention, orthostatic hypotension	Bowel movements, BP; caution patients about orthostatic hypotension
Guanabenz	Wytensin	Central-acting inhibitor of sympathetic nervous system	4 mg PO q 12 hr	Dry mouth, sedation, dizziness, headache; rebound if abruptly discontinued	BP, change in neurologic status; do not discontinue abruptly
Guanadrel	Hylorel	Peripheral-acting inhibitor, which inhibits norepinephrine release and depletes norepinephrine stores	5 mg PO q 12 hr	Diarrhea, impotence, sodium/water retention, orthostatic hypotension	Bowel movements, BP; caution patients about orthostatic hypotension

Hydralazine	Apresoline	Vasodilator	10–40 mg IM/IV q 4–6 hr; 25–75 mg PO q 4–6 hr	Sodium/water retention, anginal pain, reflex tachycardia, headache, flushing, peripheral neuropathy	ECG, BP, HR
Methyldopa	Aldomet	Central acting alpha agonist	250–500 mg PO/IV q 4–6 hr	Sodium/water retention, lethargy, depression, drug fever, hemolytic anemia, hepatitis	BP, change in neurologic status, liver function tests
Minoxidil	Loniten	Vasodilator	5–20 mg PO q 24 hr	Hypertrichosis, sodium/water retention, tachycardia, pericardial effusion and tamponade	BP, HR
Nitroprusside	Nipride	Vasodilator	0.5–10.0 μg/kg/min continuous IV infusion	Vomiting, hypotension, abdominal pain, palpitations	BP, ECG; change in neurologic status may imply toxicity
Prazosin	Minipress	Vasodilator	1–2 mg PO q 8 hr	Syncope, headache, drowsy, dizziness, fatigue, palpitations	BP, HR
Reserpine	Serpasil	Depletes norepinephrine stores in brain and peripheral sympathetic nerve endings	1–2 mg IM/PO q 24 hr	Sodium/water retention, diarrhea, peptic ulcer disease, depression, sedation, bradycardia, extrapyramidal reactions	BP, ECG, change in neurologic status
Trimethaphan	Arfonad	Ganglionic blocker	0.1–1.0 mg/min continuous IV infusion	Urinary retention, constipation, mydriasis, bradycardia, tachyphylaxis after 24–48 hr	BP, HR, urine output; head of patient's bed must be raised ~30 degrees for therapy to be effective

HR, heart rate

**See* Table B–8 for a complete review of dosage, adverse effects, and nursing parameters

ANTIMICROBIALS

Tables B–13–16 list antibiotics according to their classification. Table B–17 lists several other antibiotics that must be categorized by other tables. Tables B–18 and B–19 contain information on antifungals and antivirals.

TABLE B–13
*Antibiotics: Penicillins**

Generic name	Trade name	Dosage range	Adverse effects	Nursing parameters
Ampicillin	Polycillin-N	0.5–1.0 g IV/IM q 4–6 hr	Hypersensitivity, diarrhea, bacterial/fungal superinfection; uncommon: seizures, leukopenia	WBC, temperature, skin (for rash)
Azlocillin	Azlin	3.0 g IV q 4 hr	Hypersensitivity, diarrhea, hypokalemia, seizures, impaired platelet function	WBC, temperature, skin (for rash), serum potassium, platelet count; 2.17 mEq Na/g
Carbenicillin	Geopen	5.0 g IV/IM q 4 hr	Hypersensitivity, hypokalemia, seizures, metabolic alkalosis, impaired platelet function	WBC, temperature, skin (for rash), serum potassium, platelet count, serum bicarbonate; 4.7 mEq Na/g
Methicillin	Staphcillin	1.0 g IV/IM q 4–6 hr	Hypersensitivity, diarrhea, interstitial nephritis, leukopenia	WBC, temperature, skin (for rash), renal function tests
Mezlocillin	Mezlin	3.0 g IV/IM q 4–6 hr	Hypersensitivity, diarrhea, hypokalemia, seizures, impaired platelet function	WBC, temperature, skin (for rash), serum potassium, platelet count; 1.85 mEq Na/g

Nafcillin	Unipen	0.5–1.0 g IV/IM q 4–6 hr	Hypersensitivity, diarrhea; uncommon: seizures, leukopenia	WBC, temperature, skin (for rash)
Oxacillin	Prostaphlin	0.5–2.0 g IV/IM q 4–6 hr	Hypersensitivity, diarrhea; uncommon: hepatitis, interstitial nephritis, leukopenia	WBC, temperature, skin (for rash), serum creatinine, BUN, liver function tests
Penicillin G	—	variable	Hypersensitivity, seizures, hemolytic anemia	WBC, temperature, skin (for rash), serum potassium, change in mental status
Piperacillin	Pipracil	3.0 g IV/IM q 4 hr	Hypersensitivity, diarrhea, hypokalemia, seizures, impaired platelet function	WBC, temperature, skin (for rash), serum potassium, platelet count; 1.85 mEq Na/g
Ticarcillin	Ticar	3.0 g IV/IM q 4 hr	Hypersensitivity, diarrhea, hypokalemia, seizures, impaired platelet function	WBC, temperature, skin (for rash), serum potassium, platelet, count; 5.2 mEq Na/g

Na, sodium.
*All penicillin antibiotics act by inhibiting bacterial cell wall synthesis.

TABLE B–14

*Antibiotics: Cephalosporins**

Generic name	Trade name	Dosage range	Adverse effects	Nursing parameters
Cefamandole§	Mandol	0.5–1.0 g IV/IM q 4–8 hr	Hypersensitivity; uncommon: thrombocytopenia, neutropenia, liver function test alterations, hypoprothrombinemia	WBC, temperature, skin (for rash), PT, bleeding
Cefazolin+	Ancef Kefzol	0.5–1.0 g IV/IM q 8 hr	Hypersensitivity; uncommon: thrombocytopenia, seizures	WBC, temperature, skin (for rash)
Cefonicid§	Monocid	0.5–2.0 g IV/IM q 24 hr	Hypersensitivity, liver function test alterations; uncommon: neutropenia	WBC, temperature, skin (for rash)
Cefoperazone**	Cefobid	1.0–2.0 g IV/IM q 6–12 hr	Hypersensitivity, hypoprothrombinemia, diarrhea	WBC, temperature, skin (for rash), PT, bleeding
Ceforanide§	Precef	0.5–1.0 g IV/IM q 12 hr	Hypersensitivity; uncommon: thrombocytopenia, neutropenia	WBC, temperature, skin (for rash)
Cefotaxime**	Claforan	1.0–2.0 g IV/IM q 4–6 hr	Hypersensitivity, diarrhea; uncommon: thrombocytopenia	WBC, temperature, skin (for rash)
Cefoxitin§	Mefoxin	1.0–2.0 g IV/IM q 4–6 hr	Hypersensitivity; uncommon: hemolytic anemia, neutropenia	WBC, temperature, skin (for rash)
Ceftizoxime**	Cefizox	1.0–2.0 g IV/IM q 8–12 hr	Hypersensitivity; uncommon: thrombocytopenia, neutropenia	WBC, temperature, skin (for rash)

Cefuroxime§	Zinacef	1.5 g IV/IM q 6–8 hr	Hypersensitivity, diarrhea	WBC, temperature, skin (for rash)
Cephalothin+	Keflin	5.0–2.0 g IV/IM q 4–6 hr	Hypersensitivity; uncommon: thrombocytopenia, neutropenia	WBC, temperature, skin (for rash)
Moxalactam**	Moxam	0.5–1.0 g IV/IM q 8–12 hr	Hypersensitivity, hypoprothrombinemia	WBC, temperature, skin (for rash) PT, bleeding

PT, prothrombin time.
*All cephalosporin antibiotics act by inhibiting bacterial cell wall synthesis.
+First generation.
§Second generation.
**Third generation.

TABLE B–15

*Antibiotics: Aminoglycosides**

Generic name	Trade name	Dosage range	Adverse effects	Nursing parameters
Amikacin	Amikin	5–7.5 mg/kg IV/IM q 8–12 hr	Nephrotoxicity, ototoxicity, neuromuscular blockade	WBC, temperature, SCr, BUN, urine output, urinalysis; serum peak levels >25, trough levels >10 μg/ml associated with toxicity
Gentamicin	Garamycin	1.0—1.7 mg/kg IV/IM q 8 hr	Nephrotoxicity, ototoxicity, neuromuscular blockade	WBC, temperature, SCr, BUN, urine output, urinalysis; serum peak levels >10, trough levels >2 μg/ml associated with toxicity
Kanamycin	Kantrex	7–5 mg/kg IV/IM q 12 hr	Nephrotoxicity, ototoxicity, neuromuscular blockade	WBC, temperature, SCr, BUN, urine output, urinalysis
Neomycin	Mycifradin	1–2 g PO q 6 hr	Nephrotoxicity, ototoxicity, neuromuscular blockade	WBC, temperature, SCr, BUN, urine output, urinalysis
Netilmicin	Netromycin	1.3–2.2 mg/kg IV/IM q 8 hr	Nephrotoxicity, ototoxicity, neuromuscular blockade	WBC, temperature, SCr, BUN, urine output, urinalysis
Streptomycin	—	0.5–2.0 g IM q 24 hr	Nephrotoxicity, ototoxicity, neuromuscular blockade	WBC, temperature, SCr, BUN, urine output, urinalysis
Tobramycin	Nebcin	1.0–1.66 mg/kg IV/IM q 8 hr	Nephrotoxicity, ototoxicity, neuromuscular blockade	WBC, temperature, SCr, BUN, urine output, urinalysis; serum peak levels >10, trough levels >2 μg/ml associated with toxicity

SCr, serum creatinine.
*All aminoglycoside antibiotics act by inhibiting protein synthesis.

TABLE B–16

*Antibiotics: Tetracyclines**

Generic name	Trade name	Dosage range	Adverse effects	Nursing parameters
Doxycycline	Vibramycin	0.1 g IV/PO q 12 hr	Photosensitivity, fungal superinfection; never use during pregnancy	WBC, temperature
Minocycline	Minocin	0.1 g IV/PO q 12 hr	Fungal superinfection, vertigo, aggravation of preexisting renal insufficiency; never use during pregnancy	WBC, temperature, BUN, SCr
Tetracycline	Achromycin V	0.25–0.5 g IV/PO g 6 hr	Diarrhea, enterocolitis, antianabolism, hepatotoxicity, fungal superinfection; never use during pregnancy	WBC, temperature, BUN, SCr, liver function tests

SCr, serum creatinine.
*All tetracycline antibiotics act by inhibiting protein synthesis.

TABLE B–17

Antibiotics: Miscellaneous

Generic name	Trade name(s)	Mechanism of action	Dosage range	Adverse effects	Nursing parameters
Erythromycin	—	Inhibits protein synthesis	0.5–1.0 g IV/IM/PO q 6 hr	Diarrhea, hepatotoxicity; uncommon: ototoxicity	WBC, temperature, diarrhea, liver function tests
Chloramphenicol	Chloromycetin	Inhibits protein synthesis	0.5–1.0 g IV q 6 hr	Optic neuritis, gray baby syndrome in neonates, blood dyscrasias	WBC, temperature, platelet count, Hb, reticulocyte count, serum iron
Clindamycin	Cleocin	Inhibits protein synthesis	0.3–0.6 g IV/IM q 6–12 hr	Diarrhea, pseudomembranous colitis	WBC, temperature, diarrhea
Co-Trimoxazole	Bactrim Septra	Inhibits bacterial synthesis of folic acid	160 mg trimethoprim and 800 mg sulfamethoxazole PO/IV q 12 hr, for routine infections; for *Pneumocystis carinii,* 20 mg/kg/24 hr trimethoprim and 100 mg/kg/24 hr sulfamethoxazole PO/IV	Agranylocytosis, hemolytic anemia, cholestatic hepatitis, hypersensitivity, renal insufficiency	WBC, temperature, skin (for rash), renal function tests, fluid load (IV preparation requires large volume)
Metronidazole	Flagyl	Prevents bacterial cell wall synthesis	250–500 mg PO/IV q 6–8 hr	Peripheral neuropathy, seizures, unpleasant metallic taste	WBC, temperature, change in neurologic status
Vancomycin	Vancocin	Inhibits bacterial cell wall synthesis	500 mg IV q 6 hr; 125–500 mg PO q 6 hr	Ototoxicity, nephrotoxicity; dermal necrosis if extravasation occurs	WBC, temperature, renal function tests, changes in hearing

TABLE B–18
Antimicrobials: Antifungals

Generic name	Trade name	Mechanism of action	Dosage range	Adverse effects	Nursing parameters
Amphotericin B	Fungizone	Alters cell membrane permeability	0.5–10. mg/kg/day IV over 4–8 hr; 25–50 mg/liter CBI over 24 hr	Fever, chills, myalgias, hypotension; thrombophlebitis, nephrotoxicity, anemia, hypokalemia	Temperature, renal function tests, serum potassium
Flucytosine	Ancobon	Inhibits DNA-synthesis	50–150 mg/kg/day PO divided as q 6 hr	Bone marrow depression; CNS: headache, drowsiness, dizziness	Changes in neurologic function, CBC; must decrease dose in patients with impaired renal function
Ketoconazole	Nizoral	Alters cell membrane permeability	200–400 mg PO q 24 hr	Hepatotoxicity	Liver function tests
Miconazole	Monistat IV	Alters cell membrane permeability	600–2,400 mg/24 hr divided as q 8 hr	Thrombophlebitis, pruritus, anemia, hypokalemia	Monitor IV sites, serum sodium

CBI, continuous bladder irrigation.

TABLE B–19
*Antimicrobials: Antivirals**

Generic name	Trade name	Dosage range	Adverse effects	Nursing parameters
Acyclovir	Zovirax	5 mg/kg IV q 8 hr	CNS: delirium, confusion; thrombophlebitis	Change in mental status
Vidarabine	Vira-A	15 mg/kg/day, IV infusion over 12–24 hr	CNS: confusion, hallucination; bone marrow depression	Change in mental status, CBC; diluted in large volume of fluid—observe fluid load

*These antivirals inhibit viral DNA synthesis.

OTHER DRUGS

This group of drugs includes those medications that come from a variety of different pharmacologic classes but are frequently used in an ICU.

TABLE B–20

Drugs Commonly Used in the ICU

Generic name	Trade name	Mechanism of action	Dosage range	Adverse effects	Nursing parameters
Acetazolamide	Diamox	Carbonic anhydrase inhibitor	250–500 mg IV q 6–8 hr	Metabolic acidosis, alkalinized urine	Blood pH, PCO_2
Aminophylline	—	Bronchodilator	250–500 mg PO/IV q 6 hr; 0.5–1.0 mg/kg/hr continuous IV infusion	Nausea, vomiting, tachycardia, arrhythmias, tremor, agitation, insomnia, confusion, seizures	HR, BP, change in neurologic status; theophylline levels >20 μg/ml generally associated with toxicity
Aminrone	Inocor	Inotropic, vasodilator	0.75 mg/kg IV followed by 5–10 μg/kg/min continuous IV infusion	Thrombocytopenia, hypotension, arrhythmias	BP, HR, platelet count
Cimetidine	Tagamet	Histamine H_2 antagonist	300 mg IV/IM/PO q 6 hr	Agranulocytosis, thrombocytopenia, mental confusion, gynecomastia, bradycardia	Gastric pH, WBC, platelet count, HR, change in mental status, HCT
Heparin	—	Stimulates the action of antithrombin III; anticoagulant	500–3,500 U/hr continuous IV infusion; 5,000–10,000 U IV q 4 hr; 5,000 U SC q 8–12 hr	Hemorrhage, thrombocytopenia	BP, Hct, stool and urine for blood, APTT (or other clotting study), platelet count
Metoclopramide	Reglan	Antiemetic, increases, gastric motility	10–20 mg IV/PO q 6 hr; 2 mg/kg IV as antiemetic for chemotherapy	Extrapyramidal reactions, sedation, insomnia	Change in neurologic status

Morphine	—	Narcotic (an opiate derivative); analgesic	2–20 mg IM/SC q 2–4 hr; 2.5–15 mg IV q 2–4 hr	Respiratory depression, nausea, constipation, urinary retention, postural hypotension, addiction, miosis, sedation, CNS depression	BP, respiratory rate, change in mental status, bowel movements
Naloxone	Narcan	Narcotic antagonist	0.4–0.8 mg IV/IM/SC prn narcotic overdose or excess	Tachycardia, narcotic withdrawal, tremor	If patient is on chronic narcotic therapy, watch for signs/symptoms of narcotic withdrawal
Nifedipine	Procardia	Calcium channel blocker	10–20 mg PO q 8 hr	Headache, hypotension, flushing, weakness, peripheral edema	BP, HR, edema
Nitroglycerin	—	Vasodilator	0.5–1.0 μg/kg/min continuous IV infusion	Tachycardia, headache, hypotension	BP, HR
Pancuronium	Pavulon	Neuromuscular blocker	0.01 mg/kg (2–4 mg) IV q 1–2 hr prn	Increase heart rate and/or BP, paralysis	BP, HR, emotional support to patient
Ranitidine	Zantac	Histamine H_2 antagonist	150 mg PO q 12 hr	Headache	Gastric pH, Hct
Streptokinase	Streptase	Fibrinolytic	250,000 U IV over 30 min, then 100,000 U/hr continuous IV infusion	Hemorrhage, hypersensitivity reaction, fever	BP, Hct, stool and urine for blood, clotting studies, no IM/SC injections, avoid excessive venipunctures
Theophylline	Theolair Theo-Dur Slo-Phyllin Resbid	Bronchodilator	Theo-Dur 100–300 mg PO q 6–12 hr Slo-Phylline 100–200 mg PO q 4–6 hr	Nausea, vomiting, tachycardia, arrhythmias, tremor, agitation, insomnia, confusion, seizures	HR, BP, change in neurologic status; theophylline levels >20 μg/ml generally associated with toxicity

Generic name	Trade name	Mechanism of action	Dosage range	Adverse effects	Nursing parameters
Urokinase	Abbokinase	Fibrinolytic	4,400 U/kg over 10 min, then 4,400 U/kg/hr continuous IV infusion	Hemorrhage, hypersensitivity reaction, fever	BP, Hct, stool and urine for blood, clotting studies, no IM/SC injections, avoid excessive venipunctures
Vasopressin	Pitressin	Exogenous vasopressin, used as vasoconstrictor	0.2–0.6 U/min continuous IV infusion	Water intoxication, bradycardia, increased BP, arrhythmias, bowel infarction, decreased renal perfusion	HR, BP, ECG, renal function tests

APTT, activated partial thromboplastin time; HR, heart rate.

CORTICOSTEROIDS

TABLE B–21

Commonly Prescribed Corticosteroids

Corticosteroid	Equivalent dose	Relative anti-inflammatory potency	Sodium-retaining properties
	mg		
Cortisone	25.0	0.8	+2
Dexamethasone	0.75	30.0	0
Hydrocortisone (cortisol)	20.0	1.0	+2
Methylprednisolone	4.0	5.0	0
Prednisolone	5.0	4.0	+1
Prednisone	5.0	4.0	+1
Triamcinolone	4.0	5.0	0

Reprinted from Comer, J.B. Pharmacology in Critical Care. John Wiley & Sons, Inc., New York. 1981. p. 122.

TABLE B–22

Average Doses for Commonly Prescribed Corticosteroids

Generic name	Trade name	Use	Dose*
Dexamethasone	Decadron	Cerebral edema Neoplasms	4–6 mg q 6 hr 0.25–4 mg q 6–12 hr
Hydrocortisone	Cortef, Solu-Cortef	Severe inflammation† Adrenal insufficiency	100–200 mg q 6–12 hr
Methylprednisolone	Medrol, Solu-Medrol	Shock Severe inflammation	30 mg/kg q 6 hr 2–60 mg q 6 hr
Prednisone	Deltasone	Severe inflammation	2.5–20 mg q 6–12 hr
Prednisolone	Delta-Cortef	Severe inflammation	2.5–20 mg q 6–12 hr

*Doses are for IV and PO therapy.
†Severe inflammation: collagen vascular diseases, asthma, etc.
Reprinted from Comer, J.B. Pharmacology in Critical Care. John Wiley & Sons, Inc. New York. 1981. p 123.

COMPATIBILITY CHART

The following is a conservative chart that should be used as a quick, nonspecific reference for IV compatibilities. Ideally, two different IV medications should never be mixed together; however, this may not always be possible, and sometimes medications must be "piggybacked" or infused simultaneously.

Symbols

Blank: No data available regarding the compatibility of these two medications. Therefore they should be considered incompatible until proven otherwise.

I: Incompatible.

1. Never mix these two medications. A chemical and/or biologic incompatibility may occur without a physical and/or visual change.
2. Do not administer these two medications simultaneously through the same line. When "piggybacking" medications, flush line thoroughly between medications.
3. If two incompatible medications are administered by continuous infusion, two different infusion sites must be used (e.g., aminophylline and norepinephrine).
4. When administering two incompatible antibiotics, flush the line thoroughly after administering the first antibiotic and wait ≥15 min before administering the second antibiotic (e.g., gentamicin and carbenicillin: infuse the gentamicin, flush the line, wait 15 min, flush the line, begin the carbenicillin).

C: Compatible. No problem if these two medications are infused simultaneously through the same IV site.

Reprinted from Comer, J.B. Pharmacology in Critical Care. John Wiley & Sons, Inc., New York. 1981. App. C.

	ACETAZOLAMIDE	AMIKACIN	AMINOCAPROIC ACID	AMINOPHYLLINE	AMPICILLIN	CALCIUM CHLORIDE	CALCIUM GLUCONATE	CARBENICILLIN	CEFAMANDOLE	CEFAZOLIN	CEFOXITIN	CEPHALORIDINE	CEPHALOTHIN	CEPHAPIRIN	CEPHRADINE	CHLORAMPHENICOL	CIMETIDINE	CLINDAMYCIN	DEXAMETHASONE	DIAZEPAM	DIGOXIN	DOBUTAMINE	DOPAMINE	DOXYCYCLINE	ERYTHROMYCIN	ETHACRYNIC ACID	FOLIC ACID	FUROSEMIDE
ACETAZOLAMIDE	C										I											I						
AMIKACIN		C		I	I	C	C	I	I	I	I	I	I	I	I	C	I	C	C	I			I		I			
AMINOCAPROIC ACID			C																									
AMINOPHYLLINE		I		C	I		C			I	I		I	I		I	I	I	C	I	I	I	I	I	I			I
AMPICILLIN		I		I	C	I	I	I		I	I	I	I			I	I	I		I	I	I	I	I	I			
CALCIUM CHLORIDE		C			I	C							I	C	I	C												
CALCIUM GLUCONATE		C		C	I		C		I	I		C	I	C	I	I		I	C	I					C		I	
CARBENICILLIN		I			I			C		I	I	I				I		I		I			I		I			
CEFAMANDOLE		I					I		C								I											
CEFAZOLIN		I		I	I		I	I		C						I	I	I	I	I					I			
CEFOXITIN	I	I		I	I			I			C									I							I	
CEPHALORIDINE		I			I		C	I				C								I								
CEPHALOTHIN		I		I	I	I	I						C			I	I	I		I			I		I			
CEPHAPIRIN		I		I		C	C							C		C				I					I		I	
CEPHRADINE		I				I	I								C													
CHLORAMPHENICOL		C		I	I	C	I	I		I			I	C		C			C	I			I		I			
CIMETIDINE		I		I	I				I	I			I				C	C		I					I			
CLINDAMYCIN		C		I	I		I	I		I			I				C	C							I			
DEXAMETHASONE		C		C			C			I						C			C	I								
DIAZEPAM		I		I	I		I	I		I	I	I	I	I		I	I		I	C	I		I		I	I	I	I
DIGOXIN				I	I															I	C		I				I	I
DOBUTAMINE	I			I	I																	C					I	I
DOPAMINE		I		I	I			I					I			I				I	I		C		I	I	I	I
DOXYCYCLINE				I	I																			C				
ERYTHROMYCIN		I		I	I		C	I		I			I	I		I	I	I		I			I		C			
ETHACRYNIC ACID																				I			I			C		
FOLIC ACID							I				I			I						I	I	I	I				C	
FUROSEMIDE				I																I	I	I	I					C
GENTAMICIN		I			I			I	I	I	I	I	I	I	I	I	I	I		I			I		I			
HEPARIN		I		I	I		C			I	I	I	I	C		I	C	I	C	I	C		I	I	I			
HYDRALAZINE				I	I																I					I		I
HYDROCORTISONE		C		C	I	C	C	I		C			C	C		I		C	C	I	C		I	I	C			
INSULIN		I		I	I						I		I				C			I	I				I	I		I
IRON DEXTRAN																							I				I	
ISOPROTERENOL	I	I		I	I	C	C	I					C							I	I				I	I	I	I
KANAMYCIN		I		C	I		I	I		I	I		I	I		C	C	C	C	I			C		I			
LIDOCAINE		I		C	I	C		C			C	C	I		I	C			C	I			I	I	C			
LINCOMYCIN		C			I			I				C	C			C				I								
MAGNESIUM SULFATE							I						C		I	C		I										
MANNITOL	I	C		I	I									I									I				I	I
METARAMINOL	I	C		I	I		C						I	C		C			I		I			I	I	I	I	I
METHOXAMINE																												
METHYLDOPA	I			I	I											C					I					I	I	I
METHYLPREDNISOLONE		I		I	I		I	C		I			I			I		C		I			I		I			
MINOCYCLINE																												
MORPHINE	I			I	I																						I	I
MULTIVITAMIN	C	I		I	I						C					I			I	I					I			
NAFCILLIN	I	I		I	I										I	C	C		C		I		I		I		I	I
NITROFURANTOIN		I		I		I							I	I		I						I			C			
NITROGLYCERIN	I	I	I	I	I	I	I	I	I	I	I	I	I	I	I	I	I	I	I	I	I	I	I	I	I	I	I	I
NITROPRUSSIDE	I	I	I	I	I	I	I	I	I	I	I	I	I	I	I	I	I	I	I	I	I	I	I	I	I	I	I	I
NOREPINEPHRINE	I	C		I	I	C	I			C			I	I		I		I		I	I		C	I	I	I	I	I
OXACILLIN		I		I	I		C	C		C			I	C		I				I	I				I			
OXYTOCIN		I								C						C				I	I				I	I		I
PENICILLIN G	I	I		I	I	C	C			I			I	C		I	I	I	C	I	I		I		C		I	I
PHENYTOIN	I	I	I	I	I	I	I	I	I	I	I	I	I	I	I	I	I	I	I	I	I	I	I	I	I	I	I	I
POTASSIUM CHLORIDE	C	C		C	I		C	C		I			C	C		C	C	C	C	I	C		I	I	C			
PROCAINAMIDE		I		C			C									C				I				I	I	I		
SODIUM BICARBONATE		C		C	I	I	I	I		C			I	C		C		C	C	I	I	I	I	I	C			
TETRACYCLINE		I		I	I	I	I	I		I		I	I	I	I	I			C	I	I		C		I	I		I
TICARCILLIN		I		I	I															I					I			
TOBRAMYCIN		I			I		I	I	I	I	I	I	I	I	I			I		I	I				I			
TRIMETHAPHAN	I			I	I																						I	I
VANCOMYCIN		C		I	I		I									I			I	I	I				I	I		I
VITAMIN B WITH C		I		I	I	C	C	I		I			I	C		I	C	I	I	I	C			I	I		I	I

				I					I	I		I		I	I		I													I						I	C				I		I			I		I	I	I	I	I	I	I	I	I	I	I			I			I		GENTAMICIN
I	I		I		I		C	C	I	I	I		I	I	I	C	C		I			I		I			C	C	I	I		I	I	I	C	I				I	I	I		C	I	C	I	C	I		C	I	I	I	I			C		I	I		I		HEPARIN
									I	I				I	I												I								I	C	I		I		I					I																I	I				HYDRALAZINE
I	I				I	I	C	I	I	C	I		C	I	I		I				C	I		I				C	I			I	C	I	I					C	I	I			C	I	C	C		I		C	C			C		I	C	C	I	C		C		HYDROCORTISONE
C						I		C	I	I				I	I	I	I									I			I				C	I		I		I		I	I				I	I			C				I		I						I	I		I		INSULIN
									I					I	I																		C				I			I				I																				IRON DEXTRAN
C				C	C	I		C	I	I				I	I		I	C							I	C		I		C					I		I	I	I	I				I	I							C					I	C	C	I	I		I	I	ISOPROTERENOL
C	I		I	I	C	I			I	C		I		I	I	I	I	C						C			I		C				I		I	I				I		C			I	C	C	C	C		I	I		I	I		I	I		I	C		I		KANAMYCIN
C					C	I		C	I	C			I	I	I	C								C				C		I		I	C		C					C	I	I			I	C			C	I		I	C	C			C		C	I	C		I		LIDOCAINE
C					C				I	I				I	I													C		I							C									I				C			C	C				I			I			C		LINCOMYCIN
			I			I			I				C	I	I							C				C				C																		I		C	I		C						I							MAGNESIUM SULFATE
I			C		I			I	I		I		I	I	I							I		I	C					I		I		I				I	I					I									I								I	I		C	I	MANNITOL
C	C				C	C	C	C	I	I	C	I	I	I	I	I	I	I			I			C	I			C	C				I		I		I	I	I	I	I			I		I			C		C	I						C		I	I		C	I	METARAMINOL
									I					I	I								C																																											METHOXAMINE
C					I	C		C	I	I				I	I		I	C				C			I	C							I		I		I	I	I					I					C											I	I			I	METHYLDOPA
I	I				I	I		C	I	C			C	I	I						C			I											C							I		I			I		C		I			I			I		C	I		I	I		I		METHYLPREDNISOLONE
									I					I	I					C																																													MINOCYCLINE
						I			I					I	I	I			C																		I		I	I																					I	I			I	MORPHINE
					I			C	I	I			C	I	I		I	C				C		I					C	C										I					I	I			I					C					I	I		I	C	MULTIVITAMIN
I	I		I		I	C		C	I		I	I	I	I	I	C	C	I				I		I					I	I		I	I		C	I	I	I		I		I		I		C		C	C	I									I	I		I	I	NAFCILLIN
I	I				I				I	I		I	I	I	I	C	C		I					I				C	I			I			C				C			I					I		I	I							I		I		I		NITROFURANTOIN
I	I	I	I	I	I	I	I	I	I	I	I	I	I	I	C	I	I	I	I	I	I	I	I	I	I	I	I	I	I	I	I	I	I	I	I	I	I	I	I	I	I	I	I	I	I	I	I	I	I	I	I	I	I	I	I	I	I	I	I	I	I	I	I	I	NITROGLYCERIN
I	I	I	I	I	I	I	I	I	I	I	I	I	I	C	I	I	I	I	I	I	I	I	I	I	I	I	I	I	I	I	I	I	I	I	I	I	I	I	I	I	I	I	I	I	I	I	I	I	I	I	I	I	I	I	I	I	I	I	I	I	I	I	I	I	NITROPRUSSIDE
C					I	I		C	I	I	I	I	C	I	I	I	I	C			C			I	I	C		I					C		I		I	I	I	I	I	C		I	I		I		I		I	I			C			I	C	I	I		C	I	NOREPINEPHRINE
I			I		I			C	I	I		C	I	I	I	I	I							I								I							I				I				I	I				I			C		C	C		I	I		I		OXACILLIN
					C				I	C	C		I	I	I		I							C	I										I		I		I		I	I				I	I				C						C								I		OXYTOCIN
I	I		I	C	I	I	C	C	I	C	C	I	I	I	I	I		I			C	I		I			I	C	C	I		I	C	I	I	I	I	I		C		I		I	I	C	I	I	I		C	I			I			C	C	I	I		I	I	PENICILLIN G
I	I	I	I	I	I	I	I	I	C	I	I	I	I	I	I	I	I	I	I	I	I	I	I	I	I	I	I	I	I	I	I	I	I	I	I	I	I	I	I	I	I	I	I	I	I	I	I	I	I	I	I	I	I	I	I	I	I	I	I	I	I	I	I	I	PHENYTOIN
C	C				C	C		C	I	C		C	C	I	I		C	C			C	C		C	I			C		C		C	I		C				C	I	I		C	I	C	C	C	C		C	C	C		I		C	C		I	C		C	C	POTASSIUM CHLORIDE
C	C				C		C		I	C				I	I									C											C		C				I	I	I				I				C									C		C		I		PROCAINAMIDE
I	I				I	C		C	I	I			I	I	I		C		I		I	C		C		I		I	I		I	I						C	I	I	I	I	I	C	C		C		C	I			C		I	I	I	I	C		C		SODIUM BICARBONATE
I	C				C	I	C	C	I	I	C	I	I	I	I	I	I	I			I	I		C	I		C	C	C	C			I		I		I		I	I		C		I	I	C			I	I	I	I	I		I		I	I	I	I	I		I		TETRACYCLINE
			I	C					I	C				I	I														I	C						I				I					I														I	I		I		TICARCILLIN
			C	I					I	I		I		I	I		I								C	I			I						I				I				I	I		I			I	I	I	I	I	I	I	I		I			I		TOBRAMYCIN
		C							I					I	I																							I	I																				I	I			I	TRIMETHAPHAN
I	C				C	I	C	C	I	I				I	I	I	I				I			C					I				I		I		I		I	I				I	I	I			I									I		I	I		C		VANCOMYCIN
C	I				I	I	C	C	I	I		I	C	I	I	I	I				I	C		C	I		C	C	C	C		C	I		I		I	I		I	I			C	I	I	I	C	I		C	I			I		I	C	C	I	I		I		VITAMIN B WITH C

BIBLIOGRAPHY

Chapter 1

American Association of Critical Care Nurses Standards Committee, editors. Standards for Nursing Care of the Critically Ill. Reston Publishing Co., Inc., Reston, Va. 1981.

Carpenter, L. Nursing Diagnosis: Applications to Clinical Practice. J.B. Lippincott Co., Philadelphia. 1983.

Doenges, M., M. Jeffries, and M.F. Moorhouse. Nursing Care Plans—Nursing Diagnosis in Planning Patient Care. F.A. Davis Co., Philadelphia. 1984.

Hayne, A., and Z. Bailey. Nursing Administration of Critical Care. Aspen Systems Corp., Rockville, Md. 1982.

Hickey, M. Nursing diagnosis in the critical care unit. *Dimensions of Critical Care Nursing* (March-April 1984). 91–97.

Joint Commission on Accreditation of Hospitals. Accreditation Manual for Hospitals. Joint Commission on Accreditation of Hospitals, Chicago. 1985.

Kim, M., and D. Moritz, editors. Classification of Nursing Diagnoses. McGraw-Hill Book Co., New York. 1982.

Merkel, S. Problem-oriented recording in the intensive care unit. *Dimensions of Critical Care Nursing* (July-August 1982). 232–40.

Voorman, D. Critical care nursing: an art, a science and a spirit. *In* AACN's Clinical Reference for Critical Care Nursing. McGraw-Hill Book Co., New York. 1981. 3–7.

Weed L. Medical Records, Medical Education, and Patient Care. Case Western Reserve University Press, Cleveland. 1969.

Chapter 2

Andreoli, K. G., V. K. Fowkes, D. P. Zipes, and A. G. Wallace. Comprehensive Cardiac Care. C. V. Mosby Co., St. Louis. 1983. Fifth edition.

Braunwald, E., editor. Heart Disease. W. B. Saunders Co., Philadelphia. 1980.

Guzzetta, C. E., and B. M. Dossey. Cardiovascular Nursing: Body-Mind Tapestry. C. V. Mosby Co., St. Louis. 1984.

Horvath, P. T., editor. Care of the Adult Cardiac Surgical Patient. John Wiley & Sons, Inc., New York. 1984.

Michaelson, C. R., editor. Congestive Heart Failure. C. V. Mosby Co., St. Louis. 1983.

Saunderson, R. G., and C. L. Kurth. The Cardiac Patient: A Comprehensive Approach. W. B. Saunders Co., Philadelphia. 1983. Second edition.

Smith, J. J., and J. P. Kampine. Circulatory Physiology—The Essentials. Williams & Wilkins Co., Baltimore. 1980.

Underhill, S. L., S. L. Woods, E. S. Sivarajan, and C. J. Halpenny. Cardiac Nursing. J. B. Lippincott Co., Philadelphia. 1982.

Wells, S. J., S. A. Stokes, and K. G. Mahoney. Manual of Cardiovascular Assessment. Reston Publishing Co., Reston, Va. 1983.

Wenger, N. K., J. W. Hurst, and M. C. McIntyre. Cardiology for Nurses. McGraw-Hill Book Co., New York. 1980.

Chapter 3

Bates, D. A., P. T. Macklem, and R. V. Christie. Respiratory Function in Disease. W. B. Saunders Co., Philadelphia. 1977.

Burton, G., and J. Hodgkin. Respiratory Care: A Guide to Clinical Practice. J. B. Lippincott Co., Philadelphia. 1984.

Cherniak, R. M., L. Cherniak, and A. Naimark. Respiration in Health and Disease. W. B. Saunders Co., Philadelphia. 1972.

Comroe, J. H., R. E. Forster, A. B. Dubois, W. A. Briscoe, and E. Carlsen. The Lung: Clinical Physiology and Pulmonary Function Tests. Year book Medical Publishers, Inc., Chicago. 1974.

Cotes, J. E. Lung Function, Assessment and Application in Medicine. Blackwell Scientific Publications, Inc., Boston. 1974.

Duroux, P., G. Simmonneau, P. Petitpretz, and P. Herve. Therapeutic approach to acute pulmonary embolism. *Intensive Care Medicine* (October 1984). 99–102.

Emanuelsen, K. L., and M. J. Densmore. Acute Respiratory Care. John Wiley & Sons, Inc., New York. 1981.

Fishman, A. P. Pulmonary Diseases and Disorders. McGraw-Hill Book Co., New York. 1980.

George, R. B., R. W. Light, and R. A. Mathay. Chest Medicine. Churchill Livingstone Inc., New York. 1983.

Shoemaker, W., N. Thompson, and P. Holbrook. Textbook of Critical Care. W. B. Saunders Co., Philadelphia. 1984.

Chapter 4

Bates, B. A Guide to Physical Examination. J. B. Lippincott Co., Philadelphia. 1983. Third edition.

Chanarin, J., M. Brozovic, E. Tedmarsh, and D. A. Waters. Blood and Its Diseases. Churchill Livingstone, Inc., New York. 1976.

Eastman, R. D. Clinical Hematology. John Wright and Sons Ltd., London. 1977. Fifth edition.

Halloway, N. M. Nursing the Critically Ill Adult. Addison-Wesley Publishing Co., Menlo Park, Calif. 1979.

Mahoney, E. A., and J. P. Flynn, editors. Handbook of Medical-Surgical Nursing. John Wiley & Sons, Inc., New York. 1983.

Robbins, S., and R. S. Cotran. Pathologic Basis fo Disease. W. B. Saunders Co., Philadelphia. 1979. Second edition.

Weiss, L. The Blood Cells and Hematopoietic Tissues. McGraw-Hill Book Co., 1977.

Williams, W. J., E. Beutler, A. J. Erslew, and R. W. Runales. Hematology. McGraw-Hill Book Co., New York. 1977.

Wintrobe, M. M., G. R. Lee, D. R. Bothell, J. W. Athens, and J. Foerster. Clinical Hematology. Lea & Febiger, Philadelphia. 1981. Eighth edition.

Wyngaarden, J. B., and L. H. Smith. Cecil Textbook of Medicine. W. B. Saunders Co., Philadelphia. 1982. Sixteenth edition.

Chapter 5

Brunner, L., and Suddarth, D. The Lippincott Manual of Nursing Practice. J. B. Lippincott Co., Philadelphia. 1978. Second edition.

Connolly, R., and G. E. Zave. Update: head injuries. *Journal of Neurosurgical Nursing* (August 1981). 195–201.

Courjon, J., F. Mauguière, M. Revol, Advances in Neurology. Raven Press, New York. 1982.

Mancall, E. Essentials of the Neurologic Examination. F. A. Davis Co., Philadelphia. 1981. Second edition.

Mills, N., and H. Plasterer. Guillain-Barré syndrome: a framework for nursing care. *Nursing Clinics of North America* (June 1980). 257–264.

Robinson, J., editor. Nursing Skillbook. Coping with Neurologic Problems Proficiently. Intermed Communications, Inc., Horsham, Pa. 1979.

Perdue,P. Head injuries. *RN* (June 1981). 37–42.

Ricci, M. Intracranial hypertension: barbiturate therapy and the role of the nurse. *Journal of Neurosurgical Nursing* (December 1979). 247–252.

Tucker, C. A. Complex partial seizures. *American Journal of Nursing* (May 1981). 996–1,000.

Wilson, S. Neuro-Nursing. Springer Publishing Co., Inc., New York. 1979.

Chapter 6

Goyette, R. E., Endocrine Pathology and Pathophysiology Case Studies. Medical Examination Publishing Co., Inc., Garden City, N.Y. 1978.

Greenberg, A. Common emergencies of acid-base balance. *Topics In Emergency Medicine* (January 1984). 1–15.

Hamburger, S., D. Rush, and G. Bosker. Endocrine and Metabolic Emergencies. Robert J. Brady Co., Bowie, Md. 1984.

Kruger, J. A., and J. C., Ray. Endocrine Problems in Nursing: A Physiologic Approach. C. V. Mosby Co., St. Louis. 1976.

Luckmann, J., and K. A. Sorensen. Medical-Surgical Nursing—A Psychophysiologic Approach. W. B. Saunders Co., Philadelphia. 1980. Second edition.

Muthe, N. Endocrinology—A Nursing Approach. Little, Brown & Co., Boston. 1981.

Streck. W., and D. Lockwood, editors. Endocrine Diagnosis—Clinical and Laboratory Approach. Little, Brown & Co., Boston. 1983.

Tepperman, J. Metabolic and Endocrine Physiology. Year Book Medical Publishers Inc., Chicago. 1980.

Swartz, S. Solving antidiuretic hormone puzzles. *Patient Care* (June 30, 1982). 114–143.

Williams. R. H., editor. Textbook of Endocrinology. W. B. Saunders Co., Philadelphia. 1981.

Chapter 7

Binkley, L. S. Keeping up with peritoneal dialysis. *American Journal of Nursing* (June 1984). 729–733.

Brenner, B. M., and F. C. Rector. The Kidneys. W. B. Saunders Co., Philadelphia. 1981. Second edition.

Brundage, D. J. Nursing Management of Renal Problems. C. V. Mosby Co., St. Louis. 1980. Second edition.

Gutch, C. F., and M. H. Stoner. Review of Hemodialysis for Nurses and Dialysis Personnel. C. V. Mosby Co., St. Louis. 1979. Second edition.

Kagan, L. W. Renal Disease: A Manual of Renal Problems. McGraw-Hill Book Co., New York. 1979.

Mars, D. R., and D. Trebar. Acute tubular necrosis - pathophysiology and treatment. *Heart and Lung* (March 1984). 194–202.

Menzel, L. K. Clinical problems of electrolyte balance. *Nursing Clinics of North America* (September 1980). 559–576.

Metheny, N. M., and W. D. Snively. Nurses' Handbook of Fluid Balance. J. B. Lippincott Co., Philadelphia. 1983. Fourth edition.

Vander, A. J. Renal Physiology. McGraw-Hill Book Co., New York. 1985. Third edition.

Chapter 8

Bolt, R. J., P. E. S. Palmer, B. H. Ruebner, and D. W. Watson. The Digestive System. John Wiley & Sons, Inc., New York. 1983.

Borg, N., D. Nikas, J. Stark, and S. Williams, editors. Core Curriculum for Critical Care Nursing. W. B. Saunders Co., Philadelphia. 1981. Second edition.

Dobrilla, G., C. Liguory, and G. Misiewicz. Current Therapy of Gastrointestinal Disorders. Cortina International, Verona, Italy. 1983.

Given, B. A., and S. J. Simmons. Gastroenterology in Clinical Nursing. C. V. Mosby Co., St. Louis. 1984. Fourth edition.

Guyton, A. C. Textbook of Medical Physiology. W. B. Saunders Co., Philadelphia. 1981. Sixth edition.

Kinney, M. R., C. B. Dear, D. R. Packa, and D. M. N. Voorman, editors. AACN's Clinical Reference for Critical Care Nursing. McGraw-Hill Book Co., New York. 1981.

Orr, M. E. Acute Pancreatic and Hepatic Dysfunction. John Wiley & Sons, Inc., New York. 1981.

Schiff, L., and E. R. Schiff, editors. Diseases of the Liver. J. B. Lippincott Co., Philadelphia. 1982. Fifth edition.

Sherlock, S. Diseases of the Liver and Biliary System. Blackwell Scientific Publications, Oxford. 1981. Sixth edition.

Spiro, H. M. Clinical Gastroenterology. Macmillan Inc., New York. 1983. Third edition.

Chapter 9

Artz, C. P., J. A. Moncrief, and B. A. Pruitt, Jr. Burns: A Team Approach. W. B. Saunders Co., Philadelphia. 1979.

Barry, J., editor. Emergency Nursing. McGraw-Hill Book Co., New York. 1978.

Heimbach, D. M. Advances in burn care. *Western Journal of Medicine* (March 1981). 274

Hills, S. W., and J. J. Birmingham. Burn Care. John Wiley & Sons, Inc., New York. 1981.

Hummel, R. P., editor. Clinical Burn Therapy, A Management and Prevention Guide. John Wright PSG Inc., Littleton, Mass. 1982.

McDougal, S. W., C. L. Slade, and B. A. Pruitt, Jr. Manual of Burns. Springer-Verlag New York, Inc., New York. 1978.

National Institute of General Medical Sciences Office of Research. Special Report on Burn and Trauma Research. National Institute of General Medical Sciences, Bethesda, Md. 1982.

Wachtel, T. L., V. Kahn, and H. A. Frank. Current Topics in Burn Care. Aspen Systems Corp., Rockville, Md. 1983.

Wagner, M. M., editor. Care of the Burn Injured Patient—A Multi-Disciplinary Involvement. PSG Publishing Co., Inc., Littleton, Mass. 1981.

Chapter 10

American College of Surgeons, Committee on Trauma. Early Care of the Injured Patient. W. B. Saunders Co., Philadelphia. 1976.

Berk, J. L., and J. E. Sampliner. Handbook of Critical Care. Little, Brown & Co., Boston. 1982.

Guyton, A. C. Textbook of Medical Physiology. W. B. Saunders Co., Philadelphia. 1976.

Little, R. C. Physiology of the Heart and Circulation. Year Book Medical Publishers Inc., Chicago. 1979.

Shires, G. T. Care of the Trauma Patient. McGraw-Hill Book Co., New York. 1979.

Swan, K. G., and R. C. Swan. Gunshot Wounds: Pathophysiology and Management. PSG Publishing Co., Inc., Littleton, Mass. 1980.

Trunkey, D. D., and F. R. Lewis. Current Therapy of Trauma: 1984–1985. B. C. Decker, Inc., Philadelphia. 1984.

Way, L., editor. Current Surgical Diagnosis and Treatment. Lange Medical Publications, Los Altos, Calif. 1983.

Worth, M. H. Principles and Practice of Trauma Care. Williams & Wilkins Co., Baltimore. 1982.

Zuidema, G. D., W. F. Bullinger, and R. B. Rutherford. The Management of Trauma. W. B. Saunders Co., Philadelphia. 1979.

Chapter 11

DelRio, D., K. Williams, and B. M. Esvelt. The 1983 Handbook of Enteral Nutrition. Medical Specifics Publishing, El Segundo, Calif. 1982.

Forlaw, L., and L. M. Bayer. Symposium on nutrition. *Nursing Clinics of North America* (March 1983). 111–117.

Grant, J. Handbook of Total Parenteral Nutrition. W. B. Saunders Co., Philadelphia. 1980.

Homsy, F. N., and G. L. Blackburn. Modern parenteral and enteral nutrition in critical care. *Journal of the American College of Nutrition* (February 1983). 75–95.

Jeejbhoy, K. N. Total Parenteral Nutrition in the Hospital and at Home. CRC Press, Inc., Boca Raton, Fla. 1983.

Jensen, T. G., D. M. Englert, and S. J. Dudrick. Nutrition Assessment: A Manual for Practitioners. Appleton-Century-Crofts, Norwalk, Conn. 1983.

Luther, R. W., and T. R. Sylus. Textbook of Enteral Nutrition. Grune & Stratton, Inc., New York. 1983.

Merritt, R. J., G. C. Blackburn, and R. M. Suskind. Textbook of Pediatric Nutrition. Raven Press, New York. 1981.

Roe, D. A. Handbook: Interactions of Selected Drugs and Nutrients in Patients. The American Dietetic Association, Chicago. 1982.

Chapter 12

Brennan, J. M. Sharpening your skills for arterial sticks. *RN* (April 1984). 59–61.

Cohen, J. J., and J. P. Kassirer. *Acid-Base.* Little, Brown & Co., Inc., Boston. 1982.

Cohen, S. Blood-gas and acid-base concepts in respiratory care. Programmed Instruction. *American Journal of Nursing* (June 1976). 1–30.

Donlen, J. Interpreting acid-base problems through arterial blood gases. *Critical Care Nurse* (September-October 1982). 34–38.

DuBose, T. D. Clinical Approach to patients with acid-base disorders. *Medical Clinics of North America* (July 1983). 799–810.

Emanuelsen, K. L., and M. J. Densmore. Acute Respiratory Care. John Wiley & Sons, Inc., New York. 1981.

Filley, G. F. Acid-Base and Blood Gas Regulation. Lea & Febiger, Philadelphia. 1972.

Guenther, V. Clinical interpretation of arterial blood gases. *The Australasian Nurses Journal* (July 1980). 25.

Signor, G., and D. J. DelBueno. A sinfully easy way to interpret ABGs. *RN* (September 1982). 45–49.

Sweetwood, H. M. Nursing in the Respiratory Intensive Care Unit. Springer Publishing Co., Inc., New York. 1979. Second edition.

Chapter 13

Cherniack, R. M., and L. Cherniack. Respiration in Health and Disease. W. B. Saunders Co., Philadelphia. 1983. Third edition.

Emanuelsen, K. L., and M. J. Densmore. Acute Respiratory Care. John Wiley & Sons, Inc., New York. 1981.

Martz, K. V., J. W. Joiner, and R. M. Shepherd. Management of the Patient-Ventilator System. C. V. Mosby Co., St. Louis. 1984.

McPherson, S. P. Respiratory Therapy Equipment. C. V. Mosby Co., St. Louis. 1981.

Morrison, M. L., editor. Respiratory Intensive Care Nursing from Beth Israel Hospital, Boston. Little, Brown & Co., Boston. 1979. Second edition.

Nursing Photobook Series. Providing Respiratory Care. Intermed Communications Inc., Horsham, Pa. 1983.

Petty, T. Intensive and Rehabilitative Respiratory Care. Lea & Febiger, Philadelphia. 1982. Third edition.

Shapiro, B. A., R. A. Harrison, and C. A. Trout. Clinical Application of Respiratory Care. Year Book Medical Publisher, Inc., Chicago. 1979. Second edition.

Sweetwood, H. M. Nursing in the Intensive Respiratory Care Unit. Springer Publishing Co., New York. 1979. Second edition.

Wade, J. F. Comprehensive Respiratory Care. C. V. Mosby Co., St. Louis. 1982. Third edition.

Chapter 14

Armstrong, P. W., and R. S. Baigrie. Hemodynamic Monitoring in the Critically Ill. Harper & Row, New York. 1980.

Ford, P., and R. N. Weintraub. Intra-Aortic Balloon Pumping Manual. Beth Israel Hospital, Boston. 1974.

Gazes, P. C. Clinical Cardiology—A Bedside Approach. Year Book Medical Publishers Inc., Chicago. 1983.

Huang, S. H., L. A. Dasher, C. A. Larson, and C. D. McCulloch. Coronary Care Nursing. W. B. Saunders Co., Philadelphia. 1983.

Pierson, D. J., and L. D. Hudson. Monitoring hemodynamics in the critically ill. *Medical Clinics of North America* (November 1983). 1343–1360.

Purcell. J. A., L. Pippin, and M. Mitchell. Intra-aortic balloon pump therapy. *American Journal of Nursing* (May 1983). 775–790.

Sanderson, R. G., and C. L. Kurth. The Cardiac Patient—A Comprehensive Approach. W. B. Saunders Co., Philadelphia. 1983.

Strandness, D. E., and D. S. Sumner. Hemodynamics for Surgeons. Grune & Stratton Inc., New York. 1975.

Swan, H. J. C., and W. Ganz. Measurement of right atrial and pulmonary arterial pressures and cardiac output: clinical application of hemodynamic monitoring. Year Book Medical Publishers Inc., Chicago. 1982. 453–473.

Wenger, N. K., J. W. Hurst, and M. C. McIntyre. Cardiology for Nurses. McGraw-Hill Book Co., New York. 1980.

Chapter 15

American Heart Association. Standards and guidelines for cardiopulmonary resuscitation (CPR) and emergency cardiac care (ECC). *The Journal of the American Medical Association* (August 1, 1980). 455–509.

Bander, J. J. Defibrillation. *In* Budassi, S. A., J. J. Bander, L. Kimmerli, and K. F. Eri, editors. Cardiac Arrest and Cardiopulmonary Resuscitation. Aspen Systems Corp., Rockville, Md. 1980.

Gahart, B. L. Intravenous Medications. C. V. Mosby Co., St. Louis. 1981.

Goldman, M. R. Shock and cardiac arrest. *In* Johnson, R. A., E. Haber, and W. G. Austen, editors. The Practice of Cardiology. Little, Brown & Co., Boston. 1980.

Hawthorne, J. W., J. McDermott, and F. K. Poulin. Cardiac pacing. *In* Johnson, R. A., E. Haber, and W. G. Austen, editors. The Practice of Cardiology. Little, Brown & Co., Boston. 1980.

Hoenig, S. A., and D. H. Scott. Medical Instrumentation and Electrical Safety. John Wiley & Sons, Inc., New York. 1977.

Kaye, W. Invasive therapeutic techniques: emergency cardiac pacing, pericardiocentesis, intracardiac injections, and emergency treatment of tension pneumothorax. *Heart and Lung* (May 1983). 300–320.

Roberts, W., and S. L. Underhill. Cardiac abnormalities associated with intracranial events. *In* Underhill, S. L., S. L. Woods, E. S. Sivarajan, and C. J. Halpenny. Cardiac Nursing. J. B. Lippincott Co., Philadelphia. 1982.

Rogove, H. J. Pathophysiology of cardiac arrest. *In* Aurebach, P. S., and S. A. Budassi, editors. Cardiac Arrest and Cardiopulmonary Resuscitation. Aspen Systems Corp., Rockville, Md. 1983. Second edition.

Spodick, D. H. Acute cardiac tamponade. In Chung, E. K., editor. *Cardiac Emergency Care.* Lea & Febiger, Philadelphia. 1980.

Chapter 16

Arking, L., and L. Saravolatz. Antimicrobial treatment, a coordination challenge for nursing. *Nursing Clinics of North America* (December 1980). 689–701.

Bennett, J., and P. Brachman, editors. Hospital Infections. Little, Brown & Co., Boston. 1979.

Centers for Disease Control. Guideline for prevention of intravascular infections. Center for Infectious Diseases, U.S. Department of Health & Human Services, Atlanta, Ga. 1982.

Centers for Disease Control. Guideline for prevention of nosocomial pneumonia. Center for Infectious Diseases, U. S. Department of Health & Human Services, Atlanta, Ga. 1982.

Centers for Disease Control. Guideline for isolation precautions in hospitals. Center for Infectious Diseases, U.S. Department of Health & Human Services, Atlanta, Ga. 1983.

Craig, C., and S. Connelly. Effect of intensive care unit nosocomial pneumonia on duration of stay and mortality. *American Journal of Infection Control* (August 1984). 233–238.

Rhoades, C., M. Adcock, and J. Javanovich. Prevention of nosocomial infection in critical care units. *Nursing Clinics of North America* (December 1980). 803–815.

Roderick, M., editor. Infection Control in Critical Care. Aspen Systems Corp., Rockville, Md. 1983.

Soule, B., editor. *The APIC Curriculum for Infection Control Practice.* Association for Practitioners in Infection Control, Mundelein, Ill. 1983.

Tafuro, P., and P. Ristuccia. Recognition and control of outbreaks of nosocomial infections in the intensive care setting. *Heart & lung* (September 1984). 486–495.

Chapter 17

Beland, I. L., and J. Y. Passos. Clinical Nursing: Pathophysiological and Psychosocial Approaches. Macmillan Inc., New York. 1981. Fourth edition.

Hall, K. V. Detecting septic shock before it is too late. *RN* (September 1981). 29–32.

Holloway, N. M. The Critically Ill Adult. Addison Wesley Publishing Co., Menlo Park, Calif. 1979.

Hudak, C. M., T. Lohr, and B. M. Gallo. Critical Care Nursing. J. B. Lippincott Co., Philadelphia. 1982. Third edition.

Luckman, J., and K. C. Sorensen. Medical Surgical Nursing—A Psychophysiologic Approach. W. B. Saunders Co., Philadelphia. 1980. Second edition.

Meador, B. Cardiogenic shock—help break the vicious cycle. *RN* (April 1982). 38–42.

Robbins, S. L., and R. S. Cotran. Pathologic Basis of Disease. W. B. Saunders Co., Philadelphia. 1979. Second edition.

Rose, M. Shock—fluids restore circulation. *Monitoring Fluids and Electrolytes Precisely.* Intermed Communications, Inc., Horsham, Pa. 1978.

Shoemaker, W. C., W. L. Thompson, and P. R. Holbrook. Textbook of Critical Care. W. B. Saunders Co., Philadelphia. 1984.

Wyngaarden, J. B., and L. H. Smith. Cecil Textbook of Medicine. W. B. Saunders Co., Philadelphia. 1982. Sixteenth edition.

Chapter 18

Branch v. *Hempstead County Memorial Hospital.* 539 F. Supp. 908 (D.C. Ark. 1982).

Eichelberger v. *Barnes Hospital.* 655 S.W. 2d 699 (Mo. App. 1983).

Emmett v. *Eastern Dispensary and Casualty Hospital.* 396 F. 2d 931 (D.C. Dis. of C. 1967).

Kirby v. *Sprivey.* 307 S.E. 2d 538 (Ga. App. 1983).

Logan v. *Greenwich Hospital Assoc.* 191 Conn. 282 (1983).

Chapter 19

Albrecht, T. L. What job stress means for the staff nurse. *Nursing Administration Quarterly* (Fall 1982). 1–11.

Barry, P. D. Psychosocial nursing assessment and intervention. J. B. Lippincott Co., Philadelphia. 1984.

Bouman, C. C. Identifying priority concerns of families of ICU patients. *Dimensions of Critical Care Nursing* (September-October 1984). 313–319.

Daley, L. The perceived immediate needs of families with relatives in the intensive care setting. *Heart and Lung* (May 1984). 231–237.

Hackett, T. P., and N. H. Cassem, editors. Massachusetts General Hospital Handbook of General Hospital Psychiatry. C. V. Mosby Co., St. Louis. 1978. Chapters 10, 14, 16, 17.

Harris, J. S. Stressors and stress in critical care. *Critical Care Nurse* (January-February 1984). 84–97.

Hay, D., and D. Oken. The psychological stresses of intensive care unit nursing. *Psychosomatic Medicine* (March-April 1972). 109–118.

Kübler-Ross, E. On death and dying. Macmillan Inc., New York. 1969.

McMorrow, M. E. Managing stress in critical care nursing. *Critical Care Update* (May 1982). 39–42.

Selye, H. The stress of life. McGraw-Hill Book Co., New York. 1956.

Appendix A

Andreoli, K. G., V. H. Fowkes, A. G. Wallace, and D. P. Zipes. Comprehensive Cardiac Care. C. V. Mosby Co., St. Louis. 1979. Fifth edition.

Conover, M. B. Understanding Electrocardiography. C. V. Mosby Co., St. Louis 1984. Fourth edition.

Marriott, H. J. L. Practical Electrocardiography. Williams & Wilkins Co., Baltimore. 1981. Sixth edition.

Talkington, S. G. ECG—A Pocket Guide. Fleschner Publishing Co., Bethany, Conn. 1982.

Appendix B

Bukowskyj, M., K. Nakatsu, and P. W. Munt. Theophylline reassessed. *Annals of Internal Medicine* (July 1984). 63–73.

Comer, J. B. Pharmacology in Critical Care. John Wiley & Sons, Inc., New York. 1981.

Eliopoulous, G. M., and R. C. Moellering. Azlocillin, mezlocillin and piperacillin. *Annals of Internal Medicine* (November 1982). 755–760.

Goodman, L. S., and A. Gilman. The Pharmacological Basis of Therapeutics. Macmillan, Inc., New York. 1980. Sixth edition.

Ristuccia, A. M., and B. A. Cunha. The aminoglycosides. *Medical Clinics of North America* (January 1982). 303–313.

Rodman, J., and D. Benditt. Progress in arrhythmia therapy. *Clinical Pharmacy* (July-August 1983). 307–311.

Sonnenblicke, E., W. H. Frishman, and T. H. LeJemtel. Dobutamine: a new synthetic cardioactive sympathetic amine. *New England Journal of Medicine* (January 1979). 17–22.

Swartz, S. L., and R. R. Dluhy. Corticosteroids. *Drugs* (1978). 238–255.

Thompson, L. T. and A. J. Wright. Cephalosporin antibiotics. *Mayo Clinic Proceedings* (February 1983). 79–87.

Wollam, G. L., R. W. Gifford, and R. C. Tarazi. Antihypertensive drugs: Clinical Pharmacology and therapeutic use. *Drugs* (1977). 420–460.

INDEX

A

I